Infectious Diseases

In 30 Days

Notice

Medicine is an ever-changing science. As new research and clinical experience broaden our knowledge, changes in treatment and drug therapy are required. The authors and the publisher of this work have checked with sources believed to be reliable in their efforts to provide information that is complete and generally in accord with the standards accepted at the time of publication. However, in view of the possibility of human error or changes in medical sciences, neither the authors nor the publisher nor any other party who has been involved in the preparation or publication of this work warrants that the information contained herein is in every respect accurate or complete, and they disclaim all responsibility for any errors or omissions or for the results obtained from use of the information contained in this work. Readers are encouraged to confirm the information contained herein with other sources. For example and in particular, readers are advised to check the product information sheet included in the package of each drug they plan to administer to be certain that the information contained in this work is accurate and that changes have not been made in the recommended dose or in the contraindications for administration. This recommendation is of particular importance in connection with new or infrequently used drugs.

Infectious Diseases

In 30 Days

FREDERICK S. SOUTHWICK, M.D.

Professor of Medicine
Chief of Infectious Diseases
Vice Chairman of Medicine
University of Florida College of Medicine
Gainesville, Florida

McGraw-Hill

Medical Publishing Division

New York   Chicago   San Francisco   Lisbon   London   Madrid   Mexico City   Milan
New Delhi   San Juan   Seoul   Singapore   Sydney   Toronto

Infectious Diseases in 30 Days

1 2 3 4 5 6 7 8 9 0   DOC/DOC   0 9 8 7 6 5 4 3

ISBN 0-07-137518-X

This book was set in Garamond by Pine Tree Composition.
The editors were James Shanahan and Michelle Watt.
The production supervisor was Catherine Saggese.
Project management was provided by Hearthside Publishing Services.
The index was prepared by Deborah Tourtlotte.

RR Donnelley was printer and binder.

This book is printed on acid-free paper.

Library of Congress Cataloging-in-Publication Data

Infectious diseases in 30 days / edited by Frederick S. Southwick.
    p. ;cm.
  Includes bibliographical references and index.
  ISBN 0-07-137518-X
  1. Communicable diseases.   I. Title: Infectious diseases in thirty days.
    II. Southwick, Frederick S.
  [DNLM: 1. Communicable Diseases.   2. Bacterial Infections. WC 100 I40273 2003]
RC111 .I51265 2003
616.9--dc21
                                            2002032587

To my wife Kathie Southwick
for all her loving encouragement

Contents

Contributors

Bernard Hirschel, M.D.
Associate Professor of Medicine
Division of Infectious Diseases
University of Geneva
Geneva, Switzerland

P. Daniel Lew, M.D.
Professor of Medicine and Chief
    of Infectious Diseases
University of Geneva
Geneva, Switzerland

Reuben Ramphal, M.D.
Professor of Medicine
Division of Infectious Diseases
University of Florida College of Medicine
Gainesville, Florida

Frederick S. Southwick, M.D.
Professor of Medicine
Chief of Infectious Diseases
Vice Chairman of Medicine
University of Florida College of Medicine
Gainesville, Florida

Sankar Swaminathan, M.D.
Associate Professor of Medicine
Division of Infectious Diseases
University of Florida College of Medicine
Gainesville, Florida

Preface

The discovery of penicillin, followed by the development of ever more powerful anti-infective agents combined with the broad use of vaccines, promised a cure for all infectious diseases. However, the optimism of earlier decades has proved premature, and today's health care professional will encounter clinical challenges not faced by clinicians just 20 years ago.

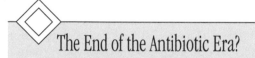

The End of the Antibiotic Era?

Time and *Newsweek* magazines have heralded the "End of the Antibiotic Era," echoing the concerns of many infectious disease and health policy experts. *The Chicago Tribune's* feature on "Unhealthy Hospitals" warns that the "overuse of antibiotics are spawning drug-resistant germs that are spreading from hospitals into the community at unprecedented rates." Newly discovered infectious diseases such as Ehrlichia, Lyme disease, and West Nile encephalitis are showing up at our doorstep. Ancient infectious diseases such as tuberculosis and malaria pose significant threats in many parts of the world. A recent bioterrorist attack launched using anthrax spores illustrates the critical need for all health providers to recognize the manifestations of this nearly forgotten pathogen and others that can be used as weapons of mass destruction. The AIDS epidemic is devastating sub-Saharan Africa, and it is spreading at an alarming rate in Asia and the former Soviet Union. HIV strains resistant to antiretroviral therapy are increasing throughout the United States and Europe. Diseases long believed to have non-infectious etiologies are now confirmed as having microbial origins. Infectious diseases have re-emerged as one of the world's top health care priorities, and to meet the needs of the 21st century, health care providers must possess a solid grounding in clinical infectious diseases.

But how does the busy clinician achieve this goal? The field of infectious diseases can be complex and daunting, and many infectious disease textbooks are thousands of pages in length. *Infectious Diseases in 30 Days* provides the health care provider with the ideal tool for attaining an efficient and complete understanding of infectious disease diagnosis and management. After reading this book, the clinician will be able to more judiciously select anti-infective agents, and will possess a new understanding of the pathogenesis, clinical manifestations, diagnosis, and treatment of the most common and important infectious diseases.

As the title suggests, the busy clinician will be able to efficiently accomplish this task within 30 days. For medical students and residents participating in a one month infectious disease elective, *Infectious Diseases in 30 Days* will provide the solid background and understanding required to explore primary literature sources and intelligently utilize more detailed reference textbooks. For medical practitioners, specialists in other fields of medicine, nurse practitioners, and physician assistant practitioners, this new book will provide an efficient, understandable, and updated foundation in the management of patients with infectious diseases.

Features of the Book

We have included many features designed to assist the reader in applying the book directly to the care of patients. Guidelines are provided as to the number of days that should be allotted for completing each chapter. Diseases are classified by anatomic site rather than by organism, because that is how the clinician encounters infectious diseases. Chapters are preceded by a series of Guiding Questions. Key Points about each disease are summarized in colored boxes to re-emphasize important facts. To further assist in clinical management, the potential severity of each infectious disease is assessed at the beginning of each section. Finally, illustrative case reports precede descriptions of the clinical manifestations to emphasize important clinical clues.

Organization of the Book

The clinician will find many of the chapters helpful in the day-to-day management of their patients. Chapter 1, Anti-Infective Therapy, provides specific strategies for designing cost-effective, efficacious anti-infective regimens, in addition to simply reviewing the antimicrobial spectrums, toxicities, and doses of each agent. Antimicrobial agents are classified by cost and spectrum, and the use of narrow-spectrum antibiotics is emphasized. Chapter 4, Pulmonary Infections, provides a concise and logical approach to community-acquired and nosocomial pneumonia. Chapter 6, Central Nervous System Infections, reviews the anatomic sites of central nervous system infection, allowing clinicians to understand the anatomic basis for subdural and epidural empyema, meningitis, brain abscess, and encephalitis as well as the physiologic sig-

nificance of the blood-brain barrier. Chapter 9, Genitourinary Tract Infections and Sexually Transmitted Diseases, contains the 2002 sexually transmitted disease treatment recommendations recently published by the Centers for Disease Control and Prevention. Chapter 12, Parasitic Infections, covers the major parasites that are likely to be encountered in general practice and includes helpful diagrams and schematic drawings that will be useful in board examination review and for assisting laboratory personnel in making the proper diagnosis. Up-to-date reviews of the evolving subjects of bioterrorism and emerging zoonotic infections are provided in Chapters 13 and 14. The final chapter, HIV Infection, written by a world-renowned HIV clinician Bernard Hirschel, covers the essential clinical facts about HIV and AIDS. This chapter provides a remarkably succinct but complete description of the basic principles of diagnosis and management of what many infectious disease specialists regard as the ultimate infectious disease challenge.

On completing *Infectious Diseases in 30 Days* the health care professional will possess a new appreciation of the evolving nature of this exciting and challenging subspecialty. Their new understanding of the epidemiology and clinical manifestations of each infectious disease will allow the earlier diagnosis of specific infections, and prevent many of the deadly complications associated with delayed therapy. A new understanding of microbial resistance and the strategic design of antibiotic regimens will allow each health care provider to prevent the "end of the antibiotic era."

Frederick S. Southwick

Acknowledgments

I wish to thank Drs. Morton Swartz and Paul Beeson who, as mentors and teachers, fostered my great love and excitement for the field of infectious diseases. My warmest appreciation goes to Dr. Tom Stossel who helped guide and support my academic career.

I also wish to thank the physicians who read sections of this book and suggested improvements: Drs. Leighton Cluff, Richard Howard, Denise Schain, Hong Nguyen, and Jennifer Janelle. Thank you to my contributors, Drs. P. Daniel Lew, Reuben Ramphal, Bernard Hirschel, and Sankar Swaminathan, for their prompt and outstanding submissions. I am also grateful to Arthur Flowers and Sony Kuruppacherry for their cheerful and steadfast office support.

A special thanks is given to Jim Shanahan of McGraw-Hill whose encouragement and insights were always helpful. Finally, I wish to acknowledge the excellent artwork of Roger Hoover.

Infectious Diseases
In 30 Days

Chapter 1

Anti-Infective Therapy

Recommended Time to Complete: 4 days

Guiding Questions

1. Are we at the end of the antibiotic era?

2. Why are "superbugs" suddenly appearing in our hospitals?

3. How do bacteria become resistant to antibiotics?

4. How can we prevent the continued selection of highly resistant organisms?

5. Is antibiotic treatment always the wisest course of action?

6. Can one antibiotic cure all infections?

7. What strategies underlie optimal antibiotic usage?

8. How is colonization distinguished from infection and why is this distinction important?

Introduction

Over the past few years the press has been publicizing the end of the antibiotic era. Some commentators have dismissed these claims as alarmist and exaggerated. However, infectious disease consultants and the Centers for Disease Control and Prevention are very concerned about the steady increase in the percentage of penicillin-resistant *Streptococcus pneumoniae*, methicillin-resistant *Staphylococcus aureus*, and vancomycin-resistant enterococcus. These developments certainly warrant sounding the alarm. The lay public must be educated that anti-infective therapy in many circumstances may do more harm than good. These agents need to be reserved for treatable infections and not used simply to calm the patient or the patient's family. Too often, patients with viral infections that do not warrant anti-infective therapy arrive at the physician's office expecting to be treated with an antibiotic. And health care workers too often prescribe antibiotics to fulfill these expectations.

Health care providers wish to establish a simple set of rules for treatment and to establish practices that maintain the highest standard of care for their patients. Sales representatives from the pharmaceutical companies understandably try to fulfill these desires. Too often, they attempt to convince physicians that their anti-infective agent should be used to treat all patients with possible infection. Many excellent broad-spectrum antibiotics can effectively treat the majority of bacterial infections without necessitating a specific etiologic diagnosis. However, overuse of empiric broad-spectrum antibiotics has resulted in the selection of highly resistant pathogens.

Unfortunately, a simplistic approach to anti-infective therapy and establishment of a fixed series of simple rules for the use of these agents is unwise and has proved harmful to patients. Physicians who are unschooled in the principles of microbiology use anti-infective agents just as they would more conventional medications such as anti-inflammatory agents, antihypertensive medications, and cardiac drugs, and the pharmaceutical industry often encourages this practice. These physicians ignore the remarkable adaptability of bacteria, fungi, and viruses. It is no coincidence that these more primitive life forms have been in existence for millions of years, far longer than the human race.

The rules for the use of anti-infective therapy are dynamic and must take into account these pathogens' ability to adapt to the selective pressures exerted by the overuse of antibiotics, antifungal agents, and antiviral agents. The days of the "shotgun" approach to infectious diseases must end, or more and more patients will become infected with multiresistant organisms that cannot be treated. Only through the judicious use of anti-infective therapy can

we hope to slow the arrival of the end of the antibiotic era.

KEY POINTS
Anti-Infective Therapy

1. Too often, antibiotics are prescribed to fulfill the patient's expectations rather than to treat a true bacterial infection.
2. A single antibiotic cannot fulfill all infectious disease needs.
3. Physicians ignore the remarkable adaptability of bacteria, fungi, and viruses at their patients' peril.
4. Anti-infective therapy is dynamic and requires a basic understanding of microbiology.
5. The "shotgun" approach to infectious diseases must end, or we may truly experience the end of the antibiotic era.

Antibiotic Resistance

Genetic Modifications Leading to Antimicrobial Resistance

To understand why antibiotics must be used judiciously, the physician needs to understand how bacteria are able to adapt to their environment. Point mutations can develop in the DNA of bacteria as they replicate. These mutations occur in the natural environment but are of no survival advantage unless the bacterium is placed under selective pressures. In the case of mutations that render a bacterium resistant to a specific antibiotic, exposure to the specific antibiotic allows the bacterial clone that possesses the antibiotic resistance mutation to grow, while bacteria without the mutation die and no longer compete for nutrients. Thus the resistant strain becomes the dominant bacterial flora. In addition to point mutations bacteria can transfer genetic material from one bacterium to another by three major mechanisms:

1. **Conjugation.** Bacteria often contain circular double-stranded DNA called plasmids. These circular strands of DNA lie outside of the bacterial chromosome (see Figure 1.1). Such plasmids often carry R or resistance genes. Through a mechanism called conjugation, plasmids can be transferred from one bacterium to another. The plasmid encodes for the formation of a pilus on the bacterium's outer surface. This pilus attaches to a second bacterium and serves as bridge for the transfer of the plasmid DNA from the donor to the recipient bacterium. By this mechanism a single resistant bacterium can transfer resistance to other bacteria.

2. **Transduction.** Bacteriophages are protein-coated DNA segments that attach to the bacterial wall and inject DNA. This process is called transduction. These infective particles can readily transfer resistance genes to multiple bacteria.

3. **Transformation.** In addition to plasmids and bacteriophages, linear segments of chromosomal DNA can be released by donor bacteria and taken up by other recipient bacteria, where the new DNA is incorporated into the recipient's chromosome. This process is called transformation, and the naked DNA that is capable of incorporating into the chromosome of recipient bacteria is called a transposon (see Figure 1.1). Natural transformation most commonly occurs in Streptococcus, Haemophilus, and Neisseria species. Transposons can transfer multiple antibiotic resistance genes as a single event and have been shown to be responsible for high-level vancomycin resistance in enterococci.

Thus bacteria possess multiple ways to transfer their DNA and promiscuously share their genetic information. This promiscuity provides a survival advantage by allowing bacteria to adapt quickly to their environment.

KEY POINTS

Antibiotic Resistance

1. Bacteria can quickly alter their genetic makeup by:
   a. Point mutations,
   b. Transfer of DNA by plasmid conjugation,
   c. Transfer of DNA by bacteriophage transduction,
   d. Transfer of naked DNA transposons by transformation.
2. The ability of bacteria to share their DNA provides a survival advantage, allowing them to adapt quickly to antibiotic exposure.
3. Biochemical alterations leading to antibiotic resistance include:
   a. Degradation of antibiotics by b-lactamases and other enzymes,
   b. Blocking antibiotic entry,
   c. Pumping antibiotics out,
   d. Modifying cell wall precursors,
   e. Modifying target enzymes,
   f. Modifying the ribosomal binding site.
4. Under the selection pressures of antibiotics, it is not a question of whether or not resistant bacteria will take over, but only a question of when.

Biochemical Mechanisms for Antimicrobial Resistance

What are some of the proteins for which these resistant genes encode and how do they work? The mechanisms by which bacteria resist antibiotics can be classified into several groups:

1. **β-Lactamases.** Many bacteria synthesize one or more enzymes called β-lactamases, which inactivate antibiotics by breaking the amide bond on the β-lactam ring. Plasmids and transposons primarily transfer β-lactamase ac-

Figure 1.1

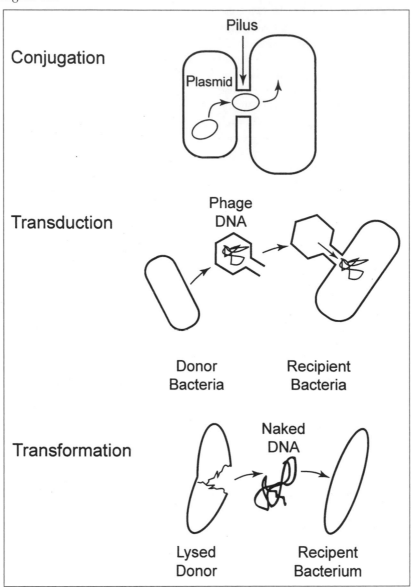

Mechanisms of bacterial transfer of antibiotic resistance genes.

tivity. There are multiple classes of β-lactamases. Some preferentially break down penicillins; others preferentially destroy specific cephalosporins or carbenicillin. Extended-spectrum β-lactamases (commonly abbreviated ESBL) readily destroy most cephalosporins. Another class of β-lactamases is resistant to clavulanate, an agent that is added to numerous antibiotics to inhibit β-lactamase activity. Finally, some bacteria are able to produce β-lactamases that are capable of inactivating imipenem and meropenem. Gram-negative bacilli produce a broader spectrum of β-lactamases then Gram-positive organisms do, and therefore infections with Gram-negative organisms more commonly arise in patients who have been treated with prolonged broad-spectrum antibiotics. In some instances β-lactamase activity is low before the bacterium is exposed to antibiotics; however, following exposure β-lactamase activity is induced. Enterobacter is a prime example. This Gram-negative bacterium may appear to be sensitive to cephalosporins on initial testing. Following cephalosporin treatment β-lactamase activity increases, resistance develops, and the patient's infection relapses. For this reason cephalosporins are not recommended for serious Enterobacter infections.

2. **Other enzyme modifications of antibiotics.** Erythromycin is readily inactivated by an esterase that hydrolyzes the lactone ring of the antibiotic. This esterase has been identified in *Escherichia coli*. Other plasmid-mediated erythromycin-inactivating enzymes have been discovered in Streptococcus species and *Staphylococcus aureus*. Chloramphenicol is inactivated by chloramphenicol acetyltransferase, which has been isolated from both Gram-positive and Gram-negative bacteria. Similarly, aminoglycosides can be inactivated by acetyltransferases. Bacteria also inactivate this class of antibiotics by phosphorylation and adenylation. These resistance enzymes are found in many Gram-negative strains and are increasingly detected in enterococci, *S. aureus*, and *S. epidermidis*.

3. **Alterations in bacterial membranes.** For an antibiotic to work, it must be able to penetrate the bacterium and reach its biochemical target. Gram-negative bacteria contain an outer lipid coat that impedes penetration of hydrophobic reagents such as most antibiotics. The passage of hydrophobic antibiotics is facilitated by the presence of porins, or small channels in the cell walls of Gram-negative bacteria that allow the passage of charged molecules. Mutations leading to the loss of porins can decrease antibiotic penetration and lead to antibiotic resistance.

4. **Production of efflux pumps.** Transposons have been found that encode for an energy-dependent pump that can actively pump tetracycline out of bacteria. Active efflux of antibiotics has been observed in many enteric Gram-negative bacteria, and this mechanism is used to resist tetracycline, macrolide, and fluoroquinolone antibiotic treatment. *Staphylococcus aureus, Staphylococcus epidermidis, Streptococcus pyogenes*, group B streptococci, and *Streptococcus pneumoniae* also can utilize energy-dependent efflux pumps to resist antibiotics.

5. **Alterations of cell wall precursors.** This mechanism is the basis for vancomycin-resistant enterococcus. Vancomycin and teicoplanin binding requires that D-alanine-D-alanine be at the end of the peptidoglycan cell wall precursors of Gram-positive bacteria. Resistant strains of *Enterococcus faecium* and *E. faecalis* contain the van A plasmid that encodes a protein that synthesizes D-alanine-D-lactate instead of D-alanine-D-alanine at the end of the peptidoglycan precursor. Loss of the terminal D-alanine markedly reduces vancomycin and teicoplanin binding, allowing the mutant bacterium to survive and grow in the presence of these antibiotics.

6. **Changes in target enzymes.** Penicillins and cephalosporins bind to specific proteins in the bacterial cell wall called penicillin-binding proteins (PBPs). Penicillin-resistant *Streptococcus pneumoniae* demonstrates decreased numbers of PBPs and/or PBPs that bind penicillin with lower affinity. Decreased penicillin binding reduces the ability of the antibiotic to kill the targeted bacteria. The basis for antibiotic resistance in methicillin-resistant *Staphylococcus aureus* (commonly abbreviated MRSA) is the production of a low-affinity PBP encoded by the mec A gene. Mutations in the target enzymes dihydropteroate synthetase and dihydrofolate reductase cause sulfonamide and trimethoprim resistance, respectively. Single amino acid mutations that alter DNA gyrase function can result in resistance to fluoroquinolones.

7. **Alterations in ribosomal binding site.** Tetracyclines, macrolides, lincosamides, and aminoglycosides all act by binding to and disrupting the function of bacterial ribosomes (see individual antibiotics below). A number of resistance genes encode for enzymes that demethylate adenine residues on bacterial ribosomal RNA, and this activity inhibits antibiotic binding to the ribosome. Ribosomal resistance to gentamicin, tobramycin, and amikacin is less common because these aminoglycosides have several binding sites on the bacterial ribosome and require multiple bacterial mutations to block their binding.

Conclusions

Bacteria can readily transfer antibiotic resistance genes from species to species. Bacteria have multiple mechanisms to destroy antibiotics, block their entry, pump them out, and interfere with their binding. Under the selective pressures of prolonged antibiotic treatment it is not a question of whether or not resistant bacteria will take over, but only a question of when.

◆ Factors That Determine Anti-Infective Agent Dosing

The characteristics that need to be considered in administering antibiotics include absorption (when dealing with oral antibiotics), volume of distribution, metabolism, and excretion. These factors determine the dose of each drug and the time interval of administration. To effectively clear a bacterial infection, serum levels of the antibiotic need to be maintained above the minimum inhibitory concentration for a significant period. The minimum inhibitory concentration (MIC) is determined for each pathogen by serially diluting the antibiotic into liquid media containing 10^4 bacteria per milliliter. Inoculated tubes are incubated overnight until broth without added antibiotic has become cloudy or turbid as a result of bacterial growth. The lowest concentration of antibiotic that prevents active bacterial growth (i.e., clear liquid media) constitutes the MIC (see Figure 1.2). For an individual pathogen, automated machinery is now capable of quickly determining the MICs for multiple antibiotics, and this data serves to guide the physician's choice of antibiotics. The mean bactericidal concentration (MBC) is determined by taking each clear tube and inoculating the solution onto a solid media plate. Plates are then incubated to allow colonies to form. The lowest concentration of antibiotic that blocks all growth of bacteria (i.e., no colonies on solid media) represents the MBC.

Successful cure of an infection depends on multiple host factors in addition to serum antibiotic concentrations. However, investigators have attempted to predict successful treatment by plotting the serum antibiotic levels versus time and determining the ratio of the area under the curve to the MIC (see Figure 1.3). Another related parameter that is thought to be helpful in

Figure 1.2

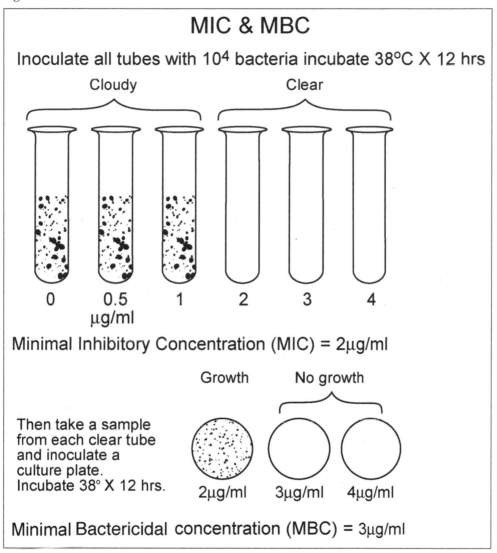

MIC & MBC

Inoculate all tubes with 10^4 bacteria incubate 38°C X 12 hrs

Cloudy   Clear

0   0.5   1   2   3   4
μg/ml

Minimal Inhibitory Concentration (MIC) = 2μg/ml

Growth   No growth

Then take a sample
from each clear tube
and inoculate a
culture plate.
Incubate 38° X 12 hrs.   2μg/ml   3μg/ml   4μg/ml

Minimal Bactericidal concentration (MBC) = 3μg/ml

Determination of minimum inhibitory concentration (MIC) and mean bactericidal concentration (MBC).

predicting successful outcome is the time above the MIC. To maximize the likelihood of a successful outcome, investigators have recommended that serum antibiotic levels be maintained above the MIC for at least 50% of the time interval. It should be kept in mind that there are few human studies to support this recommendation.

Another characteristic that may be considered is concentration-dependent killing. In vitro, tobramycin and fluoroquinolones demonstrate greater killing the more the antibiotic concentra-

Figure 1.3

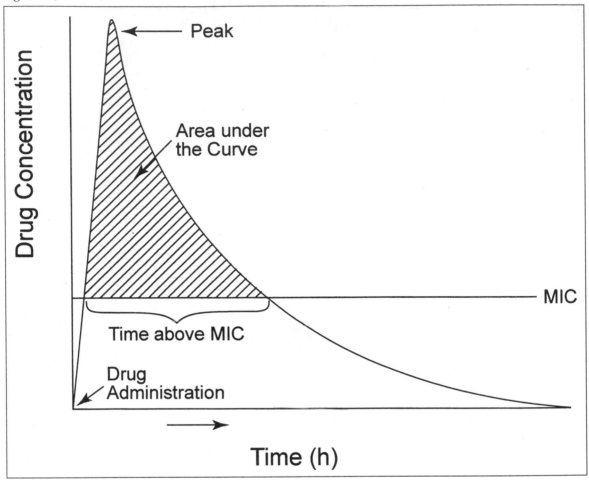

Pharmacokinetics of a typical antibiotic.

tion exceeds the MIC. For these antibiotics high peak levels may be more effective in curing infection than low peak concentrations. In vitro studies also show that some antibiotics demonstrate a postantibiotic effect. When the antibiotic is removed, there is a delay in the recovery of bacterial growth. After exposure to aminoglycosides or fluoroquinolones, Gram-negative bacteria demonstrate a delay in the recovery of active growth for 2–6 hours. Penicillins and cephalosporins demonstrate no postantibiotic effect on Gram-negative bacteria but generally cause a 2-hour delay in the recovery of Gram-positive organisms. Investigators suggest that antibiotics with significant postantibiotic effect can be dosed less frequently, while those with no postantibiotic effect should be administered by constant infusion. Although these in vitro effects suggest certain therapeutic approaches, it must be kept in mind that both concentration-dependent killing and postantibiotic effect are in vitro phenomena, and treatment strategies based on these parameters have not been substantiated by controlled human clinical trials.

KEY POINTS

Antibiotic Dosing

1. Absorption, volume of distribution, metabolism, and excretion all affect serum antibiotic levels.
2. Minimum inhibitory concentration (MIC) is helpful in guiding antibiotic choice.
3. To maximize success with β-lactam antibiotics, serum antibiotic levels should be > MIC for at least 40–50% of the time.
4. The clinical importance of concentration-dependent killing and postantibiotic effect remains to be proven in clinical trials.

Basic Strategies for Antibiotic Therapy

The choice of antibiotics should be carefully considered. A step-by-step logical approach is helpful. The clinician needs to do the following.

1. Decide Whether or Not the Patient Has a Bacterial Infection

This issue will be discussed in more detail in the subsequent chapters dealing with specific infections. One useful test that often helps to differentiate an acute systemic bacterial infection from a viral illness is the peripheral white blood cell count (WBC). In patients with serious systemic bacterial infections the peripheral WBC is often elevated and demonstrates an increased percentage of neutrophils. Often, less mature neutrophils such as band forms and occasionally metamyelocytes are observed on peripheral blood smear. Most viral infections fail to induce a neutrophil response. Viral infections, particularly Epstein-Barr virus, induce an increase in lymphocytes and/or monocytes and may induce the formation of atypical monocytes. The severity of the patient's illness should also guide the physician. Severely ill patients usually have a bacterial infection and generally warrant antibiotic treatment.

2. Make a Reasonable Statistical Guess as to the Possible Pathogens

The probability of a specific pathogen depends on the anatomic site of the primary infection. And the anatomic site of possible infection can often be determined on the basis of the patient's symptoms and signs as well as by laboratory tests. For example, burning on urination associated with pyuria on urinalysis suggests a urinary tract infection. The organisms that cause uncomplicated urinary tract infection usually arise from the bowel flora and include *E. coli*, Klebsiella, and Proteus. Antibiotic treatment needs to cover these potential pathogens. The following chapters will review the common pathogens associated with infections at specific anatomic sites and will review the recommended antibiotic coverage for these pathogens.

3. Be Aware of the Susceptibility Patterns in Your Hospital

In patients who develop infection while in the hospital, that is, a nosocomial infection, empiric therapy needs to take into account the antibiotic susceptibility patterns of the hospital and the floor where the patient became ill. Many hospitals have a high incidence of methicillin-resistant *Staphylococcus aureus*, and therefore empiric antibiotic treatment for a possible staphylococcal infection must include vancomycin pending culture results. Other hospitals have a large percentage of Pseudomonas strains that are resistant to gentamicin, eliminating this antibiotic as a consideration for empiric treatment of possible Gram-negative sepsis.

4. Take into Account Previous Antibiotic Treatment

The remarkable adaptability of bacteria makes it highly likely that the new pathogen will be resistant to the previously administered antibiotics. If the onset of the new infection was preceded by a significant interval when antibiotics were not given, the resident flora may have recolonized with less resistant flora. However, the reestablishment of normal flora can take weeks. Furthermore, patients in the hospital are likely to recolonize with highly resistant hospital flora.

5. Take into Consideration Important Host Factors

a. **The site of infection**. In some instances this will eliminate certain antibiotics from consideration. For example, patients with bacterial meningitis should not be treated with antibiotics that fail to cross the blood-brain barrier (for example, first-generation cephalosporins, gentamicin, and clindamycin).

b. **Peripheral white blood cell count**. Patients with neutropenia have a high mortality rate from sepsis. Therefore immediate broad-spectrum high-dose intravenous antibiotic treatment is recommended as empiric therapy.

c. **Age and underlying diseases (hepatic and renal dysfunction)**. Elderly patients tend to metabolize and excrete antibiotics more slowly; therefore longer dosing intervals are often required. Agents with significant toxicity, such as aminoglycosides, should generally be avoided because the elderly suffer greater toxicity. Antibiotics that are primarily metabolized by the liver should generally be avoided or reduced in patients with significant cirrhosis. In patients with significant renal dysfunction, antibiotic doses need to be modified.

d. **Duration of hospitalization**. Patients who have just arrived in the hospital tend to be col-

onized with community-acquired pathogens, while patients who have been in the hospital for prolonged periods and have received several courses of antibiotics are generally colonized with highly resistant bacteria as well as fungi. A standard empiric regimen can be used for the newly hospitalized patient. However, the empiric antibiotic regimen for the patient who has been hospitalized for a prolonged period must be carefully designed to take into account previous exposure to antibiotics, past culture results, and the common nosocomial pathogens that are found on the hospital floor.

e. **Severity of the patient's illness**. Is the patient toxic and hypotensive, or does the patient simply have a new fever without other serious systemic complaints or dysfunction? In the severely ill patient, broad-spectrum antibiotics need to be instituted immediately after cultures are obtained, while in most cases the patient with fever and no other systemic complaints may be observed off antibiotics while awaiting culture results.

6. Use the Fewest Drugs Possible

a. Multiple drugs may lead to antagonism rather than synergy. Many combination regimens have not been completely studied. Some regimens such as penicillin and an aminoglycoside for enterococcus have been shown to result in synergy. That is, the combined effects of the two antibiotics are greater than the effects of simply adding the MBCs of the two agents. In other instances certain combinations have proved to be antagonistic (for example, the use of rifampin combined with oxacillin is antagonistic in some strains of *Staphylococcus aureus*). The natural assumption that the more antibiotics are given, the more killing power there will be often does not apply.

b. Use of multiple antibiotics increases the risk of adverse reactions. Drug allergies are common, and when a patient who is on more than one antibiotic develops an allergic reaction, all antibiotics become potential offenders, and these agents can no longer be used. In some instances combination therapy can increase the risk of toxicity (for example, gentamicin and vancomycin increase the risk of nephrotoxicity).

c. Use of multiple antibiotics often increases the cost and increases the risk of administration errors. Administration of two or more intravenous antibiotics requires multiple intravenous reservoirs and multiple intravenous lines as well as pumps. Nurses and pharmacists are required to dispense each antibiotic dose, increasing labor costs. Also, the more drugs a patient receives, the higher is the probability of an administration error. Finally, the use of two or more drugs usually increases the acquisition cost.

d. Use of multiple antibiotics increases the risk of infections with highly resistant organisms. Prolonged use of broad-spectrum antibiotic coverage increases the risk of methicillin-resistant *Staphylococcus aureus*, vancomycin-resis-

tant enterococcus, multiresistant Gram-negative bacilli, and fungal infections. When multiple antibiotics are used, the spectrum of bacteria killed is increased. Killing of the majority of the normal flora in the pharynx and gastrointestinal tract is harmful to the host. The normal flora compete for nutrients, occupy binding sites that are used by pathogenic bacteria, and produce agents that inhibit the growth of competitors. Loss of the normal flora allows resistant pathogens to overgrow.

7. Switch to Narrower-Spectrum Antibiotic Coverage within 3 Days

Following the administration of antibiotics, sequential cultures of mouth flora reveal that within 3 days the numbers and types of bacteria begin to significantly change. The normal flora dies, and resistant Gram-negative rods, Gram-positive cocci, and fungi begin to predominate. The more quickly the selective pressures of broad-spectrum antibiotic coverage can be dis-

Table 1.1

Classification of Antibiotics by Spectrum of Activity

NARROW	MODERATELY BROAD	BROAD	VERY BROAD
Penicillin	Ampicillin	Ampicillin-sulbactam	Ticarcillin-clavulanate,
Oxacillin/nafcillin	Ticarcillin	Amoxicillin-clavulanate	Piperacillin-tazobactam
Cefazolin	Piperacillin	Ceftriaxone	Imipenem
Cephalexin/cephradine	Cefoxitin	Cefotaxime	Meropenem
Aztreonam	Cefotetan	Ceftizoxime	Ertapenem
Aminoglycosides	Cefuroxime-axitel	Ceftazidime	Gatifloxacin
Vancomycin	Cefaclor	Cefixime	Moxifloxacin
Macrolides	Ciprofloxacin	Cefpodoxime proxetil	
Clindamycin	Trimethoprim-	Cefepime	
Lanazolid	sulfamethoxazole	Tetracycline	
Synercid™		Doxycycline	
Metronidazole		Chloramphenicol	
		Levofloxacin	

continued, the lower is the risk of selecting for highly resistant pathogens. Broad coverage is reasonable as initial empiric coverage until cultures are available. Generally, by 3 days the pathogen or pathogens can be identified in the microbiology laboratory, and a narrower-spectrum, specific antibiotic regimen can be initiated. Table 1.1 and the sections on specific antibiotics classify each antibiotic by their spectrum of activity to assist in these choices. Despite the availability of culture results, too often the clinician continues the same empiric broad-spectrum antibiotic regimen, and this behavior is a critical factor in explaining subsequent infections with highly resistant superbugs.

8. When All Things Are Equal, Pick the Least Expensive Drug

As will be discussed in subsequent chapters, there is often more than one antibiotic regimen that can be used to successfully treat a specific infection. Given the strong economic forces driving medicine today, the physician needs to consider the cost of therapy whenever possible. Too often, new, more expensive antibiotics are

Table 1.2

Cost Ranges for Intravenous and Oral Antibiotics

Intravenous Preparations (daily cost)	
Low:	$20–60
Moderate:	$61–100
Moderately high:	$101–140
High:	$140–180
Very high:	>$180
Oral Preparations (cost for 10 days of treatment)	
Low:	$10–40
Moderate:	$41–80
Moderately high:	$81–120
High:	$121–160
Very high:	>$160

chosen over older, generic antibiotics that are equally effective. In reviewing each specific antibiotic, we have tried to classify antibiotics into cost ranges (see Tables 1.2–1.4) to assist the clinician in making cost-effective decisions.

In assessing cost, however, it is also important to factor in toxicity. For example, the acquisition cost of gentamicin is low; however, when monitoring of blood levels, the requirement to closely follow BUN and serum creatinine, and the potential of an extended hospital stay due to nephrotoxicity are factored into the cost equation, gentamicin often is not cost-effective.

KEY POINTS

The Steps Required to Design an Antibiotic Regimen

1. Assess the probability of bacterial infection. (Antibiotics should be avoided in viral infections.)
2. Be familiar with the primary pathogens responsible for infection at each anatomic site.
3. Be familiar with the bacterial flora in your hospital.
4. Take into account previous antibiotic treatment.
5. Take into account the specific host factors (age, immune status, hepatic and renal function, duration of hospitalization, severity of illness).
6. Use the minimum number and narrowest-spectrum antibiotics possible.
7. Switch to a narrower-spectrum antibiotic regimen based on culture results.
8. Take into account acquisition cost and the costs of toxicity.

Obey the 3-Day Rule. Continuing broad-spectrum antibiotics beyond 3 days drastically alters the host's normal flora, selecting for resistant organisms. After 3 days, streamline your antibiotics. Use narrower-spectrum antibiotics to specifically treat the pathogens identified by culture and Gram stain.

Table 1.3

Classification of Parenteral Anti-infectives by Cost

Low	Moderate	Moderately High	High	Very High
Penicillin	Piperacillin-	Ampicillin-	Nafcillin	Lanazolid
Ampicillin	tazobactam	sulbactam	Itraconazole	Synercid™
Oxacillin	Cefoxitin	Imipenem	Acyclovir	Amphotericin B
Ticarcillin-	Ceftizoxime	Meropenam	Aminoglycosides	lipid preparations
calvulanate	Fluconazole			Voriconazole
Cefazolin	Ganciclovir			Caspofungin
Cefotetan	Foscarnet			Cidofovir
Cefuroxime				Interferon-α
Ceftriaxone				
Cefotaxime				
Ceftazidime				
Cefepime				
Aztreonam				
Ertapenem				
Vancomycin				
Erythromycin				
Doxycycline				
Clindamycin				
Chloramphenicol				
Ciprofloxacin				
Levofloxacin				
Gatifloxacin				
Metronidazole				
Trimethoprim/				
sulfamethoxazole				
Amphotericin B				

Colonization versus Infection

◆ **CASE 1.1**

Following a motor vehicle accident, a 40-year-old white male was admitted to the intensive-care unit with four fractured ribs and a severe lung contusion on the right side. Chest X-ray (CXR) demonstrated an infiltrate in the right lower lobe. Be-

cause of a depressed mental status he required respiratory support. Initially, sputum Gram stain demonstrated few polymorphonuclear leukocytes (PMNs) and no organisms. On the third hospital day he developed a fever to 103°F (39.5°C), and his peripheral white blood cell count (WBC) increased from 8,000 to 17,500 (80% PMN, 15% band forms). CXR demonstrated extension of his right lower lobe infiltrate. Sputum Gram stain revealed abundant PMN and 20–30 Gram-positive cocci in clusters/hpf. His sputum culture grew methicillin-sensitive *Staphylococcus aureus*. Intravenous cefa-

Table 1.4

Classification of Oral Antibiotics by Cost

Low	Moderate	Moderately High	High	Very High
Penicillin-VK	Cefadroxil	Cefuroxime-	Amoxicillin-	Vancomycin
Amoxicillin	Cefaclor	axetil	clavulanate	Lanazolid
Dicloxacillin	Clarithromycin	Cefpodoxime	Itraconazole	Ganciclovir
Cephalexin	Azithromycin	Clindamycin		Voriconazole
Cephradine	Ciprofloxacin	Cycloserine		Ribavirin
Cefixime	Levofloxacin	Fluconazole		
Erythromycin	Gatifloxacin			
Tetracycline	Moxifloxacin			
Doxycycline	Rifabutin			
Metronidazole	Terbinafine			
Trimethoprim-	Valacyclovir			
sulfamethoxazole	Flucytosine			
INH				
Rifampin				
Pyrazinamide				
Ethambutol				
Ethionamide				
Griseofulvin				
Acyclovir				

zolin (1.5 gm Q8H iv) was initiated. He defervesced, and secretions from his endotracheal tube decreased over the next 3 days. On the fourth day a repeat sputum sample was obtained. Gram stain revealed moderate numbers of PMN and no organisms; however, culture grew *E. coli* resistant to cephazolin. The physician changed his antibiotic to cefepime (1 gm Q8H iv).

Case 1.1 represents a very typical example of how antibiotics are misused. The initial therapy for a probable early *Staphylococcus aureus* pneumonia was appropriate, and the patient responded (fever resolved, sputum production decreased, Gram-positive cocci disappeared from the Gram stain, and *S. aureus* no longer grew on culture). However, because the subsequent sputum culture was positive for a resistant strain

of *E. coli*, the physician switched to a broader-spectrum antibiotic. The correct decision should have been to continue cefazolin.

One of the most difficult and confusing issues for many physicians is the interpretation of culture results. Wound cultures and sputum cultures are most commonly misinterpreted. Once a patient has been started on an antibiotic, the bacterial flora on the skin and in the mouth and sputum will change. Often, these new organisms do not invade the host but simply represent new flora that has colonized these anatomic sites. Too often, physicians try to eradicate the new flora by adding new, more powerful antibiotics. The result of this strategy is to select for organisms that are multiresistant. The eventual outcome can be the selection of a bacterium that is resistant to all antibiotics.

There is no definitive method for differentiating between colonization and true infection. Several clinical findings, however, are helpful in guiding the physician. Evidence supporting the onset of a new infection include a new fever or a change in fever pattern, a rise in the peripheral white blood cell count with an increase in the percentage of PMNs and band forms (left shift), and Gram stain demonstrating an increased number of PMNs in association with a predominance of bacteria that are morphologically consistent with the culture results. In the absence of these findings, colonization is more likely, and the current antibiotic regimen should be continued.

KEY POINTS

Differentiating Colonization from Infection

> 1. Growth of resistant organisms is the rule in the patient on antibiotics.
> 2. Antibiotics should be switched only if there is evidence of a new infection.
> 3. Evidence of a new superinfection includes the following:
>   a. New fever or a worsening fever pattern,
>   b. Increased peripheral leukocyte count with left shift,
>   c. Increased inflammatory exudate at the original site of infection,
>   d. Increased PMN on Gram stain,
>   e. Correlation between Gram-stain bacterial morphology and culture.

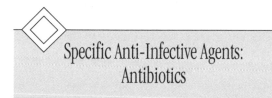

Specific Anti-Infective Agents: Antibiotics

Before prescribing a specific antibiotic, the clinician should be able to answer the following questions:

Guiding Questions

1. How does the antibiotic kill or inhibit bacterial growth?
2. What are the antibiotic's toxicities and how should they be monitored?
3. What are the indications for using each specific antibiotic?
4. How is the drug metabolized and what are the dosing recommendations? Does the dosing schedule need to be modified in patients with renal dysfunction?
5. How much does the antibiotic cost?
6. How broad is the antibiotic's antimicrobial spectrum?

The clinician should be familiar the general classes of antibiotics and their mechanisms of action, as well as their major toxicities. The differences between the specific antibiotics in each class can be subtle and often require the expertise of an infectious disease specialist to design the optimal anti-infective regimen. The general internist or physician in training should not attempt to memorize all the facts outlined below but rather should read the following pages as an overview of anti-infectives. The chemistry, mechanisms of action, major toxicities, spectrum of activity, treatment indications, pharmacokinetics, dosing regimens, and cost will be reviewed. The specific indications for each anti-infective will be covered briefly in this chapter. A more complete discussion of specific regimens will be included in the later chapters covering infections of specific anatomic sites.

When the physician prescribes a specific antibiotic, he or she should reread the specific sections on toxicity, spectrum of activity, pharmacokinetics, dosing, and cost. Because new anti-infectives are frequently being introduced, the prescribing physician should also take advantage of handheld devices, on-line pharmacology databases, and antibiotic manuals (see Further Reading at the end of this chapter) to provide up-to-date treatment. When the proper therapeutic choice is unclear, on-the-job training can also be provided by requesting an infectious disease specialist consultation. Anti-infective agents are often considered to be safe. However, the multiple potential toxicities outlined below combined with the likelihood of selecting for resistant organisms emphasize the dangers of overprescribing antibiotics.

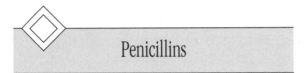

Penicillins

Chemistry and Mechanisms of Action

Penicillins have in common a central structure (Figure 1.4) consisting of a β-lactam ring (A) and a thiazoladine ring (B). The side chain attached to the β-lactam ring (R) determines many of the antibacterial and pharmacologic characteristics of the specific penicillin.

Penicillin G was the first β-lactam to be discovered. In addition to penicillins the cepha-

losporins contain a similar β-lactam ring, and these two classes of antibiotics kill bacteria by the same mechanism. The β-lactam antibiotics bind to different penicillin-binding proteins (PBPs). PBPs represent a family of enzymes that are important for bacterial cell wall synthesis, including carboxypeptidases, endopeptidases, transglycolases, and transpeptidases. Strong binding to PBP-1, a cell wall transpeptidase and transglycolase, causes rapid bacterial death. Inhibition of this transpeptidase prevents the cross-linking of the cell wall peptidoglycans, resulting in loss of the integrity of the bacterial cell wall. Without its protective outer coat the hyperosmolar intracellular contents swell, and the bacterial cell membrane lyses. Inhibition of PBP-3, a transpeptidase and transglycolase that acts at the septum of the dividing bacterium, causes the formation of long filamentous chains of nondividing bacteria as well as bacterial death. Inhibition of other PBPs blocks cell wall synthesis in other ways and activates bacterial lysis. The activity of all β-lactam antibiotics requires active bacterial growth and active cell wall synthesis. Therefore bacteria that are in a dormant or static phase will not be killed, while those in an active log phase of growth are quickly lysed. Bacteriostatic agents slow bacterial growth and antagonize β-lactam antibiotics; therefore bacteriostatic antibiotics should not be combined with β-lactam antibiotics.

Toxicity

Hypersensitivity reactions are the most common side effect associated with the penicillins. Penicillin is the most common agent to cause drug allergies; allergic reactions range from 0.7-10%. Breakdown products, particularly penicilloyl and penicillanic acid, form amide bonds with serum proteins, and these antigens elicit allergic reactions. Patients who have been sensitized by prior exposure to penicillin may develop an immediate IgE-mediated hypersensitivity reaction that can result in anaphylaxis as well as urticaria. Anaphylaxis can result in tightness of the

Figure 1.4

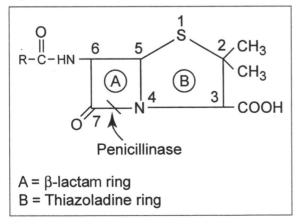

A = β-lactam ring
B = Thiazoladine ring

Basic structure of penicillins.

throat, wheezing, respiratory arrest, and shock. In the United States, penicillin-induced allergic reactions result in 400–800 fatalities per year. Because of this potential danger, patients with a history of an immediate hypersensitivity reaction to penicillin should never be given a β-lactam antibiotic, including a cephalosporin or a carbapenem. High levels of IgG antipenicillin antibodies can cause serum sickness, a syndrome resulting in fever, arthritis and arthralgias, urticaria, and diffuse edema. A macular pruritic rash involving the trunk and limbs is the most frequent allergic reaction. When this rash is first noted, penicillin should be immediately discontinued, because on rare occasions the rash can progress to exfoliative dermatitis. Stevens-Johnson syndrome has also been associated with penicillin administration. This syndrome consists of high fever, mucosal ulcerations, and erythema multiforme (target lesions on the trunk, palms, and soles followed by desquamation). Other manifestations of immune reactions to penicillin include hemolytic anemia, agranulocytosis, thrombocytopenia, nephritis, pneumonitis, and vasculitis. A less common side effect is the development of grand mal seizures. Penicillin at very high concentrations lowers the seizure threshold. Seizures are observed primarily in patients with renal failure who have a decreased ability to clear penicillin and, as a consequence, have high serum levels of penicillin.

KEY POINTS

Penicillins

1. Contain a β-lactam ring.
2. Bind to and inhibit penicillin-binding proteins, enzymes that are important for cross-linking bacterial cell wall peptidoglycans.
3. Require active bacterial growth for bactericidal action.
4. Are antagonized by bacteriostatic antibiotics.
5. Have, as principal toxicity, hypersensitivity reactions (0.7–10%).

Natural Pencillins

PENICILLIN G

PHARMACOKINETICS   Because penicillin G is rapidly inactivated at pH 2.0, oral administration is not effective. Intramuscular preparations containing procaine or benzathine and intravenous preparations of potassium or sodium penicillin G are available. Intravenous administration is associated with a peak serum level within 15–30 minutes followed by rapid renal excretion, resulting in a serum half-life of less than 30 minutes. To maintain therapeutic levels, intravenous penicillin G must be administered every 4 hours. Intramuscular procaine penicillin results in a slower release of penicillin, allowing administration every 12 hours. Benzathine results in an even more gradual release of penicillin, allowing administration every 15–20 days. Penicillin is only minimally metabolized and is primarily excreted unmodified in the urine. Probenecid slows renal excretion, and this agent can be used to sustain higher serum levels. Penicillin is well distributed in the body and is able to penetrate most inflamed body cavities. Its ability to cross the blood-brain barrier in the absence of inflammation is poor. However, in the presence of inflammation, therapeutic levels are generally achievable in the cerebrospinal fluid.

SPECTRUM OF ACTIVITY AND TREATMENT RECOMMENDATIONS   The natural penicillins have a narrow spectrum and therefore do not disturb the normal flora to the same extent that more broad-spectrum antibiotics do. As was noted above, whenever possible a narrow-spectrum antibiotic is preferred over a broad-spectrum antibiotic. Penicillin remains the treatment of choice for *Streptococcus pyogenes* (group A streptococcus) and the *Streptococcus viridans* group. This antibiotic remains the most effective agent for the treatment of infections caused by mouth flora, including *Actinomyces israelii*, *Capnocytophaga canimorsus*, and *Fusobacterium*. Penicillin G is also primarily recommended for *Clostridium perfringens*, *Clostridium tetani*, *Neisseria meningitidis*, *Erysipelothrix* *rhusiopathiae, Pasteurella multocida,* and spirochetes, including syphilis and leptospira. Penicillin G remains the primary recommended therapy ·for *S. pneumoniae* that is sensitive to penicillin (MIC: <0.1 µg/ml). However, in many areas of the United States over 30% of strains are moderately resistant to penicillin (MIC: 0.1–1 µg/ml). In these cases ceftriaxone, cefotaxime, or high-dose penicillin (≥12 million units/day) can be used. Moderately resistant strains of *S. pneumoniae* possess a lower-affinity PBP, and this defect in binding can be overcome by high serum levels of penicillin. Infections with high-level penicillin-resistant *S. pneumoniae* (MIC: ≥2 µg/ml) require treatment with vancomycin.

PENICILLIN G IN SODIUM OR POTASSIUM SALT

Dose (for moderate to severe systemic infections): 2 million to 4 million units iv Q4H
Renal dosing: For a creatinine clearance (Cr Cl) < 10 cc/min, the dose should be decreased by half. The potassium salt preparation should be avoided in patients with renal failure because of the risk of hyperkalemia.
Cost: Low
Spectrum: Narrow
See Tables 1.1 and 1.2 for classifications.

PROCAINE PENICILLIN G

Dose (moderate systemic infections): 0.6 million to 1.2 million units im QD

BENZATHINE PENICILLIN G

Dose: *Late latent syphilis*: 2.4 million units im Q1 week × 3 weeks
Streptococcus pyogenes pharyngitis: 1.2 million units im × 1 dose
Cost of both im preparations: Low
Spectrum: Narrow

PENICILLIN V-K

This preparation resists acid damage by the stomach and results in oral absorption rates of

60%. Peak levels of antibiotic are achieved 1–2 hours after ingestion. Peak concentrations are lowered and delayed to 2–3 hours if the antibiotic is taken with food. Oral penicillin can be used to treat throat infections with *Streptococcus pyogenes* and as prophylaxis for rheumatic fever.

Dose: *S. pyogenes pharyngitis*: 250–500 mg po Q6–8h × 10 days. Each dose should be taken 1 hour before meals or 2 hours after meals.
Rheumatic fever prophylaxis: 250 mg po BID
Cost: Low
Spectrum: Narrow

KEY POINTS
The Natural Penicillins

1. Very short half-life (15–30 minutes).
2. Excreted renally; excretion delayed by probenecid.
3. Narrow spectrum: indicated for *Streptococcus pyogenes, S. viridans* gp., mouth flora, *Clostridia perfringens, Neisseria meningitidis,* Pasteurella, and spirochetes.
4. Recommended for penicillin-sensitive *S. pneumoniae*; however, penicillin-resistant strains are now frequent (>30%).

Aminopenicillins

AMPICILLIN

These modifications to penicillin slightly broadened the spectrum of activity and increased the resistance to stomach acid. Ampicillin can be given orally, intramuscularly, or intravenously. The pharmacokinetics of ampicillin is similar to that of penicillin. The half-life is short (1 hour), and the drug is primarily excreted unmodified in the urine.

TREATMENT RECOMMENDATIONS   This antibiotic is recommended for treatment of *Listeria monocytogenes,* sensitive enterococci, *Proteus mirabilis,* non-β-lactamase-producing *Haemophilus influ-*

enzae, sensitive strains of nontyphoidal Salmonella, and *Shigella flexneri*. It also can be used to treat otitis media and air sinus infections.

Dose: *Oral*: 250–500 mg Q6H given 1–2 hours before food
Intravenous: Up to 14 gm/day given in Q4-6H doses
For meningitis: 2 gm Q4H is generally recommended. Dosing is modified to Q8H for a Cr Cl of 30–50 cc/min and to Q12H for Cr Cl < 10 cc/min
Cost: Low
Spectrum: Moderate

AMOXICILLIN

This preparation has excellent oral absorption: 75% compared to 40% for ampicillin. Absorption is not impaired by food. With the exception of absorption, the pharmacokinetics is similar to that of ampicillin. The higher achievable peak levels have allowed a longer dosing interval, making this a more convenient oral antibiotic than ampicillin.

TREATMENT RECOMMENDATIONS Amoxicillin is commonly used as initial outpatient therapy for acute otitis media and acute bacterial sinusitis. It must be kept in mind that amoxicillin fails to cover β-lactamase-producing *Haemophilus influenzae* as well as *Moraxella catarrhalis*, common pathogens in these two infections. If significant improvement is not observed within 3 days, the patient should be switched to a broader-spectrum antibiotic such as amoxicillin-clavulanate (see below).

Dose: 500mg Q8H or 875 mg Q12H
Renal dosing: Cr Cl < 10 cc/min, dose Q24H
Cost: Low
Spectrum: Moderate (See Tables 1.1 and 1.2 for classifications.)

AMOXICILLIN-CLAVULANATE (AUGMENTIN)

Amoxicillin combined with the β-lactamase inhibitor clavulanate significantly broadens this antibiotic's spectrum of activity. Absorption and pharmacokinetics are similar to those of amoxicillin. This agent is effective against methicillin-sensitive strains of *Staphylococcus aureus*, *Moraxella catarrhalis*, and β-lactamase producing *Haemophilus influenzae*.

TREATMENT RECOMMENDATIONS Augmentin may be used to treat otitis media and sinusitis; however, its high cost and lack of proven superiority over amoxicillin raise concerns about Augmentin's cost-effectiveness. Pediatricians often prefer this agent because of its ability to kill amoxicillin-resistant *Haemophilus influenzae*. Compared to the other oral penicillins, amoxicillin-clavulanate treatment is more frequently associated with diarrhea.

Dose: Identical to that of amoxicillin
Cost: High
Spectrum: Broad

AMPICILLIN-SULBACTAM (UNASYN)

This intravenous preparation has a spectrum identical to that of Augmentin. Sulbactam, like clavulanate, inhibits β-lactamase activity.

Dose: 1.5–2 gm Q6H not to exceed 8 gm of ampicillin or 4 gm of sulbactam per day
Renal dosing: Dosing adjustments for renal dysfunction are identical to those of ampicillin
Cost: High
Spectrum: Broad
See Tables 1.1 and 1.2 for classifications.

KEY POINTS
Aminopenicillins

1. Short half-life (1 hour), clearance similar to that of natural penicillins.
2. Slightly broader spectrum of activity.
3. Parenteral ampicillin indicated for *Listeria monocytogenes*, sensitive enterococci, *Pro-*

teus mirabilis, and non-β-lactamase-producing *Haemophilus influenzae*.

4. Ampicillin + an aminoglycoside is the treatment of choice for enterococci. Whenever possible, vancomycin should be avoided.
5. Amoxicillin has excellent oral absorption: initial drug of choice for otitis media and bacterial sinusitis.
6. Amoxicillin-clavulanate: Improved Staphylococcus, *H. influenzae*, and *M. catarrhalis* coverage, but expensive and high incidence of diarrhea. Increased efficacy versus amoxicillin not proven in otitis media. However, covers amoxicillin-resistant *H. influenzae*, a common pathogen in this disease.

Penicillinase-Resistant Penicillins

NAFCILLIN, OXACILLIN, AND METHICILLIN

The synthetic modification of penicillin to render it resistant to the β-lactamases produced by *Staphylococcus aureus* reduced the ability of these antibiotics to kill anaerobic mouth flora as well as microaerophilic streptococci and Neisseria species. These agents have the same half-life as penicillin (30 minutes) and require Q4H dosing. Methicillin is utilized for disk sensitivity testing but is rarely used for treatment because it is unstable at acid pH, is less potent, and is associated with a higher incidence of interstitial nephritis, CNS toxicity, and bone marrow suppression than other penicillins.

TREATMENT RECOMMENDATIONS These agents are strictly recommended for the treatment of methicillin-sensitive *Staphylococcus aureus*. They are also used to treat cellulitis when the most likely pathogens are *S. aureus* and *Streptococcus pyogenes*. The liver efficiently excretes nafcillin, and the dose needs to be adjusted in patients with significant hepatic dysfunction. The liver less efficiently excretes oxacillin, and adjustment is usually not required for liver disease. Because the liver can excrete these antibiotics, the doses

of nafcillin and oxacillin usually do not need to be adjusted for renal dysfunction.

Dose: Nafcillin, 0.5–2 gm iv Q4H; Oxacillin, 1–2 gm iv Q4H
Cost: Nafcillin, high; Oxacillin, low
Spectrum: Very narrow

DICLOXACILLIN AND CLOXACILLIN

Although oxacillin can also be given orally, it is less well absorbed than cloxacillin or dicloxacillin. The same oral dose of cloxacillin achieves twofold higher serum levels and dicloxacillin achieves fourfold higher serum levels than oxacillin. Food interferes with absorption.

TREATMENT RECOMMENDATIONS Because serum levels are considerably lower, these agents should not be used to treat *Staphylococcus aureus* bacteremia. They are used primarily for mild soft tissue infections or to complete therapy of a resolving cellulitis.

Dose: 0.25–1 gm po Q6H taken 1 hour before meals or 2 hours after meals
Cost: Low
Spectrum: Very narrow
See Tables 1.1 and 1.2 for classifications.

KEY POINTS

Pencillinase-Resistant Penicillins

1. Short half-life, hepatically metabolized.
2. Indicated primarily for methicillin-sensitive *Staphylococcus aureus* and cellulitis.
3. Poor anaerobic activity.

Carboxypenicillins and Ureidopenicillins

CARBENICILLIN AND TICARCILLIN

These agents are able to resist β-lactamases produced by Pseudomonas, Enterobacter, Morganella, and Proteus-Providencia species. Carbenicillin is less active than ticarcillin and is no longer recommended. Ticarcillin has two to four times the activity against Pseudomonas compared to carbenicillin. Because the half-life of ticarcillin is short (1 hour), it requires frequent dosing. Sale of ticarcillin alone may soon be discontinued in favor of ticarcillin-clavulanate.

TREATMENT RECOMMENDATIONS The combination of ticarcillin and an aminoglycoside results in synergistic killing of *Pseudomonas aeruginosa*, and this regimen is recommended as primary therapy for infections with this pathogen. At high doses ticarcillin can also kill many strains of *Bacteroides fragilis*, and this antibiotic can be used for empiric coverage of moderate to severe intra-abdominal infections.

Dose: Ticarcillin, 3 gm Q4H
Renal dosing: Cr Cl 10–50 cc/min, dose 2–3 gm
    Q6–8H; Cr Cl < 10 cc/min, dose 2 gm Q12H
Cost: Moderate
Spectrum: Moderately broad

TICARCILLIN-CLAVULANATE (TIMENTIN)

Addition of the β-lactamase inhibitor clavulanate broadens the spectrum of coverage of ticarcillin.

TREATMENT RECOMMENDATIONS This agent effectively kills methicillin-sensitive *Staphylococcus aureus* and is a reasonable alternative to nafcillin or oxacillin when Gram-negative coverage is also required. Ticarcillin-clavulanate can be used for in-hospital aspiration pneumonia to cover for both mouth flora and Gram-negative rods and can also be used for serious intra-abdominal and gynecologic infections. This agent has also been used for skin and bone infections that are thought to be caused by a combination of Gram-negative and Gram-positive organisms.

Dose: 3.1 gm Q4–6H
Renal dosing: Cr Cl 10–50 cc/min, dose Q6–8H;
    Cr Cl <10 cc/min, 2 gm Q12H
Cost: Low
Spectrum: Very broad

PIPERACILLIN

This agent effectively kills many of the enterobacteriaceae as well as streptococcal species, *Haemophilus influenzae*, and Neisseria. It has excellent anaerobic coverage and kills most strains of *Pseudomonas aeruginosa* at high doses. Piperacillin alone may soon be discontinued in favor of piperacillin-tazobactam.

TREATMENT RECOMMENDATIONS Indications are the same as those for mezlocillin and ticarcillin.

Dose: 3–4 gm iv Q4–6H
Renal dosing: Cr Cl 10–50 cc/min, 3 gm
    Q8H; Cr Cl < 10 cc/min, 3 gm Q12H
Cost: Moderate
Spectrum: Moderately broad

PIPERACILLIN-TAZOBACTAM (ZOSYN)

This agent effectively kills many of the enterobacteriaceae as well as streptococcal species, *Haemophilus influenzae*, and Neisseria. It has excellent anaerobic coverage and kills most strains of *Pseudomonas aeruginosa* at high doses. Addition of the β-lactamase inhibitor tazobactam broadens the spectrum of piperacillin, improving *Staphylococcus aureus* coverage as well as that for many other β-lactamase-producing organisms.

TREATMENT RECOMMENDATIONS This combination is similar in efficacy to ticarcillin-clavulanate and has similar treatment indications. Because Q6H dosing is recommended to prevent accumulation of tazobactam, piperacillin-tazobactam is not recommended for *Pseudomonas aeruginosa* pneumonia, since the levels of piperacillin achievable in the sputum with this dosage schedule are too low to efficiently kill this pathogen. It is also recommended that when piperacillin-tazobactam is given in combination with an aminoglycoside, the administration of piperacillin-tazobactam should be separated from the administration of the aminoglycoside by 30–60 minutes.

Dose: 3/0.375 gm iv Q6H
Renal dosing: Cr Cl 10–50 cc/min, 2/0.25 gm
  Q6H; Cr Cl <10 cc/min, 2/0.25 gm Q8H Cost:
  Moderate
Spectrum: very broad

KEY POINTS
Carboxypenicillins and Ureidopenicillins

1. More effectively resist Gram-negative β-lactamases.
2. Carboxypenicillins or ureidopenicillins combined with aminoglycosides demonstrate
   synergistic killing of *Pseudomonas aeruginosa* and are recommended as primary therapy.
3. Piperacillin more effectively kills enterobacteriaceae.
4. Ticarcillin-clavulinate and piperacillin-
   tazobactam have excellent broad- spectrum
   coverage, including methicillin-sensitive
   Staphylococcus aureus and anaerobes, and
   are useful for intra-abdominal infections,
   acute prostatitis, in-hospital aspiration pneumonia, and mixed soft tissue and bone infections.

Cephalosporins

CHEMISTRY AND MECHANISMS OF ACTION

The basic structure of cephalosporins is very
similar to that of penicillin, consisting of a four-
member β-lactam ring connected to a six-member dihydrothiazine ring. This basic structure has
been modified by substituting groups at positions 7 (R_1 substitutions) and 3 (R_2 substitutions)
(see Figure 1.5). R_1 substitutions change the antimicrobial spectrum by altering resistance to
specific β-lactamases, affecting bacterial cell wall
penetration, and changing the affinity of the antibiotic for PBPs. R_2 substitutions affect the pharmacokinetics and metabolism of the antibiotic.
These modifications have resulted in an ever-

Figure 1.5

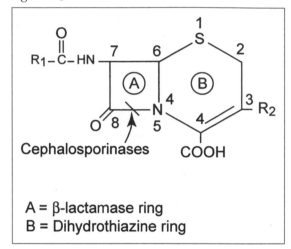

Basic structure of cephalosporins.

expanding number of cephalosporins that possess different antibacterial spectrums and pharmacokinetics.

Cephalosporins kill bacteria by the same
mechanisms as penicillin. (See above for a more
complete description.) They bind to bacterial
PBPs and block cell wall synthesis, causing lysis
and death of bacteria. Cephalosporins, like penicillins, are bactericidal and require active bacterial growth.

KEY POINTS
Cephalosporin Structure and Mechanisms of Action

1. Contain a β-lactam ring like penicillin.
2. Substitutions at the R_1 site change antibiotic
   spectrum.
3. Substitutions at the R_2 site affect pharmacokinetics.
4. Bind to penicillin-binding proteins (PBPs).
5. Block cell wall synthesis and cause cell wall
   lysis.
6. Require active bacterial growth to be bacteriocidal.

TOXICITY

Cephalosporins are considered the safest class of antibiotics. With a few unique exceptions, hypersensitivity reactions are the predominant adverse reaction associated with cephalosporin administration. However, the incidence of serious immediate IgE-mediated hypersensitivity reactions is much lower than occurs with penicillin. Delayed hypersensitivity reactions are also less common, skin rash with or without eosinophilia being reported in 1–3% of patients receiving cephalosporins. Because a significant number of patients have a history of penicillin allergy, clinicians must be concerned with the potential of cross-reactivity between cephalosporins and penicillins. Cephalosporin allergic reactions have been reported in 1–7% of patients with a history of penicillin allergy; therefore in patients with a history of immediate IgE-mediated reactions to penicillin, cephalosporins should be avoided. In patients with a history of delayed hypersensitivity reactions to penicillin, allergic cross-reactions to cephalosporins are rarely severe, and cephalosporins may be used in these patients if necessary. Hematologic manifestations of cephalosporin allergy include eosinophilia (1–7%) and, following prolonged high-dose therapy, neutropenia (<1%).

A potential concern, particularly for postoperative patients, is the development of hypoprothrombinemia in patients receiving cephalosporins with an R_2 substitution containing a methylthiotetrazole (MTT) ring (cefamandole, cefoperazone, moxalactam, cefotetan). Poor nutrition, debilitation, recent gastrointestinal surgery, and renal failure increase the risk of hypoprothrombinemia. Weekly prophylaxis with vitamin K is recommended for high-risk patients receiving MTT-bearing cephalosporins. The MTT group is similar in structure to disulfiram (Antabuse). Like disulfiram, these agents can interfere with alcohol metabolism to cause a buildup of acetaldehyde, resulting in tachycardia, hypotension, headache, flushing, nausea, and vomiting.

Gastrointestinal tract toxicities include nonspecific transaminase and alkaline phosphatase elevation that rarely requires discontinuing the cephalosporin. Nonspecific antibiotic-associated diarrhea develops in 2–5% of patients taking cephalosporins. The incidence is somewhat higher in association with cefoperazone and ceftriaxone, cephalosporins that are excreted via the biliary tract. Cephalosporins have an incidence of *Clostridium difficile* toxin–associated pseudomembranous colitis similar to that of penicillins (see Chapter 8, "Gastrointestinal and Hepatobiliary Infections"). Ceftriaxone excretion through the biliary tract has also been associated with the formation of biliary sludge in the gallbladder. Patients are usually asymptomatic but on occasion can experience symptoms of cholecystitis. Risk of biliary sludge formation is higher in children, in patients receiving high-dose ceftriaxone (>2 gm/day), and in those receiving total parenteral nutrition.

Nephrotoxicity is uncommonly associated with cephalosporin administration. Acute tubular necrosis has been reported in patients receiving higher than recommended doses of cephalosporins and in some elderly patients receiving high-dose cephalosporins. Cephalosporins also potentiate the nephrotoxicity of aminoglycosides. Therefore this antibiotic combination should be avoided in patients who are at high risk for aminoglycoside nephrotoxicity (see the discussion of aminoglycosides below). As is observed with penicillin, hypersensitivity reactions to cephalosporins on rare occasion have resulted in interstitial nephritis.

KEY POINTS
Cephalosporin Toxicity

1. Hypersensitivity reactions are most common.
2. There is 1–7% cross-reactivity in penicillin-allergic patients.

3. Cephalosporins should be avoided in patients with a history of immediate IgE-mediated hypersensitivity reactions to penicillin.
4. Allergic reactions may result in eosinophilia or neutropenia.
5. Cephalosporins can potentiate aminoglycoside toxicity.
6. Nonspecific diarrhea is observed in 2–5% of patients.

Classification of Cephalosporins

In an attempt to create some semblance of order, the cephalosporins have been classified into generations on the basis of their spectrums of activity. First-generation cephalosporins are effective predominantly against Gram-positive cocci, while second-generation cephalosporins demonstrate increased activity against aerobic and anaerobic Gram-negative bacilli but variable activity against Gram-positive cocci. The third-generation cephalosporins demonstrate even greater activity against Gram-negative bacilli but limited activity against Gram-positive cocci. Finally, fourth-generation cephalosporins demonstrate the broadest spectrum of effective activity against both Gram-positive cocci and Gram-negative bacilli. Classification of the cephalosporins by generation naturally leads to the assumption that newer, later-generation cephalosporins are better than older cephalosporins. However, it is important to keep in mind that for many infections earlier-generation, narrower-spectrum cephalosporins are preferred to the more recently developed broader-spectrum cephalosporins.

First-Generation Cephalosporins

The first-generation cephalosporins have a somewhat higher incidence of hypersensitivity reactions compared to later-generation cephalosporins. They are usually the least expensive.

CEFAZOLIN

Cefazolin is safe, well tolerated, and inexpensive. It has a longer half-life than penicillin, 1.8 hours, and like penicillin is primarily excreted by the kidneys. This antibiotic penetrates most body cavities but fails to cross the blood-brain barrier. Cefazolin is very active against Gram-positive cocci, including methicillin-sensitive *Staphylococcus aureus*, and has moderate activity against community-acquired *Klebsiella pneumoniae*, *E. coli*, *Proteus mirabilis*, and *Moraxella catarrhalis*. It is also active against oral cavity anaerobes but is ineffective for treating *Bacteroides fragilis*, *Haemophilus influenzae*, *Listeria monocytogenes*, methicillin-resistant *S. aureus* (MRSA), penicillin-resistant *Streptococcus pneumoniae*, and enterococcus.

TREATMENT RECOMMENDATIONS　This drug is an effective alternative to nafcillin or oxacillin for soft tissue infections that are thought to be caused by methicillin-sensitive *Staphylococcus aureus* or *Streptococcus pyogenes*. Cefazolin is also the antibiotic of choice for surgical prophylaxis. Because of its inability to cross the blood-brain barrier, cefazolin should never be used to treat bacterial meningitis.

Dose: 1–1.5 gm iv or im Q6–8H not to exceed 12 gm/day
Renal dosing: Cr Cl 10–50 cc/min, 0.5–1 gm Q8–12H; Cr Cl < 10 cc/min, 0.25–0.75 gm Q18–24H
Cost: Low
Spectrum: Narrow
See Tables 1.1 and 1.2 for classifications.

CEPHALEXIN AND CEPHRADINE

These drugs are very well absorbed, achieving excellent peak serum concentrations (0.5 gm results in 18 µg/ml peak). Absorption is not affected by food. The half-lives of these two drugs are short: 0.9 hour for cephalexin and 0.7 hour for cephradine.

TREATMENT RECOMMENDATIONS Commonly used to treat less severe soft tissue infections, including impetigo, early cellulitis, and mild diabetic foot ulcers.

Dose: 0.25–1 gm po Q6–8H for cephalexin and Q6H for cephradine
Cost: Low for generic forms
Spectrum: Narrow

CEFADROXIL

This antibiotic is 100% absorbed orally. The half-life is somewhat longer, 1.2 hours, than those of the above two agents, allowing a longer dosing interval.

TREATMENT RECOMMENDATIONS Treatment indications are the same as for cephalexin and cephradine.

Dose: 0.5–1 gm Q12H
Cost: Moderate
Spectrum: Narrow

KEY POINTS
First-Generation Cephalosporins

1. Higher incidence of hypersensitivity reactions than other generations.
2. Excellent Gram-positive coverage, some Gram-negative coverage.
3. Do not cross the blood-brain barrier.
4. Inexpensive.
5. Useful for treating soft tissue infections and in surgical prophylaxis. Can often be used as an alternative to oxacillin/nafcillin.

Second-Generation Cephalosporins

This category includes true cephalosporins and the cephamycins (cefoxitin and cefotetan). These agents demonstrate increased activity against *Haemophilus influenzae*, *Neisseria meningitidis*, *N. gonorrhoeae*, and *Moraxella catarrhalis* in addition to effectively treating methicillin-sensitive *Stapylococcus aureus* and nonenterococcal streptococci. Given the availability of first-, third-, and fourth-generation cephalosporins as well as the newer penicillins, second-generation cephalosporins are rarely recommended as primary therapy. Therefore a complete description of all the second-generation cephalosporins will not be included. Because cefoxitin and cefotetan demonstrate increased anaerobic coverage in addition to covering the gonococcus, these two agents are used as part of the first line therapy in pelvic inflammatory disease.

CEFOXITIN

This antibiotic demonstrates increased activity against *E. coli*, *Klebsiella*, and some strains of Proteus compared to first-generation cephalosporins. Cefoxitin has a short half life (0.8 hour) and requires frequent dosing. The major advantage of cefoxitin is its broader anaerobic spectrum. This agent kills many strains of *Bacteroides fragilis*.

TREATMENT RECOMMENDATIONS Cefoxitin has proved effective for the treatment of intra-abdominal infections. Because it effectively kills *Neisseria gonorrhoeae*, this agent is commonly recommended in combination with doxycycline for the treatment of pelvic inflammatory disease. Cefoxitin is also used in other gynecologic infections and in mixed aerobic-anaerobic soft tissue infections, including diabetic foot infections.

Dose: 1–2 gm iv or im Q4–6H not to exceed 12 gm/day
Renal dosing: Cr Cl 50–80 cc/min, 1–2 gm Q8–12H; Cr Cl 10–50 cc/min, 1–2 gm Q12–24H; Cr Cl < 10 cc/min, 0.5–1 gm Q12–48H
Cost: Moderate
Spectrum: Moderately broad

CEFOTETAN

This agent provides coverage that is similar to that of cefoxitin. Cefotetan has an MTT group; however, treatment has not been clearly shown to increase the incidence of bleeding. Vitamin K prophylaxis may be given to malnourished patients. Cefotetan has a much longer half-life than cefoxitin (3.5 hours versus 0.8 hour), allowing it to be dosed every 12 hours.

TREATMENT RECOMMENDATIONS   Cefoxitin and cefotetan can be used interchangeably.

Dose: 1–2 gm iv or im Q12H
Renal dosing: Cr Cl 10–50 cc/min, 1–2 gm
    Q24H; Cr Cl < 10 cc/min, 1–2 gm Q48H
Cost: Low
Spectrum: Moderately broad

CEFUROXIME

Cefuroxime provides excellent coverage against *Haemophilus influenzae*, Neisseria species, *Streptococcus pneumoniae*, and *S. pyogenes*. Cefuroxime effectively crosses the blood-brain barrier and has been used for the treatment of bacterial meningitis. However, a randomized trial comparing cefuroxime to ceftriaxone in the treatment of children with bacterial meningitis revealed significantly better outcomes with ceftriaxone. The half-life of this drug is 1.3 hours, allowing Q8H dosing.

TREATMENT RECOMMENDATIONS   Cefuroxime is not recommended as the first line therapy for any infection. It can be used as an alternative treatment for *Neisseria gonorrhoeae*, *Haemophilus influenzae*, or *Streptococcus pyogenes*.

Dose: 0.75–1.5 gm iv Q8H
Renal dosing: Cr Cl 10–50 cc/min, 0.75–1.5 gm
    Q12H; Cr Cl <10 cc/min, 0.75 gm Q24H
Cost: Low
Spectrum: Moderately broad

CEFUROXIME-AXETIL

Esterification of cefuroxime increases its oral absorption to 30–50%. The peak levels that are achievable orally are approximately one tenth those of intravenous administration. Food increases absorption.

TREATMENT RECOMMENDATIONS   The oral preparation can be used for mild to moderately severe infections and is effective for the outpatient treatment of uncomplicated urinary tract infections as well as otitis media. It provides the same coverage as cefuroxime; however, serum levels are lower. Other, less costly oral antibiotics effectively cover the same pathogens.

Dose: 0.25–0.5 gm Q12H
Renal dosing: Cr Cl < 10 cc/min, 0.25 gm Q24H
Cost: Moderately high
Spectrum: Moderately broad

CEFACLOR

This oral second-generation cephalosporin is absorbed similarly to cephalexin and has a similar half-life (0.8 hour). Its spectrum of coverage is somewhat broader, demonstrating moderate increased activity against *Haemophilus influenzae*, *Moraxella catarrhalis*, *E. coli*, and *Proteus mirabilis*. However, β-lactamases produced by *H. influenzae* and *M. catarrhalis* are able to inactivate cefaclor. A slow-release tablet is available; however, peak serum levels are lower with this preparation. Food interferes with absorption, and cefaclor should be taken 1 hour before meals.

TREATMENT RECOMMENDATIONS   This oral antibiotic has been recommended for otitis media; however, other oral antibiotics are generally preferred.

Dose: 0.25–0.5 gm Q8H, no requirement for adjustment in renal failure
Cost: Moderate
Spectrum: Moderately broad

KEY POINTS

Second-Generation Cephalosporins

> 1. Improved activity against *Haemophilus influenzae*, Neisseria species, and *Moraxella catarrhalis*.
> 2. Cefoxitin and cefotetan have anaerobic activity and are used in mixed soft tissue infections and pelvic inflammatory disease.
> 3. Cefotetan and cefomandole have an MTT ring that decreases prothrombin production. Vitamin K prophylaxis is recommended in malnourished patients.
> 4. Cefuroxime-axetil is a popular oral cephalosporin; however, less expensive alternative oral antibiotics are available.
> 5. Overall, this generation is of limited usefulness.

Third-Generation Cephalosporins

These agents have enhanced activity against many aerobic Gram-negative bacilli but do not cover *Serratia marcescens*, Acinetobacter, and *Enterobacter cloacae*. With the exceptions of ceftazidime and cefoperazone, third-generation cephalosporins are ineffective against *Pseudomonas aeruginosa*. These agents have excellent cidal activity against *Streptococcus pneumoniae* (including moderately penicillin-resistant strains), *S. pyogenes*, and other streptococci. With the exception of ceftazidime, they are also effective against methicillin-sensitive *Staphylococcus aureus*, *Haemophilus influenzae*, and *Moraxella catarrhalis*. *Neisseria meningitidis* and *N. gonorrhoeae* are very sensitive to all third-generation preparations. All members of this generation are ineffective for treating enterococcus, methicillin-resistant *Staphylococcus aureus*, highly penicillin-resistant pneumococcus, and *Listeria monocytogenes*. Extended-spectrum β-lactamases (ESBLs) are increasing in frequency and promise to reduce the effectiveness of the third- and fourth-generation cephalosporins. A large number of third-generation cephalosporins are available, all

with similar indications. Small deficiencies in coverage, increased toxicity, and less desirable pharmacokinetics have decreased the popularity of many of these drugs. Only those members that are commonly included in hospital formularies will be discussed.

CEFTRIAXONE

This antibiotic has superior activity against most aerobic Gram-positive cocci and modest activity against *Staphylococcus aureus*. Ceftriaxone is the most potent member of the third-generation cephalosporins against *Neisseria gonorrhoeae*, *N. meningitidis*, and *Haemophilus influenzae*. This agent has a prolonged half-life of 8 hours, allowing once-a-day administration for most infections. In meningitis Q12H dosing is generally recommended. Achievable peak levels are very high (250 µg/ml following a 2-gm dose), enhancing delivery across the blood-brain barrier as well as in other less penetrable body sites. Ceftriaxone is cleared by the kidneys and by the biliary tract. The potential for biliary sludging increases with higher doses and prolonged therapy and is higher in children.

TREATMENT RECOMMENDATIONS Ceftriaxone is recommended for the empiric treatment of community-acquired bacterial meningitis and of community-acquired pneumonia (see Chapters 4 and 6). Ceftriaxone is one of several cephalosporins that can be used in combination with other antibiotics to empirically treat the septic patient. This antibiotic is also recommended for treatment of *Neisseria gonorrhoeae*. The once-a-day dosing schedule increases the feasibility and convenience of home intravenous therapy.

Dose: 1–2 gm Q12–24H, no adjustment required for renal failure
Cost: Low to moderate depending on the dose
Spectrum: Broad

CEFOTAXIME

This antibiotic has activity very similar to that of ceftriaxone. However, its half-life is 1 hour, necessitating Q8H dosing. At high doses (2 gm Q4H) this drug reliably enters the cerebrospinal fluid and can be used for the treatment of bacterial meningitis. Cefotaxime is cleared renally and does not form sludge in the gallbladder. For this reason this agent is preferred over ceftriaxone by some pediatricians.

TREATMENT RECOMMENDATIONS   Cefotaxime has a spectrum of coverage identical to that of ceftriaxone and has the same treatment recommendations. Pediatricians prefer this agent to ceftriaxone, particularly for the treatment of bacterial meningitis for which high-dose therapy is required.

Dose: 2 gm Q6–8H, for meningitis 2 gm Q4–6H, maximum dose 12 gm/day
Renal dosing: Cr Cl 10–30 cc/min, Q8–12H; Cr Cl <10 cc/min, Q12–24H
Cost: Low to moderate, depending on dose
Spectrum: Broad

CEFTIZOXIME

This antibiotic also has a spectrum similar to that of ceftriaxone but is somewhat less effective against *Streptococcus pneumoniae*. It covers a larger percentage of *Bacteroides fragilis* than does cefotaxime or ceftriaxone. Ceftizoxime also crosses the blood-brain barrier at high doses but is not recommended as a first-line drug for meningitis.

TREATMENT RECOMMENDATIONS   Ceftizoxime is recommended for the treatment of *Klebsiella pneumoniae* and indole-positive Proteus (including *Providencia rettgeri*, *Morganella morganii*, and *Proteus vulgaris*).

Dose: 1–4 gm Q8–12H up to 12 gm/day
Renal dosing: Cr Cl 10–30 cc/min, Q12H; Cr Cl < 10 cc/min, Q24H

Cost: Moderate to high depending on dose
Spectrum: Broad

CEFTAZIDIME

This is the only third-generation cephalosporin that has excellent activity against *Pseudomonas aeruginosa*. Ceftazidime is a weak inducer of β-lactamases and binds poorly to many β-lactamases, making it a particularly effective agent for the treatment of Gram-negative bacilli. Ceftazidime has reduced activity against Gram-positive bacteria, particularly *Staphylococcus aureus*. It also has poor activity against *Bacteroides fragilis*.

TREATMENT RECOMMENDATIONS   Ceftazidime provides effective coverage for most cases of pyelonephritis. *Pseudomonas aeruginosa* is often treated with ceftazidime, although ciprofloxacin is now considered first-line therapy. It is also recommended for treatment of *Klebsiella pneumoniae*, indole-positive Proteus, and *E. coli*. Ceftazidime crosses the blood-brain barrier and is the treatment of choice for *Pseudomonas aeruginosa* meningitis.

Dose: 1–3 gm iv or im Q8H up to 8 gm/day
Renal dosing: Cr Cl 10–50 cc/min, 1 gm Q12–24H; Cr Cl < 10 cc/min, 0.5 gm Q24–48H
Cost: Low to moderate
Spectrum: Broad

CEFIXIME

An oral cephalosporin, cefixime has a long half-life of 3.7 hours, allowing once-a-day dosing. Cefixime provides effective coverage for *Streptococcus pneumoniae* (penicillin-sensitive), *S. pyogenes*, *Haemophilus influenzae*, *Moraxella catarrhalis*, Neisseria species, and many Gram-negative bacilli but is ineffective against *Staphylococcus aureus*. This agent's absorption is not affected by food.

TREATMENT RECOMMENDATIONS Potential second-line therapy for community-acquired pneumonia. It is an alternative to penicillin for the treatment of bacterial pharyngitis.

Dose: 400 mg QD or BID
Renal dosing: Cr Cl 10–30 cc/min, 300 mg QD; Cr Cl <10 cc/min, 200 mg QD
Cost: Low
Spectrum: Broad

CEFPODOXIME PROXETIL

This oral third-generation cephalosporin has an antimicrobial spectrum similar to that of cefixime and in addition has moderate activity against *Staphylococcus aureus*. Cefpodoxime proxetil has a half-life of 2.2 hours, and its absorption is enhanced by food.

TREATMENT RECOMMENDATIONS Cefpodoxime has indications similar to those of cefixime. It has also has been recommended as an alternative treatment for acute sinusitis.

Dose: 200–400 gm BID
Renal dosing: Cr Cl 10–30 cc/min, 200–400 mg 3 × per week; Cr Cl <10 cc/min, 200–400 mg 1 × per week
Cost: Moderately high
Spectrum: Broad

KEY POINTS
Third-Generation Cephalosporins

1. Improved Gram-negative coverage.
2. Excellent activity against *Neisseria gonorrhoeae*, *N. meningitidis*, *Haemophilus influenzae*, and *Moraxella catarrhalis*.
3. Ceftriaxone has a long half-life, allowing once-a-day dosing.
4. In children acalculus cholecystitis can occur with large doses.

5. Cefotaxime has a shorter half-life but identical activity to ceftriaxone but does not cause biliary sludging.
6. Ceftzidime has excellent activity against most *Pseudomonas aeruginosa* strains but reduced activity against *Staphylococcus aureus*.
7. ESBL (spectrum β-lactamases) are increasing in frequency and endangering the effectiveness of third-generation cephalosporins.

Fourth-Generation Cephalosporins

The R_2 substitution of the fourth-generation cephalosporins contains both a positively charged and a negatively charged group that together have zwitterionic properties that allow these antibiotics to penetrate the outer wall of Gram-negative bacteria and concentrate in the periplasmic space. They are resistant to most β-lactamases and only weakly induce β-lactamase activity. These agents also bind Gram-positive PBPs with high affinity.

CEFEPIME

This is the only fourth-generation cephalosporin that is available in the United States. In addition to having broad antimicrobial activity against Gram-negative bacilli, including *Pseudomonas aeruginosa*, cefepime provides excellent coverage for *Streptococcus pneumoniae*, including strains that are moderately resistant to penicillin, *Streptococcus pyogenes*, and methicillin-sensitive *Staphylococcus aureus*. Like the third-generation cephalosporins, it effectively kills *Haemophilus influenzae* and Neisseria species. Cefepime and ceftazidime provide comparable coverage for *Pseudomonas aeruginosa*. To maximize the likelihood of cure of serious *P. aeruginosa* infections, more frequent dosing (Q6H) has been recommended. Cefepime is not effective against *Listeria monocytogenes*, methicillin-resistant *Staphylococcus aureus*, or *Bacteroides fragilis*.

Compared to third-generation cephalosporins, cefepime is more resistant to β-lactamases, including the ESBLs. This drug has a half-life of 2.1 hours. Cefepime penetrates inflamed meninges and has been used effectively to treat Gram-negative meningitis.

TREATMENT RECOMMENDATIONS This agent is effective as a single agent in the febrile neutropenic patient and is an excellent agent for initial empiric coverage of nosocomial infections.

Dose: 0.5–2 gm Q8–12H
Renal dosing: Cr Cl 10–30 cc/min, 0.5–1 gm
    Q24H; Cr Cl <10 cc/min, 250–500 mg Q24H
Cost: Low to moderate
Spectrum: Broad

CEFIPIROME

This drug is not available in the United States. Cefipirome has an antimicrobial spectrum similar to that of cefepime, although it is somewhat less active against *Pseudomonas aeruginosa*. The pharmacokinetics of cefipirome is also similar to that of cefepime.

Dose: 1–2 gm Q12H
Renal dosing: Same as cefepime

KEY POINTS
Fourth-Generation Cephalosporins

> 1. Zwitterionic properties allow excellent penetration of the bacterial cell wall as well as human tissues and fluids.
> 2. Weakly induce β-lactamases.
> 3. More resistant to ESBL and chromosomal β-lactamases.
> 4. Excellent Gram-positive (including MSSA) and Gram-negative coverage (including *Pseudomonas aeruginosa*).
> 5. Excellent broad-spectrum empiric therapy. Useful in nosocomial infections.

Monobactams

AZTREONAM

This β-lactam antibiotic was originally isolated from *Chromobacterium violaceum* and subsequently modified. Aztreonam has a distinctly different structure from that of the cephalosporins. Rather than a central double ring, aztreonam has a single-ring or monocyclic β-lactam structure and has been classified as a monobactam. It is the only antibiotic in this class that is available. Aztreonam does not bind to the PBPs of Gram-positive organisms or anaerobes but binds with high affinity to PBPs, particularly PBP-3 (which is responsible for septum formation during bacterial division), of Gram-negative bacilli, including *Pseudomonas aeruginosa*. Gram-negative organisms that are exposed to aztreonam form long, filamentous structures and are killed.

Aztreonam is effective against most Gram-negative bacilli, and this agent has been marketed as a nonnephrotoxic replacement for aminoglycosides. However, unlike aminoglycosides, aztreonam does not provide synergy with penicillins for enterococcus. A major advantage of aztreonam is its restricted antimicrobial spectrum, which allows survival of the normal Gram-positive and anaerobic flora that can compete with more resistant pathogens. This monobactam penetrates body tissue well and crosses the blood-brain barrier of inflamed meninges. Aztreonam's half-life is approximately 2 hours, being primarily cleared by the kidneys.

TREATMENT RECOMMENDATIONS Aztreonam can be used for the treatment of most infections due to Gram-negative bacilli. It has been used effectively in pyelonephritis, nosocomial Gram-negative pneumonia, Gram-negative bacteremia, and Gram-negative intra-abdominal infections. It is important to keep in mind that aztreonam provides no Gram-positive or anaerobic coverage. Therefore when used for empiric treatment of the seriously ill patient, aztreonam should be combined with vancomycin, clindamycin, erythromycin, or a penicillin to treat for potential Gram-positive pathogens. Because of its unique structure, aztreonam exhibits no cross-reactivity with other β-lactam antibiotics and can be used safely in the penicillin-allergic patient.

Dose: 1–2 gm iv or im Q6H
Renal dosing: Cr Cl 10–30 cc/min, 1–2 gm
    Q12–18H; Cr Cl < 10 cc/min, 1–2 gm Q24H
Cost: Low to moderate
Spectrum: Narrow

Key Points
Aztreonam

1. A distinctly different structure than the cephalosporins.
2. No cross-reactivity with PCN.
3. Binds the PBPs of Gram-negative but *not* Gram-positive bacteria.
4. Narrow spectrum with excellent activity against aerobic Gram-negative rods.
5. Marketed as a nonnephrotoxic replacement for aminoglycosides. However, as compared to aminoglycosides:
   a. Does not result in synergy with PCNs in enterococcal infections,
   b. Not helpful for treating *S. viridens* endocarditis.
6. Excellent empiric antibiotic when combined with an antibiotic with good Gram-positive activity; useful for the treatment of pyelonephritis.

Carbapenems

These agents have a modified thiazoladine ring as well as a change in the configuration of the side chain that renders the β-lactam ring highly resistant to cleavage.

Imipenem and Meropenem

These antibiotics have a hydroxyethyl side chain that is in a *trans* rather than a *cis* conformation, and this configuration is thought to be responsible for their remarkable resistance to β-lactamase breakdown. Imipenem is combined in a 1:1 ratio with cilastatin to block rapid breakdown by renal dehydropeptidase I. Because the carbapenems have zwitterionic characteristics at physiologic pH and are the smallest β-lactam antibiotics, they readily penetrate tissues. Imipenem and meropenem are primarily cleared by the kidneys and have half-lives of 1 hour. Only minimal concentrations are secreted into the bile.

Imipenem has been associated with immediate hypersensitivity reactions, and 3–7% of penicillin-allergic patients also experience allergic reactions to imipenem. Patients with a history of immediate hypersensitivity reactions to penicillin should not receive carbapenems. Seizures are the other serious toxicity and are reported in 0.4–1.5% of patients receiving imipenem. Meropenem and ertapenem are less epileptogenic. Lesions in the central nervous system, a prior history of seizures, renal insufficiency, old age, and excessive doses all increase the risk of seizures. Nausea and vomiting occur in 4% of patients, often being associated with rapid infusion or doses of >2gm/day). Diarrhea occurs in 3% of patients (only the minority of which is due to *Clostridium difficile*).

Carbapenems bind with high affinity to the high-molecular-weight PBPs of both Gram-positive and Gram-negative bacteria. As a result they can effectively kill virtually all strains of Gram-positive and Gram-negative bacteria, including anaerobes. In addition to *Streptococcus pneumoniae*, *S. pyogenes*, and methicillin-sensitive *Staphylococcus aureus*, imipenem and meropenem are cidal against organisms that are not covered by cephalosporins, including Listeria, Nocardia, Legionella, and *Mycobacterium aviumintracellulare*. They have static activity against penicillin-sensitive enterococcus; however, many penicillin-resistant strains are resistant. Methicillin-resistant *Staphylococcus aureus,* some penicillin-resistant strains of *S. pneumonia,* and *Clostridium difficile* as well as *Stenotrophomonas maltophilia* and *Burkhodleria cepacia* are resistant to imipenem and meropenem. Resistance in Gram-negative bacilli is most often secondary to loss of an outer membrane protein called D2 that is required for intracellular penetration of imipenem. Certain Gram-negative strains can also produce a β-lactamase that can hydrolyze carbapenems.

TREATMENT RECOMMENDATIONS   Imipenem and meropenem represent one of several classes of antibiotics that can be used as empiric therapy for sepsis. These agents are particularly useful if polymicrobial bacteremia is a strong possibility. Imipenem or meropenem can also be used to treat severe intra-abdominal infections and are one of a number of alternatives that can be used to treat the seriously ill patient with pyelonephritis. Infections due to Gram-negative bacilli that are resistant to cephalosporins and aminoglycosides may be sensitive to imipenem and meropenam. These agents are recommended as the primary therapy for Serratia. In general, imipenem and meropenem should be reserved for the seriously ill patient or the patient who is infected with a highly resistant bacterium that are sensitive only to these antibiotics. Because the carbapenems have an extremely broad spectrum, they kill nearly all normal flora. The loss of normal flora increases the risk of nosocomial infections with resistant pathogens, including methicillin-resistant *Staphylococcus aureus* (MRSA), vancomycin-resistant enterococcus (VRE), Pseudomonas, and Candida. Imipenem and meropenam are therapeutically equivalent and can be used for the same indications.

Imipenem
Dose: 0.5–1 gm Q6H
Renal dosing: Cr Cl 50–80 cc/min, 0.5 gm Q6–8H; Cr Cl 10–50 cc/min, 0.5 gm Q8–12H; Cr Cl <10 cc/min, 0.25–0.5 gm Q12H
Cost: Moderately high to very high
Spectrum: Very broad

Meropenem
Dose: 1 gm iv Q8H
Renal dosing: Cr Cl 10–50 cc/min, 0.5 gm Q12H; Cr Cl <10 cc/min, 0.5 gm Q24H
Cost: Moderately high
Spectrum: Very broad

ERTAPENEM

This newly released carbapenem has a slightly narrower spectrum of activity than imipenem or meropenem. This agent has broad Gram-positive and anaerobic coverage as well as Gram-negative coverage, but does not cover *Pseudomonas aerugionsa*. The primary advantage of ertapenem is its prolonged half-life of 4 hours, allowing the drug to be dosed once per day. Like other carbapenems, it is primarily excreted by the kidneys. The indications for use of this agent are evolving. Ertapenem has been approved by the FDA for complicated intraabdominal infections; complicated skin and soft tissue infections; community-acquired penumonia due to *S. pneumoniae, Hemophilus influenza,* and *Moraxella catarrhalis;* postoperative and postpartum acute pelvic infections; and complicated urinary tract infections due to *E. coli* or *Klebsiella pneumoniae.*

Dose: 1 gram im or iv QD
Renal dosing: Cr Cl ≤30 cc/min, 500 mg QD
Cost: Low
Spectrum: Very Broad

KEY POINTS
Carbapenems

1. The β-lactam ring is highly resistant to cleavage.
2. Have zwitterionic characteristics and penetrate all tissues.
3. Frequent cross-reactivity in penicillin-allergic patients (7%).
4. Imipenem causes seizures at high doses; be cautious in renal failure patients. Meropenem and ertapenem less epileptogenic.

5. Bind PBPs of all bacteria with high affinity.
6. Impipenem and meropenem
   a. Have very broad cidal activity for aerobic and anaerobic Gram-positive and Gram-negative bacteria. Also cover *Listeria monocytogenes* and Nocardia.
   b. Are useful for empiric therapy in which a mixed aerobic and anaerobic infection is suspected or for a severe nosocomial infection, pending culture results
   c. Reserve for the severely ill patient
7. Ertapenem
   a. Does not cover *Pseudomonas aeruginosa*
   b. May be used for complicated intraabdominal infections, complicated skin and soft tissue infections, some forms of community-acquired pneumonia, postoperative and postpartum pelvic infection, and complicated UTI due *E. coli* and *Klebsiella pneumoniae*.
   c. Can be given once per day.
8. Treatment markedly alters the normal bacterial flora.

Aminoglycosides

Chemistry and Mechanism of Action

Aminoglycosides were originally derived from Streptomyces species. These agents have a characteristic six-membered ring with amino group substitutions and are highly soluble in water. At neutral pH they are positively charged, and this positive charge contributes to their antibacterial activity. Because the positive charge is reduced by low pH, aminoglycoside antimicrobial activity is reduced by acidic conditions. Their positive charge also causes aminoglycosides to bind to and become inactivated by β-lactam antibiotics. Therefore aminoglycosides should never be stored in the same solution with β-lactam antibiotics.

Aminoglycosides bind electrostatically to the bacterial outer membrane. They competitively displace magnesium and calcium, weakening lipopolysaccharide links and causing the formation of temporary holes that allow the antibiotic to enter the bacterial cytoplasm. The aminoglycoside then becomes trapped in the cytoplasm, and the positively charged antibiotic molecules interact with and precipitate DNA and other anionic components. Aminoglycoside uptake is energy dependent, requiring an electrochemical gradient of protons. The greater the transmembrane potential, the greater is the antibacterial effect of the aminoglycosides. Acid pH, an anaerobic environment, and hyperosmolar conditions lower this potential. Aminoglycosides also bind to the 30S subunit of bacterial 16S ribosomal RNA and interfere with translation. The combined effects on the bacterial outer membrane and ribosome are bactericidal.

Resistance

Bacteria are able to resist aminoglycoside action by three mechanisms. Most commonly, they produce enzymes that modify and reduce the antimicrobicidal activity of aminoglycosides. These enzymes are generally encoded by plasmids that can be transferred from one bacterial strain to another. The second mechanism of bacterial resistance consists of an alteration in the 16S ribosomal binding site, reducing the ability of the antibiotic to impair translation. Finally, bacteria can alter their aminoglycoside transport pathways and prevent high concentrations of the antibiotic from entering the bacteria.

Toxicity

The aminoglycosides have a narrow therapeutic-to-toxic ratio, and monitoring serum levels is generally required to prevent toxicity. Three major toxicities are observed:

1. **Nephrotoxicity.** Injury to the proximal convoluted tubules of the kidney leads to a decrease in creatinine clearance. The brush border cells of the proximal tubule take up aminoglycosides by endocytosis, and intracellular entry is associated with cell necrosis. Aminoglycosides cause significant reductions of glomerular filtration in 5–25% of patients. Patient characteristics associated with an increased risk of nephrotoxicity include older age, preexisting renal disease, hepatic dysfunction, volume depletion, and hypotension. Reexposure to aminoglycosides increases risk, as does the use of larger doses, more frequent dosing intervals, and treatment for more than 3 days. The risk of renal failure is also associated with coadministration of vancomycin, amphotericin B, clindamycin, piperacillin, cephalosporins, foscarnet, or furosemide. Because renal tubular cells have regenerative power, renal dysfunction usually reverses on discontinuation of the aminoglycoside. Because aminoglycosides are primarily renally cleared, aminoglycoside serum levels are useful for detecting worsening renal function. Trough aminoglycoside serum levels often rise prior to the detection of a significant rise in serum creatinine.

2. **Ototoxicity.** Aminoglycosides enter the inner ear fluid and damage outer hair cells, which are important for detecting high-frequency sound. High-frequency hearing loss occurs in 3–14% of patients treated with aminoglycosides. The risk of hearing loss is greater after prolonged treatment; most cases develop after 9 or more days of therapy. Hearing loss is irreversible and can occur weeks after therapy has been discontinued. A genetic predisposition has been observed, certain families having a high incidence of deafness after receiving aminoglycosides. The risk of hearing loss depends on the aminoglycoside; neomycin has the highest risk of toxicity, followed in decreasing frequency by gentamicin, tobramycin, amikacin, and netilmicin. Use of furosemide and vancomycin and exposure to loud noises increase the risk. Once-daily dosing reduces the toxic risk compared to frequent dosing.

    In addition to affecting hearing, aminoglycosides can impair vestibular function by damaging type I hair cells in the semicircular canals. This complication is particularly devastating for elderly patients, who often have visual deficits as well as depressed proprioception and cerebellar function. These deficits combined with loss of vestibular function can result in a loss of the ability to walk without falling. The incidence is estimated to be 4–6% in patients receiving aminoglycosides.

3. **Neuromuscular blockade.** This is a rare but potentially fatal complication. By blocking internalization of calcium into the presynaptic region of the axon, aminoglycosides interfere with presynaptic release of acetylcholine. They also can interfere with postsynaptic receptors. These effects can cause weakness of respiratory musculature, flaccid paralysis, and dilated pupils. The risk of neuromuscular blockade is higher in patients receiving curarelike agents, succinylcholine, or similar agents and is potentiated by hypocalcemia or hypomagnesemia. Paralysis is reversed by administering calcium gluconate and can be prevented by slowly infusing the aminoglycoside over 20–30 minutes.

Given the high risk of toxicity, aminoglycosides should be used only when alternative antibiotics are unavailable. When aminoglycosides are required, the duration of therapy should be as brief as possible. Pretreatment and periodic high-frequency hearing testing should be monitored in addition to following serum creatinine and aminoglycoside levels.

KEY POINTS

Aminoglycoside Toxicity

1. Very low therapeutic-to-toxic ratio.
2. Monitoring serum levels is usually required.

3. Nephrotoxicity occurs commonly, usually reversible. Higher incidence in
   a. Elderly,
   b. Preexisting renal disease,
   c. Volume depletion and hypotension,
   d. Liver disease.

   Higher incidence with vancomycin, cephalosporins, clindamycin, piperacillin, foscarnet, or furosemide.
4. Ototoxicity: high-frequency hearing loss and vestibular dysfunction, often devastating for the elderly.
5. Neuromuscular blockade.
6. Once-a-day therapy may be less toxic.

Antimicrobial Spectrum and Treatment Recommendations

The aminoglycosides are cidal for most aerobic Gram-negative bacilli, including Pseudomonas species. Streptomycin is the most effective drug for treating *Yersinia pestis*, and streptomycin or gentamicin effectively kills *Francisella tularensis*. Spectinomycin can effectively kill many strains of *Neisseria gonorrhoeae*. These agents kill rapidly, and killing is concentration-dependent; that is, the rate of killing increases as the concentration of the antibiotic increases. Once-a-day dosing takes advantage of this characteristic. Aminoglycosides also demonstrate persistent suppression of bacterial growth for 1–3 hours after the antibiotic is no longer present. The higher the concentration of aminoglycoside, the longer is the postantibiotic effect. Finally, aminoglycosides demonstrate synergy with antibiotics that act on the cell wall (β-lactam antibiotics and glycopeptides). The effect of the drug combination is greater than the sum of each individual drug's antimicrobial effect. Synergy has been achieved in the treatment of enterococci, *Streptococcus viridans*, *Staphylococcus aureus*, coagulase-negative staphylococcus, *Pseudomonas aeruginosa*, *Listeria monocytogenes*, and group JK corynebacteria.

An aminoglycoside in combination with other antibiotics is generally recommended for treatment of severely ill patients with the sepsis syndrome to ensure broad coverage for Gram-negative bacilli. An aminoglycoside combined with penicillin is recommended for empiric coverage of bacterial endocarditis. Tobramycin combined with an antipseudomonal penicillin or an antipseudomonal cephalosporin is recommended as primary treatment of Pseudomonas aeruginosa. Streptomycin or gentamicin is the treatment of choice for tularemia as well as Yersinia pestis. Gentamicin combined with penicillin is the treatment of choice for both Streptococcus viridans and Enterococcus faecalis.

1. Six-member ring, soluble in water, positively charged; never store with cephalosporins or acidic solutions.
2. Causes temporary holes in bacterial membranes, binds to ribosomal RNA and interferes with translation.
3. Killing is concentration dependent.
4. The higher the concentration, the longer is the postantibiotic effect.
5. Excellent Gram-negative coverage; streptomycin or gentamicin for tularemia and plague.
6. Synergy with penicillins in *Streptococcus viridans*, enterococcus, and *Pseudomonas aeruginosa* infections.

Pharmacokinetics

Following intravenous infusion aminoglycosides take 15–30 minutes to distribute throughout the body. Therefore to determine the peak serum level, the blood sample should be drawn one half hour after completion of the intravenous infusion. The half-life of the aminoglycosides is 1.5–3.5 hours. Proper dosing of aminoglycosides is more complicated than that of most other antibiotics and requires close monitoring. In many hospitals a pharmacist is consulted to assist in dose management. For multiple-daily-dose therapy, a loading dose is first given to rapidly achieve a therapeutic serum level, followed by maintenance doses. Doses are calculated on the basis of ideal body weight. In the setting of renal dysfunction dosing must be carefully adjusted, and peak and trough serum levels must be monitored. As renal impairment worsens, the dosage interval should be extended.

Recently, once-daily aminoglycoside dosing has been utilized. Compared to multidose therapy, once-a-day administration reduces the concentration of aminoglycoside that accumulates in the renal cortex and lowers the incidence of nephrotoxicity. The high peak levels that are achieved with this regimen also increase the rate of bacterial killing and prolong the postantibiotic effect. In addition this regimen is simpler and less expensive to administer. The regimen has not been associated with a higher incidence of neuromuscular dysfunction. To adjust for renal impairment, the daily dose should be reduced.

Monitoring of serum levels is recommended for both regimens. With multidose therapy a peak level should be drawn one half hour after intravenous infusion is completed, and a trough level should be drawn one half hour before the next dose. Peak and trough levels should be drawn after the third dose of antibiotic to ensure full equilibration with the distribution volume. In the critically ill patient a peak level should be drawn after the first dose to ensure the achievement of an adequate therapeutic level. For single-dose therapy, trough levels need to be monitored to ensure adequate clearance. Serum level at 18 hours should be <1 µg/ml. Alternatively, a level can be drawn between 6 and 14 hours, and the value can be applied to a normogram to decide on subsequent doses. In the seriously ill patient a peak level one half hour after completion of infusion should also be drawn to ensure that a therapeutic level is being achieved. Single-dose therapy is not recommended for the treatment of bacterial endocarditis and has not

been sufficiently studied in osteomyelitis, pregnancy, or patients with cystic fibrosis.

KEY POINTS
Dosing and Serum Monitoring of Aminoglycosides

1. Aminoglycosides take 15–30 minutes to equilibrate in the body.
2. For multidose therapy peak serum levels should be drawn 30 minutes after infusion.
3. Trough serum levels should be drawn one half hour before the next dose.
4. Conventionally, the aminoglycosides are given three times per day. Dosing should be based on ideal body weight.
5. Once-a-day dosing takes advantage of concentration-dependent killing and the postantibiotic effects of aminoglycosides.
6. Once-a-day dosing reduces the incidence of nephrotoxicity.
7. In most cases only trough serum values need to be monitored with once-a-day dosing. Toxicity correlates with high trough levels.
8. Once-a-day dosing is not recommended for patients with endocarditis or cystic fibrosis, or pregnant females.

Multidose Therapy

GENTAMICIN AND TOBRAMYCIN

Loading dose: 2 mg/kg; maintenance dose: 1.7 mg/kg Q8H

Renal dosing: Cr Cl 80–90 cc/min, Q12H; Cr Cl 50–80 cc/min, Q12–24H; Cr Cl 10–50 cc/min, Q24–48H; Cr Cl <10 cc/min, Q48–72H

Desired serum levels: Peak: 4–10 µg/ml; trough: 1–2 µg/ml

NETILMICIN

Loading dose: 2 mg/kg; maintenance dose: 2 mg/kg Q8H

Renal dosing: Same dosing intervals as gentamicin and tobramycin

Desired peak and trough levels: identical to those for gentamicin and tobramycin

STREPTOMYCIN

Loading dose: 7.5 mg/kg; maintenance dose: 7.5 mg/kg Q12H

Renal dosing: Same dosing intervals as gentamicin and tobramycin

Desired serum levels: peak: 15–30 µg/ml; trough: 5–10 µg/ml

AMIKACIN

Loading dose: 7.5 mg/kg; maintenance dose: 7.5 mg/kg Q12H

Renal dosing: Same dosing intervals as gentamicin and tobramycin

Desired serum levels: peak: 15–30 µg/ml; trough: 5–10 µg/ml

Once-a-Day Dosing

GENTAMICIN AND TOBRAMYCIN

Dose: 5–6 mg/kg/day, adjust dose to achieve trough levels of <0.5 µg/ml

Renal dosing: Cr Cl 60–79 cc/min, 4 mg/kg/24H; Cr Cl 50 cc/min, 3.5 mg/kg/24H; Cr Cl 40 cc/min, 2.5 mg/kg/24H; Cr Cl < 30 cc/min, use multidose regimen

AMIKACIN AND STREPTOMYCIN

Dose: 15 mg/kg/day, adjust dose to achieve trough levels of < 1 µg/ml

Renal dosing: Cr Cl 60–79 cc/min, 12 mg/kg/24H; Cr Cl 50 cc/min, 7.5 mg/kg/24H; Cr Cl 40 cc/min, 4.0 mg/kg/24H; Cr Cl < 30 cc/min, use multidose regimen

COST

Gentamicin: Low
Tobramycin: Low
Streptomycin: Low
Amikacin: Moderate

Although the acquisition costs of aminoglycosides are low, when the monitoring costs and potential costs of nephrotoxicity are taken into account these agents should be placed in the high to very high cost range.

SPECTRUM

Similar for all aminoglycosides, narrow.

Glycopeptide Antibiotics

Chemistry and Mechanism of Action

Vancomycin and teichoplanin are complex glycopeptides of approximately 1,500 Da molecular weight. These agents primarily act at the cell wall of Gram-positive organisms by binding to the D-alanine-D-alanine precursor and preventing it from being incorporated into the peptidoglycan. The binding of vancomycin to this cell wall precursor blocks both transpeptidase and transglycolase enzymes, interfering with cell wall formation and increasing permeability. These agents may also interfere with RNA synthesis. They bind rapidly and tightly to bacteria and rapidly kill actively growing organisms. They also have a 2-hour postantibiotic effect.

KEY POINTS

Glycopeptide Antibacterial Activity

1. Acts on the cell wall of Gram-positive bacteria by binding to the D-alanine-D-alanine peptidoglycan precursor.
2. Requires active bacterial growth.
3. Also interferes with RNA synthesis.
4. Has a 2-hour postantibiotic effect.

Toxicity

Early preparations of vancomycin contained a high percentage of impurities, resulting in frequent adverse reactions; however, modern highly purified preparations have proved to be much safer. The most common side effect is "red man syndrome," which occurs most often when vancomycin is infused rapidly. The patient experiences flushing of the face, neck, and upper thorax. This reaction is thought to be caused by sudden histamine release secondary to local hyperosmolality and is not a true hypersensitivity reaction. Infusing vancomycin over 1 hour usually prevents this reaction. Vancomycin frequently causes phlebitis and therefore should be given through an intravenous catheter that has been positioned in the right side of the heart. The most serious side effect is deafness. Loss of hearing is often preceded by tinnitus. This complication is infrequent when serum levels are kept below 30 µg/ml. Nephrotoxicity is uncommon but has been associated with excessively high serum levels. Renal dysfunction generally reverses when the antibiotic is discontinued. The incidence of aminoglycoside nephrotoxicity is increased by coadministration of vancomycin.

There is less experience with teichoplanin; however, this agent does not cause significant thrombophlebitis, and the skin flushing after rapid infusion is uncommon. Ototoxicity has been reported.

KEY POINTS

Vancomycin Toxicity

> 1. Rapid infusion associated with "red man syndrome."
> 2. Phlebitis is common.
> 3. Ototoxicity leading to deafness uncommon, preceded by tinnitus.
> 4. Rarely nephrotoxic, potentiates aminoglycoside nephrotoxicity.

Antimicrobial Spectrum and Treatment Recommendations

Vancomycin and teichoplanin both cover methicillin-resistant as well as methicillin-sensitive *Staphylococcus aureus* and are the recommended treatment for MRSA. These agents also kill most strains of coagulase-negative Staphylococcus and are recommended for the treatment of coagulase-negative staphylococcal line sepsis and bacterial endocarditis. For the latter infection the glycopeptide antibiotic should be combined with one or more additional antibiotics (see Chapter 7). Intermediately vancomycin-resistant strains of *S. aureus* (VIRSA) were first discovered in Japan and have also been identified in Europe and the United States. These strains have MICs of 8–16 µg/ml and are cross-resistant to teichoplanin. Recently a highly vancomycin-resistant strain (VRSA, MIC >32 µg/ml) has been identified in the United States. The increasing use of vancomycin has selected for these strains and warns us that the indiscriminate use of the glycopeptide antibiotics must be avoided.

In addition to Staphylococcus, vancomycin and teichoplanin have excellent activity against penicillin-resistant and susceptible strains of *Streptococcus pneumoniae* and are recommended for empiric treatment of the seriously ill patient with pneumococcal meningitis to cover for highly penicillin-resistant strains. The glycopeptide antibiotics also effectively treat *S. pyogenes*, GpB streptococci, *Viridans streptococci*, and *S. bovis* and are recommended for treatment of these infections in the penicillin-allergic patient. *Corynebacterium jeikeium* (previously called JK diphtheroids) is sensitive to vancomycin, and this antibiotic is recommended for treatment. Oral vancomycin clears *Clostridium difficile* from the bowel and in the past was recommended for *C. difficile* toxin–associated diarrhea. However, because of the increased risk of developing vancomycin-resistant enterococcal infection following oral vancomycin, this regimen is recommended only for cases that are refractory to metronidazole or the patient with life-threatening pseudomembranous colitis (see Chapter 8).

Vancomycin is frequently used to treat *Enterococcus faecalis* and *E. faecium*; however, an increasing number of strains have become resistant. Three gene complexes transfer resistance. The Van A gene cluster directs peptidoglycan cell wall synthesis and converts D-alanine-D-alanine (the site of action of vancomycin) to D-alanine-D-lactate, markedly reducing vancomycin and teichoplanin binding. The other two resistance gene clusters, Van B and Van C, result in vancomycin resistance but do not impair teichoplanin activity.

KEY POINTS

Treatment Recommendations for Vancomycin

1. Treatment of choice for MRSA; vancomycin-tolerant strains have been reported.
2. Treatment of choice for coagulase-negative staphylococcus.
3. Excellent activity against high-level penicillin-resistant *Streptococcus pneumoniae*.
4. In the penicillin-allergic patient, recommended for *S. pyogenes*, Gp B streptococcus, *S. viridans*, and *S. bovis*.
5. Excellent activity against some strains of enterococcus; however, Van A gene-mediated vancomycin-resistant enterococcus (VRE) is increasing in frequency.
6. Vancomycin use must be restricted to reduce the likelihood of selecting for VRE and vancomycin-tolerant *Staphylococcus aureus*.

VANCOMYCIN

The half-life of vancomycin is 4–6 hours, and it is primarily excreted by the kidneys. In the anuric patient the half-life is prolonged to 7–9 days. Peak levels should achieve concentrations of 20–50 µg/ml, and trough levels should be maintained at 10–12 µg/ml. Vancomycin penetrates most tissue spaces but does not cross the blood-brain barrier in the absence of inflammation, but therapeutic cerebrospinal fluid levels are achieved in patients with meningitis.

Dose: 1 gm iv Q12H; 125–500 mg po Q6H
Renal dosing: Cr Cl 40–60 cc/min, Q12– 24H; Cr Cl 20–40 cc/min, Q24–48H; Cr Cl 10–20 cc/min, Q48–72H; Cr Cl < 10 cc/min, Q3–7 days. Exact dosing is based on serum levels.
Cost: Low (In patients requiring serum levels the cost will be higher.)
Spectrum: Narrow
See Tables 1.1 and 1.2 for classifications.

TEICHOPLANIN

The half-life of teichoplanin is 40–70 hours, and it is primarily cleared by the kidneys. Unlike vancomycin, which is minimally bound to protein, teichoplanin is 90% protein bound, accounting for its slow renal clearance. Tissue penetration has not been extensively studied, and there is little data on penetration of bone or peritoneal or cerebrospinal fluid.

Dose: 6 mg/kg loading dose followed by 3 mg/kg QD iv or im. (Doses as high as 12 mg/kg have been given but are associated with a higher incidence of toxicity.)
Renal dosing: Cr Cl 10–50 cc/min, 1/2 dose; Cr Cl < 10 cc/min, 1/3 dose
Cost: Not available, a new antibiotic
Spectrum: Narrow

Macrolides

Chemistry and Mechanism of Action

Erythromycin, the founding member of the macrolide family, was originally purified from a soil bacterium. It has a complex 14-member macrocylic lactone ring (giving rise to the class name "macrolides") attached to two sugars. Azithromycin has a 15-membered lactone ring and a nitrogen substitution. Clarithromycin has a methoxy group modification at carbon 6 of the erythromycin molecule. These modifications enhance oral absorption and broaden the antimicrobial spectrum. The macrolides inhibit RNA-dependent protein synthesis by binding to the 50S ribosomal subunit. Binding to this site is thought to prevent translocation of the peptide chain, blocking protein synthesis. Erythromycin is a weak base, and its activity is greater at more alkaline pH.

Toxicity

This is one of the safest classes of antibiotics. The primary adverse reactions are related to erythromycin's ability to stimulate bowel motility. In fact this agent can be used to treat gastric paresis. Particularly in younger patients, abdominal cramps, nausea, vomiting, diarrhea, and gas are common. These symptoms are dose related and can occur with oral or intravenous administration of erythromycin. Gastrointestinal toxicity can be debilitating and may force the drug to be discontinued. The newer macrolides azithromycin and clarithromycin at the usual recommended doses are much less likely to cause these adverse reactions. Hypersensitivity reactions, including skin rash, fever, and eosinophilia, can occur with any of the macrolides. Estolate preparations of erythromycin have caused reversible cholestatic jaundice in adults. High doses of erythromycin have resulted in transient reversible hearing loss, particularly in elderly patients. Macrolides prolong the QT interval, and erythromycin administration has on rare occasion been associated with ventricular tachycardia.

KEY POINTS
Macrolide Chemistry, Mechanisms of Action, and Toxicity

1. Complex 14-membered lactone ring structure.

2. Inhibit RNA-dependent protein synthesis, bind to 50S ribosomal subunit.
3. Can be bacteriostatic or bacteriocidal.
4. Overall very safe.
5. Gastrointestinal irritation, particularly erythromycin, is the major toxicity.
6. Hypersensitivity reactions.
7. Transient hearing loss with high doses mainly in the elderly.
8. Prolonged QT interval, rarely causes ventricular tachycardia.

Antimicrobial Spectrum and Treatment Recommendations

ERYTHROMYCIN

Erythromycin demonstrates excellent activity against most Gram-positive organisms and some Gram-negative bacteria. It can be bacteriostatic or bactericidal. Cidal activity increases when antibiotic concentrations are high and bacteria are growing rapidly. Erythromycin is effective against many strains of *Streptococcus pneumoniae*; however, resistance to the macrolides has steadily increased and now ranges between 10% and 15%. Resistance is more likely in intermediately penicillin-resistant strains (40% macrolide resistant) and highly penicillin-resistant strains (60% macrolide resistance). In most countries, including the United States, 95% of *S. pyogenes* are sensitive to macrolides. However, in Japan, where macrolides are commonly used, 60% are resistant. Most methicillin-sensitive *Staphylococcus aureus* strains are also sensitive to macrolides. However, because one-step resistance can develop, macrolides are generally not recommended for treatment of *S. aureus*. The macrolides are effective against mouth flora, including anaerobes, but do not cover the bowel anaerobe *Bacteroides fragilis*. These agents are also effective against a limited number of Gram-negative pathogens, including *Neisseria gonor-*

rhoeae and *N. meningitidis*. They are recommended for the treatment of *Campylobacter jejuni* and *Bordatella pertussis*. The macrolides are also the treatment of choice for *Legionella pneumophila*, azithromycin and clarithromycin being more potent than erythromycin. They are the primary antibiotics used to treat *Mycoplasma pneumoniae, Ureaplasma urealyticum, Chlamydia trachomatis*, and *Chlamydia pneumoniae*. Erythromycin is also the first choice for the treatment of bacillary angiomatosis as well as diphtheria. In many instances erythromycins can be used as an alternative to penicillin in the penicillin-allergic patient.

There are multiple oral forms of erythromycin, including the stearate, ethylsuccinate, and estolate forms, all of which reach peak serum levels 3 hours after ingestion. These agents should be taken on an empty stomach. The base oral form is absorbed more erratically and peaks 4 hours after being taken. The two intravenous preparations lactobionate and gluceptate both peak within 1 hour of administration. Erythromycin penetrates most tissues, including the prostate and middle ear. It is primarily concentrated in the liver and passed into the bowel via the biliary system. A small percentage is also excreted in the urine.

Dose: Oral, 0.25–0.5 gm Q6H; intravenous, 0.5–1 gm Q6H
Renal dosing: No modifications required for renal dysfunction
Cost: Oral and iv, low
Spectrum: Narrow
See Tables 1.1 and 1.2 for classifications.

CLARITHROMYCIN

Compared to erythromycin clarithromycin is two to four times more active against *Streptococcus pneumoniae, Streptococcus pyogenes*, and methicillin-sensitive *Staphylococcus aureus*. It has equivalent activity against Legionella and somewhat greater activity against *Haemophilus*

influenzae, Moraxella catarrhalis and is recommended for the treatment of outpatient community-acquired pneumonia. *Chlamydia trachomatis, Ureaplasma urealyticum*, and *Borrelia burgdorferi* are also sensitive to this antibiotic. Clarithromycin has significant activity against *Mycobacterium leprae* and is the most active macrolide against the *Mycobacterium avium* complex. Finally, this agent demonstrates significant activity against *Toxoplasma gondii*.

Clarithromycin is well absorbed orally. The improved absorption as well as the lower incidence of gastrointestinal toxicity makes clarithromycin preferable to erythromycin in most instances if cost is not a primary issue. The half-life of the drug is approximately 4 hours, and it is primarily metabolized and cleared by the liver. However, a significant percentage is also excreted in the urine. Clarithromycin is widely distributed in tissues, achieving concentrations that are several times the peak concentrations achieved in the serum. Levels in the middle ear fluid are nearly 10 times higher than serum levels. Clarithromycin poorly penetrates the blood-brain barrier.

The indications for the use of clarithromycin are evolving. Increased use of macrolides has resulted in a rise in resistant strains of *Streptococcus pyogenes*. A significant percentage of *S. pneumoniae* strains are resistant, raising concerns about using macrolides for pharyngitis or otitis media or as a single agent for the treatment of severe community-acquired pneumonia. Clarithromycin has been recommended for these indications in the penicillin-allergic patient. It is one of the primary antibiotics used for the treatment of atypical mycobacterial infections, particularly *Mycobacterium avium* complex. It is also recommended for the treatment of *Mycoplasma pneumoniae* and *Ureaplasma urealyticum*.

Dose: 250–500 mg po Q12H
Renal dosing: Cr Cl <10 cc/min, Q24H
Cost: Moderate to moderately high
Spectrum: Narrow

AZITHROMYCIN

Compared to erythromycin, azithromycin is less active against *Streptococcus pyogenes*, *Streptococcus pneumoniae*, and *Staphylococcus aureus*. However, azithromycin demonstrates increased activity against Gram-negatives, particularly *Moraxella catarrhalis* and *Haemophilus influenzae,* and is recommended for the initial treatment of outpatient, community-acquired pneumonia. Azithromycin also demonstrates increased in vivo activity against *Legionella pneumophila* in animal studies and is the drug of choice for the treatment of patients who are well enough to take oral medications. Azithromycin in combination with other antibiotics is recommended for the treatment of *Mycobacterium avium* complex. It can be used alone for *M. avium-intracellulare* (MAI) prophylaxis in HIV-infected patients with CD4 counts below 100 cells/cc. Single high-dose azithromycin (1 gm) effectively treats chancroid as well as *Chlamydia trachomatis* urethritis and cervicitis. Single-dose therapy also cures male *Ureaplasma urealyticum* urethritis. In addition to antacid therapy, effective regimens for curing peptic ulcer disease caused by *Helicobacter pylori* include azithromycin or clarithromycin combined with bismuth salts and either amoxicillin, metronidazole, or tetracycline. Other potential roles for azithromycin include prophylaxis against chloroquine-resistant *Plasmodium falciparum* and treatment of chronic *Chlamydia pneumoniae*, which may contribute to atherosclerotic coronary artery disease.

Azithromycin is absorbed almost as well as clarithromycin; however, food interferes with absorption. Therefore this drug should be taken 1 hour before meals or 2 hours after meals. Aluminum- or magnesium-containing antacids slow absorption and should be avoided. Tissue concentrations exceed serum levels by 10-fold to 100-fold, and the average half-life in tissues is 2–4 days. Therapeutic levels of the antibiotic have been estimated to persist for 5 days after the completion of a 5-day treatment course. The majority of the drug is not metabolized, being excreted unchanged in the bile. A small percentage is also excreted in the urine.

Dose: A 5-day course oral regimen is usually recommended: a 500-mg loading dose followed by either 250 or 500 mg on days 2–5
Renal dosing: No data
Cost: Low to moderate
Spectrum: Narrow

KEY POINTS

Spectrum and Treatment Recommendations for Macrolides

1. Gram-positive coverage as well as mouth anaerobes.
2. Increased use of macrolides selects for resistant strains of *Streptococcus pyogenes* and *S. pneumoniae*. PCN-resistant strains of *S. pneumoniae* are often resistant to macrolides.
3. Not recommended for treatment of methicillin-sensitive *Staphylococcus aureus* because of rapid development of one-step resistance.
5. Recommended for the treatment of outpatient community-acquired pneumonia. Recommended for *Legionella pneumophila*, mycoplasma, ureaplasma, and chlamydia.
6. Clarithromycin and azithromycin have less gastrointestinal toxicity, greater activity against *Legionella pneumophila*. Azithromycin has increased activity against *Haemophilus influenzae*. Both are used for treatment of *Helicobacter pylori*.
7. Clarithromycin has greater activity against *Streptococcus pneumoniae* and *S. pyogenes*; one of the primary drugs for *Mycobacterium avium-intracellulare* (MAI).
8. Azithromycin accumulates in tissues and persists for 5 days, allowing a shorter course of therapy (5 days versus 10 days). The drug of choice for oral treatment of *Legionella pneumophila* and is used for prophylaxis of MAI.

Clindamycin

Chemistry and Mechanism of Action

Although this agent is structurally different from erythromycin, many of its biological characteristics are similar. Clindamycin consists of an amino acid linked to an amino sugar and was derived by modifying lincomycin. This agent binds to the same 50S ribosomal binding site as the macrolides, blocking bacterial protein synthesis.

Toxicity

Diarrhea is a major problem and is seen 20% of patients taking clindamycin. The incidence is highest with oral administration. In up to half of these patients the cause of diarrhea is pseudomembranous colitis, a disease that is caused by the overgrowth of the anaerobic bacteria *Clostridium difficile*. *C. difficile* produces a cytotoxin that damages gastrointestinal cells, causing yellow white plaques that can be seen on endoscopy. This complication can lead to toxic megacolon and death. When *C. difficile* toxin is detected or pseudomembranous colitis is suspected, it is critical that clindamycin be discontinued. Oral metronidazole is the treatment of choice for eradicating *C. difficile* (see Chapter 8). Less common side effects include allergic reactions, hepatotoxicity, neutropenia, thrombocytopenia, and hypotension.

Antimicrobial Spectrum and Treatment Recommendations

Clindamycin is similar to erythromycin in its activity against *Streptococcus pneumoniae*, *Streptococcus pyogenes*, and methicillin-sensitive *Staphylococcus aureus*. Moderately penicillin-resistant *Streptococcus pneumoniae* strains are often sensitive to clindamycin. In the penicillin-allergic patient clindamycin is a reasonable alternative for *Streptococcus pyogenes* pharyngitis. Because its activity against *Haemophilus influenzae* is limited, clindamycin is not recommended for the treatment of otitis media. Clindamycin distinguishes itself from the macrolides by possessing excellent activity against *Bacteroides fragilis* as well as most other anaerobic bacteria. This agent is used effectively in combination with an aminoglycoside, aztreonam, or third-generation cephalosporin to treat fecal soilage of the peritoneum. However, other, less toxic regimens have proved to be equally effective. Clindamycin is also effective for the treatment of anaerobic pulmonary and pleural infections. Because this agent has been shown to reduce toxin production by *Staphylococcus aureus* and *Streptococcus pyogenes*, clindamycin is often combined with a semisynthetic penicillin or cephalosporin to treat serious soft tissue infections (see Chapter 10). Finally, clindamycin has significant activity against *Toxoplasma gondii* and is recommended as alternative therapy in the sulfa-allergic patient.

Pharmacokinetics

Clindamycin is well absorbed orally. However, the drug can also be administered intravenously, and this route can achieve higher peak serum levels. It penetrates most tissues but does not enter the cerebrospinal fluid. Clindamycin has a half-life of 2.4 hours, being primarily metabolized by the liver and excreted in the bile. Therapeutic concentrations of clindamycin persist in the stool for 5 or more days after the antibiotic is discontinued, and the reduction of clindamycin-sensitive flora persists for up to 14 days. Small percentages of clindamycin metabolites are also excreted in the urine.

Dose: Oral, 150–300 mg Q6H; intravenous, 300–900 mg Q6–8H

Renal dosing: Usually no modification required. In the anuric patient the dose should be halved.

Cost: Oral, moderately high to high; intravenous, low to moderate

Spectrum: Narrow; however, kills most bowel flora anaerobes

KEY POINTS
Clindamycin

1. Binds to the same 50S ribosomal binding site as macrolides.
2. Diarrhea is a common side effect, *Clostridium difficile* toxin found in 20% of cases.
3. Pseudomembranous colitis can lead to toxic megacolon and death.
4. If *C. difficile* toxin is detected, clindamycin should be discontinued.
5. Active against most Gram-positives, including MSSA; covers many moderately PCN-resistant *Streptococcus pneumoniae* but not a first-line therapy.
6. Excellent anaerobic coverage, including *Bacteroides fragilis*.
7. Used to reduce toxin production by *Streptococcus pyogenes* and *Staphylococcus aureus*.
8. Used to treat anaerobic lung abscesses and in the sulfa-allergic patient for toxoplasmosis.

Tetracyclines

Chemistry and Mechanisms of Action

The tetracyclines consist of four six-member rings with substitutions at the 4, 5, 6, and 7 positions, which alter the pharmacokinetics of the various preparations; however, these changes have no effect on the antimicrobial spectrum.

The tetracyclines enter bacteria by passively diffusing through porins in Gram-negative bacteria. They bind to the 30S ribosomal subunit and block tRNA binding to the mRNA ribosome complex. This blockade primarily inhibits protein synthesis in bacteria but to a lesser extent also affects mammalian cell protein synthesis, particularly that of mitochondria. The inhibition of bacterial protein synthesis stops bacterial growth but does not kill most bacteria. Therefore tetracycline is termed a bacteriostatic agent.

Toxicity

Photosensitivity reactions consisting of a red rash over sun-exposed areas can develop. Hypersensitivity reactions are less common with tetracyclines than with the penicillins but do occur. Tetracyclines interfere with enamel formation, and in children teeth often become permanently discolored. Therefore these agents are not recommended for children age 8 years or younger or for pregnant women. Gastrointestinal side effects are also reported, including esophageal ulcers, nausea, vomiting, and diarrhea. Hepatotoxicity is rare, but in high doses these drugs can result in fatty changes in the liver. Because the tetracyclines inhibit protein synthesis, they increase azotemia in renal failure patients. Finally, neurologic side effects have been observed. Minocycline can cause vertigo, and this side effect has limited its use. Benign intracranial hypertension (pseudotumor cerebri) is another rare neurologic side effect.

Antimicrobial Spectrum and Treatment Recommendations

These agents are able to inhibit the growth of a broad spectrum of bacteria. However, for most conventional pathogens other agents are more effective. High concentrations of tetracyclines are achieved in the urine, and these agents can be used for uncomplicated urinary tract infections. Doxycycline combined with gentamicin is the treatment of choice for brucellosis. The tetracyclines are also useful for treating Vibrio infections. *Mycobacterium marinum* is susceptible to tetracyclines, and doxycycline is usually recommended for initial treatment. Tetracyclines are also recommended for the treatment of Lyme disease (*Borrelia burgdorferi*) and chlamydia infections (including chlamydia pneumonia, psittacosis, epididymitis, urethritis, and endocervical infections). Tetracyclines are the treatment of choice for rickettsial infections (including Rocky Mountain spotted fever, ehrlichiosis, Q fever, and typhus). They are also often used for the treatment of pelvic inflammatory disease in combination with other antibiotics.

Pharmacokinetics

Tetracycline is reasonably well absorbed (70–80%) by the gastrointestinal tract. Food interferes with its absorption. The half-life for clearance is 8 hours, and tetracycline is primarily cleared by the kidneys. Doxycycline is nearly completely absorbed in the gastrointestinal tract and has a prolonged half-life of 18 hours. The liver primarily clears doxycycline. Calcium- or magnesium-containing antacids, milk, or multivitamins markedly impair absorption of all tetracycline preparations, and simultaneous ingestion of these products should be avoided.

Dose: *Tetracycline*: 250–500 mg po BID–QID
Renal dosing: Cr Cl 50–80 cc/min, Q8–12H; Cr Cl 10–50 cc/min, Q12–24H; Cr Cl < 10 cc/min, Q24H
Cost: Low
Spectrum: Broad
Doxycycline: 100 mg po BID; no renal adjustments required
Cost: Low

Spectrum: Broad
See Tables 1.1 and 1.2 for classifications.

Chloramphenicol

Chemistry and Mechanisms of Action

The agent consists of a nitro group on a benzene ring and a side chain containing five carbons. Chloramphenicol enters bacteria by an energy-dependent mechanism and, once in the cell, binds to the larger 50S subunit of the 70S ribosome, blocking attachment of transfer RNA. This effect results in inhibition of bacterial protein synthesis, and this antibiotic is bacteriostatic, like the tetracyclines. Chloramphenicol is cidal for *Haemophilus influenzae*, *Streptococcus pneumoniae*, and *Neisseria meningitidis*.

Toxicity

Probably as a result of binding to human mitochondrial ribosomes, this agent has significant bone marrow toxicity. Two forms are observed. The first form is dose related and is commonly observed in patients receiving 4 gm or more chloramphenicol per day. The reticulocyte count decreases, and anemia develops in association with an elevated serum iron. Leukopenia and thrombocytopenia are also commonly encountered. These changes reverse when the antibiotic is discontinued. The second form of marrow toxicity, irreversible aplastic anemia, is rare but usually fatal. This complication can occur weeks to months after the antibiotic is discontinued. Patients receiving chloramphenicol require twice-a-week monitoring of their peripheral blood counts, and if the white blood cell count drops below 2500/mm³, the drug should be discontinued. Other side effects have included optic neuritis, peripheral neuritis, mental confusion, hypersensitivity reactions, nausea, vomiting, diarrhea, and bleeding secondary to vitamin K deficiency.

Antimicrobial Spectrum and Treatment Recommendations

Chloramphenicol has excellent activity against most Gram-positive organisms, with the exception of enterococci and *Staphylococcus aureus*. It also has excellent activity against *Haemophilus influenzae, Neisseria meningitidis, N. gonorrhoeae*, some strains of *E. coli*, Klebsiella, and Proteus. A high percentage of Salmonella strains, including *S. typhi*, are sensitive, as are most strains of Shigella. Chloramphenicol is very effective for treating Brucella species as well as *Bordatella pertussis*. It also has excellent anaerobic coverage, demonstrating excellent activity against Peptostreptococcus, Clostridium species, *Bacteroides fragilis*, and Fusobacterium species. Chloramphenicol is also active against spirochetes, rickettsiae, chlamydiae, and mycoplasmas.

Because of its bone marrow toxicity, chloramphenicol is not considered the treatment of choice for any infection. Alternative, less toxic agents are available for each indication. For the penicillin-allergic patient chloramphenicol can be used for bacterial meningitis. Chloramphenicol can also be used as alternative therapy for brain abscess, *Clostridium perfringens*, psittacosis, rickettsial infections including Rocky Mounted spotted fever and typhoid fever, and *Vibrio vulnificus*.

Pharmacokinetics

As a result of the much higher incidence of idiosyncratic aplastic anemia associated with oral administration as compared to intravenous administration, chloramphenicol oral preparations are no longer available in the United States. The drug is well absorbed, and therapeutic serum levels can be achieved orally. Chloramphenicol is metabolized by the liver and has a half-life of 4 hours. It diffuses well into tissues and crosses the blood-brain barrier of uninflamed as well as inflamed meninges. A serum assay is available, and serum levels should be monitored in patients with hepatic disease, maintaining the serum concentration between 10 and 25 µg/ml.

Dose: 0.25–1 gm iv Q6H
Renal dosing: No correction for renal insufficiency required. For liver failure, monitor serum levels.
Cost: Low
Spectrum: Broad
See Tables 1.1 and 1.2 for classifications.

KEY POINTS

Chloramphenicol

> 1. Binds to 50S subunit of the ribosome, blocking protein synthesis; bacteriostatic.

2. Idiosyncratic aplastic anemia has limited the use of chloramphenicol, also can cause dose-related bone marrow suppression.
3. Has a broad spectrum of activity, including Salmonella, Brucella, Bordetella, anaerobes, rickettsiae, chlamydiae, mycoplasma, and spirochetes.
4. Can be used as alternative therapy in the penicillin-allergic patient.

Quinolones

Chemical Structure and Mechanisms of Action

The quinolones all contain two six-membered rings (see Figure 1.6) with a nitrogen at position 1, a carbonyl group at position 4, and a carboxyl group attached to the carbon at position 3. Potency of the quinolones is greatly enhanced by adding fluorine at position 6, and Gram-negative activity is enhanced by addition of a nitrogen-containing piperazine ring at position 7. The quinolones inhibit two enzymes that are critical for DNA synthesis: DNA gyrase, which is important for regulating the superhelical twists of bacterial DNA, and topoisomerase IV, which is responsible for segregating newly formed DNA into daughter cells. The loss of these activities blocks DNA synthesis and results in rapid bacterial death. *E. coli* resistance is mediated by mutations in the DNA gyrase that reduce quinolone binding affinity. Resistance can also arise in Pseudomonas strains and *E. coli* as a result of changes in outer membrane proteins that interfere with antibiotic penetration. Efflux pumps expressed in both Gram-negative and Gram-positive bacteria can reduce the intracellular concentration of quinolones.

Toxicity

Quinolones rarely cause serious adverse reactions. The most common side effects are mild anorexia, nausea, vomiting, and abdominal dis-

Figure 1.6

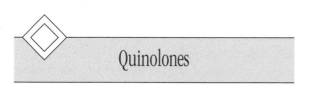

Basic structure of quinolones.

comfort. Diarrhea is less common, and pseudo-membranous colitis is rare. Mild headache, dizziness, insomnia, and seizures in association with theophylline have been reported. Allergic reactions consisting primarily of skin rash can occur but are less commonly encountered than with the penicillins or cephalosporins. Other, less frequently reported allergic reactions include fever, urticaria, serum sickness, interstitial nephritis, and anaphylactic reactions. Leukopenia and eosinophilia have been reported but are rare. Increased skin sensitivity to ultraviolet exposure can develop. Quinolones can result in arthropathy due to cartilage damage as well as tendinitis. Although rare, this complication can be debilitating, but it usually reverses weeks to months after the quinolone is discontinued. Because of concerns about cartilage damage in children, quinolones are not recommended for routine administration in pediatric patients. Mild asymptomatic elevations of serum transaminase levels have been reported. Serious hepatic toxicity was observed in several patients receiving trovafloxacin, and as a result this antibiotic is no longer marketed.

KEY POINTS
Chemistry, Mechanisms of Action, and Toxicity of Quinolones

1. Inhibit bacterial DNA gyrase, which is important for coiling DNA and topoisomerase required to segregate DNA to daughter cells; rapidly cidal.
2. Resistance mediated by mutations in the DNA gyrase, outer bacterial membranes, and efflux pumps.
3. Overall very safe antibiotics. Main side effects are nausea and anorexia. Allergic reactions are less common than with PCN or cephalosporins. Arthropathy and tendinitis. May damage cartilage. Not recommended routinely in children.

Specific Quinolones

CIPROFLOXACIN

This is the most potent quinolone for *Pseudomonas aeruginosa*. Ciprofloxacin also demonstrates excellent activity against *E. coli*, Klebsiella, *Enterobacter cloacae*, Proteus, Providencia, Salmonella, Shigella, Yersinia, Campylobacter, *Neisseria meningitidis*, *N. gonorrhoeae*, *Moraxella catarrhalis*, *Haemophilus influenzae*, and Legionella. Its activity is more variable for strains of *Serratia marcescens*, *Morganella morganii*, *Burkoderia cepacia*, Aeromonas, Acinetobacter, and Citrobacter species. Ciprofloxacin kills *Mycoplasma pneumoniae*, *Chlamydia pneumoniae*, *C. trachomatis*, and *Ureaplasma urealyticum*.

As a result of its excellent Gram-negative spectrum, ciprofloxacin is one of the primary antibiotics recommended for the treatment of urinary tract infections. This agent concentrates in the prostate and is recommended for treatment of prostatitis. For gonococcal urethritis, ciprofloxacin is a useful alternative to ceftriaxone. Ciprofloxacin has been used effectively for traveler's diarrhea, which is most commonly caused by enterotoxigenic *E. coli* and Shigella. This is the drug of choice for *Salmonella typhi* (typhoid fever) and also is recommended for treatment of Salmonella gastroenteritis when antibiotic treatment is necessary. Ciprofloxacin is the recommended treatment for cat-scratch disease caused by *Bartonella henselae*.

Ciprofloxacin is readily absorbed orally but can also be given intravenously. It has a half-life of 4 hours and is cleared primarily by the kidneys. All quinolones demonstrate similar tissue penetration, being concentrated in prostate tissue, feces, bile, and lung tissue. These drugs tend to be very highly concentrated in macrophages and neutrophils.

Dose: 250–750 mg Q12H po, 200–400 mg Q12H iv

Renal dosing: Cr Cl 10–50 cc/min, Q18H; Cr Cl < 10 cc/min, Q24H

Cost: Moderately high po, low to moderate iv
Spectrum: Moderately broad; doesn't kill anaerobes

LEVOFLOXACIN

This drug has a somewhat improved Gram-positive coverage. Activity against *Streptococcus pneumoniae* and other Streptococcus species including enterococcus, *Staphylococcus aureus*, and *Streptococcus pyogenes* is greater than that of ciprofloxacin. Levofloxacin has been recommended as one of the first-line treatments for community-acquired pneumonia in the otherwise healthy adult who does not require hospitalization. Levofloxacin can also be used in soft tissue infections when a mixed infection including both Gram-positive and Gram-negative organisms is suspected.

Levofloxacin is well absorbed orally and also is available as an intravenous preparation. The half-life of the drug is 6–8 hours, and it is excreted by the kidneys.

Dose: 500 mg 24H po and iv
Renal dosing: Cr Cl 10–50 cc/min, 250 mg Q24H; Cr Cl < 10 cc/min, 250 mg Q48H
Cost: Oral, moderately high; intravenous, low
Spectrum: Broad

GATIFLOXACIN AND MOXIFLOXACIN

Gatifloxacin is 2–4 times and moxifloxacin is 4–8 times more active than levofloxacin against *Streptococcus pneumoniae*, including strains with high-level penicillin resistance. They are effective against methicillin-sensitive *Staphylococcus aureus* but are not active against methicillin-resistant strains. Both agents also demonstrate moderate in vitro activity against anaerobes. Otherwise, their spectrums of activity are similar to that of levofloxacin. Clinically significant prolongation of the QT interval has been reported with moxifloxacin but not with gatifloxacin. The exact indications for these agents are in evolution. Given their improved *Streptococcus pneumoniae* coverage, these new agents should be considered as a first-line regimen for community-acquired pneumonia that does not require hospitalization, particularly in the elderly patient with increased risk for Gram-negative pneumonia (see Chapter 4). Both agents are absorbed well orally. An intravenous preparation is available for gatifloxacin. Moxifloxacin is partially metabolized by the liver.

Dose: *Gatifloxacin*: 400 mg Q24H po or iv
Renal dosing: Cr Cl 10–50 cc/min, 400 mg Q24–48H; Cr Cl <10 cc/min, 400 mg Q48H
Moxifloxacin: 400 mg Q24H po
Renal dosing: No adjustments required
Cost: Both moderate po; gatifloxacin iv, low
Spectrum: Very broad

KEY POINTS

Specific Quinolones

1. Ciprofloxacin:
   a. Excellent coverage of Pseudomonas. Also covers many other Gram-negatives, including *E. coli*, Salmonella, Shigella, Neisseria, and Legionella.
   b. Kills Mycoplasma, Chlamydia, and Ureaplasma.
   c. Recommended for urinary tract infections and prostatitis, gonococcal urethritis, traveler's diarrhea, typhoid fever, and Salmonella gastroenteritis; used for cat-scratch disease.
2. Levofloxacin:
   a. Somewhat improved Gram-positive coverage, equivalent Gram-negative coverage except for Pseudomonas.
   b. Recommended for community-acquired pneumonia, mixed skin infections.
3. Gatifloxacin and moxifloxacin:
   a. Greater activity against *Streptococcus pneumoniae*, covers highly PCN-resistant strains.
   b. Also cover MSSA and anaerobes.
   c. First-line therapy for community-acquired pneumonia in the elderly

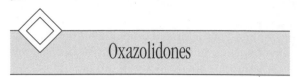

Oxazolidones

Chemistry and Mechanisms of Action

These compounds have a unique ring structure consisting of a five-membered ring containing an oxygen and nitrogen. The nitrogen connects to a six-membered ring, and each specific compound has side chains added to both rings at positions A and B (see Figure 1.7). The agents bind to the 50S ribosome at a site similar to that of chloramphenicol. However, unlike chloramphenicol these agents do not inhibit the attachment of tRNA but instead block the initiation of protein synthesis by preventing the nearby 30S subunit from forming the 70S initiation complex. The oxalidones are static against staphylococcal species and enterococci.

LINEZOLID

TOXICITY Linezolid is the only agent in this class that has been released for use. Side effects associated with this drug include discoloration of the tongue, folliculitis, headache, and diarrhea. Reversible thrombocytopenia has also been reported in association with prolonged therapy, and monitoring of the platelet count is recommended for patients receiving two or more weeks of linezolid. Leukopenia and hepatic enzyme elevations have also been reported. Because this agent is a weak inhibitor of monoamine oxidase, hypertension has been reported in association with ingestion of large amounts of tyramine. Pseudoephedrine and selective serotonin reuptake inhibitors should be prescribed with caution.

ANTIMICROBIAL ACTIVITY AND TREATMENT RECOMMENDATIONS Linezolid demonstrates activity only against Gram-positive organisms. It has bacteriostatic activity against both vancomycin-resistant *Enterococcus faecium* and *E. faecalis*. This agent is also active against methicillin-sensitive and methicillin-resistant *Staphylococcus aureus* and has activity against penicillin-resistant *Streptococcus pneumoniae*. Linezolid is recommended primarily for the treatment of vancomycin-resistant enterococcal infections.

PHARMACOKINETICS Linezolid is well absorbed orally, peak serum levels being achieved in 1–2 hours. Food slows absorption but does not lower peak levels. An intravenous preparation is also available. The drug has a half-life of 5 hours, being partly metabolized by the liver and excreted in the urine.

Dose: 600 mg Q12H both po and iv
Renal dosing: No adjustment required
Cost: Moderately high
Spectrum: Narrow

KEY POINTS
Linezolid

1. Binds to the 50S ribosome subunit like chloramphenicol, inhibits the initiation of protein synthesis.
2. Thrombocytopenia common with treatment ≥ 2 weeks, inhibitor of monoamine oxidase; avoid tyramine, pseudoephedrine, serotonin reuptake inhibitors.

Figure 1.7

Basic structure of oxazolidones.

3. Strictly Gram-positive activity, bacteriostatic activity for VRE and MRSA. Also has activity against PCN-resistant *Streptococcus pneumoniae*.
4. Recommended for the treatment of VRE.

Streptogramins

Chemical Structure and Mechanisms of Action

These agents belong to the macrolide family. They are derived from pristinamycin. Quinupristin is a peptide derived from pristinamycin IA, and dalfopristin is derived from pristinamycin IIB. A combination of 30:70 quinupristin/dalfopristin results in synergistic activity and has been named Synercid. These two agents inhibit bacterial protein synthesis by binding to the 50S bacterial ribosome. Quinupristin inhibits peptide chain elongation, and dalfopristin interferes with peptidyl transferase activity.

Toxicity

Adverse reactions include nausea, vomiting, and diarrhea; myalgias; and arthralgias. Experience with this drug remains limited.

Antimicrobial Activity and Treatment Indications

Synercid is primarily active against Gram-positive organisms. It has proved to be efficacious in the treatment of vancomycin-resistant enterococci as well as methicillin-resistant *Staphylococcus aureus*. Synercid or linazolid is the treatment of choice for vancomycin-resistant enterococcus.

Pharmacokinetics

These agents are administered intravenously and are primarily metabolized in the liver. The half-life of the drug is 1.5 hours.

Dose: 7.5 mg/kg Q8–12H iv
Renal dosing: No adjustment required
Cost: Very high
Spectrum: Narrow
See Tables 1.1 and 1.2 for classifications.

KEY POINTS
Synercid

1. A combination of two pristinamycin derivatives: quinupristin and dalfopristin. Together, they synergistically block protein synthesis. Both bind to the 50S ribosomal subunit.
2. Myalgias and arthralgias can force discontinuation of the drug. Nausea, vomiting, and diarrhea also occur.
3. Spectrum of activity primarily Gram-positive bacteria. Active against VRE and MRSA.
4. Recommended for the treatment of VRE.

Metronidazole

Chemical Structure and Mechanisms of Action

Metronidazole is a nitroimidizole and has a low molecular weight, allowing it to readily diffuse into tissues. Within the bacterium this antibiotic acts as an electron acceptor, being quickly reduced. The resulting free radicals are toxic to the bacterium, producing DNA damage as well as damage to other macromolecules. Metronidazole has significant activity against anaerobes.

Toxicity

This drug is usually well tolerated but can result in a reaction with alcohol consumption like that of disulfiram (Antabuse). Seizures, encephalopathy, cerebellar dysfunction, and peripheral neuropathy have rarely been reported. Concern about the mutagenic potential of this agent has resulted in multiple studies that overall fail to demonstrate significant DNA abnormalities in most mammalian studies. Metronidazole is not recommended in pregnancy and should usually be avoided in patients who are taking coumadin because it impairs coumadin metabolism.

Spectrum of Activity and Treatment Recommendations

Metronidazole was originally used primarily for *Trichomonas vaginitis*, being effective both topically and orally. This drug is also effective for treating amoebic abscesses and giardiasis. Metronidazole is cidal for most anaerobic bacteria and is the antibiotic of choice for covering anaerobes. Because metronidazole has no significant activity against aerobes, it is usually administered in combination with a cephalosporin for aerobic coverage. Metronidazole is the drug of choice for treatment of pseudomembranous colitis due to overgrowth of *Clostridium difficile*. Metronidazole is also recommended as part of the regime for *Helicobacter pylori* gastric and duodenal infection.

Pharmacokinetics

This agent is rapidly and completely absorbed orally but also can be given intravenously. Therapeutic levels are achieved in all body fluids, including the cerebrospinal fluid and brain abscess contents. The half-life of the drug is 8 hours, and the liver primarily metabolizes it. In patients with severe hepatic failure, doses should be reduced to one half.

Dose: Intravenous, 15 mg/kg loading dose followed by 7.5 mg Q6–8H not to exceed a

maximum daily dose of 4 gm; oral, 500 mg Q6–8H
Renal dosing: No adjustment required
Cost: Low
Spectrum: Narrow
See Tables 1.1 and 1.2 for classifications.

KEY POINTS
Metronidazole

1. An electron acceptor that produces free radicals that damage bacterial DNA.
2. Antabuse-like reaction can occur; mutagenic effects not proven in mammals, but metronidazole should be avoided in pregnancy. Impairs coumadin metabolism.
3. Excellent activity against anaerobes as well as amoeba, giardia, and trichomonas. Penetrates tissues well, including abscesses.
4. Indicated in combination with other antibiotics for mixed bacterial infections. Has no activity against aerobic bacteria.
5. Treatment of choice for *Clostridium difficile*–induced diarrhea. Used as part of combination treatment for *Helicobacter pylori*.

Sulfonamides and Trimethoprim

Chemical Structure and Mechanisms of Action

The sulfonamides all have a structure similar to that of para-aminobenzoic acid (PABA), a substrate that is required for bacterial folic acid synthesis (see Figure 1.8). All sulfonamides inhibit bacterial folic acid synthesis by competitively inhibiting PABA incorporation into tetrahydropteroic acid. These agents are bacteriostatic. A sulfonyl radical is attached to carbon 1 of the six-membered ring and increases PABA inhibi-

Figure 1.8

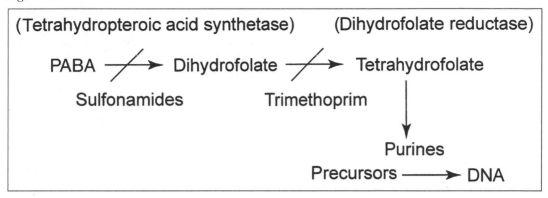

Effects of sulfonamides and trimethoprim on the bacterial folate pathway.

tion. Alterations in the sulfonyl radical determine many of the pharmacokinetic properties of the compounds.

Toxicity

Hypersensitivity reactions represent the most severe toxicity. Macular papular drug rashes, erythema multiforme and Stevens-Johnson syndrome, vasculitis including drug-induced lupus, serum sickness-like syndrome, and anaphylaxis have been reported. Other side effects include nausea, vomiting, diarrhea, headache, depression, jaundice, and hepatic necrosis. Hemolytic anemia can be associated with glucose-6-phosphate dehydrogenase deficiency (G6PD-deficiency). Agranulocytosis, thrombocytopenia, and leukopenia have also been reported. Sulfonamides should be avoided in the last month of pregnancy because they displace bilirubin bound to plasma albumin and increase fetal blood levels of unconjugated bilirubin.

Antimicrobial Spectrum of Activity and Treatment Recommendations

The sulfonamides demonstrate activity against Gram-positive and Gram-negative organisms; however, resistance in both community and nosocomial strains is widespread. The sulfonamides have significant activity against many strains of *Streptococcus pyogenes*, *Listeria monocytogenes*, and *Bacillus anthracis*, as well as some strains of *Staphylococcus aureus* and *Streptococcus pneumoniae*. Among Gram-negative strains, *E. coli*, Shigella species, *Haemophilus influenzae*, *Neisseria gonorrhoeae*, and *N. meningitidis* tend to be the most sensitive. Some strains of Klebsiella species, *Proteus mirabilis*, and Salmonella may also be treated with this agent. The sulfonamides are usually very active against *Chlamydia trachomatis* and *Nocardia asteroides*. Sulfonamides have proved to be effective for the empiric treatment of uncomplicated urinary tract infections. However, because of widespread resistance, they are rarely used as empiric therapy in other infections. Sulfonamides are the treatment of choice for *Nocardia asteroides* and are useful in combination with other agents for the treatment of *Mycobacterium kansasii*.

Pharmacokinetics

Sulfonamides are classified as short-, medium-, and long-acting, depending on their half-life. Sulfisoxazole is in the short-acting class, having a half-life of 5–6 hours. Sulfamethoxazole and sulfadiazine are medium-acting, having a half-life of 8–17 hours. Sulfadoxine is long-acting, having a half-life 100–230 hours. These agents are generally well absorbed orally. Intravenous preparations are available for some agents. They are all metabolized by the liver, undergoing acetylation and glucuronidation. These metabolites are excreted in the urine.

Dose:
Sulfisoxazole: 1–2 g po Q6H
Renal dosing: Cr Cl 10–50 cc/min, 1 g Q8–12H; Cr Cl < 10 cc/min, 1 g Q12–24H
Sulfadiazine: 0.5–1.5 g po Q4–6H
Renal dosing: Cr Cl 10–50 cc/min, 0.5–1.5 g Q8–12H; Cr Cl < 10 cc/min, 0.5–1.5 g Q12–24H
Cost: Sulfisoxazole, very low; sulfadiazine, low
Spectrum: Moderately broad, without significant anaerobic activity

TRIMETHOPRIM

Consists of two six-membered rings: one with two nitrogens and two amino groups and the other with three methoxybenzyl groups. This agent strongly inhibits dihyrofolate reductase and complements sulfonamides' inhibition of folate metabolism (see Figure 1.8). Trimethoprim's inhibition of bacterial dihydrofolate reductase is 100,000 times greater than its inhibition of the mammalian enzyme, minimizing toxicity to the patient. Trimethoprim alone is active against many Gram-positive and Gram-negative bacteria but is generally administered in combination with sulfamethoxazole. This combination often results in significant activity against *Staphylococcus aureus*, *Streptococcus pneumoniae*, *Streptococcus pyogenes*, and some strains of enterococcus. Trimethoprim-sulfamethoxazole (TMP-SMX) demonstrates excellent activity against *Listeria monocytogenes* and is the antibiotic of choice in the penicillin-allergic patient with listeriosis. This combination is generally not used for upper respiratory tract infections but is reserved for the treatment of urinary tract infections. In many cases TMP-SMX demonstrates excellent activity against the major urinary pathogens *E. coli* and

Proteus mirabilis. It has somewhat lower activity against some strains of Klebsiella. It can be used to treat a number of other Gram-negative pathogens, including Shigella species, Salmonella, *Burkholderia cepacia*, *Stenotrophomonas maltophilia*, *Yersinia enterocolitica*, and *Neisseria gonorrhoeae*. Plasmid-mediated resistance is common, and treatment for these pathogens should be initiated only after sensitivity is confirmed by microbiologic testing. This combination is highly effective for killing *Pneumocystis carinii* and is the drug of choice for treating this infection in immunocompromised hosts, including AIDS patients. TMP-SMX is commonly given in the immunocompromised patient to prevent pneumocystis pneumonia. Trimethoprim is excreted primarily by the renal tubules, and very high concentrations of active drug are found in the urine. Some trimethoprim is also excreted in the bile. The half-life of trimethoprim is 9–11 hours, matching the half-life of sulfamethoxazole. The ratio of trimethoprim to sulfamethoxazole supplied is 1:5, that is, 80 mg of trimethoprim and 400 mg of sulfamethoxazole in the single-strength tablet and 160 mg of trimethoprim and 800 mg of sulfamethoxazole in the double-strength pill.

Dose: Oral and parenteral, 1–5 mg/kg of the trimethoprim component Q6–12H
Renal dosing: Cr Cl 10–50 cc/min, half the oral dose, reduce the iv dose to 1–5 mg/kg Q12–24H; Cr Cl <10 cc min, avoid administering
Cost: Oral, low; intravenous, low to moderate
Spectrum: Moderately broad

KEY POINTS
Sulfonamides and Trimethoprim

1. Competitively inhibit PABA incorporation, blocking folic acid synthesis; trimethoprim inhibits dihydrofolate reductase, potentiating sulfonamide activity.
2. Hypersensitivity reactions, including Stevens-Johnson syndrome, common; hemolytic ane-

mia in G6PD-deficient patients. Agranulocytosis, thrombocytopenia less common.
3. Broad spectrum of activity for Gram-positive and Gram-negative bacteria, but resistance is common.
4. Used for initial therapy of uncomplicated urinary tract infections. Treatment of choice for Nocardia.
5. TMP-SMX the drug of choice for pneumocystis prophylaxis and treatment.

Antimycobacterial Agents

The principal strategies for treating mycobacteria differ somewhat from those for treating more conventional bacteria. Because mycobacteria are intracellular and grow very slowly and because dormant tuberculous organisms found in necrotic cavitary lesions are difficult to kill, antituberculous therapy must be prolonged (months). Second, because the number of mycobacterial organisms in the host is usually high, the potential for selecting resistant mycobacteria is high. To reduce this risk, treatment with two or more antimycobacterial medications is recommended. Generally, 1×10^6 organisms are resistant to isoniazid. Cavitary lesions often contain 10^9–10^{10} organisms, ensuring the survival and replication of resistant organisms. Administration of two drugs reduces the probability of selecting for a resistant organism because only 1×10^{12} organisms ($10^6 \times 10^6$) would be expected to be resistant to both antimicrobial agents. A third major consideration is the increased incidence of multidrug-resistant *Mycobacterium tuberculosis* (MDR-TB). These mycobacteria are resistant to isoniazid and rifampin and must be treated with three or more other antimycobacterial agents.

The antituberculous agents have been classified as first-line and second-line drugs. First-line medications include isoniazid (INH), rifampin, pyrazinamide, streptomycin, and ethambutol. These agents are more efficacious and less toxic than the second-line drugs. With the exception of ethambutol, first-line agents are also bactericidal. Whenever possible, first-line drugs should be employed for the treatment of *Mycobacterium tuberculosis*. Standard therapy for drug-sensitive tuberculosis is a combination of three bactericidal agents—INH, rifampin, and pyrazinamide—for six months.

KEY POINTS

Antituberculous Therapy

1. Therapy must be prolonged; *at least* six months required to kill dormant organisms.
2. Whenever possible, use first-line medications.
3. Two or more antimycobacterials are required for treatment to prevent the selection of resistant organisms. (1×10^6 mycobacteria are resistant to one drug, and 1×10^{12} are resistant to two drugs. Cavitary lesions have 10^9–10^{10} mycobacteria.)
4. The incidence of multidrug-resistant *Mycobacterium tuberculosis* is increasing.

First-Line Medications

ISONIAZID (INH)

CHEMISTRY AND MECHANISM OF ACTION This agent was synthesized in 1952 and is a hydrazide. Isoniazid's mechanism of action is not completely understood; however, it is known to inhibit mycolic acid synthesis. Mycolic acids are long-chain fatty acids found in the middle layer of the mycobacterial cell wall, and damage to this layer results in bacterial death.

TOXICITY The major toxicity associated with INH is hepatocellular damage. Ten to twenty percent of patients develop a transient rise in serum transaminase values on initiation of therapy. Levels return to normal in the majority of patients. However, in a small percentage of cases when INH was continued, hepatitis progressed and was fatal. The incidence of serious hepatitis is age-related, progressively increasing in patients over age 35. Hepatotoxicity occurs in ≤0.3% in patients under 35 years, ≤1.2% in patients age 35–49 years, and ≤2.3% in patients over age 50 years. The risk of hepatotoxicity increases in patients receiving rifampin, overusing alcohol, or taking acetaminophen. Monitoring of hepatocellular enzymes remains controversial; however, all patients should be warned to discontinue INH if they experience symptoms of early hepatitis: loss of appetite, nausea, malaise, and right upper quadrant or midabdominal pain. An increased incidence of peripheral neuropathy is observed in malnourished patients receiving INH. This drug increases pyridoxine excretion, and coadministering pyridoxine can prevent this complication. Hypersensitivity reactions and arthritic disorders are less common.

ANTIMICROBIAL SPECTRUM OF ACTIVITY AND TREATMENT RECOMMENDATIONS At low concentrations INH is inhibitory, and at higher concentrations it is cidal to actively growing mycobacteria. In active infection INH should never be given alone. INH resistance is observed in a significant percentage of primary isolates (7–8%) and is more commonly observed in large cities. Therefore three or four drug regimens are commonly recommended until sensitivity to INH can be confirmed.

PHARMACOKINETICS INH is well absorbed orally or intramuscularly. This agent penetrates all body spaces, including the blood-brain barrier. The liver metabolizes INH, and the rate of metabolism depends on the livers' capacity to acetylate INH. The half-life of INH is 3 hours in slow acetylators and 1 hour in rapid acetylators. Approximately half of American Caucasians are slow acetylators, while only 5% of Eskimos fall into this category. Using the standard regimen, both slow and rapid acetylators achieve therapeutic levels, and cure rates are similar. However, slow acetylators have a higher incidence of

neurotoxicity, while fast acetylators have a greater risk of developing hepatotoxicity.

Dose: 300 mg or 5 mg/kg po QD
Renal dosing: Cr Cl <10 cc/min, slow acetylators 1/2 dose
Cost: Low
Spectrum: Mycobacteria only

KEY POINTS
Isoniazid (INH)

1. Inhibits mycolic acid synthesis, cidal activity against mycobacteria.
2. Half of Caucasians acetylate INH slowly. Slow acetylators have an increased incidence of peripheral neuropathy. Fast acetylators have a higher incidence of hepatotoxicity.
3. Age-related hepatotoxicity is the major toxicity in patients over 35. Patients should discontinue if they experience symptoms of hepatitis.
4. Peripheral neuropathy is increased in malnourished patients, prevented by pyridoxine.
5. Primary resistance to INH 7–8%, higher in large cities.

RIFAMYCINS

CHEMICAL STRUCTURE AND MECHANISMS OF ACTION Rifamycins are macrocyclic compounds that act as zwitterions capable of diffusing through lipids. These agents inhibit DNA-dependent RNA polymerase, preventing chain initiation. They are far more active against bacterial RNA polymerase than mammalian mitochondrial polymerase.

TOXICITY Hepatotoxicity is one of the most frequent side effects, asymptomatic serum transaminase values being observed in up to 14% of patients and overt hepatitis developing in 1% in the absence of INH and in 2–3% when INH is coadministered with rifampin. The risk of hepatotoxicity increases with age, alcohol consumption, and malnutrition. As is recommended for

INH, patients need to be instructed to discontinue this medication if they experience the symptoms of early hepatitis. A rise in serum bilirubin can occur in the absence of hepatitis in the first week of therapy as a result of competitive inhibition of hepatic bilirubin metabolism. Other side effects include skin rash; gastrointestinal complaints; renal dysfunction; orange discoloration of urine, sweat, and tears; and organic brain syndrome. Rifampin is a potent inducer of hepatic enzymes and shortens the half-life of a number of therapeutic agents, including coumadin, cyclosporin, digoxin, fluconazole, anti-HIV protease inhibitors, theophylline, thyroxine, and zidovudine. Trimethoprim-sulfamethoxazole increases rifampin levels. Before rifampin or rifabutin is administered, all other medications should be reviewed, and potential interactions should be investigated.

ANTIMICROBIAL ACTIVITY AND TREATMENT RECOMMENDATIONS   Rifampin has excellent activity against *Mycobacterium tuberculosis*, as well as some activity against *M. avium-intracellulare, M. fortuitum, M. kansasii, and M. marinum.* Rifabutin, a semisynthetic derivative of rifampin, has better activity against *M. avium-intracellulare* (MAI) than rifampin does. Because the rapid development of resistance is very frequent, these agents should never be used as monotherapy and should be combined with other antimycobacterial agents. Rifabutin is the drug of choice for prevention of MAI in HIV-infected patients and also is more effective than rifampin in combination therapy for active MAI infections.

Rifampin is active against a number of nontuberculous organisms. It has excellent activity against *Neisseria meningitidis*, and rifampin is one of the antibiotics recommended for meningococcal prophylaxis. *Staphylococcus aureus* and *Staphylococcus epidermidis* as well as *Streptococcus pyogenes* are exquisitely sensitive to rifampin; however, the mutation rate for rifampin resistance is high, prohibiting monotherapy. Studies suggest that rifampin combined with vancomycin may improve the outcome of prosthetic valve endocarditis due to *Staphylococcus epidermidis*, particularly when combined with gentamicin. However, the use of a rifampin combination in *Staphylococcus aureus* bacteremia or endocarditis remains controversial. This agent demonstrates excellent activity against Legionella and Chlamydia; however, rifampin generally has not been used to treat these pathogens. Rifampin also is active against *Rhodococcus equi* and has been used in combination with vancomycin in a small number of patients.

PHARMACOKINETICS   Oral preparations are almost completely absorbed. Peak serum levels are observed in 1–4 hours. Rifampin has a half-life of 2–5 hours, and rifabutin has a half-life of 16 hours. Both drugs are taken up by the liver, deacetylated to an active metabolite, and then excreted via the biliary tract. These agents penetrate all tissues and achieve excellent intracellular levels. They also cross the blood-brain barrier.

Dose:
Rifampin: 600 mg QD po, can increase to 600 mg BID for nontuberculous infections
Renal dosing: No adjustments required
Rifabutin: 300 mg QD po
Renal dosing: No adjustments required
Cost: Rifampin, low; rifabutin, moderate
Spectrum: narrow

KEY POINTS
Rifamycins

1. Zwitterions that diffuse through lipids, inhibit bacterial RNA polymerase.
2. Symptomatic hepatitis occurs in 1% of patients; discontinue if symptoms of hepatitis occur.
3. Orange discoloration of tears, sweat, and urine.
4. Potent inducer of hepatic enzymes, shortens the half-life of many drugs.
5. Rifampin is preferred for *Mycobacterium tuberculosis*, rifabutin for MAI.

6. Rifampin is used in combination with vancomycin and gentamicin for *Staphylococcus
epidermidis* prosthetic endocarditis, in combination with vancomycin for *Rhodococcus
equi.*

PYRAZINAMIDE

Pyrazinamide (PZA) is a pyrazine analogue of
nicotinamide. Its mechanism of action is unknown. This drug is most active in an acidic environment such as the low pH of the
macrophage phagolysosome, where tubercle
bacilli are commonly found. It is cidal against
replicating *Mycobacterium tuberculosis*. This
drug should never be used as monotherapy because resistance develops rapidly. The most
common side effects are nausea and vomiting.
Hepatitis is dose related and is uncommon with
current dosing recommendations. Interstitial
nephritis, polymyalgia, rhabdomyolysis, and
photosensitivity are rare complications. PZA decreases tubular secretion of urate, and asymptomatic hyperuricemia is noted in approximately
half of patients. This drug is well absorbed and
readily distributes throughout the body, including the cerebrospinal fluid. PZA is recommended for the treatment of tuberculous meningitis. The liver is the primary pathway for
metabolism, and the kidneys primarily excrete
metabolites. The drug's half-life is 10–16 hours.

Dose: 15–30 mg/kg QD po
Renal dosing: Cr Cl < 10 cc/min, 12–20 mg/kg QD
Cost: Low
Spectrum: Narrow

KEY POINTS
Pyrazinamide

1. Most active in an acidic environment such
as the phagolysosome.
2. Hepatotoxicity is dose-related, rare at recommended doses; nausea and vomiting are

other common side effects. Asymptomatic
hyperuricemia is also common.
3. Penetrates all tissues and fluids, including
the CSF; recommended for tuberculous
meningitis.
4. Never used in monotherapy because of the
rapid development of resistance.

STREPTOMYCIN

This aminoglycoside has the same mechanism
of action as the other aminoglycosides and similar toxicities. Nephrotoxicity and hearing loss are
less common; however, the incidence of vestibular dysfunction is higher than that with other
aminoglycosides. Patients need to be warned
that if they develop tinnitus, decreased hearing,
or dizziness, they should report these symptoms
to their physician and discontinue the drug.
Streptomycin is cidal for extracellular *Mycobacterium tuberculosis* but fails to achieve therapeutic intracellular levels. This agent should
never be given alone because resistance develops rapidly with monotherapy. As is observed
with other aminoglycosides, streptomycin is excreted by the kidneys and has a half-life of 2–5
hours. The need for parenteral administration,
usually intramuscularly, causes some inconvenience for outpatient therapy.

Dose: 500 mg Q12H, im or iv
Renal dosing: Cr Cl 50–80 cc/min, 15 mg/kg
Q24–48H; Cr Cl 10–50 cc/min, 15 mg/kg
Q72–96H; Cr Cl < 10 cc/min, 7.5 mg/kg
Q72–96H
Cost: Moderate
Spectrum: Narrow

KEY POINTS
Streptomycin

1. Same mechanism of action as other aminoglycosides.
2. Increased incidence of vestibular toxicity as
compared to other aminoglycosides.

3. Discontinue if there are complaints of dizziness or tinnitus.
4. Cidal for extracellular mycobacteria but fails to penetrate cells.
5. Administered intramuscularly.

ETHAMBUTOL

CHEMICAL STRUCTURE AND MECHANISMS OF ACTION
Ethambutol is an eight-carbon noncyclic molecule that was specifically synthesized as an antituberculous agent. This agent inhibits arabinosyl transferases that are important for mycobacterial cell wall synthesis. Ethambutol is a static agent.

TOXICITY   The major toxicity of ethambutol is optic neuritis resulting in loss of visual acuity and defective red-green color vision. This toxicity is dose related, being more common with doses of 25 mg/kg than 15 mg/kg. On high-dose ethambutol and in those with baseline visual dysfunction receiving 15 mg/kg, monitoring of visual acuity and color perception every 4–6 weeks is recommended.

PHARMACOKINETICS   The drug is well absorbed orally and has a broad tissue distribution, including the CSF. It is metabolized by the liver, and the resulting metabolites are excreted by the kidneys. Ethambutol has a half-life of 3–4 hours.

Dose: 15–25 mg/kg QD po
Renal dosing: Cr Cl 50–80 cc/min, 15 mg/kg Q24H; Cr Cl 10–50 cc/min, 15 mg/kg Q24–36H; Cr Cl < 10 cc/min, 15 mg/kg Q48H
Cost: Low
Spectrum: Narrow

KEY POINTS
Ethambutol

1. Inhibits arabinosyl transferases that are important for mycobacterial cell wall synthesis.
2. A static agent.

3. Major toxicity is loss of red-green color vision and decreased visual acuity, dose-related.
4. Test vision every 4–6 weeks while on high-dose therapy (25 mg/kg).

Second-Line Medications

QUINOLONES

These agents are often cidal for mycobacteria. Ciprofloxacin and ofloxacin are frequently used for the treatment of multiresistant *Mycobacterium tuberculosis*. The recommended dose is ciprofloxacin 750 mg BID or ofloxacin 400 mg BID.

OTHER AMINOGLYCOSIDES

Capreomycin, amikacin, kanamycin, and viomycin have all been used for the treatment of multidrug-resistant *Mycobacterium tuberculosis*. Capreomycin is less toxic than other aminoglycosides and is the preferred drug in this category. Capreomycin can be given only intramuscularly and is excreted unaltered by the kidneys. Its major side effects are nephrotoxicity and ototoxicity. Multidrug-resistant strains exhibiting resistance to streptomycin are generally sensitive to capreomycin. Amikacin is the most active aminoglycoside against *M. tuberculosis*. However, the high incidence of nephrotoxicity and ototoxicity associated with prolonged therapy limits its usefulness. Kanamycin and viomycin are less commonly used because they exhibit cross-resistance to capreomycin and amikacin and are more toxic.

Dose:
Capreomycin: 1 g QD
Renal dosing: Cr Cl 10–50 cc/min, 7.5 mg/kg Q24–48H; Cr Cl < 10 cc/min, 7.5 mg/kg twice per week
Cost: Very high
Spectrum: Narrow
Amikacin: 7–10 mg/kg (not to exceed 1 g) five times per week

Renal dosing: Dose based on serum levels
Cost: Low
Spectrum: Narrow

CYCLOSERINE

This bacteriostatic agent is usually not effective against multidrug-resistant strains but has been used in primary drug-resistant *Mycobacterium tuberculosis*. Cycloserine has severe central nervous system toxicity, including seizures, somnolence, headache, and severe depression. This agent should not be given to patients with a history of seizures or depression. Cycloserine is well absorbed orally, distributes to all tissues, and readily crosses the blood-brain barrier. It is renally excreted and has a half-life of 8–12 hours.

Dose: 250–500 mg BID po
Renal dosing: Cr Cl 10–50 cc/min, 250–500 mg QD; Cr Cl < 10 cc/min, 250 mg QD
Cost: Moderately high
Spectrum: Narrow

PARA-AMINOSALICYLIC ACID (PAS)

This agent inhibits folate metabolism of tuberculous organisms and is a static agent. Its usefulness is limited by the frequent occurrence of nausea and vomiting. Other side effects include hypersensitivity reactions, including a lupuslike syndrome, lymph node hypertrophy, and hepatitis. It is incompletely absorbed orally and is excreted in the urine. The drug is available through the Centers for Disease Control and Prevention. The usual dose is 10–12 g/day in three or four divided doses.

ETHIONAMIDE

This compound is derived from isonicotinic acid and is tuberculostatic, interfering with mycolic acid synthesis. Ethionamide often causes nausea and vomiting. Neurologic side effects are common, including peripheral neuropathy and psychiatric disorders. Reversible hepato-

toxicity is also reported. Ethionamide is well absorbed orally and penetrates all tissues, including the blood-brain barrier. It is metabolized by the liver, and metabolites are excreted in the urine. The half-life of the drug is 2–4 hours.

Dose: Initial dose, 250 mg BID, increasing by 250 mg/day to reach a final dose of 500 mg BID
Renal dosing: Cr Cl < 10 cc/min, 5 mg/kg Q48H
Cost: Low
Spectrum: Narrow

KEY POINTS

Second-Line Antimycobacterial Therapy

1. Quinolones demonstrate excellent cidal activity.
2. Aminoglycosides: Amikacin is most active against *Mycobacterium tuberculosis*, but there is a high risk of nephrotoxicity. Capreomycin is less toxic. Given intramuscularly.
3. Cycloserine: A static agent. Severe CNS toxicity, including seizures, somnolence, and depression.
4. Para-aminosalicylic acid (PAS): Inhibits mycobacteria folate metabolism. A static agent. Nausea and vomiting are very common, limiting its usefulness.
5. Ethionamide: Tuberculostatic, interferes with mycolic acid synthesis. Side effects include nausea, vomiting, peripheral neuropathy, and psychiatric disturbances.

Antifungal Agents

Fungi are eukaryotes and share many of the structural and metabolic characteristics of human cells. As a result, designing agents that affect fungi without harming human cells has proved difficult. One major difference between the two cell types is the primary sterol building block that is used to form the plasma membrane. The fungal plasma membrane consists of ergesterols, while the major sterol component of the human plasma membrane is cholesterol. This difference has been exploited in the development of two classes of drugs. The polyenes act by binding to ergesterol and disrupting the fungal membrane. These agents are fungicidal. The azoles inhibit ergesterol synthesis, and lowered ergesterol levels result in fungal membrane breakdown. These agents are usually fungistatic.

KEY POINTS

The Major Difference between Mammalian and Fungal Cells

> Like mammals, fungi are eukaryotes. Drug therapy takes advantage of the fact that fungi use ergesterols rather than cholesterol as the major building block of the plasma membrane.

Agents for Treatment of Systemic Fungal Infections

AMPHOTERICIN B

CHEMICAL STRUCTURE, MECHANISMS OF ACTION, AND SPECTRUM OF ACTIVITY This long, cyclic polyene compound forms a large, rodlike structure. Multiple molecules bind to ergesterol in the fungal membrane, forming pores that result in leakage of intracellular potassium and fungal cell death. This fungicidal action is rapid and does not require active growth. This agent is effective against most fungal infections and remains the most effective agent for systemic fungal infections. Clinical resistance to amphotericin B has been demonstrated among *Candida lusitaniae*, Fusarium species, and *Pseudallescheria boydii*. *C. lusitaniae* initially is susceptible to amphotericin B but develops resistance during treatment. Alterations in sterol structure required for

amphotericin B resistance often reduce tissue invasiveness, such strains being capable of growing only on mucosal surfaces or in the urine.

KEY POINTS

The Mechanism of Action and Spectrum of Amphotericin B

> 1. A polyene compound that forms rodlike structures that bind to ergesterol in the fungal membrane and form pores, resulting in a leak of intracellular potassium.
> 2. Rapidly cidal, does not require active growth.
> 3. Effective against most fungi except *Candida lusitaniae*, Fusarium, and *Pseudallescheria boydii*.
> 4. The preferred antifungal agent for severe systemic fungal infections.

TOXICITY Nephrotoxicity is the major complication associated with the conventional deoxycholate form of the drug (amphotericin B deoxycholate, or ABD). This agent causes vasoconstriction of renal arterioles, resulting in a reduction in glomerular filtration rate. Vasoconstriction also impairs proximal and distal tubular reabsorption, causing potassium, magnesium, and bicarbonate wasting. These effects are reversible. However, permanent loss of nephrons and permanent damage to tubular basement membranes are also observed and correlate with the total dose of ABD administered. Renal dysfunction is observed in virtually all patients receiving ABD, and serum creatinine levels of 2–3 mg/dl are to be expected. Hydration with normal saline prior to infusion reduces nephrotoxicity.

Fever is commonly associated with administration of amphotericin B, and the drug can be associated with chills, fever, and tachypnea, particularly if it is infused too rapidly. Amphotericin B should be administered over a minimum of 2–3 hours. A more rapid infusion of lipid-complexed amphotericin B is required to prevent drug precipitation. Usually, fever and chills diminish with each ensuing dose. However, if these reactions persist, the patient can be premedicated with acetaminophen or by the addition of 25–50 mg of hydrocortisone to the solution. It is important to keep in mind that this febrile response does not represent an allergic reaction and should not be misinterpreted as anaphylaxis. Some physicians have advocated a 1-mg test dose prior to administration of the full dose. The helpfulness of this practice has not been proven, and use of a test dose delays achievement of therapeutic antifungal serum and tissue levels. Other side effects include nausea, vomiting, and anorexia. Phlebitis usually develops when the drug is administered by a peripheral vein. Therefore this drug should be administered by a centrally placed intravenous line.

KEY POINTS
Toxicity of Amphotericin B

1. Nephrotoxicity is observed in virtually all patients receiving amphotericin B deoxycholate (ABD). Reduced by hydrating with normal saline. Reversible in most cases. Permanent damage with prolonged therapy.
2. Fever is common with all preparations. Slow infusion (2–3 hours with ABD, <2 hours with liposomal preparations) reduces severity. Premedication with corticosteroids and/or acetaminophen often reduces fever.
3. Phlebitis is common, requiring administration by a central intravenous line.

PHARMACOKINETICS   Amphotericin B deoxycholate is insoluble in water at physiologic pH and is stored as a powder that is dispersed as a colloidal suspension in a 5% dextrose solution. The addition of electrolytes aggregates the colloids, making the solution cloudy. Following intravenous infusion, amphotericin B is bound to lipoproteins in the serum and then leaves the circulation. The drug is stored in the liver and other organs and subsequently released into the circu-

lation. Lipid-complex amphotericin B is ingested by macrophages, resulting in high intracellular levels in this cell type. This drug poorly penetrates the blood-brain barrier and brain. Therapeutic levels are detectable in inflamed pleural fluid, the peritoneum, and joint fluid. Amphotericin B is slowly degraded, and degradation is not affected by hepatic or renal dysfunction. The initial half-life of the drug is 24 hours; however, over time the half-life extends to 15 days. Serum concentrations of the drug are detectable seven weeks after therapy is discontinued.

EFFICACY OF DIFFERENT AMPHOTERICIN B PREPARATIONS   Lipid-complexed preparations of amphotericin B are now available. These preparations are very expensive and in clinical trials have efficacy comparable to that of ABD. Lipid-complexed amphotericin B markedly reduces nephrotoxicity and should be used primarily in patients with significant preexisting renal dysfunction or in patients who develop progressive renal failure (serum creatinine above 2.5 mg/dl) while being treated with ABD.

Dose:
Amphotericin B deoxycholate: 0.3–1.4 mg/kg QD
Renal dosing: No adjustment required
Amphotericin B lipid complex: 3–5 mg/kg QD
Renal dosing: No adjustment required
Cost: Amphotericin B deoxycholate, low; amphotericin B lipid complex, all three preparations, very high (liposomal preparation > $1,000/day; lipid complex preparation $270/day)

KEY POINTS
The Different Amphotericin B Preparations

1. Lipid-complexed preparations reduce nephrotoxicity.
2. Similar incidence of fever.

3. Comparable efficacy to conventional amphotericin B deoxycholate (ABD).
4. Higher doses required: 3–5 mg/kg/day, compared to 0.3–1.4 mg/kg for ABD.
5. Very high cost, recommended only for patients with significant preexisting renal dysfunction or those who develop progressive renal dysfunction on ABD (serum creatinine > 2.5 mg/dl).

AZOLES

CHEMICAL STRUCTURE AND MECHANISMS OF ACTION
These agents were chemically synthesized. Five azoles are currently licensed in the United States: two imidazoles (miconazole and ketoconazole) and three triazoles (fluconazole, itraconazole, and voriconazole). The imidazoles are rarely used for systemic infections, being reserved primarily for topical treatment of superficial fungal infections. Because they are better absorbed orally and have excellent toxicity profiles, the triazoles are the class of azoles that are preferred for systemic fungal infection. The azoles all inhibit a cytochrome P450–dependent demethylation system that results in decreased production of ergesterol and accumulation of intermediate sterols. The loss of ergesterol results in altered fungal membrane permeability, disturbed activity of membrane surface enzymes, and retention of metabolites. These agents have broad antifungal activity but demonstrate fungistatic rather than fungicidal activity. Itraconazole can antagonize amphotericin B activity by reducing its binding target, ergesterol.

KEY POINTS
Mechanism of Action of Azoles

1. Inhibit the cytochrome P450–dependent demethylation, resulting in decreased ergesterol production and altered fungal membrane permeability.

2. Azoles are usually fungistatic.
3. Itraconazole can antagonize amphotericin B activity by reducing its binding target.

TOXICITY   Ketoconazole not only interferes with fungal sterol metabolism, but at higher doses also interferes with testosterone and cortisone production. Gynecomastia and loss of libido are commonly observed. Nausea and vomiting are common, as are asymptomatic increases in serum transaminase levels. Severe hepatitis can develop, and patients should be alerted to the need to discontinue this medication if they experience the symptoms of hepatitis (anorexia, malaise, nausea, and vomiting). As a result of its many toxicities, ketoconazole is rarely prescribed today. Fluconazole demonstrates minimal toxicity. Side effects include headache, anorexia, reversible alopecia, and asymptomatic increases in serum transaminase levels. Itraconazole also has an excellent toxicity profile. The most common complaints associated with this drug are nausea and abdominal discomfort. Hypokalemia, mild hypertension, and edema are reported in association with daily doses of 400 mg or higher. Voriconazole infusion is associated with transient loss of light perception. This symptom resolves with subsequent doses. Visual hallucinations occur less commonly.

KEY POINTS
Azole Toxicity

1. Ketoconazole: Interferes with testosterone and cortisone production, resulting in gynecomastia and loss of libido; hepatitis can be severe; ketoconazole should be discontinued when symptoms of hepatitis develop, and liver function test should be drawn.
2. Fluconazole: Rare side effects include headache, anorexia, and asymptomatic elevation of serum transaminases.

3. Itraconazole: Excellent toxicity profile, can cause nausea and abdominal pain.
4. Voriconazole: Transient loss of light perception.

SPECTRUM OF ACTIVITY AND TREATMENT RECOMMENDATIONS

Fluconazole   This agent has no activity against Aspergillus species, and some strains of Candida demonstrate natural resistance to fluconazole, including *Candida glabrata* and *C. krusei*. Any Candida species can develop resistance to fluconazole owing to increased production of demethylase as well as increased drug efflux. Fluconazole is recommended for the treatment of oropharyngeal candidiasis as well as vulvovaginal candidiasis. Intravenous fluconazole has proved therapeutically equivalent to amphotericin B in uncomplicated candidemia in the nonimmunocompromised host. However, for the immunocompromised (including neutropenic) host and for seriously ill patients with deep tissue Candida infection, amphotericin B remains the treatment of choice.

Fluconazole is also effective for the completion of treatment of cryptococcal meningitis in AIDS patients. After initial therapy with amphotericin B with or without flucytosine for two weeks, fluconazole (400 mg QD) treatment is recommended for two months, followed by daily fluconazole maintenance therapy (200 mg QD). The role of fluconazole in non-AIDS patients with cryptococcal infection has not been defined. The use of fluconazole for the prevention of fungal infections has been explored in neutropenic allogeneic bone marrow transplant patients and was found to reduce mortality and the incidence of invasive Candida infections but had no effect on the incidence of Aspergillus infections.

Fluconazole prophylaxis of leukemia patients also reduced the incidence of invasive Candida infections but did not affect mortality. This antifungal agent is frequently used in surgical intensive-care unit patients in hopes of preventing candidemia. To date, such prophylaxis has not been proven to significantly reduce Candida infections. Furthermore, this practice increases the prevalence of fluconazole-resistant fungi, including *Candida krusei* and *C. glabrata*. Because of the risk of selecting resistant fungi, fluconazole prophylaxis is not recommended in HIV-infected patients.

KEY POINTS

The Spectrum of Activity and Indications for Fluconazole

1. No activity against Aspergillus. Active against *Candida albicans*, but natural resistance to *C. glabrata* and *C. krusei* is common. Active against *Cryptococcus neoformans*.
2. Drug resistance can develop in Candida species with prolonged treatment.
3. Treatment of choice for oral candidiasis and Candida vulvovaginitis.
4. Can be used for uncomplicated *Candida albicans* fungemia in the nonimmunocompromised patient.
5. After an initial course of amphotericin B, can be used to complete therapy of cryptococcal meningitis in HIV patients.
6. Prophylaxis reduces Candida infections in neutropenic patients. The role of prophylaxis in other settings remains controversial because of the risk of selecting resistant strains.

Itraconazole   This agent has improved activity against histoplasmosis, coccidiomycosis, blastomycosis, and sporotrichosis compared to fluconazole. Itraconazole can be used for acute and chronic vaginal candidiasis and HIV-associated oral and esophageal candidiasis. This agent has been used in the treatment of invasive Aspergillus and phaeohyphomycosis. It is the preferred agent for the treatment of lymphocutaneous sporotrichosis and nonmeningeal, non-life-threatening histoplasmosis, blastomycosis, and coccidiomycosis. The clinical efficacy in candidemia and deeply invasive Candida infection has not been systematically investigated. For disseminated histoplasmosis and coccidiomycosis, amphotericin B remains the treatment of choice. Itraconazole is recommended as primary prophylaxis and for the prevention of relapse of histoplasmosis in AIDS patients.

KEY POINTS

The Spectrum of Activity and Indications for Itraconazole

1. Improved activity against histoplasmosis, coccidiomycosis, blastomycosis, and sporotrichosis.
2. Used in less severe cases of histoplasmosis and coccidiomycosis.
3. Used to prevent relapse of disseminated histoplasmosis in AIDS patients.
4. Absorption of the drug is erratic.

Voriconazole   This azole is the newest of the azoles. This agent has increased activity against Aspergillus. In patients with neutropenia and persistent fever, voriconazole is a suitable alternative to amphotericin B for empiric antifungal therapy, and it is associated with fewer side effects.

KEY POINTS

The Spectrum of Activity and Indications for Voriconazole

1. Increased activity against aspergillus.
2. Comparable to amphotericin B in febrile neutropenic patients.
3. Both intravenous and oral forms available.
4. Metabolism increased by drugs that induce the cytochrome P450 system.

PHARMACOKINETICS   Fluconazole is well absorbed orally, and serum levels after ingestion of the oral preparation are comparable to those for intravenous administration. Penetration into tissues and body fluids, including the cerebrospinal fluid, is excellent. The drug is excreted primarily in the urine, smaller amounts being released into the feces. The half-life of this agent is 27–34 hours. Itraconazole is more variable in its oral absorption and requires stomach acidity for adequate absorption. Capsule absorption is enhanced by food and reduced by agents that reduce stomach acidity. Itraconazole penetrates most tissues but does not cross the blood-brain barrier and minimally enters ocular fluids. Itraconazole is primarily metabolized by the liver, and the metabolites are excreted in the feces. The half-life of this drug is 20–60 hours. Voriconazole is well absorbed orally and has a half-life of 6 hours. Voriconazole serum levels are reduced by drugs that induce the cytochrome P450 system (examples: rifampin, carbamazepine, phenobarbital). In patients with significant cirrhosis hepatic metabolism of voriconazole is impaired, and the maintenance intravenous dose should be decreased to 4 mg/kg QD.

Dose:
Fluconazole: Oral, 100–400 mg QD; intravenous, 100–400 mg QD
Renal dosing: Cr Cl 10–50 cc/min, reduce dose by 50%; Cr Cl <10 cc/min, 25–50 mg QD
Itraconazole: Oral, 200–400 mg QD; intravenous, 200 mg QD
Renal dosing: No adjustment required
Voriconazole: Oral, 200–400 mg Q12H; intravenous, 6 mg/kg Q12H first day, followed by 4 mg/kg Q12H
Renal dosing: Intravenous form contraindicated if Cr Cl < 50 cc/min
Cost:
Oral fluconazole: Moderately high to very high, depending on dose
Intravenous fluconazole: Moderate to moderately high
Oral itraconazole: High to very high, depending on dose
Intravenous itraconazole: High to very high
Oral and intravenous voriconazole: Very high

FLUCYTOSINE

CHEMICAL STRUCTURE AND MECHANISMS OF ACTION
Flucytosine, or 5-fluorocytosine (5-FC), is a fluorine analogue of cytosine. After a multistep conversion requiring deamination and phosphorylation, the resulting product, 5-fluorouracil (5-FU), acts as an inhibitor of thymidylate synthetase, impairing DNA and RNA synthesis. 5-FC is not toxic in humans because they lack the deaminase that is required for conversion to 5-FU.

TOXICITY The major toxicity is bone marrow suppression leading to neutropenia, anemia, and thrombocytopenia. This side effect is dose related and usually occurs when serum levels exceed 125 μg/ml. Patients with diminished bone marrow reserve, such as AIDS patients and patients receiving cancer chemotherapy, are more likely to suffer this complication. Commonly, 5-FC is administered in combination with amphotericin B. As was discussed above, amphotericin B impairs renal function, and reductions in renal function reduce 5-FC clearance. Monitoring of peak (2 hours after oral administration) and trough (just prior to the next dose) levels is recommended in patients with renal dysfunction. Doses should be adjusted to maintain serum levels between 20 and 100 μg/ml. Other side effects include nausea and vomiting, diarrhea, abdominal pain, and hepatitis.

SPECTRUM OF ACTIVITY AND TREATMENT RECOMMENDATIONS Most strains of *Candida albicans* and *Cryptococcus neoformans* are sensitive to 5-FC. Native resistance varies from geographical area to area. About 15% of *Candida albicans* strains and 3–5% of *Cryptococcus neoformans* strains demonstrate resistance. This agent is also active against chromomycosis. 5-FC is usually fungistatic and has inferior activity compared to amphotericin B. It should never be used alone because resistance rapidly develops with monotherapy. The combination of 5-FC and amphotericin B demonstrates additive or synergistic activity in cryptococcal infections. In cryptococcal menin-gitis, amphotericin B and 5-FC sterilize the CSF faster than does amphotericin B alone. In vitro testing and animal testing also suggest that combination therapy for Candida may be of benefit; however, efficacy has not been proven in patients. Results of combination therapy for Aspergillus have been variable.

PHARMACOKINETICS This drug is well absorbed orally. Because it is a small molecule, 5-FC penetrates tissues well and crosses the blood-brain barrier. Therapeutic levels can be achieved in the cerebrospinal fluid, aqueous humor, joint fluid, and respiratory secretions. 5-FC is cleared by the kidneys and has a half-life of 3–5 hours.

Dose: 25 mg/kg Q6H po
Renal dosing: Cr Cl 10–50 cc/min, 25 mg/kg Q12–24H; Cr Cl < 10 cc/min, adjust dose using serum levels (see above)
Cost: Moderate (See Table 1.2.)

KEY POINTS

5-Fluorocytosine (5-FC)

1. Impairs fungal DNA and RNA synthesis, fungistatic.
2. Cleared by the kidneys, penetrates all tissues and fluids including the CSF.
3. High levels cause bone marrow suppression. In patients with renal failure, doses should be adjusted and serum levels should be monitored.
4. Never use as monotherapy. In cryptococcal meningitis the combination of amphotericin B and 5-FC sterilizes the CSF faster than amphotericin B alone. In animal studies, combination therapy is beneficial for Candida infections, but efficacy has not been proven in humans.

CASPOFUNGIN

CHEMICAL STRUCTURE AND MECHANISMS OF ACTION
Caspofungin is derived from echinocandin B

and is a semisynthetic lipopeptide that blocks synthesis of β-(1,3)-D-glucan. This polysaccharide is a critical component of the cell wall of many pathogenic fungi.

TOXICITY Fever, rash, nausea, vomiting, and phlebitis have been reported. Flushing of the face has also been observed during infusion. Experience with this agent is limited, and additional toxicities may become apparent. One case of anaphylaxis has been reported. Plasma levels are increased by coadministration of cyclosporin. Agents that may reduce serum levels include efavirenz, nelfinavir, Dilantin, Tegretol, rifampin, and dexamethasone. Caspofungin reduces serum levels of tacrolimus but does not interact with mycophenolate mofetil (Cell Cept), amphotericin B, or itraconazole.

SPECTRUM OF ACTIVITY AND TREATMENT INDICATIONS
This agent is active against Aspergillus and Candida species, including isolates that are resistant to other antifungal agents. It is less effective against *Candida parapsolosis* in vitro and is not active against cryptococcus. Caspofungin has been approved for the treatment of invasive aspergillosis in patients who fail or are unable to tolerate amphotericin B or itraconazole. Clinical trials have been limited, and only about half the patients treated have demonstrated partial or complete responses to this treatment. Caspofungin can also be used to treat oral candidiasis that is refractory to azole or amphotericin B therapy.

PHARMACOKINETICS This agent is not absorbed by the gastrointestinal tract and must be administered intravenously. It is metabolized by the liver and has a half-life of 9–11 hours.

Dose: 70 mg first day, followed by 50 mg QD iv; infused over 1 hour
Renal dosing: No adjustment required. Moderate hepatic failure: reduce dose to 35 mg QD
Cost: Very high (See Table 1.2.)

KEY POINTS
Caspofungin

1. Blocks synthesis of a cell wall polysaccharide that is vital to many pathogenic fungi.
2. Active against Aspergillus and Candida, including isolates that are resistant to other antifungal agents. Not active against Cryptococcus.
3. Toxicities tend to be mild.
4. Experience with this drug is limited.
5. Recommended for the treatment of invasive Aspergillus in patients who have failed or cannot tolerate amphotericin B and for oral and esophageal candidiasis that is refractory to azoles and amphotericin B.

Agents for Treatment of Superficial Fungal Infections

Both topical and oral medications are available for the treatment of superficial fungal infections. Topical medications are generally useful in superficial infections of the feet and hands and discrete truncal lesions, while oral medications are generally required for nail infections, extensive infections of the trunk, ringworm of the scalp, and infections in heavily keratinized skin.

KEY POINTS
Treatment of Superficial Fungal Infections

1. Topical medications are used for superficial infections of the feet and hands and discrete truncal lesions.
2. Oral medications are recommended for nail infections, ringworm of the scalp, infections of heavily keratinized skin, and diffuse truncal infection.

TOPICAL PREPARATIONS

The choice of topical agent depends on the nature of the fungal lesion. For fissures, inflamed areas under breast tissue, or lesions in the groin or axilla, creams or liquid solutions are preferred. Powders are recommended only for mild lesions and to prevent recurrence. The number of available topical agents is very large, and preparations are constantly changing. Controlled clinical trials comparing various agents often have not been performed. Only the agents that are thought to have significant efficacy will be covered, and these are summarized in Table 1.5. Topical products are similar in their efficacy; therefore selection of a specific agent should be based on cost, patient preference, and availability.

AZOLES   These agents demonstrate minimal toxicity and have a broad spectrum of activity, being effective against most dermatophytes, with the exception of tinea capitis. The imidazoles are most commonly used and include clotrimazole (Lotrimin, Mycelex, Fungoid) and miconazole (Micatin, Monistat). Both of these agents are available without a prescription. Other agents that are less commonly used include oxiconazole, econazole, ketoconazole, and sulconazole.

POLYENES   These agents are primarily effective against Candida and are used primarily for oral and vaginal candidiasis. Nystatin throat lozenges have proved less effective than systemic fluconazole for oral candidiasis. Nystatin vaginal troches require more prolonged treatment compared to azole topical preparations: 14 days versus 7 days.

OTHER AGENTS   Terbinafine (Lamisil) and naftifine (Naftin) are topical allylamines that act on squalene epoxidase to block ergosterol synthesis and have excellent activity against the dermatophytes. Tolnaftate (Aftate, NP-27, Tinactin, Ting) is a thiocarbamate compound that has limited activity against dermatophytes. Undecylenic acid is widely used in nonprescription powders and creams (Cruex, Desenex) but has minimal efficacy.

KEY POINTS
Topical Antifungal Agents

1. There are many preparations available; many have limited efficacy.

Table 1-5
Treatment for Superficial Fungal Infections

DRUG	SPECTRUM OF ACTIVITY
Azoles	
Miconazole (topical)	*Candida albicans, Malassezia furfur*, all common dermatophytes, not *Aspergillus* species
Fluconazole (oral)	Candida species, not Aspergillus species
Itraconazole (oral)	Candida species, Aspergillus species, *Blastomyces dermatitidis*, Trichophyton species
Polyene macrolides	
Amphotericin B (topical)	Candida species, Aspergillus species, other filamentous fungi, *Blastomyces dermatitidis*
Nystatin (topical)	Candida species, Aspergillus species
Allylamines	
Terbinafine (oral and topical)	Candida species, Aspergillus species, dermatophytes, dimorphic fungi

2. Topical azoles (clotrimazole and miconazole) are effective against most dermatophytes.
3. Polyenes (nystatin) are primarily effective against Candida. Require longer treatment than azoles for cure.
4. Topical allylamines (terbinafine and naftifine) block ergosterol synthesis and have excellent activity against dermatophytes.
5. Tolfanate has limited activity against dermatophytes.

ORAL PREPARATIONS

Topical therapy for scalp and nail infections is generally ineffective. The primary oral antifungals that are used for superficial fungal infections are fluconazole, itraconazole, terbinafine, and griseofulvin.

FLUCONAZOLE This agent is highly effective against superficial candidal infections. A single 150-mg dose is as effective as topical azole therapy. Systemic therapy should be avoided in pregnancy because craniofacial and cardiac anomalies have been reported in association with fluconazole administration. Doses of 100–200 mg QD are recommended.

ITRACONAZOLE This agent is effective against pityriasis and dermatophytes, including tinea versicolor (truncal dermatophyte infection), nail bed infection, and ringworm. Despite its higher cost, this agent is preferred over ketoconazole because of its lower toxicity profile and better absorption. For nail bed infections, itraconazole is effective when given daily 200 mg po or as pulsed therapy, 200 mg po BID for one week per month.

TERBINAFINE This allylamine is effective for the treatment of dermatophytes. It is comparable in efficacy to itraconazole for nail bed infections. Side effects associated with this drug are minimal and include indigestion and taste complaints. Hepatitis is rarely encountered. Terbinafine is highly protein bound and accumulates in the skin, nails, and fat. It is metabolized in the liver, having an initial half-life of 12 hours. However, as a result of fat accumulation and subsequent release, with continued therapy the half-life extends to 200–400 hours. Terbinafine persists in the plasma for 4–8 weeks after it is discontinued.

Dose: 250 mg QD po
Cost: Moderate (See Table 1.2.)

GRISEOFULVIN Griseofulvin is used primarily for tinea capitis (ringworm of the scalp) and is an alternative therapy after itraconazole or terbinafine for nail bed infections. Griseofulvin has activity against most dermatophytes but has no activity against Candida species. This drug has few side effects, the primary one being headache, which generally resolves over the first week of therapy. Gastrointestinal complaints, photosensitivity, and allergic reactions are uncommonly reported. Microcrystals are absorbed orally, reaching the skin and hair after ingestion. Absorption is enhanced by fatty foods. Griseofulvin is metabolized by the liver and has a half-life of 24–36 hours.

Dose: Microsize preparations: 500 mg–1 g QD po
Ultramicrosize preparation: 330–750 mg QD po
Cost: Low for both preparations

KEY POINTS
Oral Medications for Superficial Fungal Infections

1. Fluconazole is highly effective against superficial Candida infections.
2. Itraconzole is useful for truncal dermatophyte infections, nail bed infections, and ringworm.
3. Terbinafine can be used in nail bed infections. The drug persists in the plasma for 4–8 weeks.

4. Griseofulvin remains the treatment of choice for ringworm (tinea capitis) and can be used for nail bed infections.

Antiviral Drugs (Other than Antiretroviral Agents)

Most antiviral agents target viral nucleic acid synthesis. Because these agents tend to act at a single step in viral replication, resistance may develop during treatment. The development of resistance is favored by a high viral load, a high intrinsic viral mutation rate (more common in RNA than DNA viruses), and a high degree of selective pressure (i.e., prolonged antiviral therapy or repeated courses of treatment). A second method for controlling viral infection is by modifying the host immune response. Infusions of antibody preparations and treatment with interferon have proved efficacious in several viral infections.

KEY POINTS
Antiviral Therapy

1. Usually targets viral nucleic acid synthesis.
2. Development of resistance is common and is favored by:
   a. High viral load,
   b. High intrinsic viral mutation rate (RNA viruses > DNA viruses),
   c. Prolonged or intermittent antiviral therapy.

ACYCLOVIR AND VALACYCLOVIR

CHEMICAL STRUCTURE AND MECHANISMS OF ACTION
Acyclovir is a synthetic analogue of guanine in which a side chain has been substituted for a sugar moiety. Acyclovir is phosphorylated in viral-infected cells by viral thymidine kinase, forming a monophosphate compound. Host cell kinases then add two additional phosphates, allowing acyclovir triphosphate to add to replicating DNA. The acyclic side chain prevents the addition of subsequent nucleic acids to DNA, causing premature termination. In addition, acyclovir triphosphate selectively inhibits viral DNA polymerase. Because acyclovir requires viral thymidine kinase for its initial phosphorylation step, the concentrations of acyclovir triphosphate are 40–100 times higher in infected cells than in uninfected cells. Acyclovir resistance is most commonly caused by a reduction in viral thymidine kinase. The loss or reduction in viral thymidine kinase activity impairs acyclovir phosphorylation and renders the virus resistant to penciclovir and ganciclovir, agents that also require activation by viral thymidine kinase. Other, less common mechanisms of resistance include alterations in viral thymidine kinase substrate specificity (phosphorylates thymidine but not acyclovir) and mutations in viral DNA polymerase.

TOXICITY Acyclovir toxicity is generally minimal. Rarely, patients develop rash, hematuria, headache, and nausea. Neurotoxicity may occur in 1–4% of patients receiving intravenous acyclovir and can result in lethargy, obtundation, coma, hallucinations, seizures, and autonomic instability. Most patients who suffer these complications have renal dysfunction resulting in high acyclovir serum levels. Coadministration of zidovudine and acyclovir increases the risk of developing lethargy. Intravenous administration can also cause crystalluria and crystalline nephropathy, particularly if the patient is dehydrated. Cyclosporin increases the risk of nephrotoxicity. Although acyclovir has mutagenic activity in vitro, administration has not proven to be carcinogenic or teratogenic in animal studies.

ANTIVIRAL ACTIVITY AND TREATMENT RECOMMENDATIONS Acyclovir has excellent activity against herpes simplex types 1 and 2. Topical acyclovir has not proven to be as effective as oral or intravenous administration and is rarely used. Oral acyclovir is recommended for treatment of genital herpes and is used to prevent recurrent herpes genitalis. Acyclovir is also recommended for the treatment and prevention of recurrent ocular herpes simplex. Intravenous acyclovir has reduced the mortality of herpes simplex encephalitis and is the treatment of choice for this disorder. Acyclovir also has significant activity against varicella; however, higher drug concentrations are required to kill this virus. Intravenous acyclovir is recommended for the treatment of varicella and herpes zoster in the immunocompromised host and for treatment of varicella pneumonia or encephalitis in the previously healthy adult. Acyclovir demonstrates some activity against Epstein-Barr virus but is generally not recommended for therapy. This agent also demonstrates modest protection against cytomegalovirus when used for prophylaxis in allogeneic bone marrow and renal and liver transplant recipients; however, ganciclovir has proved to be more efficacious.

PHARMACOKINETICS The oral absorption of acyclovir is limited, only 15–20% of the drug being bioavailable. Absorption tends to be even poorer in transplant patients, necessitating higher oral dosing. A newer prodrug preparation, valacyclovir, is also available. It is rapidly and completely converted to acyclovir by hepatic and intestinal valacyclovir hydrolase. Oral valacyclovir achieves acyclovir serum levels that are 3–5 times higher than those for oral acyclovir. Acyclovir is widely distributed in tissues and fluids. Therapeutic levels can be achieved in cerebrospinal fluid, saliva, vaginal secretions, and the aqueous humor. Acyclovir is primarily excreted unchanged in the urine and has a mean half-life of 2.5–3 hours. Probenecid reduces renal clearance and increases the half-life.

Oral acyclovir:
Dose: 200–800 mg 3–5 × per day (See specific infections for dosing.)

Renal dosing: Cr Cl 10–50 cc/min, 800 mg Q8H maximal dose; Cr Cl < 10 cc/min, 200 mg Q12H; for varicella infection, 800 mg Q12H
Cost: Low to very high depending on dose
Oral valacyclovir:
Dose: 500–1000 mg BID to TID
Renal dosing: Cr Cl 10–50 cc/min, 500–1000 mg Q12–24H; Cr Cl < 10 cc/min, 500 mg QD
Cost: Moderate to high depending on dose (See Table 1.2.)
Intravenous acyclovir:
Dose: 5–10 mg/kg Q8H
Renal dosing: Cr Cl 10–50 cc/min, 5–12 mg/kg Q12–24H; Cr Cl < 10 cc/min, 2.5–6 mg/kg Q24
Cost: Very high

KEY POINTS
Acyclovir and Valacyclovir

1. Require viral thymidine kinase phosphorylation for activity.
2. Bind to the replicating viral DNA, causing premature chain termination; also inhibit viral DNA polymerase.
3. Resistance is most commonly mediated by a reduction in viral thymidine kinase.
4. Toxicity is minimal. Intravenous administration can cause lethargy, obtundation, hallucinations, and seizures.
5. Valacyclovir is rapidly converted to acyclovir, results in higher acyclovir levels compared to oral preparations of acyclovir.
6. Excellent activity against herpes simplex types 1 and 2. Oral preparations are recommended for the treatment and prophylaxis of genital herpes and ocular herpes. Intravenous acyclovir is recommended for herpes simplex encephalitis.
7. Moderate activity against varicella-zoster virus; intravenous acyclovir is recommended for the immunocompromised host and for varicella pneumonia or encephalitis in the normal host.

PENCICLOVIR AND FAMCICLOVIR

CHEMICAL STRUCTURE AND MECHANISMS OF ACTION
Famciclovir is the diacetyl ester of penciclovir, and this prodrug is quickly converted to penciclovir following oral absorption. Penciclovir is an acyclic guanosine analogue similar to acyclovir and has similar mechanisms of action. However, penciclovir is not a DNA chain terminator, acting primarily as a viral DNA polymerase inhibitor. Although it is a less potent inhibitor than acyclovir, the concentrations of penciclovir in virally infected cells are much higher and persist for a longer time than acyclovir, explaining penciclovir's potent antiviral effect. Penciclovir requires viral thymidine kinase for activity, and acyclovir-resistant strains, owing to deficient thymidine kinase, demonstrate cross-resistance to penciclovir.

TOXICITY   Oral famciclovir has side effects that are similar to those of oral acyclovir, including headache, nausea, and vomiting. Hallucinations and confusion can occur in the elderly. Neutropenia and elevated serum transaminase levels have also been reported.

ANTIVIRAL SPECTRUM AND TREATMENT RECOMMENDATION   Famciclovir has antiviral activity comparable to that of acyclovir. Like acyclovir, it has excellent activity against herpes simplex types 1 and 2, good activity against varicella-zoster virus, and limited activity against cytomegalovirus. This oral agent is comparable to oral acyclovir for the treatment and prophylaxis of genital herpes and for the treatment of herpes zoster in the normal and immunocompromised host. In addition, famciclovir has been shown to reduce hepatitis B viral DNA and serum transaminase values in patients with chronic hepatitis B. Its effects are additive when it is combined with interferon. Famciclovir has also been used to treat recurrent hepatitis B following liver transplantation. A topical 1% penciclovir cream is available and has been shown to shorten recurrent orolabial herpes simplex healing by 0.5–1 day in otherwise healthy patients.

PHARMACOKINETICS   Famciclovir is well absorbed orally. In the liver and intestine its purine is quickly deacetylated and oxidized to form penciclovir. Penciclovir demonstrates excellent tissue penetration. This agent is primarily excreted by the kidneys and has a half-life of 2–3 hours. Famciclovir has no significant drug interactions.

Dose: 250 mg Q12H po for herpes simplex and 500 mg Q8H po for varicella-zoster

Renal dosing: Cr Cl 10–50 cc/min, 125 mg Q24H for herpes simplex and 500 mg Q12–24H for varicella-zoster; Cr Cl < 10 cc/min, 125 mg Q48H for herpes simplex and 250 mg Q48H for varicella-zoster

Cost: Moderate to very high depending on dose (See Table 1.2.)

KEY POINTS

Famciclovir and Penciclovir

1. Famciclovir is a prodrug that is quickly converted to penciclovir.
2. Similar mechanism of action to acyclovir.
3. Requires viral thymidine kinase for activation, and acyclovir-resistant viral strains are also resistant to famciclovir.
4. Similar spectrum of activity and treatment indications to acyclovir.
5. Topical penciclovir shortens the course of herpes labialis by 0.5–1 day.
6. Famciclovir also used for the treatment of hepatitis B virus.

GANCICLOVIR

CHEMICAL STRUCTURE AND MECHANISMS OF ACTION
Ganciclovir, like acyclovir, is a guanine analogue. Ganciclovir has an additional hydroxymethyl group on the acyclic side chain. This analogue is converted to the monophosphate form by viral thymidine kinase followed by host cell kinase phosphorylation to produce the active triphosphate form. Ganciclovir triphosphate

competitively inhibits viral DNA polymerase incorporation of guanosine triphosphate into elongating DNA but does not act as a chain terminator. Intracellular concentrations of ganciclovir triphosphate are tenfold higher in infected cells compared to acyclovir triphosphate, and once in the cell, ganciclovir triphosphate persists, having an intracellular half-life of 16–24 hours. The resulting higher intracellular concentrations may account for its greater activity against cytomegalovirus. Ganciclovir is also active against herpes simplex, varicella-zoster, and Epstein-Barr virus. Because ganciclovir requires viral thymidine kinase activity for conversion to the active triphosphate form, acyclovir-resistant viral strains with decreased thymidine kinase activity are also less sensitive to ganciclovir. Mutations that alter the structure of the viral DNA polymerase also confer ganciclovir resistance, and these mutants often demonstrate reduced sensitivity to foscarnet and cidofovir.

TOXICITY Significant concentrations of ganciclovir triphosphate accumulate in uninfected cells. Bone marrow progenitor cells are particularly sensitive to this agent. The triphosphate form can incorporate into cellular DNA and block host cell DNA replication. Neutropenia and thrombocytopenia are commonly observed in AIDS patients receiving ganciclovir, and these patients require close monitoring of their white blood cell and platelet counts during therapy. The risk is lower but significant in transplant patients. Coadministration of zidovudine increases the risk of bone marrow suppression. Discontinuation of treatment is recommended if the absolute neutrophil count drops below 500 cells/mm^3. Central nervous system side effects are also common and include headache, confusion, psychosis, coma, and seizures. Other, less common adverse reactions include rash, fever, phlebitis, and abnormal liver function tests.

SPECTRUM OF ACTIVITY AND TREATMENT INDICATIONS Of the guanine analogues, ganciclovir has the highest activity against cytomegalovirus (CMV).

Ganciclovir is the treatment of choice for CMV infections, including retinitis, pneumonia, and colitis. Ganciclovir is also used for prophylaxis of CMV in transplant patients. Finally, in AIDS patients with persistently low CD4 lymphocyte counts, ganciclovir maintenance therapy is required to prevent relapse of CMV infection after the treatment of active infection has been completed.

PHARMACOKINETICS Oral absorption is poor (5–9% bioavailability); however, low therapeutic serum levels are achievable by this route. Absorption is improved by taking the medication with food. Intravenous administration is recommended for active CMV infection, oral administration being reserved for maintenance and prophylaxis. Ganciclovir readily penetrates all tissues and fluids, including the brain and cerebrospinal fluid. The drug is primarily excreted unmodified in the urine, having a half-life of 2–4 hours in individuals with normal renal function.

Dose:
Oral: 1000 mg TID
Renal dosing: Cr Cl 50–80 cc/min, 500 mg TID; Cr Cl 10–50 cc/min, 500 mg QD; Cr Cl < 10 cc/min, 3 × per week
Intravenous: Treatment, 5 mg/kg Q12H; maintenance, 5 mg/kg QD
Renal dosing: Cr Cl 50–80 cc/min: treatment, 2.5 mg/kg Q12H; maintenance, 2.5 mg/kg QD; Cr Cl 10–50 cc/min: treatment, 2.5 mg/kg QD; maintenance, 1.25 mg/kg QD, Cr Cl < 10 cc/min: treatment, 1.25 mg 3 × per week; maintenance, 0.6 mg/kg 3 × per week
Cost: Oral, very high; intravenous, moderate

KEY POINTS
Ganciclovir

1. A guanine analogue that primarily inhibits viral DNA polymerase.

2. Like acyclovir and penciclovir, requires viral thymidine kinase for activation. Acyclovir-resistant strains are often resistant to ganciclovir.

3. Bone marrow suppression is a common toxicity, particularly in AIDS patients. The drug should be discontinued if the neutrophil count drops to <500 cells/mm^3.

4. CNS complaints including confusion, psychosis, coma, and seizures may occur.

5. Most active guanine analogue against cytomegalovirus (CMV). Also active against herpes simplex types 1 and 2, varicella-zoster, and Epstein-Barr virus.

6. Recommended for CMV retinitis, pneumonia, and colitis. Useful for prophylaxis of immunocompromised transplant patients. Following treatment of active infection in AIDS patients with low CD4 counts, oral or intravenous ganciclovir given to prevent relapse.

CIDOFOVIR

CHEMICAL STRUCTURE AND MECHANISMS OF ACTION
Cidofovir is an analogue of deoxycytidine monophosphate that inhibits viral DNA synthesis. This agent does not require viral kinase for activity, being converted by cellular enzymes to its active diphosphate form. It acts as a competitive inhibitor of viral DNA polymerase and also adds to DNA, substituting for deoxycytidine triphosphate (dCTP) and causing premature chain termination. Viral thymidine kinase mutants do not impair cidofovir activity. Resistance is conferred through viral DNA polymerase mutations, and such mutations can result in cross-resistance to ganciclovir and less commonly to foscarnet.

TOXICITY   Cidofovir is highly nephrotoxic, causing proteinuria in half of patients as well as azotemia and metabolic acidosis in a significant number. Vigorous saline hydration and coadministration of probenecid reduce nephrotoxicity. The drug should be discontinued if proteinuria of 3+ or higher develops or if the serum creatinine increases by >0.4 mg/dl. Neutropenia is also commonly encountered.

Other side effects include nausea, vomiting, diarrhea, rash, anterior uveitis, and headache. This drug has activity against many DNA viruses: CMV, herpes simplex, herpesvirus 6 and 8, varicella-zoster, poxviruses including smallpox, papilloma viruses, polyoma viruses, BK virus and adenoviruses.

TREATMENT RECOMMENDATIONS   This agent is approved only for the treatment of CMV retinitis in AIDS patients. Given its highly toxic profile, parenteral use of this drug in other viral infections is likely to be limited. Topical therapy may prove efficacious in acyclovir-resistant HSV infections in AIDS patients, and it is being studied for the treatment of anogenital warts.

PHARMACOKINETICS   Cidofovir is cleared by the kidneys and has a half-life of 17–65 hours.

Dose: 5 mg/kg iv Q 2 weeks; contraindicated in patients with Cr Cl < 50 cc/min
Cost: Very high (See Table 1.2.)

KEY POINTS
Cidofovir

1. An analogue of deoxycidine monophosphate causes premature chain termination of viral DNA and inhibits viral DNA polymerase.

2. Does not require viral thymidine kinase for conversion to its active form. Acyclovir-resistant strains are usually not resistant to cidofovir.

3. Highly nephrotoxic, causing proteinuria, azotemia, and metabolic acidosis in nearly half of patients. Neutropenia is also common.

4. Broad spectrum of antiviral activity, including CMV, herpes simplex, herpesvirus 6 and 8, varicella-zoster virus, poxviruses, papilloma virus, polyoma viruses, BK virus and adenoviruses.

5. Approved for CMV retinitis in AIDs patients. Other indications are currently being explored. However, the usefulness of cidofovir is likely to be limited because of renal and bone marrow toxicity.

FOSCARNET

CHEMICAL STRUCTURE AND MECHANISM OF ACTION Foscarnet is an inorganic pyrophosphate analogue of trisodium phosphonoformate that reversibly blocks the pyrophosphate binding site of viral DNA polymerase. Foscarnet binding inhibits the polymerase from binding deoxynucleotide triphosphates. Mutations to the viral DNA polymerase are primarily responsible for viral resistance; however, resistance among clinical isolates is rare.

TOXICITY Nephrotoxicity is the most common serious side effect, resulting in azotemia, proteinuria, and rarely acute tubular necrosis. Renal dysfunction usually develops during the second week of therapy and in most cases reverses when the drug is discontinued. Dehydration increases the incidence of nephrotoxicity, and saline loading is of benefit in reducing this complication. Metabolic abnormalities are frequent. Hypocalcemia is most common and is the result of chelation by foscarnet. Reductions in ionized calcium can cause CNS disturbances, tetany, paresthesias, and seizures. Other metabolic abnormalities include hypophosphatemia, hypomagnesemia, and hypokalemia as well as hypercalcemia and hyperphosphatemia. To minimize these metabolic derangements, intravenous infusion should not exceed 1 mg/kg/min. Electrolytes, magnesium, phosphate, and calcium should be closely monitored. Other common side effects include fever, headache, nausea, vomiting, and abnormal liver function tests.

SPECTRUM OF ACTIVITY AND TREATMENT RECOMMENDATIONS Foscarnet is active against cytomegalovirus, herpes simplex, varicella-zoster virus, Epstein-Barr virus, and herpesvirus 8. This drug is approved for the treatment of cytomegalovirus retinitis and for acyclovir-resistant mucocutaneous herpes simplex.

PHARMACOKINETICS Foscarnet is poorly absorbed orally and is administered intravenously. This drug penetrates all tissues and fluids, achieving excellent levels in the cerebrospinal fluid and vitreous humor. Foscarnet is primarily excreted by the kidneys unmodified and has a half-life of 4–8 hours.

Dose: Treatment, 60 mg/kg Q8H iv; maintenance, 90–120 mg/kg QD

Renal dosing: Cr Cl 50–80 cc/min: treatment: 40–50 mg/kg Q8H; maintenance, 60–90 mg/kg QD; Cr Cl 10–50 cc/min: treatment: 20–30 mg/kg Q8H; maintenance, 50–80 mg/kg QD; Cr Cl < 10 cc/min: contraindicated for both treatment and maintenance

Cost: High for treatment, moderate for maintenance (See Table 1.2.)

KEY POINTS

Foscarnet

1. Blocks binding of deoxynucleotide triphosphates to viral DNA polymerase.
2. Nephrotoxicity is common, usually developing during the second week of therapy. Reduced by saline hydration. Usually reversible.
3. Also causes abnormalities in serum calcium, magnesium, and phosphate.
4. Active against CMV, herpes simplex, varicella-zoster virus, Epstein-Barr virus, and herpesvirus 8.
5. Approved for the treatment of CMV retinitis and acyclovir-resistant mucocutaneous herpes simplex.

RIBAVIRIN

CHEMICAL STRUCTURE AND MECHANISMS OF ACTION Ribavirin is a guanosine analogue that contains the D-ribose side chain. It inhibits both DNA and RNA viruses. The mechanisms of inhibition are complex and not completely understood. Ribavirin is phosphorylated to the triphosphate form by host cell enzymes, and the triphosphate form interferes with viral messenger RNA formation. The monophosphate form interferes with guanosine triphosphate synthesis, lowering nucleic acid pools in the cell.

TOXICITY   Systemic ribavirin results in dose-related red blood cell hemolysis and at high doses suppresses the bone marrow. The resulting anemia reverses when the drug is discontinued. Other side effects include rash, pruritus, nausea, cough, and depression. Intravenous administration is not approved in the United States but is available for patients with Lassa fever and some other forms of hemorrhagic fever. Aerosolized ribavirin is associated with conjunctivitis and with bronchospasm that can result in deterioration of pulmonary function. A major concern for health care workers who are exposed to aerosolized ribavirin is the teratogenic and embryotoxic effects that have been noted in some animal studies. Pregnant health care workers should not administer this drug.

SPECTRUM OF ACTIVITY AND TREATMENT RECOMMENDATIONS   Ribavirin is active against a broad spectrum of DNA and RNA viruses, including respiratory syncytial virus (RSV), influenza and parainfluenza virus, herpes, adenovirus, poxviruses, bunyavirus, and arenaviruses. It is approved in the United States for the aerosol treatment of RSV bronchiolitis and pneumonia in hospitalized patients. Oral ribavirin in combination with interferon is approved for the treatment of chronic hepatitis C.

PHARMACOKINETICS   Approximately one third of orally administered ribavirin is absorbed. The drug penetrates all tissues and body fluids. Ribavirin triphosphate becomes highly concentrated in erythrocytes (40 × plasma levels) and persists for prolonged periods in red blood cells.

The drug is cleared by both the kidneys and liver and has a prolonged half-life of 300 hours. Aerosolized ribavirin results in high levels in the respiratory secretions that have a half-life of up to 2.5 hours. A special aerosol generator is required for proper administration.

Dose: Oral, 1.0–1.2 gm QD
Renal dosing: Cr Cl < 10 cc/min, not recommended
Cost: Very high (See Table 1.2.)

KEY POINTS
Ribavirin

1. A guanosine analogue that interferes with viral messenger RNA formation and reduces guanosine triphosphate synthesis, lowering nucleic acid pools in the cell.
2. Systemic drug causes red blood cell hemolysis. Intravenous administration is not approved in the U.S. Aerosolized form causes conjunctivitis and bronchospasm.
3. Teratogenic and embryotoxic. Pregnant health care workers should not administer.
4. Active against DNA and RNA viruses, including respiratory syncytial virus (RSV), influenza and parainfluenza virus, herpesviruses, adenovirus, poxviruses, bunyavirus, and arenaviruses.
5. Approved for aerosolized treatment of RSV bronchiolitis and pneumonia.
6. Approved for oral administration in combination with interferon for chronic hepatitis C.

INTERFERONS

CHEMICAL STRUCTURE AND MECHANISMS OF ACTION
The interferons (IFNs) are 16–27,000 Da molecular weight proteins synthesized by eukaryotic cells in response to viral infections. These cytokines in turn stimulate host antiviral responses. Interferon receptors regulate approximately 100 genes and, in response to INF binding, cells rapidly produce dozens of pro-

teins. A wide variety of RNA viruses are susceptible to the antiviral actions of IFNs, while most DNA viruses are only minimally affected.

TOXICITY Side effects tend to be mild when doses of less than 5 million units are administered. Doses of 1–2 million units given subcutaneously or intramuscularly are associated with an influenzalike syndrome that is particularly severe during the first week of therapy. This febrile response can be reduced by premedication with antipyretics such as aspirin, ibuprofen, and acetaminophen. Local irritation at injection sites is also frequently reported. Higher doses of interferon result in bone marrow suppression, causing granulocytopenia and thrombocytopenia. Neurotoxicity resulting in confusion, somnolence, and behavior disturbances is also common when high doses are administered. Hepatoxicity and retinopathy are other common side effects with high-dose therapy.

SPECTRUM OF ACTIVITY AND TREATMENT RECOMMENDATIONS The effectiveness of INFs has been limited by the frequent side effects associated with therapeutic doses. Interferons are approved for the treatment of chronic hepatitis C, chronic hepatitis B, Kaposi's sarcoma, and other malignancies, as well as condyloma acuminatum.

PHARMACOKINETICS INF-α is well absorbed intramuscularly and subcutaneously; other interferons have more variable absorption. Essays for biologic effect demonstrate activity that persists for 4 days after a single dose. Pegylated forms result in slow release and result in more prolonged biologic activity, allowing once-per-week administration.

Dose:
IFN-α 2A or 2B: 3 million units 3 × per week (hepatitis C); 30–35 million units per week (hepatitis B); 30–36 million units 3–7 × per week (Kaposi's sarcoma); 1 million units in-

tralesional 3 × per week (condyloma acuminatum)
Peginterferon-α *2B*: Pegintron, 1.5 μg/kg SC Q 1 wk + ribovirin; Pegasys, 180 mg SC Q 1 wk + ribovirin (both for treatment of hepatitis C)
Cost: Very high (See Table 1.2.)

KEY POINTS
Interferon

1. Binding to host cell interferon receptors upregulates many genes responsible for the production of proteins with antiviral activity.
2. RNA viruses are more susceptible to the antiviral actions of IFNs.
3. The most common side effect is an influenzalike syndrome. At doses > 5 million units, bone marrow suppression and neurotoxicity may develop. Hepatotoxicity and retinopathy are commonly associated with high doses.
4. Approved for chronic hepatitis C, chronic hepatitis B, and Kaposi's sarcoma. Intralesional injection approved for condyloma acuminata.

Anti-Influenza Viral Agents

AMANTADINE AND RIMANTADINE

MECHANISM OF ACTION These agents are effective only against influenza A. Amantadine and rimantadine bind to and inhibit the M2 protein. This viral protein is expressed on the surface of infected cells and is thought to play an important role in viral particle assembly.

TOXICITY Amantadine causes moderate CNS side effects, especially in the elderly. Insomnia, inability to concentrate, and dizziness are most commonly reported. Amantadine also increases the risk of seizures in patients with a past history of epilepsy. Rimantadine causes CNS side effects less frequently.

TREATMENT RECOMMENDATIONS Treatment must be instituted within 48 hours of the onset of symptoms to be effective. Efficacy has been proven in healthy adults; however, trials have not been performed in high-risk patients.

Amantadine treatment:
Dose: 200 mg po QD × 3–5 days
Renal dosing: 100 mg QD in patients with renal impairment and in the elderly
Cost: Low

Rimantadine treatment:
Dose: 200 mg po QD × 3–5 days
Renal dosing: 100 mg QD in patients with renal impairment and in the elderly
Cost: Moderate

NEURAMINIDASE INHIBITORS

MECHANISMS OF ACTION These agents are sialic acid analogues that inhibit neuramidase activity and have activity against both influenza A and B.

TOXICITY Zanamivir is given by inhaler and commonly causes bronchospasm, limiting its usefulness.

TREATMENT RECOMMENDATIONS The neuraminidase inhibitors must also be given within 48 hours of the onset of symptoms to be effective.

Dose:
　Zanamivir = 10 mg QD intranasally for 5 days
　Oseltamivir = 75 mg po QD for 5 days (well absorbed orally)
Cost: Moderate for both preparations

Amantadine, rimantadine, or oseltamivir can be given for longer duration, as prophylaxis in patients at risk of serious complications from influenza during an epidemic. Influenza vaccine is preferred for prophylaxis.

Additional Reading

Antibiotic Handbooks
Bartlett, J.G. *Pocket Book of Infectious Disease Therapy*. Lippincott Williams and Wilkins, Philadelphia, 2001.
Gilbert, D.N., Moellering R.C., Jr., and Sande, M.A. *Sanford Guide to Antimicrobial Therapy*. Antimicrobial Therapy, Inc., Hyde Park, Vermont, 2001.

PDA Sources
EPocrates and ePocrates ID. Web address: www.epocrates.com
Johns Hopkins Division of Infectious Diseases Antibiotic Guide. Web address: www.hopkins-abxguide.org

Other
The choice of antibacterial drugs. *The Medical Letter*, 41:95–104, 1999.
Hardman, J.G., and Limbird, L.E. *Goodman & Gilman's The Pharmacological Basis of Therapeutics*. McGraw-Hill Medical Publishers, New York, 2001.
Mandell, G.L., Bennett, J.E., and Dolin, R. (Eds.) *Principles and Practice of Infectious Diseases*, 5th edition. Churchill Livingston, Philadelphia, 2000.

Reuben Ramphal, M.D.

The Sepsis Syndrome

Recommended Time to Complete: 1 day

Guiding Questions

1. How is the sepsis syndrome defined and what is SIRS?

2. Do all episodes of bacteremia cause the sepsis syndrome and are all sepsis syndromes due to bacteremia?

3. Which bacterial products can produce the sepsis syndrome?

4. What is a "superantigen" and which bacteria produce them?

5. What host cells are most important in the sepsis syndrome and how do they mediate sepsis?

6. What clinical clues suggest preshock and why is this syndrome important to recognize?

7. What therapeutic measures need to be instituted in patients with the sepsis syndrome?

Potential Severity: The sepsis syndrome is a life-threatening syndrome that must be recognized and treated quickly to prevent progression to irreversible shock.

Prevalence of the Sepsis Syndrome

Sepsis, or severe infection leading to organ dysfunction, is a problem of increasing magnitude in the United States. Estimates of the occurrence of this syndrome range from 300,000 to 500,000 cases per year. Mortality associated with this syndrome has been reported to be between 15% and

60%, governed by factors such as underlying diseases, age, infecting organism, and the appropriateness of empiric anti-infective therapy. Most cases of sepsis syndrome are due to bacterial infection, but it should be appreciated that this syndrome is seen in viral infections (e.g., dengue fever) and fungal infections (e.g., candidemia) and is due to noninfectious diseases such as pancreatitis. For purposes of this chapter sepsis is presumed to be due to bacterial agents and their products.

KEY POINTS
Prevalence and Definitions of the Sepsis Syndrome

1. Prevalence is 300,000–500,000 cases per year in the United States.
2. Mortality ranges from 15% to 60%.
3. The sepsis syndrome is the systemic inflammatory response syndrome (SIRS) caused by microbial products.
4. SIRS can also be caused by viruses (dengue fever), fungi (candida), and noninfectious diseases (pancreatitis, tissue ischemia, severe trauma).
5. Severe sepsis is defined as SIRS caused by microbial products that is associated with organ dysfunction.
6. Septic shock is shock associated with sepsis that is unresponsive to volume replacement.
7. Bacteremia does not always cause sepsis, and the sepsis syndrome is not always caused by bacteremia.

Definitions of Sepsis

Sepsis is best defined as the "systemic inflammatory response syndrome caused by microbial products." This definition acknowledges that a systemic inflammatory response syndrome (SIRS) may be produced by entities other than infec-

tion and that microbial products in the absence of viable organisms are capable of producing this clinical picture. Severe sepsis is defined as sepsis with organ dysfunction and represents progression of SIRS with more severe pathophysiologic disturbances. Septic shock is hypotension due to sepsis that has become unresponsive to initial attempts at volume expansion. The type of infection that is often colloquially called sepsis indicates the presence of an infectious agent and should not be considered synonymous with sepsis syndrome. Bacteremia is often called sepsis, and while some bacteremias result in the sepsis syndrome, not all sepsis syndromes are caused by bacteremia. In fact, in earlier clinical trials of biologic agents in the sepsis syndrome, using the best possible definitions and available laboratory studies, fewer than 40% of patients have had proven infection.

Pathogenesis of the Sepsis Syndrome

The systemic inflammatory response syndrome (SIRS) results from the activation of cellular pathways that lead to a triggering of innate immune responses and coagulation mechanisms. The pathways are linked to ancient defense mechanisms that respond to tissue injury or the presence of microbial products in order to defend the host. This innate immune response eventually leads to a classic adaptive immune response characterized by the production of antibodies, activated T cells, and memory of antigens. Much is now known about the microbial triggers of this system, the majority of information having been obtained with a portion of the Gram-negative cell wall, the lipopolysaccharide molecule (LPS), or endotoxin. However, it is clear that Gram-positive cell wall material, specifically peptidoglycans and lipotechoic acid, toxins that are produced by

Gram-positive bacteria, and fungal cell walls are also recognized by a family of molecules on the surfaces of target cells. This recognition leads to the synthesis of molecules that trigger both inflammation and coagulation pathways.

Cell Wall Factors

In Gram-negative bacteria the cytoplasmic bilayer is covered with a layer of peptidoglycan. Overlying this is an outer membrane, into which endotoxin is inserted. Endotoxin is the most carefully studied microbial substance implicated in sepsis syndrome and shock. There is compelling evidence that endotoxin plays a key role in the pathogenesis of Gram-negative sepsis. It has a common structural organization in all Gram-negative bacteria. From the outside going inward, it consists of an O side chain that is joined to a core that is connected to the "business end" of the molecule, the lipid A portion.

Lipid A is anchored into the outer membrane. It is believed that the triggering of the inflammatory and coagulation systems begins with the interaction of LPS with cellular receptors on macrophages and mononuclear leukocytes. The structure of lipid A is remarkably well conserved in most common Gram-negative bacteria, irrespective of the species from which it is obtained. Indeed, the clinical features of sepsis caused by *Escherichia coli* are similar to the features of that caused by Klebsiella or Enterobacter species. The infusion of LPS or lipid A into animals results in a sepsislike picture.

Endotoxin can be found in the blood of patients with Gram-negative sepsis. In some cases, such as meningococcemia, there is a good correlation between the plasma level of endotoxin and the outcome; even in more general types of Gram-negative infection the presence of endotoxemia correlates with more severe physiologic variables.

In addition to LPS, fungal cell walls, Gram-positive cell walls, and possibly bacterial flagellins are also capable of interacting with macrophages to trigger the sequence of events leading to sepsis and shock. Endotoxin is not present in Gram-positive bacteria. Instead, the cell wall contains a thick layer of peptidoglycan on its surface. In capsular strains the peptidoglycan lies directly beneath the capsule. Embedded in the peptidoglycan are molecules of lipoteichoic acid. Several in vitro studies have demonstrated that these structural components of Gram-positive cell walls are able to mimic some of the properties of endotoxin, such as their ability to induce proinflammatory cytokines from mononuclear cells.

Secreted Factors

In addition to factors that are integral parts of the cell wall, secreted factors from Gram-positive bacteria are believed to cause septic shock. The prototypical factor is toxic shock syndrome toxin-1 (TSST-1), produced by some strains of *Staphylococcus aureus*. This syndrome was first described in menstruation-associated staphylococcal infection of young women. Fever and profound shock were often followed by conjunctival and palmar hyperemia and desquamation. This condition proved to be associated with the production of an exotoxin, TSST-1. Another secreted factor responsible for shock due to Gram-positive bacteria was discovered in strains of *Streptococcus pyogenes* and called streptococcal pyrogenic exotoxin A (SPEA). Clinically, the action of this toxin has been identified in necrotizing fasciitis due to *Streptococcus pyogenes* associated with shock. It is hypothesized that infection leads to local or systemic release of toxins, massive lymphocyte activation, and release of cytokines, resulting in cellular injury and organ failure. This mechanism bypasses the macrophage, and the cytokine cascade is triggered at the level of T cells. This bypassing of the macrophage has given rise to the term "superantigen" to describe toxins that are able to activate lymphocytes directly as compared to conventional antigens that require processing by macrophages and dendritic cells.

Bacterial Products that Cause the Sepsis Syndrome

1. Gram-negative bacteria have lipopolysaccharide (LPS), also called endotoxin, linked to their outer membrane.
   a. This product alone can produce the syndrome.
   b. Endotoxin (LPS) is found in the bloodstream of patients with Gram-negative bacteremia.
   c. Endotoxin (LPS) blood levels correlate with the clinical severity of the sepsis syndrome.
2. Gram-positive bacteria produce peptidoglycans, and lipoteichoic acid can mimic endotoxins.
3. Gram-positive bacteria also secrete exotoxins.
   a. *Staphylococcus aureus* can secrete toxic shock syndrome toxin-1 (TSST-1).
   b. *Streptococcus pyogenes* secretes streptococcal pyrogenic exotoxin A (SPEA).
   c. Called "superantigens," bypass macrophages and directly stimulate T cells.

Host Cell Receptors for Bacterial Products

A detailed discussion of the physiologic host responses to bacteria is beyond the scope of this chapter. There is good evidence that in Gram-negative infections, it is the monocyte-macrophage that is the first cell to respond to endotoxin. Endotoxin first binds to LPS-binding protein, an acute-phase protein produced by the liver. The LPS-protein complex acts as the ligand for CD14 (a cell surface receptor on mononuclear cells) and to Toll-like receptors (TLR) on these cells. There are a number of TLRs that recognize different substances regardless of microbial origin; for example, TLR2 recognizes peptidoglycans, mannans, and lipoteichoic acids; TLR4 recognizes LPS; and TLR5 recognizes bacterial flagellin. TLR receptors and coreceptors bind the foreign stimulant and internalize it.

This results in signal transduction and cell activation, leading to cytokine release.

Cytokines and Other Inflammatory Mediator Cascades

The activation of monocytes leads to the production of the proinflammatory (i.e., stimulating inflammation) cytokines, particularly tumor necrosis factor-α (TNF) and IL-1. Infection also activates other host pathways, including the complement and coagulation pathways, and the production of reactive oxygen intermediates. Many studies have been conducted in animals in which cytokines have been measured in response to both purified bacterial components and, perhaps more informatively, live bacterial infection. Intravenous injection of live *E. coli* in mice, rabbits, or baboons results in a consistent picture in which proinflammatory cytokines, such as IL-1, IL-6, IL-8, and TNF-α, are released in a well-ordered sequence, followed by interferon-γ and then counterregulatory cytokines, such as IL-10. This picture is similar to that seen when endotoxin is injected into humans.

How Infection Leads to Septic Shock

A simple diagram of the pathways leading to septic shock is shown in Figure 2.1. It must be realized that these events represent a continuum, and they progress at speeds that have not been characterized. However, it is generally believed that the larger the inoculum of the challenge molecule, LPS, or Gram-positive toxins, the more likely the process is to progress rapidly. Additionally, there are likely to be differences in the intrinsic potencies of the various cell wall products to stimulate the innate immune system. For example, clinical observation suggests that endotoxin is a more powerful stimulant than the cell walls of enterococci or coagulase-negative staphylococci because of the remarkable tolerance humans have for bacteremia due to these organisms.

KEY POINTS
Host Cells' Roles in the Sepsis Syndrome

1. Monocyte-macrophages are the first cell to respond to endotoxin (LPS).
2. Endotoxin binds to LPS-protein in the serum, and this complex binds to CD14 receptors and Toll-like receptor 4 (TLR-4) on mononuclear cells.
3. TLR-2 binds peptidoglycans and lipoteichoic acids found in Gram-positive bacteria and mannans found on fungi, and TLR-5 binds bacterial flagellin.
4. Receptor binding stimulates monocyte-macrophages to release:
   a. Cytokines TNF and IL-1, stimulating inflammation (proinflammatory),
   b. Toxic oxygen by-products,
   c. Products that activate the complement and coagulation cascades.

Clinical Manifestations of the Sepsis Syndrome

◆ **CASE 2.1**

A 66-year-old Causasian female underwent elective thoracoabdominal aneurysm repair. Three days after surgery she became confused and developed a new fever. She had no cough, no dysuria, and no abdominal pain. A surgical drain was noted to be leaking increasing amounts of serous fluid. She was receiving vancomycin for operative prophylaxis.

Physical examination: Temperature 39°C, pulse 143, blood pressure 110/70, intubated on a respirator. She appeared toxic and somewhat lethargic. Skin: No lesions noted; respiratory, cardiac, and abdominal examination were unremarkable. Her extremities were warm to touch.

Laboratory findings: CXR revealed no infiltrates. Peripheral WBC dropped from 11.6 the day before to 1.4 (24% PMN, 37% bands, 9% metamyelocytes). Hct 30, Bun 41, S Creat 1.0, HCO_3 26. Blood cultures and culture of the surgical drain

Figure 2.1

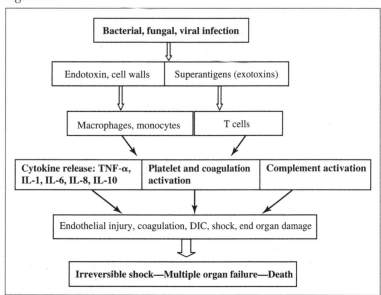

Pathophysiology of the sepsis syndrome.

subsequently grew *E. coli*. CT scan of the abdomen failed to reveal an abscess.

She was initially treated with intravenous cefepime and subsequently switched to ceftriaxone. Except for a brief bout of hypotension requiring intravenous saline and dopamine, she fully recovered and was subsequently discharged from the hospital.

Fever

As was noted in Case 2.1, fever is usually the first and most common manifestation of sepsis. In general the higher the temperature, the more likely a patient is to be bacteremic. However, it should be stressed that hypothermia and normal body temperature are seen in patients who are bacteremic. In fact, there is good reason to believe that hypothermia is a poor prognostic indicator in bacteremic patients, indicating an inability to mount an adequate inflammatory response.

Hemodynamic Changes

Tachycardia is a concomitant finding with fever and is to be expected. Case 2.1 had marked sinus tachycardia associated with her bacteremia. Bradycardia, on the other hand, is unusual and has been reported in patients with specific bacterial infections, such as typhoid fever and brucellosis. Of the easily measurable hemodynamic changes, hypotension is the most important one that determines outcome. Failure to reverse hypotension in its early stages results in serious end organ damage that might not be reversed by antibiotics or other therapy. The stage at which hypotension is reversible is called preshock. The preshock stage is often characterized by warm skin, diminished mentation (often worse in the elderly), and oliguria. Persistent hypotension leads to well-recognized findings in septic shock such as cool skin, acute renal failure, and, on occasion, hepatic injury.

Acid-Base Disturbances

Reduced tissue perfusion requires a change from aerobic to anaerobic metabolism and causes lac-

tic acid accumulation. Lactic acid and elevated cytokine levels stimulate the respiratory center, resulting in hyperventilation, and initially produce a respiratory alkalosis. This is the first pronounced and diagnostic change that is seen in impending shock and is usually seen at a time when the hemodynamic changes are reversible with fluid resuscitation. Therefore the recognition of this early stage is vital to any improvements in the management of a patient with the sepsis syndrome. Metabolic acidosis can develop just prior to hypotension or can accompany it and signals the beginning of a fatal downward spiral. Case 2.1 was recognized and treated before the development of acidosis, a fact that explains her rapid recovery.

Respiratory Changes

Tachypnea is a common feature of sepsis, generated by central nervous stimulation by cytokines, elevated body temperature, and the accumulation of lactic acid. In addition to hyperventilation, severe depression of oxygenation is often seen. The adult respiratory distress syndrome (ARDS) commonly develops in septic shock and can be experimentally induced by endotoxin. Endotoxin is thought to activate neutrophils that become trapped in the small vessels of the lung and cause vessel wall damage and leakage of fluid into the alveoli. ARDS is diagnosed by chest X-ray changes that mimic cardiac pulmonary edema and is accompanied by severe hypoxemia.

However, patients with sepsis may also demonstrate pneumonia on chest X-ray, and infection of lungs can be accompanied by bacteremia and the sepsis syndrome (see Chapter 4, "Pulmonary Infections").

KEY POINTS
Clinical Manifestations of the Sepsis Syndrome

> 1. Fever usually present:
>   a. The higher the fever, the more likely the patient is to be bacteremic.

b. Hypothermia or normal temperature in association with bacteremia is a bad prognostic sign.
2. Hemodynamic changes:
   a. Tachycardia in association with fever is the rule, pulse slower in typhoid fever and brucellosis.
   b. Hypotension is the most important determinant of outcome, failure to reverse early, warm preshock leads to irreversible organ damage and death.
3. Acid-base balance:
   a. Initially, respiratory alkalosis develops in response to anaerobic metabolism and lactic acid buildup. Critical to recognize this preshock syndrome.
   b. Failure to treat leads to metabolic acidosis and an increased likelihood of death.
4. Respiratory changes:
   a. Hyperventilation occurs early.
   b. Hypoxia and adult respiratory distress syndrome are common. Chest X-ray reveals pulmonary edema.

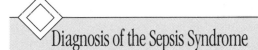

Diagnosis of the Sepsis Syndrome

The diagnosis of the sepsis syndrome is perhaps the greatest challenge encountered in designing clinical trials for new therapeutic agents. If fever, tachycardia, and tachypnea with or without leukocytosis are used to define SIRS, this definition includes other causes in addition to infection. Therefore evidence of actual infection must be sought. The most prevalent sites of infection are the lungs, bloodstream, abdomen, and wounds. Even with a positive bacterial culture from any of these sites, one is still unsure whether patients fitting the broad definitions of SIRS have sepsis. In fact, most patients with pneumonia would fit this definition of the sepsis syndrome, although they often do not require intensive care.

The strictest criteria should include the presence of a positive blood culture, preferably two, and should exclude most cases of coagulase negative staphylococci that are common skin contaminants. Exceptions to a positive blood culture would have to be made in patients in whom there is clear clinical evidence of an intra-abdominal infection such as peritonitis. Adjunctive information should also include the presence of hypotension that is not due to hypovolemia or a recent cardiac event.

Critical diagnostic tools that are not currently available include a means to rapidly diagnose the presence of bacteria in the blood and a method to rapidly quantify the inflammatory response (infection produces more inflammation than noninfectious causes). These tests would enable the physician to decide whether or not to initiate antibiotics as well as activated protein C (see below). In addition, a method for detecting early organ damage would be helpful for determining the severity of SIRS. Currently, one must rely on clinical assessment of severity of the illness and supportive bacteriologic studies that usually do not become available for 24–48 hours.

The presence of other abnormalities such as thrombocytopenia, evidence of fibrinogen consumption, and clot lysis are helpful and, when accompanied by hypotension, increased cardiac output, and changes in peripheral vascular resistance, may serve to define infection as the cause of SIRS. However, these findings are more likely to be seen in the more severe cases, in which the diagnosis of infection is already clinically apparent. Case 2.1 had a marked drop in her peripheral WBC with a marked shift to the left, with a high percentage of immature granulocyte forms indicating marked consumption of granulocytes. This finding served as a useful warning that sepsis had developed and precipitated the administration of broad-spectrum antibiotic coverage.

Common clinical and laboratory findings that are indicative of sepsis include the following:

1. Temperature < 36°C or > 38°C
2. Pulse rate > 90/min
3. Respiratory rate > 20/min

4. $PaCO_2 < 32$ with $pH > 7.45$ (early sepsis)
5. WBC $< 4,000/mm^3$ or $> 12,000/mm^3$ with a band count $> 10\%$
6. Chills, lethargy, hemorrhagic skin lesions

Laboratory studies that are recommended in patients with suspected sepsis syndrome include the following:

1. Two blood cultures, urine culture and sputum culture, if a patient has chest X-ray abnormalities
2. Complete blood count with differential and platelet count
3. Coagulation studies to include INR, fibrinogen, and D-dimers or fibrin split products
4. Blood gases and metabolic panels

KEY POINTS
Diagnosis of the Sepsis Syndrome

1. Early diagnosis is difficult and is based on clinical findings.
2. Fever, tachycardia, and hypotension need to be accompanied by documented bacteremia.
3. Tests to quickly demonstrate bacteremia, to accurately assess the extent of inflammation, and to assess organ ischemia are not currently available.
4. Thrombocytopenia and evidence of fibrinogen consumption and clot lysis, combined with hypotension, increased cardiac output, and reduced peripheral vascular resistance, suggest the diagnosis.

Treatment of the Sepsis Syndrome

Antibiotic Therapy of Patients with Sepsis

The outcome for patients with sepsis, in particular those with bacteremia, is governed by both host and microbial factors. In some studies, certain organisms have been suggested to carry a higher mortality rate. These include *Pseudomonas aeruginosa*, Candida species, and polymicrobial bacteremia. Therefore if the clinical situation is epidemiologically consistent with the isolation of these pathogens, consideration must be given to covering these possibilities empirically. The other microbial factor of significance is the susceptibility of the pathogen to empiric therapy. Patients with Gram-negative bacteremia that is treated empirically with antibiotics to which their organism is resistant have significantly higher mortality rates. Therefore empiric therapy should be embarked on with a knowledge of local susceptibility patterns, and in situations in which a bacterium was previously isolated from a suspicious site, empiric therapy should cover its susceptibility pattern. Aside from these considerations there may be other factors that may help in choosing empiric therapy for sepsis. In patients presenting with sepsis and a petechial skin rash, consideration must be given to meningococcemia, gonococcemia, *Staphylococcus aureus* bacteremia, localized *Staphylococcus aureus* infection, streptococcal bacteremia, or localized *Streptococcus pyogenes* infection. The preferred approach is to direct therapy to the most probable site of origin of the infection and cover the most likely pathogens from that site (see Table 2.1). It must be recognized that coverage for every possible pathogen is not possible and that certain pathogens in certain locations are unlikely to be responsible for life-threatening sepsis. Such organisms include enterococci at most sites and *Staphylococcus aureus* in the respiratory tract. These recommendations are made with the assumption that 90% of the organisms are sensitive to the drugs chosen, except for hospital-acquired pathogens. Certain hospitals may have specific resistance problems with any given pathogen. In these cases empiric therapy must be adjusted to reflect antibiotic sensitivities of the local bacterial flora. The regimens suggested in Table 2.1 will cover most other pathogens that are isolated at these sites in significant numbers. In 24–48 hours after blood culture results become available, the antibiotic regimen needs to be adjusted, and narrower-spectrum antibiotics should be utilized whenever possible to reduce the likelihood of selecting for highly resistant pathogens.

Management of Patients with Signs of Severe Sepsis

Management of patients with sepsis syndrome requires the prompt administration of antibiotics and volume expansion, initially with normal saline. If there is a drainable site of infection in the abdomen or pelvis or if these are the possible sources of infection, immediate surgical consultation must be sought (see Chapter 8, "Gastrointestinal and Hepatobiliary Infections"). Similarly, the presence of gas in soft tissues or

clinical evidence of a necrotizing infection mandates surgical consultation and possibly intervention (see Chapter 10, "Skin and Soft Tissue Infections"). Any intravascular catheter that is in place must be removed and cultured (see Chapter 7, "Cardiovascular Infections"). The following measurements are suggested in patients who are initially stable and kept on a conventional ward:

1. Hourly measurements of vital signs and urine output
2. Two-hourly measurements of arterial blood pH, $PaCO_2$, and PaO_2
3. Blood lactate and coagulation parameters initially and perhaps every 4–6 hours until there is a clear sense of how the patient is progressing

Failure of the patient to respond to fluids and antibiotics as indicated by a persistent fall in

Table 2.1

Empiric Antibiotic Therapy for the Sepsis Syndrome

SITE OF INFECTION	PATHOGENS TO BE COVERED	ANTIBIOTICS
Lung (hospital acquired)	*Pseudomonas aeruginosa*	Cefepime or ticarcillin/clavulanate
	Enterobacter	Piperacillin/tazobactam + aminoglycoside
Abdomen	Gram negative rods	Ticarcillin/clavulanate or piperacillin/
Pelvis	Anaerobes	tazobactam + aminoglycoside
		Imipenem or meropenem
Urinary tract	*E. coli*	Ciprofloxacin
	Klebsiella	Ceftriaxone
	Proteus	
Skin	*Staphylococcus aureus*	Oxacillin or vancomycin
	Streptococcus pyogenes	Ticarcillin/clavulanate
	Mixed aerobic/ anaerobic	Piperacillin/tazobactam
	Necrotizing fasciitis	Imipenem or meropenem
Bacteremia of unknown source (hospital acquired)	*Staphylococcus aureus* (MRSA)	Cefepime + vancomycin
	Gram-negative rods	
Bacteremia of unknown source (community acquired)	*Staphylococcus aureus*	Vancomycin + ceftriaxone or
	Streptococcus pneumoniae	cefepime
	E. coli	
	Klebsiella	
	Proteus	

blood pressure, the accumulation of lactate, increasing hypoxemia, and laboratory signs suggesting a coagulopathy dictates that the patient be moved to an intensive-care unit for closer monitoring and more aggressive hemodynamic support. There are no proven superior therapies at this time. Judicial use of vasopressors is generally recommended, beginning with dopamine and progressing to norepinephrine. Aggressive fluid resuscitation is continued with specific attention to central venous pressures and pulmonary vascular congestion. Further management needs to be deferred to the intensive-care specialists.

KEY POINTS

Treatment of the Sepsis Syndrome

1. Empiric antibiotic therapy must take into account:
   a. The presumed primary anatomic site of infection leading to bacteremia,
   b. Local hospital antibiotic sensitivities,
   c. Sensitivities for bacteria previously grown from possible sites of bacteremia.
   d. Empiric therapy must be readjusted on the basis of blood culture results.
2. Volume expansion with normal saline must be initiated emergently.
3. Surgical consultation is required for possible intra-abdominal sepsis and for cases of potential necrotizing fasciitis.
4. Potentially infected intravascular catheters must be removed.
5. Patients on conventional wards need:
   a. Q1H vital signs,
   b. Q2H arterial blood gases,
   c. Q4-6H serum lactate measurements.
   d. Deterioration of these parameters warrants transfer to an ICU.

Adjunctive Therapies

A large number of different substances have been used to reverse the persistent hypotension and associated end organ damage of the sepsis syndrome. Most of these adjunctive measures have failed to improve mortality in large studies. Given our current knowledge of the pathogenesis of sepsis, one is likely to see additional trials in the future. Some of potential therapies that to date have not proved beneficial are the following:

1. Anti-inflammatory agents such as corticosteroids and ibuprofen and even narcotic antagonists have not proved to be of value in large-scale studies.
2. Monoclonal antibody against the core of the endotoxin molecule has not been conclusively shown to be beneficial.
3. Antibody against TNF and the TNF receptor have failed.
4. Studies utilizing IL-1 receptor antagonists have been inconclusive.
5. Platelet-activating factor antagonists have failed.

Drotrecogin Alpha

Investigations of sepsis have shown that protein C levels are low and that septic patients are unable to activate this substance. Protein C plays a key role in inhibiting coagulation and may be an important inhibitor of monocyte activation. Animal studies have shown that the infusion of activated protein C reduces the mortality in lethal *E. coli* infections. Clinical trials in humans have subsequently shown that there is a modest reduction of mortality in septic shock when patients are treated with activated protein C. This agent, now called Drotrecogin alpha, has been approved by the FDA for the treatment of severe sepsis as an adjunct to standard therapy. Drotrecogin alpha reduced mortality from 30.8% in placebo-treated patients to 24.7% over 28 days, a statistically significant reduction. Because of the complexity of patient inclusion criteria, very high costs, and potential for bleeding complications, this agent is reserved for use by intensive-care and infectious disease specialists.

The major contraindication for this agent is recent surgery, the risk of bleeding complications being prohibitively high in this patient population.

KEY POINTS
Adjunctive Therapies for the Sepsis Syndrome

1. Multiple clinical trials have failed to document efficacy for:
   a. Anti-inflammatory agents,
   b. Monoclonal antibody against endotoxin,
   c. Anti-TNF antibodies,
   d. IL-1 antagonists,
   e. Platelet-activating factor antagonists.
2. Activated protein C (Drotrecogin alpha) is of limited efficacy (6% reduction in mortality):
   a. Extremely expensive,
   b. Should only be given by intensive care or infectious disease specialists,
   c. Contraindicated in postoperative patients because of bleeding complications.

Conclusions

First, the physician needs to make an immediate decision about the severity of the illness, and with clinical experience most physicians become skilled at recognizing the sickest patients. Among the severely ill, patients with sepsis syndrome have the highest mortality and morbidity. Early recognition and efforts to remove the precipitating cause of sepsis, aggressive fluid and vasopressor therapy, optimal supportive care for organ dysfunction, and empiric antimicrobial therapy for the most likely microbial pathogens remain the standard of care for sepsis. It is important that the physician reassess empiric an-tibiotic coverage in 48 hours when culture results have returned. The organisms grown on blood culture can help to identify the site of primary infection and also often allow the physician to narrow the spectrum of antibiotic coverage, reducing the likelihood of colonization with highly resistant bacterial flora (see Chapter 1, "Anti-Infective Therapy"). Activated protein C is of modest benefit, but not all patients are candidates for this agent. However, it is likely that more effective agents of this type will be developed in the future as we learn more about the mechanisms involved in the progression of sepsis.

Additional Reading

Balk, R.A. Sepsis and septic shock: Definitions, epidemiology and clinical manifestations. *Critical Care Clinics*, 16:179–192, 2000.

Bernard, G.R., Vincent, J.L., Laterre, P.F., LaRosa, S.P., Dhainaut, J.F., Lopez-Rodriguez, A., Steingrub, J.S., Garber, G.E., Helterbrand, J.D., Ely, E.W., and Fisher, C.J., Jr. Efficacy and safety of recombinant human activated protein C for severe sepsis. *New England Journal of Medicine*, 344:699–709, 2001.

Kreger, B.E., Craven, D.E., and McCabe, W.R. Gram-negative bacteremia IV: Reevaluation of clinical features and treatment in 612 patients. *American Journal of Medicine*, 68:344–355, 1980.

Pittet, D., Li, N., Woolson, R.F., and Wentzel, R.P. Microbiological factors influencing the outcome of nosocomial bloodstream infections: A 6 year validated, population based model. *Clinical Infectious Diseases*, 24:1068–1078, 1997.

Wheeler, A.P., and Bernard, G.R. Treating sepsis. *New England Journal of Medicine*, 340:207–214, 1999.

Young, L.S. Sepsis syndrome. Chapter 63 in Mandell, G.L., Bennett, J.E., and Dolin, R. (Eds.), *Principles and Practice of Infectious Diseases*, 5th edition. Churchill Livingstone, Philadelphia, 2000.

The Febrile Patient

Chapter 3

Recommended Time to Complete: 1 day

Guiding Questions

1. What region of the brain is primarily responsible for temperature regulation?
2. Does core temperature vary at different times of the day?
3. Is fever beneficial?
4. How and when should fever be treated?
5. How do aspirin and acetaminophen act to reduce fever?

Temperature Regulation and Fever

Temperature Regulation

Body temperature is regulated by the anterior hypothalamus in combination with many other neural structures, including the brain stem, spinal cord, and sympathetic ganglia. The region of the hypothalamus near the optic chiasm is thought to be primarily responsible for maintaining the body's core temperature. A distinct temperature set point is established, and when the body's core temperature drops below this set point, the nervous system increases body metabolism and stimulates shivering and chills. When the core temperature exceeds this set point, the nervous system increases peripheral blood flow and sweating. The "normal" body temperature averages 98.6°F or 37°C but varies from individual to individual, following a normal distribution. Therefore some individuals have a lower set point while others have a higher set point than the mean "normal" temperature. Furthermore, in each person the core temperature varies during the day, being lower in the morning and increasing in the evening. Before the physician decides that a patient has a fever, it is critical that he/she be familiar with the individual patient's normal set point and diurnal variation in core temperature.

Mechanisms Underlying the Febrile Response

Fever is a consequence of the anterior hypothalamus responding to inflammatory mediators. Among the mediators that are thought to stimulate a rise in the normal core temperature set point are interleukin-1 (IL-1), tumor necrosis factor alpha (TNF-α), interleukin-6 (IL-6), and interferon-gamma (IFN-γ). These cytokines are released primarily by monocytes and macrophages in response to the invasion by various pathogens as well as by other inflammatory stimuli (see Chapter 2). Investigators speculate that these cytokines stimulate the circumventricular organs near the optic chiasm activating phospholipase A_2, which in turn stimulates the cyclooxygenase pathway to produce increased levels of prostaglandin E_2. This small molecule crosses the blood-brain barrier and stimulates the neurons within the anterior hypothalamus and brain stem responsible for thermal regulation.

Benefits and Harmful Effects of Fever

In addition to serving as a warning sign for the onset of infection, fever is thought to be beneficial. The growth of some viruses, bacteria, fungi, and parasites is inhibited by a rise in temperature above 37°C. Fever has also been shown to enhance the ability of macrophages and neutrophils to kill foreign pathogens and to improve cell-mediated immune function. Depending on the individual patient, fever may also have harmful effects. Patients with heart disease may suffer cardiac ischemia due to the increase in heart rate and oxygen demands associated with fever. Similarly, patients with severe pulmonary disease may be unable to compensate for the increased oxygen demands associated with fever. Elderly patients with limited mental capacity may develop confusion and lethargy in response to fever, complicating their care. Finally, children can suffer from seizures in association with high fever. However, to date there is no proof that reducing fever prevents febrile seizures.

KEY POINTS

Fever

1. Body temperature is regulated by the hypothalamus, and prostaglandin E_2 acts on this region to stimulate fever.
2. Fever most commonly occurs in the evening as a consequence of the diurnal variation of body temperature.
3. Fever may be protective and should be reduced only in patients with ischemic heart disease, patients with pulmonary disease, the elderly, and children who have a history of febrile seizures.
4. Aspirin, NSAIDs, and acetaminophen, agents that reduce prostaglandin E_2 production, are the preferred method for reducing fever and need to be given on a regular schedule.

Treatment of Fever

The primary treatment for fever is to treat the underlying cause. The role of lowering body temperature while trying to determine the primary cause of fever remains controversial. On the basis of our present understanding of thermal regulation, direct cooling of the body using ice, cold water, or a cooling blanket should be considered only in conjunction with medicines that reset the thermal set point. Otherwise, the central nervous system will respond to such measures by inducing chills and shivering, increasing the patient's discomfort.

Use of antipyretics is probably warranted in patients with heart disease or pulmonary disease and in elderly patients with mental dysfunction in association with fever. The pharmacologic agents that are used to reset the thermal set point all inhibit prostaglandin synthetase activity and reduce prostaglandin E_2 production. Aspirin, nonsteroidal anti-inflammatory drugs (NSAIDs), and acetaminophen are all effective. Aspirin should probably be avoided in children because of the increased risk of Reye's syndrome (a deadly syndrome consisting of fatal hepatic and renal failure), and acetaminophen should be avoided in patients with serious underlying liver disease. NSAIDs have been associated with coronary artery vasoconstriction and therefore probably should not be used in patients with ischemic heart disease. To avoid repeated shifting of the thermal set point and recurrent shivering and chills, these antipyretic agents must be administered on a regular basis until the primary cause of fever has been treated.

Fever of Undetermined Origin (FUO)

Guiding Questions

1. What are the criteria used to define fever of undetermined origin (FUO)?

2. What diseases are most commonly associated with FUO?

3. What diseases are most commonly associated with FUO in the elderly?

4. What basic diagnostic tests should be ordered in cases of FUO?

5. What is Sutton's law and how is this law applied to FUO?

6. Should empiric antibiotics be started in cases of FUO?

7. What is the prognosis in patients with FUO?

Potential Severity: A chronic disorder that requires a thoughtful diagnostic approach.

Definition of FUO

In many cases, at the time the patient first visits the physician with complaints of fever the cause is not apparent. Some physicians label such individuals as having fever of undetermined origin (FUO). However, the term "fever of undetermined origin" carries with it specific criteria and should not be loosely applied. As first defined in 1961, FUO requires that the patient have (1) an illness that has lasted at least three weeks, (2) fever of over 101°F or 38.3°C on several occasions, and (3) no diagnosis after routine workup for 3 days in hospital or after three or more outpatient visits. A duration of three weeks or longer was chosen to eliminate self-limited viral illnesses, which are generally difficult to diagnose and resolve within this time period. A temperature greater than 38°C was chosen to eliminate those individuals at the far right of the normal temperature distribution curve who normally may have a slightly higher core temperature set point and an exaggerated diurnal temperature variation. Because the majority of patients with FUO in the present era of managed care are now diagnosed and managed as outpatients, the third criterion has been modified to include outpatient in addition to in hospital diagnostic testing.

KEY POINTS
Definition of FUO

1. Fever must persist for ≥ 3 weeks in order to exclude self-limited viral illnesses.
2. Temperature must be > 101° F or 38.3°C to exclude normal variations in core body set point.
3. No diagnosis after 3 days of testing

Before launching a complex and expensive series of diagnostic tests, the physician must carefully document that the patient fulfills the criteria for FUO. Most important is the documentation of true fever. The patient should be instructed to measure both 6:00 A.M. and 6:00 P.M. temperatures to rule out an exaggerated circadian rhythm. Second, an electronic thermometer should always be used to exclude the possibility of factitious fever (see below). The exact pattern of fever generally is not helpful in identifying the etiology of fever. Exceptions to this rule are the following:

1. **Cyclic neutropenia**. This is a disease of bone marrow stem cells that results in neutropenia in 21-day cycles. The nadir in neutrophils is often associated with fever. In such patients weekly peripheral white blood cell counts with differential will identify this unusual disorder.
2. **Malaria**. Periodic fever primarily occurs in patients with *Plasmodium vivax*, *P. ovale*, and *P. malaria*. Plasmodium generally take one to two weeks to synchronize the lysis of red blood cells by the trophozoites. When synchronized, red blood cell lysis occurs at 2- to 3-day intervals and is associated with high fever, sweats, chills, and malaise.
3. **Hodgkin's disease**. In Stage B Hodgkin's disease abnormal T cells intermittently release pyrogens, causing fever at irregular intervals, followed by periods of normal body temperature. This pattern has been called Pel-Ebstein fever.

Causes of FUO

Many diseases can initially present with the primary manifestation of prolonged fever (see Table 3.1). Etiologies can be classified into three major categories ("the big three"): infections, neoplasms, and autoimmune disorders. There are numerous miscellaneous etiologies; among the most common are six diseases ("the little six"): granulomatous diseases, regional enteritis, familial Mediterranean fever, drug fever, pulmonary emboli, and factitious fever.

Table 3.1

Major Causes of FUO

Big 3:
1. Infection
2. Neoplasm
3. Autoimmune diseases

Little 6:
1. Granulomatous diseases
2. Regional enteritis
3. Familial Mediterranean fever
4. Drug fever
5. Pulmonary emboli
6. Factitious fever

◆ CASE 3.1

A 19-year-old white male, university sophomore, presented with a three-week history of fevers to 104°F, fatigue, and anorexia. He was evaluated in the school infirmary and given intravenous fluids for dehydration. He was empirically treated with penicillin and clarithromycin. Despite this treatment his fevers persisted.

Epidemiology: No recent travel.

Review of systems: Negative other than 1–2 loose bowel movements per day for the week prior to admission.

Physical examination: Temperature 39.2°C, pulse 88, respirations 20, blood pressure 122/60. Mildly ill appearing. His physical exam was completely normal, including absence of palpable lymph nodes, no skin rashes, no cardiac murmurs, a benign abdominal exam without organomegaly, and normal joint and extremity exam.

Laboratory findings: WBC 11.6K (93% PMN), Hct 35, Plts 228K, BUN 6, Alb 3.0, total protein 6.2, alkaline phosphatase 327, ALT 107, ESR 105, blood cultures negative × 2, CXR within normal limits.

Because of his persistent fever and anorexia an abdominal CT scan was performed that demonstrated a 9-cm-diameter hepatic abscess in the right lower lobe of the liver. Echinoccocal serum titer was negative. Cutaneous aspiration demonstrated thick pus, and culture grew methicillin-sensitive *Staphylococcus aureus*.

Comment: Other than a mildly elevated alkaline phosphatase there were no clinical clues indicative of liver abscess. On further review of his past medical history he reported having intermittent furunculosis. It is likely that his skin was the initial portal of entry, resulting in transient bacteremia and seeding of the liver.

In patients under the age of 65 infection remains the most common cause of FUO (see Table 3.2). Common infectious causes of FUO include abscesses, particularly abdominal abscesses that may persist for prolonged periods before being diagnosed. Improvements in imaging techniques (see below) have enhanced our ability to locate and drain occult pyogenic collections. Osteomyelitis, particularly of the vertebral bodies, mandible, and air sinuses, can also present as FUO. A bone scan is particularly helpful in identifying such infections.

In earlier series subacute bacterial endocarditis (SBE) was a major cause of FUO. However, improved culture techniques, including prolonged incubation of blood cultures to identify more fastidious slow-growing pathogens such as the HASEK organisms (see Chapter 7, "Cardiovascular Infections"), and drawing large volumes of blood for culture have improved the sensitivity of blood cultures and reduced the number of undiagnosed cases of SBE. Transesophageal echocardiography has also improved our ability to identify vegetations. As a result of these advances, in more recent reports SBE has become a less common cause of FUO. Patients with SBE in almost every case have an audible murmur, emphasizing the importance of careful physical exam during the initial evaluation of the FUO patient.

Finally, the physician must keep in mind that if the patient has received antibiotics, the utility of blood cultures is markedly reduced. Administration of antibiotics prior to obtaining blood cultures temporarily sterilizes the bloodstream. Antibiotics must be discontinued for 7–10 days before blood cultures become positive. Biliary

system infections also can present as FUO. Such patients often have no right upper quadrant pain and no right upper quadrant tenderness. Subacute pyelonephritis can also present with a prolonged fever in the absence of dysuria, frequency, or flank pain.

In cases of FUO miliary tuberculosis must always be considered. This potentially lethal disease is most common in the elderly and immunocompromised patients, particularly HIV patients and patients on high-dose glucocorticoids. Bone marrow culture is particularly helpful in making this diagnosis. A chest X-ray may demonstrate micronodular (millet seed) interstitial changes; however, this radiologic finding may be absent in the elderly. If appropriate antituberculous therapy is not initiated promptly, these patients usually deteriorate over two to

Table 3.2

Infections Causing FUO

1. Abscesses
2. Osteomyelitis (vertebral, mandible, sinuses)
3. Subacute bacterial endocarditis (murmur usually present, beware of previous antibiotics)
4. Biliary system infections (may have no RUQ tenderness)
5. Urinary tract infections (absence of UTI symptoms)
6. Tuberculosis (especially miliary disease)
7. Spirochetal infection (leptospirosis, borrelia)
8. Brucellosis (animal exposure, unpasteurized cheese)
9. Rickettsial infection
10. Chlamydia
11. Epstein-Barr virus, cytomegalovirus
12. Fungal infection (cryptococcus, histoplasmosis)
13. Parasites (malaria, toxoplasmosis, trypanosomiasis)

three weeks and die (see Chapter 4, "Pulmonary Infections") Leptospirosis can cause persistent fever and is difficult to diagnose. A combination of appropriate epidemiology (animal exposure, contaminated soil or water exposure), conjuctival suffusion, aseptic meningitis, liver enzyme abnormalities, and renal dysfunction should alert the clinician to this possibility. Other spirochetal diseases that are reported to cause persistent fever include Lyme disease and relapsing fever. Animal exposure, particularly the skinning of wild boar, should raise the possibility of brucellosis. This disease can also be contracted by eating unpasteurized cheese (see Chapter 13, "Zoonotic Infections").

Rickettsial infections can also cause FUO. Epidemiology plays a critical role in alerting the clinician to this group of pathogens. A history of camping, hunting, or other outdoor activities in areas where these infections are endemic should raise the possibility of rickettsial infection. Rickettsia species are tick borne; however, a history of tick bite is not always obtained (see Chapter 13). Chlamydia is another intracellular pathogen that on occasion can cause prolonged fever. *Chlamydia psittaci* in particular can result in a syndrome that resembles mononucleosis. This organism is usually contracted from birds, including pigeons, members of the parrot family (parakeets, macaws, and cockatoos), finches (canaries, goldfinches), and poultry. Epstein-Barr virus and cytomegalovirus can both cause a mononucleosis-like syndrome resulting in sore throat, lymphadenopathy, splenomegaly, and prolonged fever (see Chapter 15, "Serious Adult Viral Illnesses other than HIV"). In addition to bacteria and viruses, fungi can occasionally result in FUO, cryptococcosis and histoplasmosis being the two most common fungal diseases reported (see Chapter 4). Finally, parasites can cause prolonged fever. Malaria (nonfalciparum forms), toxoplasmosis, and trypanosomiasis are the most commonly reported parasitic diseases associated with FUO (see Chapter 12, "Parasitic Infections").

KEY POINTS

Infectious Causes of FUO

1. The most common cause of FUO in patients < 65 years of age.
2. Epidemiology (animal exposure, insect bites, outdoor camping, travel, exposure to infected humans) is helpful.
3. Physical exam may provide useful clues, particularly skin, nail beds, fundi, and cardiac auscultation.
4. Abdominal abscess, miliary tuberculosis, and disseminated fungal infections can be fatal.
5. Prior antibiotic administration interferes with diagnosis.

Neoplastic disorders represent the second major category of diseases associated with FUO (see Table 3.3). In elderly patients neoplasia is the most frequent cause of FUO, and in this category lymphomas are the most commonly reported cause of fever. Hodgkin's lymphomas intermittently produce pyrogens. One week the patient may be afebrile, followed by a week of hectic fevers. This fever pattern has been termed a Pel-Ebstein fever and, when present, raises the possibility of Hodgkin's lymphoma. Patients with non-Hodgkin's lymphoma may also present with fever. In some cases fever can be high and

Table 3.3

Neoplastic Causes of FUO

1. Lymphoma (especially Hodgkin's, Pel-Ebstein fever)
2. Leukemia (aleukemic or preleukemic phase)
3. Hypernephroma (high ESR)
4. Hepatoma (generally not metastatic liver disease)
5. Atrial myxoma

mimic sepsis. Patients with leukemia may also present with fever. Older patients in the aleukemic or preleukemic phase of their disease may have little or no evidence of leukemia on peripheral smear. In earlier series hypernephroma was noted to cause FUO; however, examination of a large series of patients with hypernephroma has demonstrated that this solid tumor is rarely associated with fever. The solid tumor that is most frequently reported as a cause of FUO is primary hepatoma, while tumors that metastasize to liver rarely cause fever. Finally, atrial mxyoma is a rare disorder that is associated with fever and can mimic subacute bacterial endocarditis. Small pieces of the atrial tumor can break off and embolize to the periphery, causing small infarcts similar to those observed in bacterial endocarditis.

KEY POINTS
Neoplastic Causes of FUO

1. Lymphoma is the most common neoplasia causing FUO.
2. Pel-Ebstein fever strongly suggests Hodgkin's lymphoma.
3. Preleukemia can present as FUO in the elderly.
4. Primary hepatoma can be associated with FUO; however, metastatic liver disease usually does not cause fever.
5. Renal cell carcinoma uncommonly causes FUO.
6. Atrial myxoma can mimic subacute bacterial endocarditis.

◆ CASE 3.2

A 27-year-old Asian male presented with a chief complaint of fevers of two weeks' duration. Two weeks prior to arrival he began experiencing fever associated with weakness, malaise, shoulder and neck weakness, as well as muscle tenderness. He also noted a sore throat. He was admitted to a hospital in Puerto Rico, where a CXR demonstrated diffuse pulmonary infiltrates and sputum Gram stain Gm+ cocci. WBC 16,000. He was treated with intravenous mezlocillin and gentamicin and later switched to ampicillin. He failed to improve, remaining febrile, and came to the University Hospital.

Epidemiology: No pets, does not drink unpasteurized milk, without allergies, does not eat raw meat, no swimming in fresh water, no exposure to TB, no history of gonorrhea or syphilis. No exposure to tuberculosis or other infectious diseases.

Travel other than his trip to Puerto Rico was unremarkable

Social history: Occasional alcohol, single, worked as a cook.

Past medical history: At age 9 he had an acute febrile episode associated with a rash, severe joint swelling, and high fever. The illness spontaneously subsided.

Physical examination: Temp 101°F, chest clear, liver edge was palpated 2 cm below right costal margin, slightly tender. His left upper quadrant was also tender. Skin: macular rash over the chest where he had applied rubbing ointment.

Laboratory findings: WBC 20,400, 94% PMN, 4% L, 2% M, platelets 354K, Hgb 12.9, ABG pO$_2$ 69, pCO$_2$ 33, HCO$_3$ 24, U/A negative. LFTs: Total bilirubin 2.8, ALT 108, AST 98, GGT 42.

CXR: LLL infiltrate.

Ceftriaxone and erythromycin were started; however, his fevers persisted from 101°F to 105°F. Subsequent laboratory analysis included an ESR > 100 and peripheral WBC 35,000 and Hgb 9.1.

After 4 days of persistent fever his antibiotics were switched to tetracycline followed by 3 days of naprosyn. Additional tests at that time included PPD 4 mm, AFB stains of sputum negative; abdominal ultrasound and CT scan negative with the exception of consolidation seen in the left and right lung bases; bronchoscopy negative for pneumocystis and Legionella; transbronchial biopsy consistent with focal pneumonitis; lumbar puncture: CSF glucose 89 mg/100 ml, total protein 11 mg/ml, WBC 0; thick and thin malaria smears negative; stool for ova and parasites negative on three separate samples; hepatitis B surface Ab +, core Ab +, surface antigen negative; ASLO 1:185; ANA and rheumatoid factor negative, RPR negative;

blood cultures × 8 negative; mono spot negative; repeat transaminase values, ALT 94, AST 64; alkaline phosphatase 403, GGT 180.

He continued to have fevers. A liver biopsy demonstrated nonspecific inflammation. He suffered continued weight loss, and his erythrocyte sedimentation rate and WBC remained elevated. After 8 days in the hospital he developed a swollen left wrist and swollen right elbow. He was treated with high-dose oral salicylates. Within 24 hours of initiation of therapy he defervesced, and over the next two weeks his symptoms completely resolved. On the basis of his past medical history, clinical presentation, and response to salicylate he was discharged with the diagnosis of Still's disease.

Autoimmune diseases are the third major category of diseases causing FUO (see Table 3.4). In early series of FUO cases systemic lupus erythematosus (SLE) was a frequent etiology. However, with the improvement in antinuclear and anti-DNA markers, these sensitive tests readily identify cases of SLE, and therefore the diagnosis is now usually made within three weeks. Still's disease, or juvenile rheumatoid arthritis in the adult, is one of the most frequent autoimmune diseases resulting in FUO in younger patients. Key clinical features of this disease include an evanescent macular rash, arthralgias, and a sore throat. Patients with Still's disease often have high fevers associated with a high peripheral white blood cell count, and this combination frequently causes the physician to begin antibiotic therapy for a presumed bacterial infection. However,

Table 3.4

Autoimmune Diseases Causing FUO

1. Systemic lupus erythematosus
2. Still's disease
3. Hypersensitivity angiitis
4. Polymyalgia rheumatica/temporal arteritis
5. Polyarteritis nodosa
6. Mixed connective tissue disease
7. Subacute thyroiditis

fever fails to subside after initiation of antibiotics. There is no specific test for Still's disease. Serum ferritin levels are generally markedly elevated, as is the erythrocyte sedimentation rate (ESR).

In elderly patients polymyalgia rheumatica can present as FUO. This disease results in proximal muscle weakness and a high ESR. Temporal headaches and visual complaints are present with temporal arteritis, which is commonly associated with polymyalgia rheumatica.

Other autoimmune diseases that are reported to cause FUO include polyarteritis nodosa, hypersensitivity angiitis, and mixed connective tissue disease. Subacute thyroiditis may present with prolonged fever. On examination the thyroid is often tender, and serum antithyroid antibodies are elevated. Recently, Kikuchi's disease, also called histiocytic necrotizing lymphadenitis, has been reported to cause prolonged fever. This self-limited autoimmune disorder occurs in young Asian females and is associated with generalized lymphadenopathy. Diagnosis is made by lymph node biopsy.

KEY POINTS
Autoimmune Causes of FUO

1. Still's disease is associated with high fevers, evanescent skin rash, arthralgias, sore throat, leukocytosis, high serum ferritin, and elevated ESR.
2. Polymyalgia rheumatica/temporal arteritis is found in the elderly and causes proximal muscle weakness, visual symptoms, and a high ESR.
3. Subacute thyroiditis should be considered if the thyroid is tender.
4. Kikuchi's disease often presents with fever and lymphadenopathy in young Asian females.

In addition to the big three categories, the clinician must also consider the little six. First is granulomatous diseases of unclear etiology. This group of diseases presents with fever and malaise and generally involves the liver. Liver function tests generally demonstrate mild abnormalities in alkaline phosphatase, and liver biopsy reveals granulomas. The second disease in the little six is regional enteritis. This disease can present with prolonged fever in the absence of gastrointestinal complaints. For this reason contrast studies of the GI tract are generally recommended to exclude this diagnosis. Third is familial Mediterranean fever. As the name implies, this is a genetic disorder associated with recurrent serositis primarily of the abdominal cavity but can also result in pleuritis and pericarditis. A family history is critical in raising this possibility. The fourth disorder in this group is drug fever, one of the most frequently encountered causes of FUO. Table 3.5 lists the most common drugs that cause fever. The antiseizure medication dilantin is probably the most frequent drug to cause allergic reactions, including fever. Quinidine, procaine amide, and penicillins are other major offenders. When a patient presents with FUO, all medications should be discontinued or switched to exclude this possibility. Fifth is pulmonary emboli. Prolonged bed rest increases the risk of thrombus formation in the calves. When emboli are small, they might not result in respiratory complaints and may simply present as fever. In all patients who are at risk for thrombophlebitis and FUO, pul-

monary emboli need to be excluded. The final disorder in the little six is factitious fever. In earlier series patients often manipulated the mercury thermometer to fool the physician; however, with the advent of the electronic thermometer this maneuver is no longer possible. Patients usually inject themselves with saliva or stool, causing polymicrobial bacteremia and fever. This disorder occurs almost exclusively in females. A medical background is also the rule. In the absence of any clear cause for fever a history of health care training should raise the clinician's suspicion, particularly if the patient takes great interest in her illness and has a medical textbook at the bedside. The diagnostic test of choice is often a search of the patient's room seeking a syringe used for self-injection.

KEY POINTS
Other Causes of FUO

1. Regional enteritis can present with fever in the absence of gastrointestinal symptoms.
2. Pulmonary emboli can present with fever in the absence of respiratory symptoms.
3. Discontinue all medications in the patient with FUO.
4. Consider factitious fever in the female health care worker with a medical textbook at the bedside and recurrent polymicrobial bacteremia.

History for FUO

History can play a critical role in narrowing the differential diagnosis and in deciding on the most appropriate diagnostic tests. A review of all symptoms associated with the illness needs to be periodically updated. Symptoms often are transient and are recalled by the patient only after repeated questioning. In FUO patients a comprehensive history is critical. The patient's past medical history often provides useful clues.

Table 3.5
Drugs Causing FUO

Aldomet	Iodides
Antihistamines	Mercaptopurine
Barbiturates	Nitrofurantoin
Chlorambucil	Penicillins
Dilantin	Procaine amide
Hydralazine	Quinidine
Ibuprofen	Salicylates
INH	Thiouracil

History of tuberculosis, tuberculosis exposure, or a positive PPD should be included. Family history must also be thoroughly reviewed to exclude genetic disorders such as cyclic neutropenia and familial Mediterranean fever. Epidemiology history needs to include animal exposure (pets and other domestic as well as wild animals), home environment, and occupational exposure. Travel history should explore travel to areas endemic for malaria, other parasites, typhoid, coccidiomycosis, histoplasmosis, and tick-borne illnesses. Travel in Third World countries, the Southwest, and the Ohio River valley are of particular interest. Finally, a list of all medications, including over-the-counter and natural organic remedies, must be compiled to exclude the possibility of drug fever.

KEY POINTS

The History for FUO

> 1. A review of symptoms should be repeated frequently.
> 2. Past medical history of infectious diseases should be carefully reviewed.
> 3. Family history needs to be carefully reviewed.
> 4. Epidemiologic history should include animal exposure, outdoor camping, insect bites, and travel in Third World countries, the Southwest, and the Ohio River valley.
> 5. All medications must be reviewed.

Physical Examination for FUO

In addition to a careful history, careful repeat physical examination is frequently helpful. Particular attention should be paid to the skin exam, looking for embolic or vasculitic lesions or evidence of physical manipulation. Particular attention should be paid to the nail beds, where small emboli can become trapped in the distal capillaries of the fingers and toes, resulting in small, splinter-shaped infarcts. Joint motion and the presence of effusions should be looked for. Careful eye exam should be repeated, looking for conjunctival petechiae, conjunctivitis, punctate corneal lesions, uveitis, optic nerve changes, and retinal or choroidal abnormalities. Thorough palpation of all lymph nodes needs to be repeatedly performed, with documentation of the consistency, size, and tenderness of nodes in the femoral, axillary, epitrochlear, supraclavicular, and neck regions. Cardiac exam should be repeated daily, listening for cardiac murmurs and pericardial rubs. The abdomen also should be palpated daily to detect new masses, areas of localized tenderness, and hepatomegaly or splenomegaly.

KEY POINTS

Physical Examination for FUO

> 1. Thoroughly examine skin for embolic lesions.
> 2. Palpate all lymph nodes.
> 3. Perform a complete joint examination.
> 4. Listen carefully for cardiac murmurs.
> 5. Abdominal exam should assess liver and spleen size and palpate for masses and areas of tenderness.

Laboratory Studies for FUO

An algorithm can be helpful in guiding the initial workup of the patient with FUO (see Figure 3.1), and all patients with FUO should receive a series of basic diagnostic tests (see Table 3.6). However, because each case is different, a series of yes/no branch points is not possible for guiding the subsequent diagnostic approach to FUO. In recent years rather than ordering insufficient studies, clinicians have erred on the side of excessive and uninformative testing. Each patient's diagnostic workup must be tailored to that patient's history and physical findings. A cookbook approach sub-

Figure 3.1

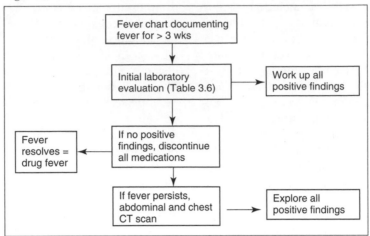

Algorithm for initial workup of FUO.

jects the patient to undue and costly testing and stress. Often "tincture of time" and repeated history and physical exam allow the physician to apply Sutton's law. Willy Sutton was a famous bank robber who, when finally captured, was asked by newspaper reporters, "Willy, why do you rob banks?" Willy replied, "That's where the money is." Clinicians need to focus on diagnostic tests that are likely to have a high yield. They need to go for "where the money is."

Table 3.6

Preliminary Tests Recommended For FUO

1. Complete history
2. Careful physical exam
3. CBC with differential
4. Giemsa and Wright stain blood smears
5. Liver function tests
6. ANA and rheumatoid factor
7. ESR
8. Urinalysis
9. Blood cultures
10. Urine culture
11. PPD skin test
12. Chest X-ray and air sinus films
13. Upper GI with small bowel follow-through
14. Renal and gallbladder ultrasound

KEY POINTS

Diagnostic Workup for FUO

1. Physicians usually err by overtesting.
2. A cookbook approach should be avoided.
3. Sutton's law should be applied: "Go for where the money is." Tests should be directed to specific complaints and abnormalities found on preliminary testing.

Diagnostic tests are most easily classified by category:

1. **Skin tests.** An intermediate-strength PPD should be performed in all patients with FUO who do not have a previously documented positive PPD. An anergy panel is no longer recommended, but it should be kept in mind that in the malnourished chronically ill patient a negative PPD does not exclude the

possibility of tuberculosis. The use of skin tests to detect histoplasmosis and coccidiomycosis is not generally recommended, biopsies and cultures being the preferred methods for diagnosing these potential causes of FUO.

2. **Cultures.** Blood cultures should be part of the initial workup of all patients with significant prolonged fever. Yield for subacute bacterial endocarditis is usually maximized by drawing three blood cultures (see Chapter 7, "Cardiovascular Infections"). In general no more than six blood cultures should be drawn. They may be repeated periodically or if there is a significant change in the fever pattern. Because of the possibility of fastidious slow-growing bacteria, all blood cultures should be held for three weeks. Multiple urine cultures should be obtained and cultured for tuberculosis in addition to more conventional bacteria. In patients with respiratory complaints or chest X-ray abnormalities sputum should be cultured, and in patients undergoing bone marrow biopsy, culture is an important component of the marrow analysis. Cerebrospinal fluid (CSF) culture may be obtained in cases with specific neurologic complaints. All biopsy specimens need to be cultured. Aerobic, anaerobic, mycobacteria, and fungal cultures should be ordered on virtually all culture samples. Viral cultures may also be considered in specific cases in which cytomegalovirus or Epstein-Barr virus is suspected.

3. **Smears.** Peripheral blood smears using Giemsa and Wright stains are critical for making the diagnosis of malaria, trypanosomiasis, and relapsing fever. In addition to a peripheral white blood cell count, Wright stain with differential cell count is often helpful in determining the nature of the inflammatory response associated with fever and should be performed in all patients with FUO. Viral illnesses tend to have lower peripheral white blood cell counts and a predominance of lymphocytes and monocytes. Patients with Epstein-Barr virus often have atypical lymphocytes and monocytes. Patients with Still's disease and patients with acute bacterial infections usually have elevated peripheral white blood cell counts with a predominance of neutrophils and band forms. Patients with cyclic neutropenia develop fever at the time when their total neutrophil count is low, and this finding in association with the classic fever pattern should raise the possibility of this inherited disease. CSF India ink smear and cryptococcal antigen are very helpful in making the diagnosis of cryptococcal meningitis. However, with the exception of patients with HIV this is a rare cause of FUO. Stool smears for ova and parasites are usually less helpful, since gastrointestinal parasites rarely present as FUO.

4. **Other peripheral blood tests.** Antibody titers should be considered when specific pathogens are part of the differential diagnosis. To prove active infection, rising antibody titers are required. Therefore two samples need to be drawn separated by three to four weeks. A single titer simply demonstrates a past history of exposure, while a rising titer indicates recent infection. Antibody titers are particularly useful in cytomegalovirus, Epstein-Barr virus, toxoplasma, rickettsia, chlamydia, and brucella infections. Tests that should be considered in the majority of cases of FUO to diagnose connective tissue disease are antibody titers to human tissue, including antinuclear antibodies (ANA), anti-DNA antibodies, rheumatoid factor, and immune complexes. An ESR should be performed in all cases of FUO. A very high ESR is seen in polymyalgia rheumatica/temporal arteritis and Still's disease. A normal ESR virtually excludes these diagnoses as well as subacute bacterial endocarditis.

5. **Imaging studies.**
A. Tests commonly performed during the initial diagnostic workup: All patients with FUO should initially undergo a chest X-ray looking for mediastinal enlargement (suggestive of

lymphoma), micronodular interstitial changes (millet seed pattern, suggestive of miliary tuberculosis), nodular lesions, or infiltrates (can be seen in many infectious diseases, connective tissue diseases, and neoplasms). Air sinus films or sinus CT scans are required to exclude occult sinus infection and tooth abscess. Upper gastrointestinal barium study with small bowel follow-through should be ordered to exclude regional enteritis. Ultrasound of the gallbladder and/or an oral cholecystogram should be ordered to exclude cholecystitis or an enlarged gangrenous gallbladder. A barium enema should be considered in older patients; however, the yield of this procedure is likely to be low in FUO. An intravenous pyelogram is often performed looking for changes consistent with renal tuberculosis, renal stones, polycystic kidney disease, and renal cell carcinoma.

B. *Tests that should be ordered depending on the patient's symptoms and signs:* X-rays of all joints should be ordered in any patient with persistent joint complaints to document anatomic defects. In patients who are suspected of having a chronic infection, radionuclide scans may be helpful in localizing the site of infection. A gallium scan may be useful in patients with chronic infection because this agent accumulates in areas of inflammation; however, an indium white blood cell scan tends to be more specific. The indium white blood cell scan also has a higher positive yield for identifying occult intra-abdominal infection in comparison to abdominal CT scan. [(18)F]fluorodeoxyglucose (FDG) represents another tracer molecule that accumulates in areas of inflammation and in malignant tumors. Unlike other scans that require that the patient be scanned over 24–36 hours, the FDG positron emission tomography (PET) scan is completed within a few hours. In preliminary studies, this test has proved more sensitive and specific than gallium scan. For the assessment of osteomyelitis as well as tumor metastasis to bone (exceptions being

prostate cancer and multiple myeloma) technetium scan is the most sensitive and specific scanning technique. Total-body CT scan is an expensive test that is commonly performed in patients without specific complaints despite prolonged observation and has up to a 10% yield. This study has proved helpful in identifying abdominal abscesses, mediastinal nodes, and defects in abdominal organs. Because of its significant yield, abdominal and chest CT should be considered if preliminary testing proves unrevealing (see Figure 3.1). In patients with a heart murmur and persistent fever, cardiac echocardiography should be considered. Transesophageal echocardiography is the test of choice, having a greater than 90% sensitivity for detecting cardiac vegetations, and is also helpful in detecting myocardial abscess as well as atrial myxoma. Ultrasound of the lower abdomen may be helpful in cases in which pelvic lesions are suspected. Abdominal CT is not as sensitive in this region because of reflection artifacts generated by the pelvic bones.

6. **Invasive procedures.** Liver biopsy is recommended if all noninvasive tests prove to be negative to exclude the possibility of granulomatous hepatitis. Laparoscopic guided biopsy improves the yield by allowing the biopsies to be taken of areas where abnormalities in the external capsule are seen. Bone marrow aspiration and biopsy are also recommended as routine invasive tests if all noninvasive studies are negative. Leukemia in its early stages may be detected as well as stage IV lymphoma. It is critical that the bone marrow be appropriately cultured (see above) because disseminated tuberculosis, histoplasmosis, and coccidiomycosis as well as other fungal and mycobacterial infections often seed the bone marrow. Other invasive procedures will depend on other diagnostic findings, history, and physical findings. In the elderly patient with a high ESR and persistent fever temporal artery biopsy is generally recommended. It should be kept in mind that be-

cause skip lesions are common in temporal arteritis, a long sample of the temporal artery should be obtained, and multiple arterial sections should be examined. In early series of FUO, diagnostic laparotomy was frequently recommended. However, with the advent of new abdominal imaging techniques this invasive procedure is now rarely performed but may be considered in selected cases. In addition to a complete series of cultures, all biopsy specimens should undergo Brown-Brenn, Ziehl-Neelsen, methenamine silver, PAS, and Dieterle silver staining in addition to routine hematoxylin and eosin staining. Frozen sections should be obtained for immunofluorescence staining, and the remaining tissue block should be saved for additional future studies.

It should be emphasized that when symptoms, signs, or a specific diagnostic abnormality is found, all other scheduled diagnostic tests should be delayed, and Sutton's law should be applied. For example, if an abnormal fluid collection is found on abdominal CT, all other diagnostic procedures can be halted, and a needle aspiration of the potential abscess can be performed. If the result proves to be positive, additional investigations are unnecessary. The "money" has been found. There is no need to order tests for completeness' sake. Overtesting is common in FUO and causes excessive discomfort for the patient as well as excess cost. When in doubt about performing additional tests, tincture of time often proves the wisest course of action. Over time the patient's fever may spontaneously resolve, or new manifestations may develop, helping to identify the etiology of fever.

Treatment of FUO

In the past many clinicians discouraged the use of antipyretics in FUO because these agents mask the pattern of fever. However, as was noted earlier, with rare exceptions the pattern of

fever has not proved to be helpful in determining the etiology of FUO. Fever is commonly associated with chills, sweating, fatigue, and loss of appetite. Therefore once true fever has been documented, in most cases of FUO antipyretics can be administered to relieve some of the patient's symptoms as the diagnostic workup is pursued. To avoid repeated shifting of the thermal set point and recurrent shivering and chills, aspirin, NSAIDs, or acetaminophen must be administered at the proper time interval to maintain therapeutic levels. Otherwise, antipyretics will exacerbate rather than reduce the symptoms of fever.

KEY POINTS
Treatment of FUO

1. Once the pattern of fever has been documented, fever can be lowered by using NSAIDs, aspirin, or acetaminophen.
2. Empiric antibiotics are contraindicated.
3. Glucocorticoids should be used only when infection has been excluded.

As was discussed in Chapter 1, physicians often overprescribe antibiotics. In cases of FUO there is a great temptation to institute an empiric trial of antibiotics. This temptation should be avoided. Antibiotics are contraindicated until a specific diagnosis has been made. Use of an empiric antibiotic trial often delays diagnosis and is rarely curative. Because infections that are susceptible to conventional antibiotics represent a small percentage of the diseases that cause FUO, in the majority of cases antibiotic treatment will have no effect. In cases of occult bacterial infection empiric antibiotics may mask the manifestations of the infection and delay appropriate treatment. The majority of infections causing FUO require prolonged antibiotic treatment and surgical drainage. In the absence of a specific diagnosis clinicians have difficulty justifying a prolonged course of antibiotics; therefore antibiotics are often discontinued after one to two weeks, allowing the infection to relapse. This all too common circumstance would therefore serve to delay diagnosis and appropriate treatment even in patients with conventional bacterial infections as the cause of their FUO.

When a connective tissue disease appears to be the most likely explanation for FUO, empiric use of systemic glucocorticoids is often considered. These agents are very effective in treating temporal arteritis and polymyalgia rheumatica and may be helpful in Still's disease and are used for specific complications in lupus erythematosus. However, because these agents markedly reduce inflammation and impair host defense, administration of glucocorticoids can markedly exacerbate bacterial, mycobacterial, fungal, and parasitic infections. Therefore before considering an empiric trial of glucocorticoids such as prednisone, dexamethasone, or solumedrol, the physician must convincingly rule out infection. The physician must also keep in mind the many potential side effects of prolonged glucocorticoid use (Cushingoid faces, osteoporosis, aseptic necrosis of the hip, diabetes mellitus, and opportunistic infections) before committing the FUO patient to a prolonged course of systemic steroid treatment.

Prognosis

Delay in diagnosis worsens the outcome in cases of intra-abdominal abscess, miliary tuberculosis, disseminated fungal infections, and pulmonary emboli. However, if these diseases are carefully excluded, the lack of a diagnosis after an extensive diagnostic workup is associated with a five-year mortality rate of only 3%. The prognosis is somewhat worse in the elderly patient because of the increased risk of malignancy. Therefore once the clinician has completed the above FUO diagnostic battery and serious life-threatening diseases have been ex-

cluded, additional diagnostic study is not warranted. If fever persists for an additional four to six months, a complete series of diagnostic studies should then be repeated.

FUO in the HIV-Infected Patient

Primary HIV infection can present with prolonged fever, and in patients with the appropriate risk profile (see Chapter 17, "HIV Infection") this diagnosis needs to be considered. Serum markers are negative in the early stages of HIV infection; therefore quantitative PCR for HIV is the diagnostic test of choice. Fever is a common manifestation of opportunistic infection in the later stages of HIV infection. In order of frequency the most common causes of FUO in AIDS patients are mycobacterial infections (*Mycobacterium tuberculosis*, *M. avium-intracellulare*, other atypical mycobacteria), other bacterial infections, cytomegalovirus, pneumocystis, toxoplasmosis, cryptococcus, and histoplasmosis. In HIV patients coming from endemic areas, visceral leishmaniasis also needs to be considered. Noninfectious causes include non-Hodgkins lymphoma and drug fever. Additional tests that are warranted in the HIV patient include mycobacterial blood culture, cryptococcal serum antigen, and cytomegalovirus serum antigen. Disseminated histoplasmosis may be difficult to detect and in our experience is most readily diagnosed by bone marrow culture.

KEY POINTS
FUO in HIV-Infected Patients

1. Can be a manifestation of primary HIV infection.

2. Often the first symptom of an opportunistic infection.
3. Mycobacteria are the most common infectious cause.
4. CMV is also common, as are cryptococcus and toxoplasma.
5. Non-Hodgkin's lymphoma is the most common noninfectious cause.

Fever in Surgical Intensive-Care and Medical Intensive-Care Patients

One of the most common problems encountered by the infectious disease consultant is the evaluation of fever in patients residing in the surgical or medical intensive-care unit. These patients are usually severely ill and have multiple potential causes for fever.

In the postoperative patient wound infection must be excluded. All surgical wounds need to be carefully examined, looking for purulent discharge, erythema, edema, and tenderness. In the immediate postoperative period (24–48 hours) group A streptococci can result in septic shock and severe bacteremia with only minimal purulence at the operative site. A Gram stain of serous exudate usually demonstrates Gram-positive cocci in chains. In the later postoperative period *Staphylococcus aureus* as well as nosocomial pathogens such as Pseudomonas, Klebsiella, and *E. coli* are associated with wound infection. Appropriate antibiotic therapy is generally guided by culture and Gram stain. Empiric antibiotic therapy should include Gram-positive and Gram-negative coverage. In patients who have suffered bowel perforation, the development of intra-abdominal abscess is a common cause of fever, and an abdominal CT scan should be ordered to exclude this possibility.

Because most intensive-care patients are intubated, bacteria colonizing the nasopharynx can more readily gain entry to the bronchi and pulmonary parenchyma, causing bronchitis and pneumonia. As will be outlined in more detail in Chapter 4, sputum Gram stain is critical for differentiating colonization from true infection. The presence of a single organism on Gram stain combined with >10 neutrophils per high power field strongly suggests infection. Sputum culture identifies the offending organism as well as its sensitivities to antibiotics. Other parameters that are helpful in differentiating colonization from true infection are chest X-ray and arterial blood gases. The presence of a new infiltrate supports the diagnosis of pneumonia, as does a decrease in arterial pO_2.

Patients in the intensive-care unit usually have one or two intravenous catheters in place as well as an arterial line. These lines are always at risk of becoming infected, and line sepsis is a common cause of fever in the intensive-care setting. At the onset of new fever, all intravenous and arterial lines should be examined for erythema, warmth, and exudate. Particularly in the patient who has developed shock, all lines should be replaced, and appropriate empiric antibiotic coverage should be instituted. *Staphylococcus aureus*, *S. epidermidis*, and Gram-negative rods are the primary causes of line sepsis, and initial antibiotic coverage should include vancomycin and a third-generation cephalosporin. Empiric antibiotic coverage must be individualized to take into account the prevailing bacterial flora in each intensive-care unit as well as the patient's history of antibiotic usage.

Another major infectious cause of fever in the intensive-care unit patient results from prolonged bladder catheterization. The bladder catheter bypasses the urethra, and despite the use of closed urinary collecting systems, within 30 days nearly all patients with bladder catheters develop urinary tract infections (see Chapter 9, "Genitourinary Tract Infections and Sexually Transmitted Diseases"). Therefore urinalysis and urine cultures need to be part of the fever workup in all patients with urinary catheters.

In patients with nasogastric tubes or patients who have been intubated through the nasal passage, the ostea draining the air sinuses can become occluded. This condition can lead to sinusitis and fever. Therefore the fever workup in these patients needs to include sinus films. If sinusitis is discovered, the tube needs to be removed from the nasal passage and appropriate antibiotic coverage instituted (see Chapter 5, "Eye and Ear, Nose, and Throat Infections").

Noninfectious causes of fever also need to be considered. As was noted for FUO patients, pulmonary emboli may present with fever. Intensive-care unit patients are usually on a large number of medications and therefore are at higher risk of developing drug fever. All medications need to be reviewed, and when possible, medications should be discontinued or changed. Another cause of persistent low-grade fever is undrained collections of blood. These collections can be identified by CT scan and generally do not require drainage but take time to fully resorb.

Fever in the ICU patient requires a systematic diagnostic approach and the judicious use of antibiotics. Too often, patients are covered unnecessarily for prolonged periods on broad-spectrum antibiotics. This condition leads to the selection of highly resistant bacterial pathogens and also predisposes patients to candidemia as well as *Clostridium difficile* colitis. Empiric antibiotic coverage needs to be streamlined once culture data is available. Close communication between the intensive-care unit staff and the infectious disease consultant is critical to achieve the best care for the febrile intensive-care unit patient.

KEY POINTS
Fever in the ICU Patient

1. Fever is extremely common in ICU patients.
2. A systematic approach to diagnosis is critical.
3. Key sites of infection include:
   a. Pulmonary infection (critical to differentiate colonization from infection),
   b. Intravenous and intra-arterial lines,
   c. Urinary tract at high risk secondary to prolonged bladder catheterization,
   d. Wounds, particularly in the early postoperative period,
   e. Sinusitis in patients with nasotracheal tubes.
4. Noninfectious causes: pulmonary emboli, drug fever, and old hemorrhage.
5. Empiric antibiotics need to be streamlined on the basis of culture results.
6. Prolonged broad-spectrum antibiotic coverage predisposes to colonization with highly resistant bacteria, fungemia, *Clostridium difficile* colitis, and drug allergies.

Additional Reading

Blockmans, D., and Knokaert, D. Clinical value of [(18)F]fluorodeoxyglucose positron emission tomography for patients with fever of unknown origin. *Clin Infect Dis*, 32:191–196, 2001.

Bujak, J.S., Aptekar, R.G., Decker, J.L., and Wolff, S.M. Juvenile rheumatoid arthritis presenting in the adult as fever of unknown origin. *Medicine* (Baltimore), 52:431–444, 1973.

Ghose, M.K., Shensa, S., and Lerner, P.I. Arteritis of the aged (giant cell arteritis) and fever of unexplained origin. *Am J Med* 60:429–436, 1976.

Larson, E.B., Featherstone, H.J., and Petersdorf, R.G. Fever of undetermined origin: Diagnosis and follow-up of 105 cases, 1970–1980. *Medicine* (Baltimore), 61:269–292, 1982.

Marik, P.E. Fever in the ICU. *Chest*, 117:855–869, 2000.

Mayo, J., Collazos, J., et al: Fever of unknown origin in the setting of HIV infection: Guidelines for a rational approach. *AIDS Patient Care STDS*, 12:373–378, 1998.

Petersdorf, R.G., and Beeson, P.B. Fever of unexplained origin: Report of 100 cases. *Medicine*, 40:1–30, 1961.

Chapter 4

Pulmonary Infections

Recommend Time to Complete: 3 days

Guiding Questions

1. What factors predispose the host to develop pneumonia?

2. How useful is sputum Gram stain and what parameters are used to assess the adequacy of a sputum sample?

3. How should the clinician interpret the sputum culture and should sputum cultures be obtained in the absence of sputum Gram stain?

4. What symptoms, signs, and diagnostic tests help to differentiate viral from bacterial pneumonia?

5. What are some of the difficulties that are encountered in trying to determine the cause of acute pneumonia?

6. How helpful is the chest X-ray in determining the specific cause of pneumonia?

7. How often should the chest X-ray be repeated and how long do the radiologic changes associated with acute pneumonia persist?

8. What antibiotic regimens are recommended for empiric therapy of community acquired pneumonia and why?

Potential Severity: Acute pneumonia is a potentially life-threatening illness requiring rapid diagnosis and treatment. A delay in antibiotic treatment increases the risk of a fatal outcome.

General Considerations

Prevalence

Two to three million cases of pneumonia are reported annually in the United States. In the United States it has been estimated that pneumonia is responsible for over 10 million physician visits, 500,000 hospitalizations, and 45,000 deaths per year. An estimated 258 persons per 100,000 require hospitalization for pneumonia; among those over age 65 years, 962 persons per 100,000 require hospitalization for pneumonia. Pneumonia occurs most commonly during the winter months.

Pathogenesis and Pathology

Under normal conditions the tracheobronchial tree is sterile. The respiratory tract has a series of protective mechanisms that prevent pathogens from gaining entry:

1. The nasal passages contain turbinates and hairs that trap foreign particles.
2. The epiglottis covers the trachea and prevents secretions or food from entering the trachea.
3. The tracheobronchial tree contains cells that secrete mucin. Mucin contains a number of antibacterial compounds, including IgA antibodies, defensins, lysozyme, and lactoferrin. Mucin also is sticky and traps bacteria or other foreign particles that manage to get past the epiglottis.

4. Cilia lining the inner walls of the trachea and bronchi beat rapidly and act as a conveyer belt to move mucin out of the tracheobronchial tree to the larynx.
5. When significant volumes of fluid or large particles gain access to the trachea, the cough reflex is activated and quickly forces the unwanted contents out of the tracheobronchial tree.
6. If pathogens are able to bypass all of the above protective mechanisms and gain entry into the alveoli, they encounter a space that under normal circumstances is dry and relatively inhospitable. The presence of an invading pathogen induces the entry of neutrophils and alveolar macrophages that ingest and kill infecting organisms. Immunoglobulins and complement are also found in this space.
7. The lymphatic channels adjacent to the alveoli serve to drain this space and transport fluid, macrophages, and lymphocytes to the mediastinal lymph nodes.

KEY POINTS
The Protective Mechanisms of the Lung

1. Normally, the tracheobronchial tree is sterile.
2. The nasal turbinates trap foreign particles, and the epiglottis covers the trachea.
3. Mucin possesses antibacterial activity, and cilia transport mucin out of the lung.
4. Coughing expels foreign material that enters the tracheobronchial tree.
5. Alveoli can deliver PMNs, macrophages, immunoglobulins, and complement to destroy invading pathogens.
6. Lymphatics drain macrophages and PMNs to the mediastinal lymph nodes.

Bacterial pathogens usually gain entry into the lung by aspiration of mouth flora or inhalation of small, aerosolized droplets (<3 μm in diameter) that can be transported by airflow to the alveoli. Once the pathogen takes hold, a series of inflammatory responses is triggered. These responses have been most carefully studied in pneumonia due to *Streptococcus pneumoniae*. First there is an outpouring of edema fluid into the alveoli, which serves as an excellent culture medium for further bacterial growth. As fluid accumulates, it spills over to adjacent alveoli through the pores of Kohn and via terminal bronchioles, resulting in the centrifugal spread of infection. Coughing and the physical motion of respiration further enhance spread. Next polymorphonuclear leukocytes (PMNs) and some red blood cells begin to accumulate in the alveolar space, eventually filling the region and forming a zone of consolidation. Next macrophages enter the lesions and assist PMNs in clearing the infection. Histopathology reveals zones of varying age. The most distal regions represent the most recent areas of infection, where edema fluid, PMNs, and red blood cells predominate. On lower-power microscopy the region has an appearance similar to the architecture of the liver and has been termed "red hepatization." Older, central regions have more densely packed PMNs and macrophages. This region has a grayer color and forms the zone of "gray hepatization."

The various pulmonary pathogens demonstrate marked differences in the invasiveness and ability to destroy lung parenchyma. *Streptococcus pneumoniae* causes minimal tissue necrosis and is associated with little or no scar formation. Full recovery of pulmonary function is the rule. *Staphylococcus aureus* releases a number of proteases that permanently destroy tissue. Gram-negative rods and anaerobic bacteria also cause permanent tissue destruction.

KEY POINTS

The Pathogenesis of Pneumonia

1. Pathogens are aspirated or inhaled as small, aerosolized droplets.

2. Bacterial invasion of the alveoli induces:
   a. Edema fluid that spreads to other alveoli through the pores of Kohn,
   b. PMNs and red blood cells followed by macrophages.
3. Centrifugal spread of infection:
   a. Newer regions in the periphery appear red (red hepatization),
   b. Older regions are central and appear gray (gray hepatization).
4. *Streptococcus pneumoniae* does not cause permanent tissue destruction.
5. *Staphylococcus aureus*, Gram-negative rods, and anaerobes cause permanent damage.

Predisposing Factors

The majority of bacterial pneumonias are preceded by a viral upper respiratory infection. Influenza virus is well known to predispose to *Streptococcus pneumoniae* and *Staphylococcus aureus* pneumonia. Viral infections of the upper respiratory tract can damage the bronchial epithelium and cilia. Virus-mediated cell damage also results in the production of serous fluid that can pool in the pulmonary alveoli, serving as an excellent culture media for bacteria. The low viscosity of this fluid, combined with depressed ciliary motility, enables the viral exudate to carry nasopharyngeal bacteria past the epiglottis into the lungs. Smoking also damages the bronchial epithelial cells and impairs mucociliary function. As a consequence, smokers have an increased risk of developing pneumonia. Patients with congenital defects in ciliary function such as Kartagener's syndrome as well as diseases resulting in highly viscous mucous such as cystic fibrosis are predisposed to recurrent pneumonia. An active cough and normal epiglottis function usually prevent nasopharyngeal contents from gaining access to the tracheobronchial tree. However, drugs such as alcohol, sedatives, and anesthetics can depress the level of consciousness and impair these functions, predisposing the patient to pneumonia. The elderly, particularly after a cerebrovascular accident, often develop impairments in swallowing function, predisposing them to aspiration. In addition the elderly demonstrate reduced humoral and cell-mediated immunity, rendering them more susceptible to viral and bacterial pneumonia. Patients with impairments in immunoglobulin production, T and B cell function, and neutrophil and macrophage function are also at greater risk for developing pneumonia. Organ transplant patients on immunosuppressive agents as well as AIDS patients have a greater likelihood of developing pneumonia. Chronic diseases have been associated with an increased risk of pneumonia, including multiple myeloma, diabetes, chronic renal failure, and sickle-cell disease. Finally, cold weather is thought to contribute to the development of pneumonia. Cold, dry weather can alter the viscosity of mucus and impair bacterial clearance. Second, cold weather encourages people to remain indoors, a condition that enhances person-to-person spread of respiratory infections.

KEY POINTS

Factors That Predispose to Pneumonia

1. Viral infections damage cilia and produce serous exudate that can transport nasopharyngeal bacteria into the alveoli.
2. Smoking damages bronchial epithelial cells and impairs cilia function.
3. Alcohol and other drugs depress coughing and epiglottis function.
4. Elderly patients have impaired swallowing owing to strokes as well as reduced humoral and cell-mediated immunity.
5. Patients on immunosuppressive agents and patients with AIDS have depressed humoral and cell-mediated immunity.
6. Patients with chronic diseases are at increased risk for pneumonia.
7. Cold weather dries mucous membranes and increases person-to-person spread of infection.

Symptoms and Signs

◆ CASE 4.1

A 55-year-old woman was first seen in the emergency room in December complaining of a nonproductive cough, nasal stuffiness, and fever. She also noted diffuse severe muscle aches and joint pains as well as a generalized headache.

Epidemiology: She had recently seen her grandchildren, who all had high fevers and were complaining of muscle aches.

Physical examination, positive findings: Temperature 103°F (39°C). Throat erythematous, clear nasal discharge. Her muscles were diffusely tender. CXR: Within normal limits.

Clinical course: Three days into her illness she noted some improvement in her cough, muscle aches, and joint pains; however, on the fourth day she developed a high fever (104°F) preceded by a teeth-chattering chill.. That day her cough became productive of rusty-colored opaque sputum, and she began feeling short of breath.

Physical examination: Temperature 105°F, respiratory rate 36. General appearance: Very ill-appearing, anxious woman gasping for air. Lungs: Mild dullness to percussion, E to A changes, rales and rhonchi localized to the right middle lung.

Laboratory findings: Peripheral WBC 16,000, 68% PMNs, 20% immature forms (bands and metamyelocytes), 8% lymphocytes, 4% monocytes. Sputum Gram stain: Many Gram-positive lancet-shaped diplococci, many PMNs (>10/high-power field), no squamous epithelial cells.

Chest X-ray: Dense right middle lobe, lobar infiltrate (see Fig 4.1).

In Case 4.1 the patient's initial symptoms suggested a viral illness involving the upper respiratory tract (rhinitis and nonproductive cough), central nervous system and/or air sinuses (headache), and musculoskeletal system (myalgias and arthralgias). Such symptoms are generally attributed to an influenzalike illness. A number of viruses can explain these symptoms, including influenza, parainfluenza, adenovirus,

Figure 4.1

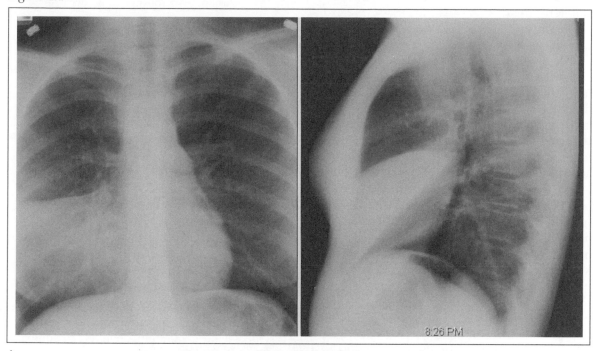

A

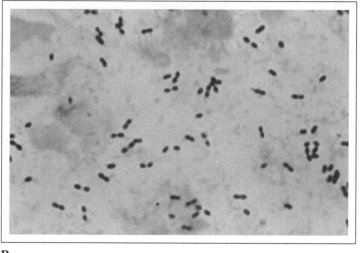

B

Lobar pneumonia due to *Streptococcus pneumoniae*. **(A)** Chest X-ray demonstrating a classic right middle lobe infiltrate. (Courtesy of Dr. Pat Abbitt, University of Florida College of Medicine.) **(B)** Sputum Gram stain showing *S. pneumoniae*. Note that the Gram-positive diplococci come to a slight point at each end, explaining the term "lancet-shaped." See Figure 4.1B on Color Plate 1.

respiratory syncytial virus (more common in children), rhinoviruses (usually less severe), and enteroviruses. Subsequently, within a 24-hour period she experienced the abrupt onset of a new constellation of symptoms. The onset of her new illness can be classified as acute. An illness is termed acute when symptoms and signs develop over 24–48 hours. Symptoms developing over 3 days to one week are generally classified as subacute, and symptoms progressing more slowly over three weeks to several months are classified as chronic.

In generating a potential list of etiologic agents, the infectious disease specialist frequently uses the pace of illness to narrow the possibilities. Pneumonias are generally classified into two groups: acute and chronic pneumonia. Most bacterial and viral pneumonias develop quickly, while fungal and mycobacterial pulmonary infections tend to develop at a slower pace. Acute pneumonia can be further classified as typical or atypical pneumonia. Typical pneumonia is characterized by the more rapid onset of symptoms, more severe symptomatology, a productive cough, and dense consolidation on chest X-ray, as observed in Case 4.1. Atypical pneumonia tends to be slower in onset (often subacute), symptoms tend to be less severe, cough is productive of minimal sputum, and a chest X-ray usually reveals a patchy or interstitial pattern. Finally, pulmonary infections are separated into community-acquired and nosocomial infection. Community-acquired infection is defined as an infection developing in a patient who has not recently (≥14 days) been hospitalized or resided in a chronic-care facility.

KEY POINTS

The Classification of Pneumonia

Pneumonias are classified by:
1. Pace of illness:
   a. Acute: Symptoms develop over 24–48 hours.
   b. Chronic: Symptoms progress over three weeks or longer.
2. Specific constellations of symptoms:
   a. Typical: Rapid onset, more severe symptoms, productive cough, dense consolidation on chest X-ray.
   b. Atypical: Somewhat slower onset, less severe symptoms, nonproductive cough, patchy interstitial pattern on chest X-ray.
3. Environment where the pneumonia was acquired:
   a. Community-acquired: Patient not recently (≥14 days) in the hospital or chronic-care facility.
   b. Nosocomial: Patient in the hospital at the time the infection developed.

Although considerable overlap in symptoms, signs, and chest X-ray findings are observed in cases of acute community-acquired pneumonia, certain key clinical characteristics are helpful in guiding the physician in determining the most likely etiologies (see Table 4.1). Generation of a logical differential list of potential pathogens guides the choice of diagnostic tests and narrows the possible treatment regimens. Important symptoms that need to be reviewed include the following:

1. **Cough**. Frequency of the cough, production of sputum, and color of the sputum should be documented. A nonproductive cough or a cough that is productive of scanty sputum suggests an atypical pneumonia, while a cough that is productive of rusty-colored sputum raises the possibility of *Streptococcus pneumoniae*. Thick, red, currant jelly sputum has been reported in cases of *Klebsiella pneumoniae*, while green-colored sputum is more frequently encountered in patients with *Haemophilus influenzae* and *Pseudomonas aeruginosa* pneumonia (typically a nosocomial pathogen or found in patients with cystic fibrosis). Frank hemoptysis is observed in

Table 4.1

Clinical Characteristics of Acute Community-Acquired Pneumonia Classified by Etiology

ETIOLOGIC AGENT	CLASSIC SYMPTOMS	TYPICAL CHEST X-RAY FINDINGS
Streptococcus pneumoniae	Rusty-colored sputum, rigors, pleuritic chest pain	Lobar infiltrate, air bronchograms
Aspiration pneumonia	After loss of consciousness poor gag, abnormal swallowing, foul-smelling sputum	Dense consolidation RLL > LLL, posterior segment of upper lobes, later lung abscess and empyema
Actinomycosis	Poor dental hygiene, spontaneous fistula formation, sulfa granules	Same distribution as aspiration, pleural involvement common
Nocardiosis	Associated with inhalation of soil particles, often immunocompromised host, can mimic lung cancer with brain metastasis	Multiple abnormalities including cavitary disease, nodules, diffuse infiltrate, can be associated with brain abscess
Haemophilus influenzae	More gradual onset, smokers with COPD	Lobar or patchy infiltrates
Staphylococcus aureus	Follows influenza pneumonia, rapidly progressive acute disease	Bronchopneumonia, lung abscess, pneumothorax, and empyema
Legionella pneumophila	Nonproductive cough, GI symptoms, confusion	Lobar pneumonia, cavities in immunocompromised host
Atypical pneumonia	Mild to moderate symptoms, nonproductive cough, pulmonary exam often normal	Patchy lower lobe bronchopneumonia

cavitary tuberculosis, lung abscess, and lung carcinoma. It should be emphasized that there is considerable overlap in the sputum characteristics of the various forms of pneumonia, and these observations cannot be considered specific.

2. **Chest discomfort**. Pleuritic chest pain (pain associated with deep inspiration) is classically described in patients with *Streptococcus pneumoniae*. Pain is usually sharp and stabbing. Because the pulmonary parenchyma has no pain-sensing nerves, the presence of chest pain indicates inflammation of the parietal pleura. When the diaphragm becomes inflamed, the pain can mimic that of cholecystitis or appendicitis and on occasion has

precipitated exploratory laparotomy. Anaerobes, *Streptococcus pyogenes*, and *Staphylococcus aureus* are other pathogens that can spread to the pleura and cause chest pain. Pleuritic pain is also characteristic of pleurodynia, a pain syndrome caused by the enteroviruses Coxsackievirus and Echovirus.

3. **Rigors**. Mild chills are encountered in most febrile illnesses. However, a teeth-chattering, bed-shaking chill indicative of a true rigor is usually associated with bacteremia. This symptom is very prominent, and patients often can report the exact time of their first rigor. A single rigor is the rule in pneumococcal infection, while multiple rigors are more typical of *Staphylococcus aureus*, anaerobes,

Klebsiella species, and *Streptococcus pyog-enes*. *Haemophilus influenzae* rarely causes rigors.

4. **Shortness of breath**. When the patient reports increased shortness of breath, this symptom suggests poor alveolar oxygen exchange, indicative of severe infection. Some patients experience shortness of breath as a result of pleuritic chest pain that limits their ability to breathe deeply. To avoid pain, patients may breath quickly and shallowly, and this breathing pattern may be interpreted as shortness of breath.

A careful epidemiologic history is often helpful. A number of environmental factors predispose to pneumonia. Animal exposure must be carefully reviewed, including contact with wild game, birds, bats, and rodents (see Chapter 13, "Zoonotic Infections"). Exposure to outside air-conditioning units or construction sites should be identified (possible sources of Legionnaire's disease). A travel history may be helpful. For example, travel to the U.S. Southwest raises concerns about coccidiomycosis, while travel to the Ohio River valley raises the possibility of histoplasmosis. Because many respiratory illnesses spread from person to person, a history of exposure to family members or friends with illnesses should be ascertained. Finally, an occupational and sexual history should be elicited.

KEY POINTS

The History in Pneumonia

> 1. Cough: Frequency, production of sputum, color and thickness of sputum.
> 2. Chest pain: Pain on deep inspiration, usually sharp = pleural involvement. Seen in *Streptococcus pneumoniae*, *S. pyogenes*, *Staphylococcus aureus*, anaerobes, and coxsackievirus and echovirus.
> 3. Rigors: Bed-shaking chill, one rigor in *S. pneumonia*, more than one in *S. aureus*,

> *Klebsiella* species, *S. pyogenes*, and anaerobes.
> 4. Shortness of breath: A worrisome symptom, may be due to pleuritic chest pain rather than poor gas exchange.
> 5. Epidemiology: Travel history, animal exposure, exposure to people with respiratory illnesses, occupational and sexual history.

A thorough physical examination should be performed during the initial evaluation for possible pneumonia. Vital signs are helpful in determining the severity of illness. A respiratory rate of >30 breaths/minute, a systolic blood pressure of <90 mm Hg, a pulse of >125, and a temperature of <35°C or >40°C are all bad prognostic signs, as is a depressed mental status. Ear, nose, and throat examination may reveal vesicular or crusted lesions consistent with herpes labialis, an infection that may reactivate as a consequence of the stress of the primary illness. Neck stiffness in association with depressed mental status may indicate the development of bacterial meningitis, a potential complication of pneumococcal pneumonia. Pulmonary auscultation often fails to detect the extent of infection; when pneumonia is being considered, the physical exam should be followed by a chest X-ray. Asymmetry of chest movements may be observed, movement being diminished on the side with pneumonia. When infection has progressed to consolidation, as in Case 4.1, filling of the lung parenchyma with exudate alters sound conduction. Air flow from the bronchi is conducted through this fluid to the chest wall, resulting in bronchial or tubular breath sounds. When the patient is asked to say "E," an "A" is heard on auscultation (this is known as egophony). Percussion of the chest wall also demonstrates dullness to percussion in the areas of consolidation. Dullness to percussion in association with decreased breath sounds suggests the presence of a pleural effusion. A "leathery" friction rub may be heard over the site of consolidation and indicates pleural inflammation.

KEY POINTS

The Physical Examination in Pneumonia

1. A respiratory rate > 30/min, BP < 90 mm Hg, pulse > 125/min, and temp < 35°C or > 40°C are bad prognostic findings.
2. Depressed mental status and stiff neck suggest bacterial meningitis.
3. Pulmonary auscultation often underestimates the extent of pneumonia:
   a. Bronchial breath sounds and egophony suggest consolidation.
   b. Dullness to percussion indicates consolidation or a pleural effusion.
   c. Pleural effusion is accompanied by decreased breath sounds and in some cases a friction rub.

Laboratory Findings

A physical exam is unreliable for making the diagnosis of pneumonia. If pneumonia is a potential diagnosis, a chest X-ray must be performed to confirm or exclude this diagnosis. The radiologic pattern can serve as a rough guideline as to possible etiologic agents. However, the use of immunosuppressive agents, resulting in neutropenia, decreased cell-mediated immunity, and depressed macrophage function, can greatly alter the typical radiologic appearance of specific pathogens. Patients with AIDS also present with atypical chest X-rays. Five classic patterns have been described:

1. **Lobar pneumonia**. This refers to a homogeneous radiologic density that involves a distinct anatomic segment of the lung. Infection originates in the alveoli. As it spreads, this form of infection respects the anatomic boundaries of the lung and does not cross the fissures. Lobar pneumonia is most commonly seen in *Streptococcus pneumoniae*, *Haemophilus influenzae*, and Legionella.

2. **Bronchopneumonia**. This form of pulmonary infection originates in the small airways and spreads to adjacent areas. Infiltrates tend be patchy, involving multiple areas of the lung, and are not confined by the pulmonary fissures. Bronchopneumonia is commonly observed with *Staphylococcus aureus*, Gram-negative bacilli, Mycoplasma, Chlamydia, and respiratory viruses.

3. **Interstitial pneumonia**. Infections causing inflammation of the lung interstitium result in a fine, diffuse granular infiltrate. Influenza and cytomegalovirus commonly present with this chest X-ray pattern. In AIDS patients *Pneumocystis carinii* infection results in interstitial inflammation combined with increased alveolar fluid that can mimic cardiogenic pulmonary edema. Miliary tuberculosis commonly presents with micronodular interstitial infiltrates.

4. **Lung abscess**. Anaerobic pulmonary infections often cause extensive tissue necrosis, resulting in loss of lung tissue and formation of cavities filled with inflammatory exudate. *Staphylococcus aureus* also causes tissue necrosis and can form cavitary lesions.

5. **Nodular lesions**. Histoplasmosis, coccidiomycosis, and cryptococcosis can present as multiple or single nodular lung lesions on chest X-ray. Hematogenous pneumonia due to right-sided endocarditis commonly presents with "cannonball" lesions that can mimic metastatic carcinoma.

KEY POINTS

Chest X-ray in Pneumonia

1. If pneumonia is being considered, a chest X-ray should always be performed.
2. Chest X-ray patterns may be atypical in patients receiving immunosuppressants and in patients with AIDS.

3. Five typical chest X-ray patterns are described:
   a. Lobar pattern: *Streptococcus pneumoniae*, *Haemophilus influenzae*, and Legionella.
   b. Bronchopneumonia pattern: *Staphylococcus aureus*, Gram-negatives, Mycoplasma, Chlamydia, and viral.
   c. Interstitial pattern: Influenza and cytomegalovirus, pneumocystis, and miliary TB.
   d. Lung abscess: Anaerobes, *S. aureus*.
   e. Nodular lesions: Fungal (histoplasmosis, coccidiomycosis, cryptococcosis) and right-sided endocarditis.
4. Chest X-ray patterns are only rough guides. Considerable overlap between different pathogens has been observed.

The role of high-resolution chest CT scan is evolving, and this test has proved helpful for more clearly demonstrating interstitial infiltration, pulmonary cavities, nodules, and pleural fluid collections.

Patients with an infiltrate who are 50 years of age or younger, have none of five important co-morbid conditions (neoplastic disease, liver disease, congestive heart failure, cerebrovascular disease, or renal disease), and have normal mental status as well as normal or only mildly deranged vital signs (termed risk Class I by the Pneumonia Patient Outcome Research Team, PORT) can be treated as outpatients. Sputum Gram stain and culture are optional in these patients, as are any additional tests.

In more severely ill patients who are being considered for hospitalization, additional tests need to be ordered to assess the severity of the patient's illness. A complete blood cell and differential count should be ordered. Patients with bacterial pneumonia usually have an elevated peripheral white blood cell count (WBC) and a left shift. When pneumococcal pneumonia is accompanied by a low peripheral WBC (<6,000), a fatal outcome is more likely. The finding of anemia

(Hct < 30%), usually indicative of chronic underlying disease, is also associated with a worse prognosis. Blood oxygenation also needs to be assessed. O_2 saturation should be determined, and if it is at all depressed, an arterial blood gas should be obtained. Systemic acidosis (pH < 7.35) and an arterial partial pressure of <60 mm Hg are bad prognostic signs. A significant depression in oxygenation reflects loss of alveolar function and lack of oxygen transfer to alveolar capillaries. Deoxygenated blood passes from the right side of the heart to the left side, creating a physiologic right-to-left shunt. Other metabolic parameters also need to be assessed. A blood urea nitrogen of >30 reflects hypoperfusion of the kidneys and/or dehydration and is a negative prognostic finding. A serum sodium of <130 mEq/l reflects increased antidiuretic hormone secretion in response to decreased intravascular volume as well as severe pulmonary disease and is another negative prognostic finding, as is a serum glucose of >250 mg/dl. Two blood cultures should be drawn prior to the institution of antibiotics. Positive blood cultures definitively identify the etiology. Blood cultures are positive in 1–16% of cases of community-acquired pneumonia.

KEY POINTS
Blood Tests in Pneumonia

1. With the exception of patients ≤50 years of age without underlying disease and normal vital signs, multiple blood tests are used to assess the severity of disease.
2. A peripheral WBC < 6,000/mm³ in *Streptococcus pneumoniae* is a bad prognostic finding.
3. Anemia (Hct < 30%), BUN > 30, Serum Na < 130 mEq/l, and glucose > 250 mg/dl are associated with a worse prognosis.
4. Arterial blood O_2 < 60 mm Hg and pH < 7.35 worsen prognosis.
5. Two blood cultures should be drawn and are positive in up to 16% of patients.

The sputum requires careful analysis and frequently provides helpful clues to the probable diagnosis. Sputum samples often become contaminated with bacteria and cells from the nasopharynx, making interpretation of cultures difficult. Ideally, the physician should supervise the acquisition of sputum to ensure that the patient coughs deeply and brings up the sample from the tracheobronchial tree, rather than simply expectorating saliva from the mouth. The adequacy of the sample should be determined by low-power microscopic analysis of the sputum Gram stain. The presence of more than 10 squamous epithelial cells per low-power field (lpf) indicates significant contamination from the nasopharynx, and the sample should be discarded. The presence of more than 25 PMNs/lpf, as well as the presence of bronchial epithelial cells, provides strong evidence that the sample originated from the tracheobronchial tree. Despite originating from deep within the lungs, sputum samples usually become contaminated with some normal throat flora as they pass through the nasopharynx. Gram stain can be helpful in differentiating normal flora (mixed Gram-positive and Gram-negative rods and cocci) from the offending pathogen. The predominance of a single type of bacteria suggests that it is the primary pathogen. For example, the presence of more than 10 lancet-shaped Gram-positive diplococci per high-power field provides strong evidence that *S. pneumoniae* is the cause of the pneumonia (approximately 85% specificity, 65% sensitivity) (see Figure 4.1). In reviewing bacterial morphology, the observer must assess the adequacy of decolorization. In the ideally stained regions the nucleus and cytoplasm should be Gram-negative, and a mixture of Gram-positive and Gram-negative organisms should be seen. A Gram-positive nucleus indicates underdecolorization, and the presence of only Gram-negative bacteria, including cocci, suggests overdecolorization. In addition to examining bacterial morphologies, the sputum Gram stain is helpful for assessing the inflammatory response.

The presence of many PMNs suggests a bacterial etiology, while the predominance of mononuclear cells is more consistent with Mycoplasma, Chlamydia, or viral infection.

KEY POINTS
Sputum Gram Stain and Culture

1. Ideally, the physician should supervise sputum collection.
2. Adequacy of the sample is assessed by low-power microscopic analysis:
   a. > 10 squamous epithelial cells = extensive mouth flora contamination.
   b. > 25 PMNs/lfp and/or bronchial epithelial cells = adequate sample.
3. Perform a sputum Gram stain in all seriously ill patients with pneumonia:
   a. Adequate decolorization should be assessed.
   b. Predominance of single organism = probable pathogen.
   c. Predominance of PMNs suggests bacterial pneumonia.
   d. Predominance of mononuclear cells suggest Mycoplasma, Chlamydia, or virus.
4. Sputum culture:
   a. Should never be ordered without an accompanying Gram stain.
   b. Should not be the sole basis for antibiotic treatment.
   c. A positive sputum culture in the intubated patient often represents colonization rather than infection.
   d. Insensitive because mouth flora can overgrow the pathogen.
   e. Helpful for determining antibiotic sensitivity of pathogens identified by Gram stain.

Sputum culture is less helpful than Gram stain because contaminating normal flora frequently overgrow, preventing identification of the true pathogen. To reduce overgrowth, samples should be inoculated on culture media quickly. Rapid processing has been shown to increase the yield for *Streptococcus pneumoniae.* Sputum cultures are falsely negative approximately half the time. Because of the potential problems with sampling error, as well as the inability to accurately quantify bacteria in sputum cultures, sputum should never be cultured in the absence of an accompanying Gram stain. The culture is most helpful in determining the antibiotic sensitivity of potential pathogens. The combination of sputum Gram stain and antibiotic-sensitivity testing may allow the clinician to narrow the spectrum of antibiotic coverage and reduce the likelihood of selecting for highly resistant pathogens. In the intubated patient sputum culture alone should never be the basis for initiating antibiotic therapy. Sputum culture will almost always be positive and often simply represents colonization rather than true infection (see Chapter 1).

Additional methods for analysis of sputum are being developed. The polymerase chain reaction (PCR) is being used to amplify specific strands of DNA from pathogens. This method will be particularly helpful in identifying organisms that normally are not part of the mouth flora and that are difficult to culture: *Legionella pneumophila, Mycoplasma pneumoniae, Chlamydia pneumoniae,* and *Pneumocystis carinii.* When Legionella pneumonia is a consideration (see below), urinary antigen for *L. pneumophila* serogroup 1 (the most common pathogenic serogroup) should be performed. This test is moderately sensitive and highly specific. Therefore a positive test is diagnostic; a negative test does not exclude the diagnosis.

More invasive procedures are usually not required in community-acquired pneumonia but may be considered in the severely ill patient when an adequate sputum sample cannot be obtained. Invasive procedures are more commonly required in the immunocompromised patient (see Chapter 16). In the past transtracheal

aspiration was utilized; however, several deaths have been reported as a consequence of bleeding, and this diagnostic procedure has fallen out of favor. Fiber-optic bronchoscopy with protected brushing or lavage is usually sensitive and specific. The sheath surrounding the brush reduces but does not eliminate contamination by mouth flora. Quantitative cultures are required to differentiate infection from contamination, growth of $>10^3$–10^4/ml indicating infection. Lavage of a lung segment with sterile fluid samples a larger volume of lung and is particularly useful for diagnosing *Pneumocystis carinii* pneumonia in AIDS patients (see Chapter 17). In addition to *P. carinii,* bronchoscopy has been shown to be particularly useful in diagnosing mycobacterial infections and cytomegalovirus.

Empiric Treatment and Outcome

The mainstay of treatment is the administration of antibiotics (see Table 4.2). Antibiotic treatment should not be delayed because of difficulties with sputum collection. Therapy should be started within 6 hours of diagnosis. Delays beyond this time period have been associated with increased mortality. In cases requiring hospitalization for acute community-acquired pneumonia, cefotaxime or ceftriaxone (covers *Streptococcus pneumoniae, Haemophilus influenzae, Staphyloccus aureus,* Klebsiella species, some Gram-negatives, and aerobic mouth flora) combined with a macrolide, either erythromycin, azithromycin, or clarithromycin (covers Legionella, Mycoplasma, Chlamydia), is a reasonable initial choice pending culture results, antibiotic susceptibilities, and clinical response. If aspiration pneumonia is suspected, metronidazole can be added. In the severely ill patient in whom highly resistant *Streptococcus pneumoniae* is suspected, vancomycin may be administered. In ambulatory patients either a macrolide in the form of azithromycin or clarithromycin or a fluoroquinolone possessing good Gram-positive activ-

Table 4.2

Empiric Treatment of Pneumonia (IDSA, 2000)

DRUG	DOSE	RELATIVE EFFICACY	COMMENTS
COMMUNITY-ACQUIRED OUTPATIENT			
Clarithromycin ·	500 mg po BID	First line	
Azithromycin	500 mg po followed by 250 mg po/QD	First line	Low serum levels, high levels in macrophages, preferred for Haemophilus influenzae
Erythromycin	500 mg QID	First line	GI toxicity is common
Gatifloxacin	400 mg po QD	First line	Levofloxacin-resistant *Streptococcus pneumoniae* reported in Canada. Preferred for nursing home residents
Levofloxacin	500 mg po QD		
Moxifloxacin	400 mg po QD		
Doxycycline	100 mg po BID	First line	A bacteriostatic agent
Amoxicillin-clavulanate	875/125 mg po BID	Alternative	Useful if *S. pneumoniae* or *H. influenzae* is suspected
2nd generation cephalosporin		Alternative	Useful if *S. pneumoniae* or *H. influenzae* is suspected
Cefuroxime	500 mg po BID		
Cefpodoxime	400 mg po BID		
Cefprozil	500 mg po BID		
COMMUNITY-ACQUIRED INPATIENT			
Cetriaxone (or)	1 gm iv or im QD	First line	Add vancomycin if penicillin-resistance *S. pneumoniae* is suspected
Cefotaxime (+)	1 gm iv Q8H		
Macrolide (+)	(same doses as above)		
Vancomycin (if seveely ill)	1 gm iv Q12H		
Fluoroquinolone alone		Alternatives	If severely ill, first-line regimen is preferred.
Gatifloxacin	400 mg iv QD		
Levofloxacin	500 mg iv QD		
ASPIRATION (COMMUNITY)			
Penicillin G	2 million iv Q4H	First line	Covers usual mouth flora
Clindamycin	600 mg iv Q8H	First line	Shown to be slightly more effective than PCN for lung abscess
ASPIRATION (IN HOSPITAL)			
Ceftriaxone + metronidazole	1 gm iv QD 500 mg iv Q8H	First line	Regimen used by the author
Fluoroquinolone + metronidazole	(same doses above) 500 mg iv Q8H	First line	
Piperacillin-tazobactam	3/0.375 gm iv Q6H	Second line	Requires a large fluid load
Ticarcillin-clavulainate	3.1 gm iv Q4–6H		

ity such as gatifloxacin, moxifloxacin, or levofloxacin is considered equally efficacious. Erythromycin is the least expensive macrolide and can also be used as first-line empiric therapy. However, the higher incidence of gastrointestinal complaints as well as poor coverage for *H. influenzae* makes erythromycin somewhat less efficacious. Concerns have been raised about the development of resistance to fluoroquinolones, and many experts recommend that this class of antibiotics be reserved for older patients with underlying disease. In addition to the standard causes of community-acquired pneumonia these patients also have an increased incidence of Gram-negative bacilli that will be covered by these fluoroquinolones.

The appropriate duration of treatment has not been systematically studied. For *Streptococcus pneumoniae* patients are generally treated for 72 hours after they become afebrile. For infections with bacteria that cause necrosis of the lung (*Staphylococcus aureus*, Klebsiella, and anaerobes), therapy should probably be continued for two weeks or more. Treatment for two weeks is generally recommended for *Mycoplasma pneumoniae*, *Chlamydia pneumoniae*, and Legionella in the immunocompetent patient. Patients on intravenous antibiotics can generally be switched to oral antibiotics when their clinical condition is improving, they are hemodynamically stable, their gastrointestinal tract is functioning normally, and they are capable of taking medications by mouth. In many cases these criteria are met within 3 days. When possible, the oral antibiotic should be of the same antibiotic class as the intravenous preparation or, if this is not possible, should have a similar spectrum of activity.

The response to treatment can be assessed by monitoring temperature, respiratory rate, pO_2 and oxygen saturation, peripheral white blood cell count, and the frequency of the cough. Chest X-ray changes often persist for several weeks despite clinical improvement. Although chest X-ray is not helpful for assessing improvement, conventional films in combination with pulmonary CT scan can be used to assess the development of complications such as pneumothorax, cavitation, empyema, and adult respiratory distress syndrome (ARDS), as well as to document continued progression of infiltrates despite therapy.

In the United States there are 45,000 deaths per year due to pneumonia. The overall mortality rate ranges from 2% to 30% in hospitalized patients. Mortality from pneumonia and influenza is particularly high in individuals over the age of 65, causing 150–250 deaths per 100,000. Mortality is also higher in individuals with underlying diseases. Five comorbid illnesses have been identified that result in statistically significant increases in mortality: neoplastic disease, liver disease, congestive heart failure, cerebrovascular disease, and renal disease.

KEY POINTS

Treatment and Outcome in Pneumonia

1. Treatment must be instituted within 6 hours of diagnosis. Delays are associated with increased mortality.
2. Empiric therapy:
   a. Hospitalized patient: A third-generation cephalosporin (ceftriaxone or cefotaxime) combined with a macrolide (azithromycin or clarithromycin).
   b. Outpatient: A macrolide (azithromycin or clarithromycin); elderly can consider a fluoroquinolone (gatifloxacin, moxifloxacin, levofloxacin).
   c. If possible aspiration: Add metronidazole.
   d. In the very ill: Penicillin-resistant *Streptococcus pneumoniae* should be covered: vancomycin or a fluoroquinolone. (Experts are concerned about development of fluoroquinolone resistance.)
3. Monitoring improvement by chest X-ray is not recommended. (Chest X-ray can take several weeks to clear.) Useful for documenting worsening or the development of complications.

4. Outcome: Mortality ranges from 2% to 30%. Mortality higher if >65 years of age, neoplastic disease, liver disease, congestive heart failure, cerebrovascular accident, and renal disease.

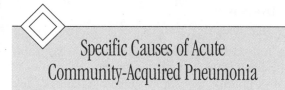

Specific Causes of Acute Community-Acquired Pneumonia

There is great overlap among the clinical manifestations of the pathogens associated with acute community-acquired pneumonia. However, constellations of symptoms, signs, and laboratory findings serve to narrow the possibilities. The ability to focus on a few pathogens or to identify a specific pathogen allows the clinician to better predict the clinical course of pneumonia as well as to narrow antibiotic coverage.

Streptococcus Pneumoniae

PATHOGENESIS

Pathogenic strains of *Streptococcus pneumoniae* contain a thick capsule that prevents PMN binding and blocks phagocytosis. Deletion of the gene that is responsible for capsular polysaccharide production markedly reduces the ability of the pneumococcus to cause disease. Certain capsular types account for most cases (types 1, 3, 4, 7, 8, and 12 in adults and types 3, 6, 14, 18, 19, and 23 in children). These capsular types more effectively resist phagocytosis by macrophages and PMNs. Type 3 has the thickest polysaccharide capsule and is the most virulent strain, being associated with the worst prognosis. Immunoglobulins that specifically recognize the capsule are able to link the bacterium to the

PMN surface through Fc receptors, enabling PMNs and macrophages (classified as phagocytes) to efficiently ingest and kill the pneumococcus. Similarly, the complement product C3b enhances phagocytosis of bacteria by the same mechanism. Immunoglobulins and C3b are called opsonins or products that enhance foreign particle ingestion by phagocytes. In addition to the polysaccharide capsule *S. pneumoniae* possesses a number of other virulence factors that enhance adherence to epithelial cells, resist phagocytosis, and activate complement. *S. pneumoniae* does not produce significant quantities of proteases. Disease manifestations are primarily the consequence of the host's inflammatory response. As a result, permanent tissue damage is rare, and spread across anatomic boundaries such as lung fissures is uncommon.

KEY POINTS

The Pathogenesis of *Streptococcus pneumoniae*

1. The thick outer capsule blocks phagocytosis. Type 3 has the thickest capsule.
2. Immunoglobulins and complement are important opsonins that allow phagocytes to ingest invading pneumococci.
3. Does not produce protease and rarely destroys lung parenchyma.
4. Does not cross anatomic barriers such as lung fissures.
5. Disease manifestations are primarily caused by the host's inflammatory response to the organism.

PREVALENCE AND PREDISPOSING FACTORS

Streptococcus pneumoniae remains the most common etiology of acute community-acquired pneumonia, representing two thirds of the cases in which a specific pathogen is identified. Because opsonins are required for efficient phagocytosis of this encapsulated organism, patients with hypogammaglobulinemia and multiple myeloma are at increased risk for developing this infection, as are patients with deficiencies in complement (C1, C2, C3, C4). Patients with HIV infection also have defects in antibody production and have a higher incidence of pneumococcal infection. Patients with splenic dysfunction have a higher risk of overwhelming *S. pneumoniae* sepsis because the spleen plays a vital role in clearing *S. pneumoniae* from the bloodstream, particularly in the absence of specific antipneumococcal capsule antibody. Other chronic diseases are also associated with greater risk of pneumococcal infection, including cirrhosis, nephrotic syndrome, congestive heart failure, chronic obstructive pulmonary disease, and alcoholism.

KEY POINTS

Streptococcus pneumoniae Prevalence and Predisposing Factors

1. The most common form of community-acquired bacterial pneumonia.
2. Patients with deficiencies in opsonin production have a higher risk:
   a. Hypogammaglobulinemias,
   b. Complement deficiencies,
   c. HIV patients.
3. Splenic dysfunction increases the risk of fatal pneumococcal bacteremia.
4. Patients with chronic diseases are at increased risk:
   a. Cirrhosis,
   b. Alcoholism,
   c. Nephrotic syndrome,
   d. Congestive heart failure,
   e. Chronic obstructive pulmonary disease.

UNIQUE CLINICAL CHARACTERISTICS

Classically, pneumococcal pneumonia has a very abrupt onset that begins with a single severe rigor. Because *Streptococcus pneumoniae*

invasion of the lung leads to capillary leakage of blood into the alveolar space, sputum can become rusty in color. Pneumococcal infection frequently infects the peripheral lung and spreads quickly to the pleura. As a result, pleuritic chest pain is a common complaint.

DIAGNOSIS

SPUTUM GRAM STAIN A careful analysis of the sputum is best performed by a knowledgeable physician. Areas with significant numbers of PMNs/hpf and a predominance of Gram-positive lancet-shaped diplococci suggests the diagnosis (see Figure 4.1). If pneumococci are found within the cytoplasm of a PMN, this finding strongly supports invasive infection.

SPUTUM CULTURE *Streptococcus pneumoniae* is catalase negative and bile soluble and, like *S. viridans*, demonstrates alpha (green) hemolysis on blood agar plates. The propensity of normal mouth flora, in particular *S. viridans*, to overgrow frequently interferes with the identification of *S. pneumoniae*. The Optochin disk inhibits *S. pneumoniae* growth but not *S. viridans* and is used to differentiate the two organisms. Another problem with sputum culture arises from the fact that *S. pneumoniae* can be present as normal mouth flora in up to 60% of healthy people. Therefore a positive sputum culture in the absence of a positive Gram stain or a positive blood culture may simply represent sputum contamination with saliva.

BLOOD CULTURES Some reports have claimed that 25% of patients with pneumococcal pneumonia develop positive blood cultures; however, the denominator required to calculate this percentage is uncertain. Even in the absence of a positive sputum Gram stain, a positive blood culture in combination with the appropriate symptoms and chest X-ray findings is interpreted as true infection. A urine test for pneumococcal polysaccharide antigen is available; however, data in children indicate that the test is unable to differentiate between nasopharyngeal colonization and active infection.

CHEST X-RAY The chest X-ray usually reveals a single area of infiltration involving one or more segments of a single lobe. Involvement of an entire lobe is less common. This organism respects the confining fissures of the lung and rarely extends beyond these boundaries, a feature that explains the classic lobar radiologic pattern (see Figure 4.1). Air bronchograms are found in the minority of cases. This radiologic finding is the consequence of inflammatory fluid filling the alveoli and outlining the air-containing bronchi. Pleural fluid may be detected in up to 40% of cases. In most instances the volume of fluid is too small to sample by thoracentesis, and if antibiotic treatment is prompt, only a small percentage go on to develop true empyema. The radiologic improvement of pneumococcal pneumonia is slow. Despite rapid defervescence and the resolution of all symptoms, X-ray changes often persist for 4–6 weeks. Therefore if the patient is improving clinically, follow-up chest X-rays are not recommended during this time period.

KEY POINTS

Clinical Manifestations and Diagnosis of Pneumococcal Pneumonia

1. Three classic features may be found:
   a. Abrupt onset accompanied by a single rigor,
   b. Rusty-colored sputum,
   c. Pleuritic chest pain.
2. Sputum Gram stain is often helpful; >10/hpf Gram-positive lancet-shaped diplococci = pneumococcal pneumonia.
3. Sputum culture insensitive, plate quickly, alpha hemolytic, Optochin-sensitive.
4. Blood cultures should always be drawn; up to 25% may be positive.

5. Urine pneumococcal antigen test may prove helpful but may be positive in patients who are simply colonized with *Streptococcus pneumoniae*.
6. Chest X-ray classically a lobar pattern, small pleural effusions common, true empyema rare. Abnormalities persist for four to six weeks after cure.

TREATMENT AND OUTCOME

In the early antibiotic era *Streptococcus pneumoniae* was highly sensitive to penicillin (MIC < 0.06 µg/ml). However, over the past decade isolates have become increasingly resistant in the United States, 25–35% demonstrating intermediate resistance (MIC 0.1–1 µg/ml) and a small percentage demonstrating high-level resistance (MIC ≥ 2 µg/ml). In some areas of Europe and South Africa higher percentages of resistant strains have been observed. In the Netherlands and Germany, where strictly limited antibiotic usage is the standard of care, the prevalence of resistant strains is lower. At the present time many intermediate strains remain sensitive to the third-generation cephalosporins ceftriaxone and cefotaxime (MIC ≤ 1 µg/ml); however, resistance to these antibiotics is increasing. For intermediate-resistant strains amoxicillin is more active then penicillin V-K and is the preferred oral antibiotic. Because penicillin resistance is due to a decrease in the affinity of penicillin-binding proteins, intermediate-level but not high-level resistance can be overcome by raising the concentration of penicillin. With the exception of the central nervous system, where the blood-brain barrier limits antibiotic penetration, standard doses of penicillin are effective in curing infections due to intermediately resistant pneumococci. Penicillin resistance is usually associated with resistance to many other classes of antibiotics, including the tetracyclines, macrolides, and clindamycin. Imipenem is inactive against highly resistant strains. The fluoroquinolones that possess good Gram-positive activity (levofloxacin, gatifloxacin, and moxifloxacin), and vancomycin usually retain excellent activity against all resistant strains. Several cases of pneumonia due to levofloxacin-resistant *S. pneumoniae* have recently been reported; however, the overall percentage of pneumococcal strains that are resistant to fluoroquinolones remains low.

For penicillin-sensitive strains, penicillin G or amoxicillin remains the preferred treatment. In the penicillin-allergic patient vancomycin or a fluoroquinolone with Gram-positive activity (levofloxacin, gatifloxacin, or moxifloxacin) can be used (for doses, see Chapter 1). For penicillin-resistant strains vancomycin combined with ceftriaxone or cefotaxime or a fluoroquinolone with Gram-positive activity is recommended. For cases in which meningitis is suspected, a fluoroquinolone should not be used because of poor cerebrospinal fluid (CSF) penetration.

In the preantibiotic era the mortality rate for pneumococcal pneumonia was 20–40%. In the antibiotic era the mortality rate has been reduced to approximately 5%. Prognosis is adversely influenced by (1) age, patients over 65 years of age and infants having a worse outcome; (2) delayed treatment; (3) infection with capsular type 2 or 3; (4) involvement of more than one lobe of the lung; (5) WBC < 6,000; (6) bacteremia, as well as shock or the development of meningitis; (7) jaundice; (8) pregnancy; (9) the presence of other underlying diseases (heart disease, cirrhosis, diabetes); and (10) alcohol intoxication. Mortality is increased by threefold in patients infected with penicillin-resistant pneumococci and sevenfold in patients infected with ceftriaxone-resistant pneumococci.

KEY POINTS

The Treatment, Outcome, and Prevention of Pneumococcal Pneumonia

1. A significant percentage of *Streptococcus pneumoniae* species are resistant to penicillin:

   a. 25–35% intermediate resistance (MIC 0.12–1 μg/ml),

   b. A smaller percentage demonstrate high level resistance (MIC ≥ 2 μg/ml).

2. Penicillin or ampicillin remains the treatment of choice for PCN-sensitive strains.

3. High-dose parenteral penicillin, a third-generation cephalosporin, or oral amoxicillin is used for intermediate-sensitivity strains, except for meningitis.

4. Vancomycin or a fluoroquinolone (gatifloxacin, moxifloxacin, or levofloxacin) is used for high-level resistant strains. Avoid fluoroquinolones in meningitis.

5. Mortality approximately 5%, worse prognosis if >65 years old, infant, treatment delayed, capsular type 2 or 3, multilobar pneumonia, bacteremia or meningitis, jaundice, pregnant, underlying disease, or alcohol intoxication.

6. The 23-valent pneumococcal vaccine is safe and efficacious. Should be given to patients who are >65 years old, have a chronic disease, are asplenic, are immunocompromised, or are alcoholic.

PREVENTION

Despite the use of antibiotics, the mortality rate during the first 36 hours of hospitalization has not changed. To prevent early mortality and reduce the incidence of *Streptococcus pneumoniae* infection (both penicillin-sensitive and -resistant strains), vaccination is strongly recommended for all patients with chronic illnesses or over the age of 65 years.

The generation of specific antibodies directed against the bacterial cell wall confers protection by allowing PMNs and macrophages to quickly ingest the invading pathogen. The generation of increased levels of specific opsonins prevents or reduces the severity of disease. Polyvalent vaccine containing antigens to 23 capsular types is available and is effective (approximately 60% reduction of bacteremia in immunocompetent adults). Efficacy decreases with age and is not measurable in immunocompromised patients. The vaccine has proved to be safe and inexpensive and should be widely used.

Aspiration Pneumonia

◆ **CASE 4.2**

A 35-year-old white male arrived in the emergency room complaining of right-sided chest pain for the past 4 days. Eight days earlier he began drinking large quantities of alcohol. He vaguely recalled passing out on at least two occasions. Four days before admission he developed a persistent cough, productive of green sputum. At that time he also began experiencing right-sided chest pains on deep inspiration (pleuritic pain). Initially, these pains were dull; however, over the next few days they became increasingly sharp.

Physical examination: Temperature 100.4°F, respiratory rate 42/min. A disheveled man, looking older than his stated age, breathing shallowly and rapidly, in obvious pain. Throat: Good gag; extensive dental caries, several loose teeth, severe gingivitis; foul-smelling breath and sputum. Lungs: Decreased excursion of the right lung, dullness to percussion right lower lung field; bronchovesicular breath sounds heard diffusely (inspiratory and expiratory breath sounds of equal duration); moist, medium rales heard in the right lower and left lower lung fields; E to A changes (egophony) as well as whispered pectoriloquy were also heard in these areas.

Laboratory findings: Hct 50, WBC 21,400, 79% PMNs, 7% bands, 1% lymphocytes, 13% monocytes, ABG pH 7.46, pO$_2$ 56, pCO$_2$ 36. Sputum Gram stain: many PMNs, mixture of Gram-positive cocci, Gram-positive rods, and Gram-negative rods. Chest X-ray: dense right lower lobe infiltrate.

While on antibiotics he continued to complain of chest pain and developed decreased breath sounds in the right lower lobe associated with dullness to percussion. A chest CT scan demonstrated a large right pleural effusion (see Figure 4.2), and thoracentesis revealed >100,000 PMNs/mm^3, pleural fluid pH 7.0, and total protein 3.4 mg/ml, and Gram stain showed a mixture of Gram-positive cocci and Gram-positive and Gram-negative rods.

Aspiration pneumonia should be suspected in patients with a recent history of depressed consciousness and in patients with a poor gag reflex or an abnormal swallowing reflex. In Case 4.2 the patient's heavy consumption of alcohol led to depression in consciousness. The elderly patient who has suffered a stroke is particularly susceptible to aspiration. Three major syndromes are associated with aspiration:

1. **Chemical burn pneumonitis**. Aspiration of the acidic contents of the stomach can lead to a chemical burn of the pulmonary parenchyma. Aspiration of large quantities of fluid can result in the immediate opacification of large volumes of lung. Acid damage causes pulmonary capillaries to leak fluid, release cytokines, and infiltrate with PMNs. In some patients noncardiogenic pulmonary edema or ARDS develops. Onset of symptoms occurs immediately after aspiration.

2. **Bronchial obstruction due to aspiration of food particles**. The inhalation of solid particles results in mechanical obstruction and interferes with ventilation, and the patient becomes immediately tachypneic.

3. **Pneumonia due to a mixture of anaerobic and aerobic mouth flora**. Onset of this form of pneumonia develops several days after the aspiration of mouth flora. Patients with severe gingivitis have higher colony counts of bacteria in their mouth and aspirate a higher inoculum of organisms, increasing the likelihood of a symptomatic pneumonia. Case 4.2 had poor dental hygiene and severe gingivitis, predisposing him to this form of pneumonia. Often the sputum is putrid smelling as a result of the high number of anaerobes. Necrosis of tissue is common in this infection, resulting in lung abscess formation. Infection often spreads to the pleura, re-

Figure 4.2

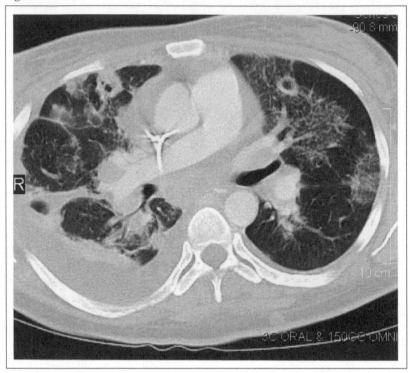

Empyema following aspiration pneumonia. CT scan showing a large right pleural effusion as well as discrete rounded cavitary lesions in the lung parenchyma of both the left and right lower lobes. (Courtesy of Dr. Pat Abbitt, University of Florida College of Medicine.)

sulting in pleuritic chest pain as experienced in Case 4.2. Pleural effusions filled with bacteria and PMNs can develop as observed in this case. An effusion containing bacteria and large numbers of PMNs is called an empyema. Necrosis of the pleural lining and lung parenchyma can result in the formation of a fistula tracking from the bronchus to the pleural space. The development of a bronchopleural fistula prolongs hospitalization and eventually may require surgical repair.

DIAGNOSIS

Sputum is often foul smelling as a result of the high numbers of anaerobic bacteria. Sputum Gram stain reveals many PMNs and a mixture of Gram-positive and Gram-negative organisms. Sputum culture usually grows normal mouth flora. When aspiration occurs in the hospitalized patient, the mouth often is colonized with more resistant Gram-negative organisms as well as *Staphylococcus aureus*. In these patients a predominance of Gram-negative rods or Gram-positive cocci in clusters may be seen on Gram stain, and Gram-negative rods or *S. aureus* may be cultured from the sputum. Chest X-ray reveals infiltrates in the dependent pulmonary segments. When aspiration occurs in the upright position, the lower lobes are usually involved, the right lower lobe being more commonly involved than the left. This difference has an anatomic explanation. The right bronchus takes off from the trachea at a straighter angle than the left mainstem bronchus, increasing the likelihood that aspirated material will flow to the right lung. When aspiration occurs in the recumbent position, the superior segments of the lower lobes or the posterior segments of the upper lobes usually become opacified.

TREATMENT

Clindamycin and penicillin are both effective antibiotic coverage for community-acquired aspiration pneumonia because they kill both aerobic and anaerobic mouth flora. In cases in which lung abscess has developed, clindamycin has been shown to be slightly superior. In nosocomial aspiration broader coverage is generally recommended, with a third-generation cephalosporin combined with metronidazole. Alternatively, a semisynthetic penicillin combined with a β-lactamase inhibitor (ticarcillin-clavulanate or piperacillin-tazobactam) or a carbapenem (imipenem or meropenem) can be used. If aspiration of a foreign body is suspected, bronchoscopy is required to remove the foreign material from the tracheobronchial tree.

KEY POINTS
Aspiration Pneumonia

1. Occurs if there is loss of consciousness, a poor gag reflex, or difficulty swallowing.
2. Three forms of aspiration:
   a. Aspiration of gastric contents: Leads to a pulmonary burn and noncardiogenic pulmonary edema;
   b. Aspiration of an obstructing object: Atelectasis and immediate respiratory distress;
   c. Aspiration of mouth flora: Associated with poor dental hygiene, foul-smelling sputum, mixed mouth aerobes and anaerobes; can lead to lung abscess and empyema. Hospital-acquired aspiration

causes Gram-negative and *Staphylococcus aureus* pneumonia.
3. Treatment:
   a. Penicillin or clindamycin for community-acquired,
   b. Third-generation cephalosporin and metronidazole for hospital-acquired,
   c. Bronchoscopy for obstructing foreign bodies.

Actinomycosis

This microaerophilic or anaerobic Gram-positive rod can be part of the polymicrobial flora associated with aspiration pneumonia, particularly in patients with poor oral hygiene. Disease is most commonly caused by *Actinomyces israelii*. Actinomycosis pulmonary infection is often indolent and slowly progressive. Lung parenchymal lesions are usually associated with pleural infection, resulting in a thickened pleura and empyema. This organism can break through fascial planes. Spontaneous drainage of an empyema through the chest wall should strongly suggest the possibility of actinomycosis. "Sulfur granules" are often found in purulent exudate and consist of clusters of branching Actinomyces filaments. Gram stain reveals branching forms that are weakly Gram-positive. These forms can be differentiated from Nocardia by modified acid-fast stain, Actinomyces being acid-fast negative and Nocardia being acid-fast positive. The organism should be cultured under anaerobic conditions and grows slowly; colonies usually require a minimum of 5–7 days to be identified. Growth can take up to four weeks. High-dose intravenous penicillin (18–24 million units iv QD) is recommended for two to six weeks followed by oral penicillin therapy for six to twelve months. Therapy must be continued until all symptoms and signs of active infection have resolved. Other antibiotics that have been successfully used to treat actinomycosis include erythromycin, tetracyclines, and clindamycin.

KEY POINTS
Actinomycosis

> 1. Branching Gram-positive bacteria, micro-
>   aerophilic or anaerobic, slow growing,
>   modified acid-fast negative.
> 2. Associated with poor oral hygiene.
> 3. Slowly progressive infection, breaks through
>   fascial planes, causes pleural effusions and
>   fistula tracks, forms sulfur granules.
> 4. Alert clinical microbiology laboratory to
>   hold anaerobic cultures.
> 5. Treatment must be prolonged: high-dose IV
>   penicillin for 2–6 weeks, followed by 6–12
>   months of oral penicillin.

Nocardia

This aerobic Gram-positive filamentous bacterium often has to be differentiated from Actinomyces. Nocardia is ubiquitous in the environment, growing in soil, organic matter, and water.
Pneumonia occurs as a consequence of inhaling
soil particles. *Nocardia asteroides* is the most
common species to cause disease. Infection
more commonly develops in patients who are
immunocompromised. However, 40–50% of
cases occur in otherwise normal individuals. Patients with AIDS, organ transplant, alcoholism,
or diabetes are at increased risk of developing
nocardiosis. In addition to pulmonary disease
these patients are at increased risk of developing disseminated infection. Patients with chronic
pulmonary disorders, in particular patients with
alveolar proteinosis, have an increased incidence of pulmonary Nocardia infection.

Onset of pulmonary disease is highly variable. In some cases onset is acute, while in others onset is gradual. Symptoms are similar to
those of other forms of pneumonia. Chest X-ray
may reveal cavitary lesions, single or multiple
nodules, a reticular nodular pattern, an interstitial pattern, or a diffuse parenchymal infiltrate.
Nocardia pulmonary infection often seeds the
bloodstream and forms abscesses in the cerebral

cortex. The combination of a lung infiltrate combined with a central nervous system lesion or lesions is often mistaken for lung carcinoma with
central nervous system metastasis. Diagnosis is
made by sputum examination or lung or cerebral cortex biopsy. Gram stain demonstrates
weakly Gram-positive branching filamentous
forms that are acid-fast on modified acid-fast
stain. On tissue biopsy organisms are demonstrated on Brown-Brenn or methenamine silver
stain. The organism is slow growing and is frequently overgrown by mouth flora on conventional plates. The clinical microbiology laboratory should be alerted to the possibility of
Nocardia so that they incubate bacteriologic
plates for a prolonged period and use selective
media. Nocardia species are sensitive to sulfonamides and trimethoprim. Trimethoprim-sulfamethoxazole is generally accepted as the treatment of choice, with a daily dose of 2.5–10
mg/kg of the trimethoprim component. High-
dose therapy should be continued for at least
six weeks, followed by lower doses for six to
twelve months. High doses of other sulfonamide
preparations are also effective (6–12 gm QD in
four to six divided doses). Nocardia is often sensitive to amikacin, imipenem, third-generation
cephalosporins, minocycline, and dapsone.
However, only anecdotal case reports support
their use.

KEY POINTS
Nocardiosis

> 1. Gram-positive branching bacteria, aerobic,
>   slow growing, modified acid-fast.
> 2. Ubiquitous organism found in the soil.
> 3. Inhalation of soil particles leads to pneu-
>   monia.
> 4. Infects:
>   a. Immunocompromised patients, causes
>   disseminated disease in AIDS,
>   b. Normal hosts,
>   c. Patients with alveolar proteinosis.

5. Pulmonary infection can lead to bacteremia and brain abscess. Can mimic metastatic lung carcinoma.
6. Alert clinical microbiology laboratory to use selective media and to hold cultures.
7. Treatment must be prolonged. High-dose parenteral trimethoprim-sulfamethoxazole for at least six weeks, followed by oral treatment for six months to one year.

2. Nontypable strains more common in the elderly and in smokers with COPD.
3. Clinically similar to *Streptococcus pneumoniae*, somewhat slower onset.
4. Treatment of hospitalized patients: parenteral ceftriaxone or cefotaxime. Multiple oral regimens: amoxicillin-clavulanate, newer macrolides, fluoroquinolones, and extended-spectrum cephalosporins.

Haemophilus influenzae

Both Group B and nontypable *Haemophilus influenzae* can cause community-acquired pneumonia. Infection with nontypable *H. influenzae* is more common in the elderly and in smokers with chronic obstructive pulmonary disease. The onset of symptoms tends to be more insidious in comparison to *Streptococcus pneumoniae* but otherwise is clinically indistinguishable. Chest X-ray can demonstrate lobar or patchy infiltrates, and sputum Gram stain reveals small Gram-negative pleomorphic coccobacillary organisms. Because of their small size and similar color to background material, this pathogen may be missed by the inexperienced diagnostician. For the patient who requires hospitalization, intravenous ceftriaxone or cefotaxime is recommended. For oral antibiotic treatment amoxicillin-clavulanate is effective. However, a number of other oral antibiotics also are active against this organism, including trimethoprim-sulfamethoxazole, the newer macrolides (azithromycin and clarithromycin), the fluoroquinolones, and the extended-spectrum cephalosporins (cefpodoxime, cefixime).

KEY POINTS

Haemophilus influenzae Pneumonia

1. A Gram-negative, small, pleomorphic coccobacilli, aerobic. May be mistaken for background material on sputum Gram stain.

Staphylococcus aureus

Fortunately, community-acquired pneumonia due to *Staphylococcus aureus* is rare. The most common predisposing factor is a preceding influenza infection. An increase in the incidence of *S. aureus* pneumonia is often a marker for the onset of an influenza epidemic. *S. aureus* pneumonia is also more common in intravenous drug abusers and in AIDS patients in association with *Pneumocystis carinii* pneumonia. The clinical manifestations of this infection are similar to those of other forms of bacterial pneumonia. However, the illness is often severe, being associated with high fever and a slow response to conventional therapy. Chest X-ray can demonstrate patchy infiltrates or dense diffuse opacifications. *S. aureus* produces multiple proteases, allowing this bacterium to readily cross the lung fissures and simultaneously involve multiple lung segments, a fact that explains the typical bronchopneumonia pattern seen on chest X-ray (see Figure 4.3). The rapid spread and aggressive destruction of tissue also explain the greater tendency *of S. aureus* pulmonary infections to form lung abscesses and to induce pneumothorax by destroying the parenchymal pleura. Spread of this infection to the pleural space can result in empyema (seen in 10% of patients). Sputum Gram stain reveals sheets of PMNs and an abundance of Gram-positive cocci in clusters and tetrads (see Figure 4.3), and culture readily grows *S. aureus*. Blood cultures may also be positive. The treatment of choice for methicillin-

Figure 4.3

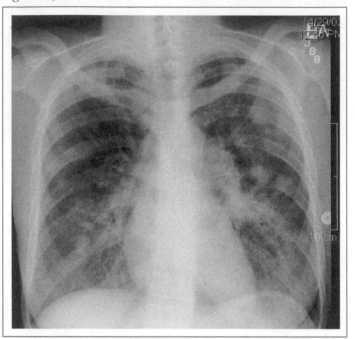

A

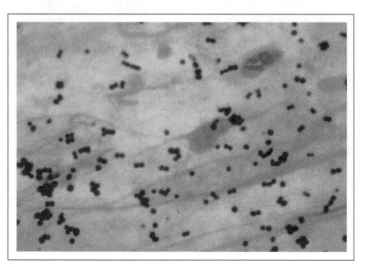

B

Bronchopneumonia due to *Staphylococcus aureus*. **(A)** Chest X-ray demonstrating diffuse macronodular infiltrates of both lung fields in a classic bronchopneumonia pattern. (Courtesy of Dr. Pat Abbitt, University of Florida College of Medicine.) **(B)** Sputum Gram stain showing large Gram-positive cocci in clusters and tetrads. See Figure 4.3B on Color Plate 1.

sensitive *S. aureus* is high-dose intravenous naf-cillin or oxacillin.

KEY POINTS

Staphylococcus Aureus Pneumonia

1. A large Gram-positive aerobic coccus, forms tetrads and clusters.
2. Most commonly follows influenza, seen in AIDS patients and IV drug abusers.
3. Destructive bronchopneumonia, complicated by:
   a. Lung abscesses,
   b. Pneumothorax,
   c. Empyema.
4. Treatment: Parenteral nafcillin or oxacillin for methicillin-sensitive *S. aureus*.

Legionella pneumophila

Legionella species are found throughout the environment in standing water and soil. Infection most commonly results from the inhalation of water droplets contaminated with Legionella. Cooling towers or showerheads are most commonly found to be responsible for aerosolizing contaminated water. Less commonly, nosocomial infection has resulted from the use of unsterilized tap water in respiratory therapy devices. Outbreaks of Legionella pneumonia have also been associated with soil excavation. Immunocompromised patients, smokers, and the elderly are most susceptible to this infection.

Clinically, Legionella causes symptoms that are typical of other acute community-acquired pneumonias, including high fever, cough, myalgias, and shortness of breath. In comparison to other bacterial pneumonias, cough usually produces only small amounts of sputum. Gastrointestinal symptoms and confusion are more frequently encountered in patients with Legionella. Laboratory findings are similar to other acute pneumonias. The only distinctive finding may be hyponatremia noted in approximately one third of patients. Chest X-ray frequently demonstrates a lobar pneumonia. In the immunocompromised host cavitary lesions may be seen. Small pleural effusions are also commonly found.

Diagnosis requires a high index of suspicion because sputum Gram stain reveals only acute inflammatory cells. The clinical microbiology laboratory must be alerted to the possibility of Legionella species to ensure that sputum samples are cultured on buffered charcoal yeast extract agar with added suppressive antibiotics. Legionella can also be identified by direct fluorescent antibody staining; however, the sensitivity of this technique is low (30–50%). Polymerase chain reaction amplification of Legionella DNA from sputum samples is available in certain reference laboratories. For *Legionella pneumophila* serogroup 1, the most common cause of Legionella pneumonia in the United States (>80% of cases), a urinary antigen test is commercially available and is highly sensitive and specific. The antigen is excreted early in the illness and persists for several weeks.

Originally, high-dose intravenous erythromycin was considered the treatment of choice. However, erythromycin treatment is often associated with severe nausea and vomiting, and treatment failures have been reported. Maximum doses of intravenous azithromycin or a fluoroquinolone (ciprofloxacin or levofloxacin) are now recommended for hospitalized patients. In transplant patients a fluoroquinolone is preferred because the macrolides interfere with cyclosporin or tacrolimus metabolism. In the immunocompetent patient therapy should be continued for 5–10 days with azithromycin and 10–14 days with a fluoroquinolone. In the immunocompromised patient, therapy needs to be prolonged for 14–21 days to prevent relapse. Mortality is high in Legionnaires' disease, being 16–30% in community-acquired disease and up to 50% in hospitalized patients.

1. Does not take up Gram stain, aerobic bacteria.
2. Found in soil and standing water. Aerosolized by cooling towers and showerheads. Also contracted after soil excavation.
3. Elderly, smokers, and immunocompromised at increased risk.
4. Similar to other acute pneumonias. Somewhat unique characteristics include:
    a. Minimal sputum production,
    b. Confusion,
    c. GI symptoms,
    d. Hyponatremia.
5. Diagnosis:
    a. Culture on buffered charcoal yeast extract agar,
    b. Direct fluorescent antibody stain (low sensitivity),
    c. PCR available in some areas,
    d. Urinary antigen to serotype I (causes 80% of infections) sensitive and specific, persists for several weeks.
6. Treatment: Azithromycin or a fluoroquinolone is the treatment of choice. In transplant patients fluoroquinolones are preferred. Mortality is high: 16–50%.

Atypical Pneumonia

This form of pneumonia tends to be subacute in onset, patients reporting up to 10 days of symptoms before seeking medical attention. Second, atypical pneumonia is associated with a nonproductive cough. Finally, clinical manifestations tend to be less severe than in other forms of pneumonia. It is important to keep in mind that there is significant overlap in the clinical manifestations of this group of infections and the more typical forms of pneumonia associated with purulent sputum production.

Mycoplasma pneumoniae is one of the most frequent causes of "walking pneumonia." This infection is primarily seen in patients under age 40 years and is an uncommon cause of pneumonia in the elderly. This disease is seasonal, the highest incidence of mycoplasma being in the late summer and early fall. Sore throat is usually a prominent symptom, and bullous myringitis is seen in 5% of cases. The presence of this abnormality is highly suggestive of mycoplasma. Tracheobronchitis results in a hacking cough that is often worse at night and persists for several weeks. An exam may reveal some moist rales; however, radiologic abnormalities classically are more extensive than is predicted by physical exam. Chest X-ray findings consist of unilateral or bilateral patchy lower-lobe infiltrates in a bronchial distribution. The clinical course is usually benign. Fever, malaise, and headache usually resolve over one to two weeks; however, cough can persist for three to four weeks. The peripheral WBC is usually <10,000, and sputum Gram stain and culture reveal only normal mouth flora and a moderate inflammatory response.

Diagnosis is made by history and clinical manifestations. An epidemiologic history of contact with a person having similar symptoms is particularly helpful. At the present time there is no definitive test. PCR of the sputum is under development. Cold agglutinin titers of ≥1:64 support the diagnosis and correlate with severity of pulmonary symptoms. Complement fixation antibody titers begin to rise 7–10 days after the onset of symptoms. Because a reliable rapid diagnostic test is not currently available, therapy is usually empiric. A macrolide or tetracycline is the treatment of choice; alternatively, a fluoroquinolone can be administered. The duration of treatment should be two to three weeks to prevent relapse.

Chlamydia pneumoniae is another important cause of atypical pneumonia, and is a common cause of community-acquired pneumonia, representing 5–15% of cases. The disease occurs sporadically and presents similarly to mycoplasma, with sore throat, hoarseness, and headache in addition to a nonproductive cough. Radiologic findings are also similar to those in mycoplasma.

No rapid diagnostic test is widely available, and treatment is empiric. A tetracycline is considered the treatment of choice. However, the macrolides and fluoroquinolones are also effective.

The final major etiologic group causing atypical pneumonia is the respiratory viruses: influenza A and B, adenovirus, parainfluenza virus, and respiratory syncytial virus. This last virus primarily infects young children, the elderly, and the immunocompromised host. These viruses can all present with a nonproductive cough, malaise, and fever. Auscultatory findings are minimal, and lower-lobe infiltrates are generally observed on chest X-ray. The clinical virology laboratory can culture each of these viruses from sputum or nasopharyngeal swab.

Rapid commercial tests (Quick View, Flu O1A, and Zstatflu) are available for detection of influenza. They take 10–20 minutes and have a sensitivity of 57–77%, and all three can distinguish between type A and type B. If Influenza A virus is diagnosed, early treatment of the virus with amantadine or rimantadine is recommended. Neuraminidase inhibitors are also available, and these agents have activity against both influenza A and B. The influenza vaccine is safe and efficacious and should be given annually in October through early November to patients 65 years of age or older, individuals with serious underlying diseases, nursing home residents, and health care workers.

KEY POINTS
Atypical Pneumonia

1. Tend to be subacute in onset.
2. Cough is nonproductive.
3. Illness is often less severe than other community-acquired pneumonias; "walking pneumonia."
4. Chest X-ray usually worse than the physical findings.

5. Three primary causes:
   a. *Mycoplasma pneumoniae*,
   b. *Chlamydia pneumoniae*,
   c. Respiratory viruses: Influenza, adenovirus, parainfluenza, and respiratory syncytial virus.
6. Treatment with a macrolide or tetracycline is recommended. If influenza is diagnosed, give amantadine, ranitidine, or a neuraminidase inhibitor within 48 hours of the onset of illness.

Nosocomial Pneumonia

Pneumonia is the second most common form of nosocomial infection, accounting for 13–19% of all nosocomial infections. Nosocomial pneumonia is a very serious complication and represents the leading infectious-related cause of death in the hospital, the mortality being roughly one out of three cases. The development of pneumonia in the hospital prolongs hospitalization by more than a week.

The condition that most dramatically increases the risk of nosocomial pneumonia is endotracheal intubation. This tube bypasses the normal protective mechanisms of the lung and increases the risk of pneumonia by twentyfold. It has been estimated that the risk of pneumonia while on a ventilator is 1–3% per day. Other factors that increase the risk of pneumonia include age greater than 70 years; central nervous system dysfunction, particularly coma, leading to an increased likelihood of aspiration; other severe underlying diseases; malnutrition; and metabolic acidosis. Patients on sedatives and narcotics have depressed epiglottal function and are also at increased risk of aspiration. Corticosteroids and other immunosuppressants reduce normal host defenses and allow bacteria to more readily invade the lung parenchyma.

Aerobic Gram-negative bacteria account for over half the cases of nosocomial pneumonia. *Escherichia coli*, Klebsiella, Serratia, and Enterobacter as well as Pseudomonas species represent the most common Gram-negative rods. *Staphylococcus aureus* is the most common Gram-positive pathogen, causing 13–40% of nosocomial pneumonias. The risk *of S. aureus* is higher in patients with wound infections or burns and is also higher in intubated patients with head trauma and post neurosurgery. Anaerobes are often isolated in nosocomial pneumonia but are thought to be the primary agent in only 5% of cases. *Streptococcus pneumoniae* rarely causes pneumonia in patients who have been hospitalized for more than 4 days.

Diagnosis of true pneumonia is often difficult in the intubated patient. In the elderly patient with chronic bronchitis and congestive heart failure or ARDS it is often impossible to prove definitively whether or not the patient has infection. Differentiating infection from colonization represents a critical branch point in appropriately managing antibiotics (see Case 1.1). Once antibiotics have been initiated, the mouth flora and flora colonizing the tracheobronchial tree will change within 3–5 days. Therefore a change in the organisms growing on sputum culture is to be expected and does not, by itself, indicate that the patient has a new infection. This change simply documents that the patient is now colonized with resistant flora. For example, in a high percentage of patients receiving broad-spectrum antibiotics *Candida albicans* begins to grow in sputum cultures as a result of the reduction in the competing bacterial mouth flora. However, this organism does not invade the lung and almost never causes airborne pneumonia. Therefore antifungal coverage is not required unless the patient has developed symptomatic thrush.

Evidence supporting the onset of a new infection include a new fever or a change in fever pattern, a rise in the peripheral white blood cell count with an increase in the percentage of PMNs and band forms (left shift), Gram stain demonstrating increased number of PMNs in as-sociation with a predominance of bacteria that are morphologically consistent with the culture results, increased purulent sputum production from the endotracheal tube, reduced arterial pO_2 indicating interference with alveolar-capillary oxygen exchange, and enlarging infiltrate on chest X-ray. These findings all support the existence of a new infection. When infection is likely or the patient is extremely ill and a new pulmonary infection cannot be convincingly ruled out, the antibiotic regimen will need to be changed to cover for antibiotic-resistant bacteria. In the absence of these findings, colonization is more likely, and the antibiotic regimen should not be changed. Indiscriminate modifications of antibiotic therapy eventually select for highly resistant pathogens that are difficult or in some cases impossible to treat. Switches to broader-spectrum, more powerful antibiotics should be undertaken cautiously and should be initiated only when convincing evidence of a new infection is present. In the patient who is deteriorating clinically, once blood, urine, and sputum cultures and Gram stains are obtained, broader-spectrum coverage can be temporarily instituted. The three-day rule should then be applied (see Chapter 1), and the antibiotic regimen should be modified within 3 days on the basis of the culture results to prevent colonization with even more highly resistant bacteria. The following regimens are recommended for nosocomial pneumonia:

1. Third-generation cephalosporin (ceftriaxone, cefotaxime, ceftizoxime, or ceftazidime)
2. Cefepime
3. Ticarcillin-clavulanate or piperacillin-tazobactam
4. Imipenem or meropenem

These may be given with or without an aminoglycoside (gentamicin, tobramycin, or amikacin). If *Pseudomonas aeruginosa* is suspected, cefepime, imipenem, or meropenem is preferred. If *Staphylococcus aureus* is suspected, vancomycin should be added. Specific anaerobic coverage is usually not required.

KEY POINTS

Nosocomial Pneumonia

1. One of the most common nosocomial infections.
2. Risk factors:
   a. Endotracheal intubation, 20 × increased risk, 1–3% incidence/day,
   b. Age > 70 years,
   c. Depressed mental status,
   d. Underlying disease and malnutrition,
   e. Metabolic acidosis.
3. Gram-negative bacilli and *Staphylococcus aureus* primary causes.
4. Difficult to differentiate colonization from infection. Factors that favor infection:
   a. Worsening fever and leukocytosis with left shift,
   b. Sputum Gram stain: Increased PMNs, predominance of one organism,
   c. Decreasing pO_2 indicative of pulmonary shunting,
   d. Expanding infiltrate on chest X-ray.
5. Broad-spectrum empiric therapy can be initiated after cultures but should be adjusted on the basis of culture results and clinical response.

Empyema

Etiologies

Infection of the pleural space most commonly is the consequence of spread of pneumonia to the parietal pleura. Over half of cases of empyema are associated with pneumonia. The most common pathogens in this setting are *Streptococcus pneumoniae, Staphylococcus aureus, Streptococcus pyogenes,* and anaerobic mouth flora. Empyema is also a complication of trauma and surgery. When these are the inciting factors

Staphylococcus aureus and aerobic Gram-negative bacilli predominate. In the immunocompromised patient fungi and Gram-negative bacilli are most commonly encountered.

Pathophysiology

Pleural effusions occur in approximately half of all pneumonias; however, only 5% of pneumonias develop true empyema. Because pleural fluid is deficient in the opsonins, IgG, and complement, if bacteria can find their way to this culture media, PMNs ineffectively phagocytose the invading pathogens. As PMNs break down in this closed space, they release lysozyme, bacterial permeability-increasing protein, and cationic proteins. These products slow the growth of bacteria, lengthening doubling times by 20- to 70-fold. The slow growth of bacteria renders them less sensitive to the cidal effects of antibiotics. The pH of the empyema cavity is low, impairing white blood cell function and inactivating some antibiotics, in particular aminoglycosides.

Clinical Manifestations

Persistent fever despite appropriate antibiotic treatment for pneumonia should always raise the possibility of an enclosed pleural infection. Fever is often accompanied by chills and night sweats. Pleuritic chest pain is a common complaint, as is shortness of breath. A physical exam is helpful in detecting large effusions. As was noted in Case 4.2, the area where fluid is collecting is dull to percussion, and breath sounds are decreased. At the margin between the fluid and aerated lung, egophony as well as bronchial breath sounds are commonly heard, reflecting areas of pulmonary consolidation or atelectasis.

On chest X-ray fluid collections as small as 25 ml can alter the appearance of the hemidiaphragm on the PA view, while on lateral views, 200 cc of fluid is generally required to blunt the posterior costophrenic angle. A lateral decubitus view with the pleural effusion side down can demonstrate layering of 5–10 ml of free fluid. Ultrasound is very useful in determining the dimensions of the effusion and is the most effective method for guiding thoracentesis. Septations are readily visualized by this technique and indicate the development of a loculated collection that requires drainage. Contrast-enhanced chest CT is particularly helpful in differentiating lung abscess from empyema and demonstrates the full extent of the effusion and the degree of pleural thickening.

When empyema is a strong consideration, a thoracentesis should be performed under ultrasound guidance. Ultrasound guidance of thoracentesis is strongly recommended because of the associated decreased incidence of complicating pneumothorax. The fluid should be analyzed for cellular content, and Gram stain, fungal stain, AFB stain, aerobic, and anaerobic cultures should be obtained. If the fluid is frankly purulent, the pleural space should be completely drained. If the fluid is not overtly purulent, the fluid should also be analyzed for pH, glucose, LDH, and total protein. A pleural fluid pH of <7.2, a glucose of <40 mg/dl, and an LDH of ≥1000 IU/l are consistent with empyema and justify pleural fluid drainage to prevent loculation, pleural scarring, and restrictive lung disease.

Treatment

Antibiotic therapy for the offending pathogen is of primary importance, and antibiotic coverage depends on the pathogen identified by sputum or pleural fluid Gram stain and culture. When a significant pleural fluid collection is apparent, a more prolonged course of antibiotics is generally required, two to four weeks. Parapneumonic effusions that move freely and are less than 1 cm in width on lateral decubitus film can be managed medically and don't require thoracentesis. If the collection is larger and/or does not flow freely, thoracentesis should be per-

formed. If biochemical evidence for empyema is present, chest tube drainage is recommended. Repeated thoracentesis is rarely successful in completely draining the pleural fluid collection unless the fluid has a thin viscosity and is present in small volumes. Closed chest tube drainage is usually successful, with smaller effusions occupying up to 20% of the hemithorax, but often is ineffective when the volume of fluid occupies ≥40% of the hemithorax. Interventional radiology is required to place French catheters precisely at sites of loculation and to break up areas of adhesion under CT guidance. If tube drainage proves ineffective after 24 hours, intrathoracic urokinase (125,000 units diluted in 50–100 cc of sterile normal saline) should be instilled in the pleural space, left for 2 or more hours, and then removed. This treatment breaks down intrapleural fibrin and allows free drainage of infected fluid. If thoracentesis and urokinase are unsuccessful, the chest surgeon must be called. Video-assisted thoracoscopy has proved to be an effective method for decorticating areas of pleural scarring and thickening and allows reexpansion of trapped lung. Empyema is a serious complication and is associated with an 8–15% mortality rate in young, previously healthy patients and a 40–70% mortality rate in elderly patients and those with significant underlying disease. Patients with nosocomial pathogens and polymicrobial infection also have a worse prognosis. Delay in diagnosis and in appropriate drainage increases the need for surgical resection of the pleura and manual reexpansion of the lung.

KEY POINTS

Empyema

1. Suspect if fever persists despite appropriate antibiotic treatment of pneumonia.
2. Most common with *Streptococcus pneumoniae*, *Staphylococcus aureus*, *Streptococcus pyogenes*, and mouth anaerobes.

3. Chest X-ray with lateral decubitus is sensitive; CT scan can also be helpful.

4. If empyema is being considered, an ultrasound guided thoracentesis should be performed.

5. pH < 7.2, glucose < 40 mg/dl, and LDH > 1000 strongly suggest empyema.

6. Tube drainage initially; if continuing to loculate, urokinase can be given. May require surgical intervention.

7. Early diagnosis and drainage prevent lung and pleural compromise.

8. Mortality associated with empyema is high: 8–15% in the young and 40–70% in the elderly.

Chronic Pneumonias

Tuberculosis

The miliary form of disease can be fatal. Clinicians must maintain a high index of suspicion for tuberculosis in immigrants, the indigent, the elderly, and patients with AIDS.

◆ CASE 4.3

A 73-year-old African American male, retired bartender, came to the emergency room complaining of increasing shortness of breath and worsening cough over the past three weeks. Five months earlier he began noting night sweats that drenched his pajamas. This was followed by the development of a nonproductive cough. One month ago he began bringing up small quantities of yellow sputum. Also at this time he began experiencing increased shortness of breath following even mild exertion (walking two blocks to the grocery store). Over the past several months he has felt very tired and has lost 10 lb despite a "good" diet.

Epidemiology: Lives in the city. Visits with a number of old drinking buddies. He denied exposure to anyone with tuberculosis and had no family history of tuberculosis.

Past medical history: He was noted to have an abnormal chest X-ray 20 years earlier and had been treated at Bellevue Hospital in NYC with isoniazid (INH) and para-aminosalicylic acid (PAS) for 1 year.

Social history: Bartender for 35 years. Recently retired. Lives alone in a one-bedroom apartment. Supported by Social Security.

Habits: Former smoker, 1/2 pack per day × 28 years. Drinks 1/2 pint/day.

Physical examination: Temperature 100.4°F, respiratory rate 18. A thin male breathing comfortably. Aside from mild clubbing of his nail beds his physical findings (including lung exam) were within normal limits.

Laboratory workup: Hct 39, WBC 6,000, 55% PMNs, 30% lymphocytes, 15% monocytes. Sputum Gram stain: Many PMNs, few Gram-positive cocci, and rare Gram-negative rods. Chest X-ray: Bilateral upper-lobe cavitary lesions (see Figure 4.4). Acid-fast stain of the sputum revealed multiple acid-fast bacilli per high-power field (see Figure 4.4).

PATHOGENESIS

Mycobacterium tuberculosis is an aerobic, nonmotile bacillus with a waxy, lipid-rich outer wall containing high concentrations of mycolic acid. This waxy outer wall fails to take up Gram stain. To visualize mycobacteria, they must be heated to melt the outer wall to allow penetration and binding of the red dye fuchsin. The lipids in the cell wall bind this dye with high affinity and resist acid-alcohol decolorization. The acid-fast bacillus is small and appears beaded (see Figure 4.4). The high lipid content allows mycobacteria to survive in the external environment and resist drying as well as many chemical disinfectants. This unique cell wall also allows the bacterium to resist killing by macrophages and PMNs and to survive for many years within the body. The rate of growth is very slow, being about 1/20th of the growth rate of most conventional bacteria. The slow rate of growth may also be ex-

Figure 4.4

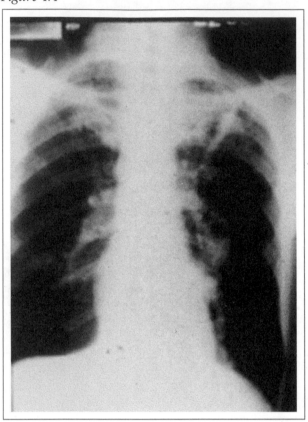

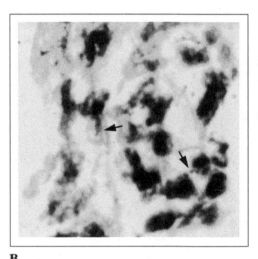

A   **B**

Bilateral apical infiltrates due to *Mycobacterium tuberculosis*. **(A)** Chest X-ray demonstrating bilateral upper lobe cavitary lesions. **(B)** AFB sputum smear showing small beaded-appearing acid-fast bacilli. See Figure 4.4B on Color Plate 1.

plained by the waxy cell wall, which limits access to nutrients.

As mycobacteria survive and grow in macrophages, they induce a profound chronic inflammatory response that accounts for the clinical manifestations of tuberculosis. This inflammatory response takes approximately one month to develop. On gaining entry into the lungs, the organisms are ingested by alveolar macrophages and transported to the hilar lymph nodes. Here macrophages and dendritic cells present tubercular antigens to T cells, inducing a cell-mediated immune response. Helper T cells (CD4+) then activate macrophages to kill the

mycobacteria and control the infection. Accumulation of one of the cell wall waxes, cord factor, stimulates the formation of granulomas that contain clusters of epithelioid cells, giant cells, and lymphocytes. Over time the centers of the granulomas become necrotic, forming cheesy debris that is termed caseous necrosis. Caseating granuloma are the hallmark lesion of tuberculosis. This pathologic finding is only rarely found in other diseases. If intracellular growth of *Mycobacterium tuberculosis* continues, increasing numbers of macrophages are activated to produce multiple cytokines. Interleukin-1 stimulates the hypothalamus to raise core body temperature, causing fever. Tumor necrosis factor interferes with lipid metabolism and causes severe weight loss. These cytokines are primarily responsible for the symptoms of fever, night sweats, and weight loss described in Case 4.3.

KEY POINTS

The Pathogenesis of Tuberculosis

1. Slow-growing, aerobic rod, not seen on Gram stain. The lipid-rich outer wall binds the red dye fuchsin and is not removed by acid, making the bacterium acid-fast.
2. The lipid wall also allows the bacterium to resist drying and many disinfectants. In addition, it allows the bacterium to survive within macrophages for years.
3. Macrophages carry the mycobacterium to the lymph nodes, where a cell-mediated immune response is generated.
4. Caseating granulomas are formed as a consequence of the cell-mediated immune response and the accumulation of lipid-rich bacteria.
5. Increased levels of IL-1 cause fever, and increased levels of tumor necrosis factor cause weight loss.

EPIDEMIOLOGY

The human is the only reservoir for *Mycobacterium tuberculosis*. Person-to-person spread of infection is almost exclusively caused by the inhalation of droplet nuclei that have been aerosolized by coughing or sneezing. The likelihood of inhaling infectious droplets is greatly increased in a closed, crowded environment. A single cough has been estimated to form 3,000 infectious droplets; sneezing produces even higher numbers. The infectiousness of an individual patient can be estimated by AFB smears; the higher the number of organisms per microscopic field, the greater is the infectious potential. Patients with laryngeal tuberculosis are particularly infectious and can release large

numbers of organisms while speaking. Patients with AIDS and tuberculosis often harbor large burdens of organisms. Finally, patients with large pulmonary cavities tend to intermittently release large numbers of infectious particles. Repeated exposure and close contact are generally required to contract this disease. Respiratory isolation and rapid treatment of infected persons are the primary ways to prevent spread of infection. Because this infection is spread by aerosolization, the sterilization of dishes, eating utensils, and clothing has no significant impact on the spread of disease.

Despite the availability of antituberculous agents, tuberculosis remains a leading cause of death worldwide. Crowded living conditions and the existence of immunologically naïve populations continue to allow rapid person-to-person spread, particularly in underdeveloped countries. In the United States after a surge in cases during the mid-1980s due to the AIDS epidemic, the number of cases has steadily declined, reaching the lowest level ever recorded in 1997: 7.4 cases per 100,000. This steady decline among permanent U.S. residents contrasts with the steady increase in the percentage of tuberculosis cases among individuals immigrating to the United States. Immigrants now account for nearly 40% of all reported cases in the United States. Individuals immigrating from underdeveloped countries have higher rates of infection. For example, Vietnamese immigrants have rates of 120 per 100,000 person years, and Haitian immigrants have a rate of 133 per 100,000, while those immigrating from established market economies such as Western Europe have a rate of only 5.4 per 100,000.

Tuberculosis occurs more frequently in single males, alcoholics, intravenous drug abusers, the urban poor (particularly the homeless), migrant farm workers, and prison inmates. The elderly are more likely to develop secondary tuberculosis because cell-mediated immunity wanes in the later years. There is a genetic predisposition for the development of active tuberculosis. Individuals with a European heritage tend to be more resistant, probably as a consequence of the devastating effects of the tuberculosis epidemic during the Industrial Revolution. At that time tuberculosis was responsible for one fourth of the deaths in Europe, killing off a significant percentage of the population who possessed a reduced immune response to mycobacteria. African Americans, Hispanics, Asian Pacific Islanders, and Native Americans suffer a five to ten times higher incidence of tuberculosis compared to Caucasians. AIDS patients are particularly susceptible to tuberculosis, and this population has been responsible for spreading this infection to others. Therefore areas and demographic groups where AIDS is most prevalent have a higher incidence of tuberculosis. The patient in Case 4.3 had a number of the epidemiologic characteristics that increased his risk for tuberculosis: He was a single male, African American, possibly alcoholic, and elderly.

KEY POINTS
The Epidemiology of Tuberculosis

1. Humans are the only reservoir of the disease.
2. Person-to-person spread via aerosolized infectious droplets following sneezing or coughing.
   a. Laryngeal tuberculosis is highly infectious.
   b. HIV patients release large numbers of organisms.
   c. Large cavitary lesions are also highly infectious.
3. Persons at increased risk:
   a. Immigrants from developing countries,
   b. Alcoholics,
   c. Urban poor,
   d. Single males,
   e. IV drug abusers,
   f. Migrant farm workers,
   g. Prison inmates,
   h. The HIV infected,
   i. The elderly.
4. A genetic predisposition: African Americans, Hispanics, Asian Pacific Islanders, and Native Americans 5–10 times higher incidence than Caucasians.

CLINICAL MANIFESTATIONS

PRIMARY TUBERCULOSIS   There are two forms of human infection: primary tuberculosis and secondary tuberculosis. Primary disease occurs when a patient inhales infectious *Mycobacterium tuberculosis* droplets for the first time. A flulike illness usually follows; however, some individuals experience no symptoms. Within four to eight weeks of exposure the human host usually mounts a cell-mediated immune response. Activated macrophages control the spread and growth of the organisms. Pulmonary lesions heal spontaneously and form areas of fibrosis or calcification called Ghon lesions. A Ghon lesion in combination with hilar adenopathy is called a Ranke complex. In addition to transporting organisms to the hilum and mediastinum, infected macrophages may gain access to the thoracic duct, enter the bloodstream, and spread throughout the body. *M. tuberculosis* grows best in regions with high oxygen tension, including the kidneys, long bone epiphyses, and vertebral bodies. This organism most commonly infects the apices of the lung, which are the regions of the lung with the highest oxygen content. Because the capillaries extracting oxygen from the apices are above the heart, blood transport and oxygen extraction from the alveoli are less efficient in this region of the lung.

Although infection is brought under control, the bacilli usually are not completely eradicated. Organisms can survive for decades, being held in check by the host immune response. However, any condition that subsequently depresses cell-mediated immunity can free *Mycobacterium tuberculosis* to grow and cause symptomatic secondary tuberculosis.

KEY POINTS

Primary Tuberculosis

1. Represents the first exposure to inhaled infectious particles.
2. Followed by a flulike illness.
3. Spread controlled over 4–8 weeks by the development of cell-mediated immunity.
4. Ghon complex is cluster of calcified lung lesions at the site of the primary infection.
5. Bacteremia develops and seeds the kidneys, epiphyses of the long bones, and vertebral bodies. These areas contain high oxygen content and can later reactivate.
6. Apical infection is most common; reduced capillary extraction of oxygen from the alveoli makes this the most favorable area for *Mycobacterium tuberculosis* survival.

MILIARY TUBERCULOSIS In a minority of individuals initial exposure to *Mycobacterium tuberculosis* fails to induce cell-mediated immunity, or the immune response is not robust enough to control the infection. Under these conditions mycobacteria continue to multiply and disseminate, causing miliary tuberculosis. The very young and the very old are at higher risk of developing disseminated disease, as are patients receiving immunosuppressants and patients with HIV infection. Underlying medical conditions are often associated with miliary tuberculosis, including alcoholism, malignancy, connective tissue diseases, renal failure, and pregnancy. However, it must be emphasized that absence of an underlying disease does not exclude the possibility of miliary tuberculosis.

Children usually present to the physician with high fever, night sweats, weight loss, hepatosplenomegaly, and lymphadenopathy. However, in adults, particularly the elderly, the clinical manifestations may be subtle. Patients usually have nonspecific complaints of fever, malaise, anorexia, weakness, and weight loss. Night sweats are also common. A physical exam usually reveals a chronically ill patient with no specific findings. In some patients lymphadenopathy may be detected. Funduscopic exam should be carefully performed following pupillary dilation in all patients and may reveal choroid tubercles in up to 50% of cases. The diagnosis is often missed, and in up to 20% of cases the diagnosis is made postmortem. The peripheral WBC is usually normal; however, some patients develop extremely high white blood cell counts (30,000–40,000 WBC), also termed a leukemoid reaction, which can be mistaken for leukemia. Pancytopenia can also develop. Liver function abnormalities are common, an elevated alkaline phosphatase and moderate increases in transaminase values being found in most patients. Serum sodium may be low as a consequence of adrenal insufficiency (a well-known complication of miliary tuberculosis) or inappropriate antidiuretic hormone secretion. Serum A.M. and P.M. cortisol levels should be measured to exclude adrenal insufficiency. In approximately two thirds of patients the chest X-ray reveals small nodules (0.05–1 mm in diameter) that resemble millet seeds (the basis for the name "miliary"); however, a negative chest X-ray in the elderly and in patients with HIV does not exclude this diagnosis. In a minority of patients ARDS may develop, causing complete opacification of the lungs.

The key to the diagnosis of miliary tuberculosis is a high index of suspicion. Sputum smears are positive in the minority of patients. Therefore samples from enlarged lymph nodes, liver biopsy, and bone marrow samples should be sought for histopathology (may reveal granulomas and acid-fast bacilli) and culture. Transbronchial biopsy can yield the diagnosis in a large percentage of patients. Blood cultures for mycobacteria should be drawn and are commonly positive in AIDS patients. If central nervous system symptoms are noted, a lumbar puncture should also be performed, although smears are usually negative. A delay in treatment can have fatal consequences. Therefore if miliary tuberculosis is high on the clinician's differential diagnosis, empiric antituberculous therapy should be initiated once cultures have been obtained. A four-drug regimen consisting of INH, rifampin, pyrazinamide, and ethambutol is the preferred regimen. Patients usually defervesce within 7–14 days.

KEY POINTS

Miliary Tuberculosis

1. Develops in the very young and very old and in HIV-infected patients.
2. Also associated with alcoholism, malignancy, connective tissue diseases, renal failure, and pregnancy.
3. In children presents with high fever, night sweats, weight loss, hepatosplenomegaly, and lymphadenopathy.
4. In adults usually presents with moderate to low-grade fever, night sweats, malaise, anorexia, weakness, and weight loss.
5. Look for choroid tubercles in the fundi (present in up to 50%).
6. Leukemoid reaction, anemia, hyponatremia, abnormal liver function tests. May also have adrenal insufficiency.
7. Chest X-ray: Micronodular interstitial pattern, may be negative in the elderly and in HIV-infected patients.
8. Blood cultures, transbronchial, bone marrow, and liver biopsy may all yield positive cultures.
9. Early treatment for all suspected cases with INH, rifampin, ethambutol, and pyrazinamide.

SECONDARY TUBERCULOSIS The reactivation of tuberculosis after primary disease occurs in 10–15% of patients. In half of the cases the infection reactivates within two years of exposure. In past decades reactivation most commonly occurred in the elderly; however, in the United States the majority of secondary cases are now reported in middle-aged adults (age 30–50 years). Early in the course of reactivation patients are often asymptomatic, and evidence of reactivation is found only by chest X-ray. However, if the infection is not detected, symptoms slowly develop and worsen over several months. The gradual onset of symptoms often causes the patient to delay seeing a physician. The patient in Case 4.3 had the typical symptoms of secondary tuberculosis: progressively worsening cough with sputum production, low-grade fever, night sweats, fatigue, and weight loss. Other symptoms that suggest more advanced disease are hemoptysis (indicating erosion of a tuberculous cavity into an arteriole) and pleuritic chest pain (suggesting pleural involvement and probable tuberculous pleural effusion).

A physical exam is often unrevealing, as was observed in Case 4.3. Despite the presence of extensive pulmonary disease, auscultation may be normal. Fine rales may be heard in the apices after a short cough and quick inspiration or after full expiration followed by a cough and rapid inspiration (posttussic rales). Decreased breath sounds and dullness to percussion at one or both bases are present with tuberculous pleural effusions.

The hallmark of secondary pulmonary disease is the presence of apical cavitary lesions on chest X-ray. Lesions usually develop in posterior segments of the upper lobes just below the clavicle. Less frequently, infiltrates are noted in the apex of the lower lobe, which is usually obscured by the heart shadow. In addition to routine chest PA and lateral films, an apical lordotic view is often helpful in visualizing upper-lobe apical lesions. Chest CT scan is helpful for assessing the extent of disease as well as for defining the size of the cavities. Unlike conventional lung abscess, tuberculous cavities uncommonly have air fluid levels. In patients with AIDS, infiltrates may be in any region of the lung and may not cavitate. Therefore any HIV-infected patient with a new pulmonary infiltrate should be considered to have tuberculosis until proven otherwise.

Individuals with cavitary disease are potentially very infectious. Cavities may contain 10^9–10^{10} organisms. Patients should be placed in respiratory isolation while sputum AFB smears and cultures are obtained. The number of organisms seen on smear directly correlates with infectiousness; the higher the number of organisms per microscopic field, the higher is the likelihood of infecting others.

KEY POINTS
Secondary Tuberculosis

1. Reactivation occurs in 10–15% of patients, half within 2 years of primary disease.
2. Most commonly occurs in males 30–50 years old.
3. Symptoms slowly progress over several months; worsening cough with sputum production, low-grade fever, night sweats, fatigue, and weight loss.
4. Hemoptysis or pleuritic pain indicates severe disease.
5. Physical exam usually has minimal findings, posttussic rales.
6. Chest X-ray: Apical cavities (without fluid), order an apical lordotic view; CT scan often helpful.
7. Cavitary disease very infectious, cavities contain 10^9–10^{10} organisms. Isolate all patients. In HIV, chest X-ray often does not show cavities, and all AIDS patients with pneumonia are considered to have tuberculosis until proven otherwise.

DIAGNOSIS

The classic test for making the diagnosis of pulmonary tuberculosis is the Ziehl-Neelsen acid-fast sputum smear. Morning sputum samples tend to have the highest yield. A single negative smear should not delude the clinician into a false sense of security. Three sputum smears are recommended because in cavitary disease the release of infectious droplets is intermittent. Only after three smears are negative should the patient be declared to be at low risk for spreading infection. Negative smears do not definitively exclude tuberculosis.

To be smear-positive, the sputum must contain 1×10^4 organisms per milliliter. A fluorochrome stain using auramine-rhodamine is more sensitive and allows sputum to be examined at low magnification (20 or 40×), compared to conventional AFB smears, which must be examined at high magnification (100×). Sputum smear has only a 60% sensitivity in comparison to sputum culture. PCR can effectively detect as few as 10 organisms in a clinical specimen. Two assays, one using mycobacterial RNA as its initial template and the other using mycobacterial DNA, are commercially available. Sensitivity and specificity are greater than 95% in smear-positive cases, and specificity in smear-negative cases is high. False-negative and false-positive results are common in less experienced laboratories, and at this time nucleic acid amplification assays are recommended only to complement traditional methods. Furthermore, PCR cannot differentiate killed from actively growing organisms in patients on antituberculous therapy.

Culture remains the most accurate method for diagnosing *Mycobacterium tuberculosis*. In patients who fail to produce sputum, aspiration of the gastric contents in the morning prior to arising from bed is useful for obtaining samples for culture. In patients with suspected disseminated disease, blood cultures in which all cells are lysed to release intracellular mycobacteria should be collected. This bacterium grows at about 1/20th the rate of more conventional bacteria and takes three to six weeks to grow on Lowenstein Jensen media. Living mycobacteria can be more quickly detected in blood, sputum, pleural fluid, or CSF using the BACTEC radiometric culture system, which is designed to detect mycobacteria metabolism within 9–16 days. Drug susceptibilities can also be reliably tested by using this method.

The Diagnosis of Tuberculosis

1. Ziehl-Neelsen acid-fast stain can detect 1×10^4 organisms/ml, 60% sensitivity.
2. Release of acid-fast bacilli from cavitary lesions is intermittent. Need three negative smears to ensure low infectivity.
3. Culture remains the most sensitive and specific test:
   a. *Mycobacterium tuberculosis* grows at 1/20th the rate of conventional bacteria.
   b. Automated techniques can detect bacteria within 9–16 days.
   c. Conventional Lowenstein Jensen media in 3–6 weeks.
4. PCR is available but should be performed only by experienced laboratories.

TREATMENT

The principles of antituberculous therapy as well the specific first-line and second-line antituberculous agents are described in Chapter 1. Prolonged therapy is required to kill dormant organisms in necrotic lesions. Second, because the number of mycobacterial organisms in the host is high, particularly in cavitary pulmonary disease, the potential for selecting drug-resistant mycobacteria is high. To prevent the development of resistance, therapy should always include two or more antituberculous medications. For example, if INH alone were used to treat active infection, 1×10^6 organisms would be expected to be naturally resistant to INH. Therefore in cavitary lesions containing 10^9–10^{10} organisms, 100–1,000 organisms would be expected to survive initial exposure to INH, multiply, and continue to cause disease. Administration of two drugs should kill all the organisms because the probability of selecting for a resistant organism is predicted to be 1×10^{12} organisms ($10^6 \times 10^6$) for two-drug therapy. These calculations assume that the tuberculous organism is sensitive to both drugs. However, this assumption is not always true, particularly

in large urban areas, where INH-resistant *Mycobacterium tuberculosis* is found in over 10% of cases. Resistance to two or more drugs, termed multidrug-resistant *M. tuberculosis* (MDR-TB), may also be encountered. MDR-TB was a major concern in the early 1990s in the United States, particularly in New York state, where in 1991, 12.9% of *M. tuberculosis* cases were resistant to both INH and rifampin. By 1998 improved infection control measures and the use of four-drug regimens as well as directly observed therapy had reduced the incidence of MDR-TB to 2% in New York City. Resistant tuberculosis strains that are cultured from patients who were previously treated for drug-sensitive tuberculosis are said to be secondarily resistant. Secondary resistance is a major problem among the homeless, illicit drug users, and AIDS patients. Primary resistance is defined as infection with a resistant strain in a patient who has never received antituberculous drugs.

Outside the United States the percentage of strains that are resistant to INH and MDR varies widely. The worldwide median frequency of primary INH resistance is estimated to be 7.3%, with higher levels being observed in Asia, Africa, and Latin America and low levels being observed in Europe and Oceania. The worldwide incidence of primary MDR-TB is 1.4%. However, rates of secondary MDR-TB are high, 13%, being particularly high in countries where tuberculosis control programs have deteriorated (e.g., Latvia, South Korea, and Russia).

The recommended treatment of pulmonary tuberculosis where a drug-sensitive infection is most likely is a four-drug regimen pending sensitivity tests: INH, rifampin, pyrazinamide, and ethambutol or streptomycin. This regimen is recommended for two months followed by INH, rifampin, and pyrazinamide for four months. If MDR-TB is suspected, extensive susceptibility testing should be performed, and expert advice should be sought to design an appropriate regimen. Treatment should consist of at least three drugs to which the organism has proven to be susceptible. Fluoroquinolones combined with aminoglycosides are particularly useful for treating MDR-TB. In patients who are deemed to be unreliable, directly observed therapy (DOT) should be instituted. Poor adherence greatly increases the risk of secondary MDR-TB, and with the institution of DOT in these patients the emergence of resistance is minimized. DOT is recommended for all patients with INH- or rifampin-resistant organisms. One commonly accepted DOT regimen is outlined in Table 4.3.

KEY POINTS
Antituberculous Therapy

1. A four-drug regimen is recommended pending sensitivity testing:
   a. One out of every 10^6 organisms is naturally resistant to one drug.
   b. Cavitary lesions have 10^9–10^{10} organisms.
   c. A minimum of two effective drugs are needed to prevent resistance $10^6 \times 10^6 = 10^{12}$.
   d. Primary INH resistance is common; therefore to reliably prevent resistance, treat with INH, rifampin, pyrazinamide, and ethambutol pending sensitivities.
2. INH-resistance is 10% in the Unites States, 7.5% worldwide; higher in Asia, Africa, and Latin America.
3. Multidrug resistance (resistance to more than one drug) is 2% in NYC, 13% in parts of Eastern Europe.
4. Secondary resistance occurs in patients who do not reliably take their medications.
5. Directly observed therapy (DOT) is now recommended for unreliable patients and for those with INH- or rifampin-resistant strains.

PREVENTION

Tuberculosis is strictly spread from person to person. Identification of individuals who have been exposed to tuberculosis and preventing them from developing active disease is a major public health goal. The PPD is a very helpful

Table 4.3
Typical Directly Observed Therapy (DOT) Regimen

First two weeks, once daily:
INH 300 mg
Rifampin 600 mg
Pyrazinamide 1.5 gm ≤ 50 kg, 2 g 51–74 kg, 2.5 gm > 74 kg body weight
Streptomycin 750 mg ≤ 50 kg or 1 gm > 50 kg body weight

Weeks 3–8, twice a week:
INH 15 mg/kg body weight
Rifampin 600 mg
Pyrazinamide 3 gm ≤ 50 kg, 3.5 gm 51–74 kg, 4.0 gm ≥ 75 kg body weight
Streptomycin 1 g < 50 kg, 1.25 gm 51–74 kg, 1.5 gm ≥ 75 kg body weight

Weeks 9–26, twice a week:
IHN 15 mg/kg body weight
Rifampin 600 mg

skin test for assessing exposure to tuberculosis. PPD is the abbreviation for "purified protein derivative," which is produced by acid-precipitating tubercle bacilli proteins. The 5-tuberculin unit (TU) dose has been standardized and is administered as a 0.1-ml subcutaneous injection on the volar aspect of the forearm. The injection should produce a discrete raised blanched wheal. Deeper injection is ineffective because tuberculous proteins can be removed by blood flow and produce a false-negative result. The test is read 48–72 hours after injection; however, the reaction usually persists for 1 week. The diameter of induration is measured, and a diameter of ≥10 mm induration is defined as positive. Ninety percent of people with a PPD reaction of 10-mm diameter are infected with tuberculosis, and essentially 100% are infected if the reaction is >15 mm. A positive test simply indicates that at some time in the past the individual was exposed to active tuberculosis; however, this finding does not indicate active disease. The conversion from negative to positive in an individual who is tested annually indicates exposure to tuberculosis during that time interval. Tuberculin skin tests are useful in otherwise healthy individuals but cannot be relied on to determine exposure in HIV patients with low CD4 counts, in patients receiving immunosuppressants, or in patients with severe malnutrition.

Individuals with a positive PPD should have a chest X-ray, and if pulmonary lesions are noted, three sputum samples should be obtained. Prophylaxis should be given only if all sputum samples prove negative for tuberculosis. Because the risk of developing active disease is highest within two years of exposure, all individuals who have converted from a negative to a positive test within two years should receive INH prophylaxis. A positive test when associated with other specific risk factors (HIV diseases, known recent exposure to tuberculosis, abnormal chest X-ray, intravenous drug abuse, and certain underlying diseases) also warrants preventive therapy. In other individuals with a positive PPD, the risk of INH hepatotoxicity must be balanced against the likelihood of preventing the development of active disease. In individuals age 35 years or older the risk of hepatotoxicity outweighs the potential benefit of INH prophylaxis, and preventive treatment is not recommended. In individuals under age 35 years with a PPD of ≥10 mm, prophylaxis is recommended for immigrants from endemic areas, medically underserved populations, and residents of long-term care facilities. Finally, all individuals under the age of 35 with a PPD of ≥15 mm should receive prophylaxis. The recommended prophylactic regimen for most individuals is INH 300 mg QD × 6 months. Twelve months of INH prophylaxis is recommended for HIV-infected patients.

KEY POINTS
Tuberculosis Prophylaxis

1. PPD 5TU is carefully standardized:
   a. ≥10 mm induration at 48 hours, 90% have *Mycobacterium tuberculosis*.

   b. ≥ 15 mm induration, 100% have *M. tuberculosis*.
2. Positive = exposure sometime in the past. Negative to positive = conversion and indicates exposure during the time interval between tests.
3. INH prophylaxis (300 mg QD 6 months) if:
   a. Conversion less than 2 years, negative chest X-ray,
   b. Positive PPD in high-risk patients (HIV infected, INH for 12 months), known recent exposure to tuberculosis, chronic underlying disease),
   c. Positive PPD and abnormal chest X-ray must have three sputums for AFB to exclude active disease. If sputums are negative, should receive prophylaxis,
   d. Positive PPD ≥15 mm and age < 35 years,
   e. Positive PPD ≥10 mm and age < 35 years who is an immigrant, medically underserved, or a resident of a long-term care facility.

Atypical Mycobacteria

Atypical mycobacteria are found throughout the environment in soil and water. These organisms have a low virulence and usually do not cause pulmonary disease in otherwise healthy individuals. In patients with underlying pulmonary disease these organisms can be inhaled and cause pulmonary infection. *Mycobacterium avium* complex is the most common of the atypical mycobacteria to infect the lung. A cavitary upper-lobe lesion is the usual manifestation of this disease. The cavities tend to be somewhat smaller and thinner-walled than in *M. tuberculosis*. *M. avium* complex pulmonary infection is seen primarily in male smokers in their early fifties who abuse alcohol. Infection of the lungs is also seen in women age 60 or older with no apparent underlying disease and most commonly involves the right middle lobe or lingula. *M. kansasii*, *M. fortuitum*, and *M. abscessus* can also infect the lungs, causing chronic cavitary disease. Because these organisms are found throughout the environment and may colonize as well as infect patients with chronic lung diseases, elaborate criteria for differentiating colonization from infection have been established. Therapy for atypical mycobacterial infection must be prolonged and is based on sensitivity testing. Often these organisms respond poorly to therapy, and resection of the infected lung segment may be required for cure. Management of these patients is complex and requires the supervision of an experienced pulmonary or infectious disease specialist.

KEY POINTS

Atypical Mycobacterial Pulmonary Infection

1. Atypical mycobacteria are found in soil and water.
2. Infects males older than 50 years who are smokers or alcoholics or who have chronic lung disease or upper lobe cavitary disease.
3. Infects females older than 60 years without apparent underlying disease, RML, or lingular disease.
4. *Mycobacterium avium* most common; *M. kansasii, M. fortuitum,* and *M. abscessus* rarer.
5. Management is complex and requires a pulmonary or infectious disease specialist.

Histoplasmosis

EPIDEMIOLOGY

Histoplasma capsulatum is one of the more common causes of chronic pneumonia in the midwestern and southeastern United States. This organism survives in moist soil in temperate climates and is most commonly reported in the Ohio and Mississippi River valleys. The development of histoplasmosis is generally associated with construction or excavation of *H. capsulatum*–contaminated soil. Infection is also reported in spelunkers, who contract the infection by disturbing dried bat guano containing high concentrations of infectious particles. Exposure to infectious particles can also occur after the renovation of old buildings that were previously inhabited by birds or bats.

PATHOGENESIS

Histoplasma capsulatum is a fungus that exists in two forms: as mycelia or yeast. In the moist soil of temperate climates the organism exists in the mycelial form existing as macroconidia (8–15 μm is size) and microconidia (2–5 μm). When infected soil is disturbed, microconidia float in the air and can be inhaled into the lung. Once in the lung, microconidia are ingested by alveolar macrophages and neutrophils. In the intracellular environment of these phagocytes the mycelia transform to rounded, encapsulated yeast cells. During this transformation multiple genes are upregulated, including a gene that increases production of a calcium-binding protein important for acquiring calcium (an essential ion for yeast survival) from the intracellular environment. The expression of this calcium-binding protein may explain the frequent finding of calcifications in infected tissues.

Just as observed in tuberculosis, infected macrophages transport yeast forms to the hilar lymph nodes where histoplasma antigens are presented to T cells. Within several weeks cell-mediated immunity develops, and CD4 T cells activate macrophages to produce fungicidal products.

KEY POINTS

The Epidemiology and Pathogenesis of Histoplasmosis

1. Found primarily in the Midwest and Southeast.
2. Grows in moist soil in temperate zones, Ohio and Mississippi River valleys.
3. Found in caves and old buildings; bat guano is a concentrated source.

4. Mycelial form in soil, macroconidia, and microconidia. Microconidia are readily aerosolized.
5. Inhaled microconidia ingested by macrophages and neutrophils convert to yeast forms and upregulate many genes, including a gene for calcium-binding.
6. Yeast is transported to hilar nodes, where cell-mediated immunity is induced.

CLINICAL MANIFESTATIONS

In over 90% of patients infection is controlled. In many patients primary exposure is asymptomatic or results in a mild influenzalike illness. The very young, the elderly, and patients with compromised immune systems are more likely to develop active disease. Usually, symptoms develop within 14 days of exposure and may include high fever, headache, nonproductive cough, and dull, nonpleuritic chest pain. This form of chest pain is thought to be due to mediastinal node enlargement. In other patients chest pain may be sharper and may be made worse by lying down, reflecting the development of pericarditis (observed in approximately 6% of cases). On chest X-ray, during acute disease patchy infiltrates may be seen that subsequently calcify, producing a "buckshot" appearance. Healed histoplasmosis is also the most common cause of calcified lesions in the liver and spleen. In acute disease, mediastinal lymphadenopathy may be prominent and may mimic lymphoma or sarcoidosis. A history of exposure to a site where soil was excavated is particularly important in trying to differentiate among these different possibilities. Rarely mediastinal nodes can become massively enlarged, reaching diameters of 8–10 cm. Severe mediastinal fibrosis is rare but can lead to impingement and obstruction of the superior vena cava, bronchi, and esophagus.

Chronic cavitary histoplasmosis develops in about 8% of patients. This complication is more common in males over the age of 50 years who have chronic obstructive pulmonary disease. The symptoms and chest X-ray findings associated with chronic pulmonary histoplasmosis are indistinguishable from cavitary tuberculosis. In fact in the past, patients in the midwestern and southeastern United States with chronic pulmonary histoplasmosis were frequently misdiagnosed as having pulmonary tuberculosis and were mistakenly confined to tuberculosis sanatoriums. Spontaneous resolution of cavitary disease occurs in 10–60% of cases.

Progressive disseminated histoplasmosis occurs in about 10% of symptomatic primary infections. Progressive dissemination also develops as a consequence of reactivation of old disease. In the immunosuppressed individual this is the most likely pathway for disseminated disease. Onset of symptoms is usually abrupt. Fever and malaise are followed by nonproductive cough, weight loss, and diarrhea. Hepatosplenomegaly usually develops, and lymphadenopathy may be detected. Anemia, thrombocytopenia, and leukopenia are observed in a high percentage of patients. Meningitis may develop, resulting in CSF lymphocytosis as well as a low CSF glucose. A chest X-ray may show a reticulonodular pattern or scattered nodular opacities; however, chest X-ray is normal in nearly one third of cases. Mortality is high if treatment is not initiated.

KEY POINTS

The Clinical Manifestations of Histoplasmosis

1. 90% brief, self-limited, flulike illness or asymptomatic.
2. Elderly, very young, and immunocompromised can develop disease.
3. 14 days post exposure:
   a. High fever, headache, nonproductive cough, and dull, nonpleuritic chest pain.
   b. Chest X-ray: Patchy infiltrates later convert to "buckshot" calcifications.

c. Mediastinal lymphadenopathy may mimic lymphoma or sarcoidosis.

d. Progressive mediastinal fibrosis is a rare complication.

4. Cavitary disease is clinically similar to tuberculosis, males >50 years old with COPD are at higher risk.

5. Disseminated disease develops in 10% of symptomatic primary disease:

a. Increased likelihood in the very old, very young, AIDS patients, and immunosuppressed.

b. Meningitis with lymphs and low glucose may develop.

c. Reticulonodular pattern on chest X-ray in most, but chest X-ray normal in one third.

DIAGNOSIS

Histoplasma capsulatum can be readily grown from tissue samples and body fluids using brain-heart infusion media containing antibiotics and cylcoheximide (inhibits the growth of saprophytic fungi). Mycelial growth can usually be detected within 7 days and confirmed using a DNA probe. The clinical microbiology lab must be notified that *H. capsulatum* represent the possible pathogen because these culture methods are not employed on routine samples. A single sputum culture has only a 10–15% yield; however, collection of multiple sputum cultures increases the yield. Bronchoscopy has proved useful for providing good sputum samples, yielding positive cultures in 90% of HIV patients with pulmonary histoplasmosis. Bone marrow and blood cultures should also be obtained and are positive in up to 50%. The lysis-centrifugation blood culture technique, which is also used to culture mycobacteria, is the most sensitive method. The most effective method for detecting progressive disseminated histoplasmosis is the urine and serum polysaccharide antigen test. Antigen is detected in up to 90% of patients with disseminated disease and also is positive in 40% of patients with cavitary pulmonary diseases and

20% with acute pulmonary histoplasmosis. A PCR method for identifying *H. capsulatum* has also been developed but is available only on an experimental basis. Histopathologic examination of infected tissue also allows rapid diagnosis. Noncaseating or caseating granulomas may be seen. An excessive fibrotic reaction may be seen in some patients. Silver stains are most effective for identifying the typical yeast forms in tissue biopsies. Organisms are poorly visualized by hematoxylin-eosin staining but can often be seen on periodic acid-Schiff stain.

KEY POINTS

The Diagnosis of Histoplasmosis

1. Sputum culture is often positive:

a. Requires selective media (brain heart infusion with antibiotics and cyclohexamide).

b. Not a routine method, clinical microbiology lab must be notified.

c. Bronchoscopy improves yield (90% in HIV patients).

2. Bone marrow is positive in 50%.

3. Blood cultures: Lysis centrifugation method positive up to 50%.

4. Polysaccharide urine and serum antigen test most sensitive, positive:

a. 90% of disseminated disease,

b. 40% cavitary disease,

c. 20% acute pulmonary disease.

5. Histopathology: Noncaseating or caseating granulomas; silver stain best for identifying the yeast forms, periodic acid-Schiff may identify, not seen on hematoxylin-eosin.

TREATMENT

Itraconazole is the most effective azole for oral treatment. In patients with acute pulmonary histoplasmosis who fail to improve over the first week, itraconazole 200 mg QD for four to six weeks is recommended. If the patient is unable to tolerate azoles or cannot take oral medications, amphotericin B 0.4–0.5 gm/kg can be administered intravenously until symptoms subside. In patients with extensive mediastinal involvement itraconazole, 200 mg QD, can be given for three to six months. If rapid resolution of symptoms is necessary, amphotericin B is preferred. Patients with severe mediastinal fibrosis may also require surgical intervention to correct vascular and airway obstruction. In cavitary pulmonary disease progression of lesions over two to three months or persistent cavities associated with declining respiratory function warrant treatment with itraconazole 400 mg QD for a minimum of 6 months. Amphotericin B may be required if lesions fail to improve on itraconazole therapy. In acute life-threatening progressive disseminated histoplasmosis amphotericin B should be given in high doses, 0.7–1 mg/kg/day. Once the patient has defervesced, the dosage can be lowered to 0.4–0.5 mg/kg, or the patient can be switched to itraconazole 400 mg QD.

KEY POINTS
The Treatment of Histoplasmosis

1. Itraconazole the oral agent of choice. Recommended for treatment of:
   a. Acute pulmonary disease that fails to improve over 7 days,
   b. Extensive mediastinal involvement,
   c. Progressive cavitary disease.
2. Amphotericin B used for more severe disease:
   a. Primary pulmonary disease if unable to take oral medications,
   b. Cavitary disease that fails to improve on itraconazole,
   c. Progressive disseminated disease.

Coccidioidomycosis

EPIDEMIOLOGY

Like *Histoplasma capsulatum*, *Coccidioides immitis* survives and grows in soil. The ideal conditions for *C. immitis* survival are dry, alkaline soil; hot summers; and winters with few freezes. These conditions exist in central California in the San Joaquin Valley and in the southern regions of Arizona, New Mexico, and Texas. *C. immitis* is also found in Mexico, Central America, and South America. Infections are most commonly reported in the summer months when the soil is dry and more readily forms dust particles. Epidemics have been associated with disruption of soil by archeological excavation, earthquakes, and dust storms. In recent years the incidence of coccidioidomycosis has increased as a consequence of the increased number of people living in endemic areas.

PATHOGENESIS

Also like *Histoplasma capsulatum*, *Coccidioides immitis* is a dimorphic fungus existing as mycelia in soil that can form small arthroconidia (5-μm barrel-shaped structures). Arthroconidia can become airborne and then inhaled by humans, where they become lodged in the terminal bronchioles. In the warm, moist environment of the lung the arthroconidia transform to spherules. As spherules mature, their outer walls become thinner, and they release endospores that are ingested by macrophages. As is observed in histoplasmosis and tuberculosis, macrophages transport these infectious particles to the hilar lymph nodes, the lymphatic system, and the bloodstream, resulting in dissemination. Cell-mediated immunity is critical for the control of infection.

KEY POINTS
The Epidemiology and Pathogenesis of Coccidioidomycosis

1. Grows in soil, preferably dry, arid soil.
2. Prefers hot summers and mild winters with few freezes.
3. Found primarily in central California, southern Arizona, New Mexico, and Texas. Also found in Mexico, Central America, and South America.
4. Contracted during the summer, dust storms, excavations, and earthquakes.

5. Inhaled arthroconidia transform to spherules (yeast forms) that release endospores.
6. Ingested by macrophages and transported to hilar lymph nodes, lymphatics, and bloodstream.
7. Cell-mediated immunity critical for control of infection.

CLINICAL MANIFESTATIONS

Approximately two thirds of patients who have been exposed to arthroconidia have minimal symptoms. When symptoms are noted, they usually develop 7–21 days after exposure. Nonproductive cough and fever are most frequent. Pleuritic chest pain, shortness of breath, headache, and fatigue are also commonly reported. Skin manifestations may include erythema nodosum (red, painful nodules on the anterior shins), erythema multiforme (targetlike lesions involving the entire body, including the palms and soles), or a nonpruritic papular rash. Arthralgias may develop in association with erythema nodosum. Eosinophilia is commonly observed on peripheral blood smear. Chest X-ray is abnormal in half of patients, most commonly demonstrating unilateral infiltrates, pleural effusions, and hilar adenopathy. In patients with depressed cell-mediated immunity, primarily patients with AIDS and CD4 counts of <100/mm^3, the infection can disseminate, causing diffuse opacification of the lungs and severe respiratory failure. Meningitis, skin lesions, bone infection, and arthritis may also develop as a consequence of dissemination. In some patients pulmonary infection can persist, causing progressive destruction of lung parenchyma associated with a productive cough, chest pain, and weight loss. Chest X-ray may demonstrate areas of fibrosis, nodules, and/or cavitary lesions. An isolated nodule can persist in approximately 4% of pulmonary cases and can be differentiated from neoplasm only by biopsy. Unlike histoplasmosis, lesions rarely calcify. A chronic pleural effusion can result from the rupture of a peripheral cavitary lesion into the pleural space. This com-

plication is most commonly reported in otherwise healthy, young, athletic males.

KEY POINTS

The Clinical Manifestations of Coccidioidomycosis

1. 7–21 days after inhalation, 1/3 are symptomatic; nonproductive cough, fever, pleuritic chest pain, shortness of breath, headache, and fatigue.
2. Skin manifestations are common: erythema nodosum, erythema multiforme, or nonpruritic papular rash.
3. Eosinophilia may be noted on peripheral blood smear.
4. Abnormal chest X-ray frequent: Unilateral infiltrates, pleural effusions, hilar adenopathy.
5. AIDS patients with CD4 < 100 mm^3 can disseminate, causing diffuse lung opacification, meningitis, bone infection, and arthritis.
6. Chronic lung disease can lead to fibrosis, nodules, or cavities.
7. Isolated pulmonary nodules are not calcified, differentiated from neoplasm by biopsy.
8. Chronic pleural effusions most commonly develop in young, healthy, athletic males.

DIAGNOSIS

Travel to, or past residence in, an endemic area should alert the clinician to the possibility of coccidioidomycosis. Examination of induced sputum or sputum obtained by bronchoscopy may reveal spherules. The fungus is not seen on Gram stain but can be detected by silver stain. Biopsies of infected tissue should be obtained and usually reveal caseating or noncaseating granuloma as well as spherules. The organism readily grows as a white mold on routine mycology media as well as bacterial media under aerobic conditions.

Multiple serologic tests are available and often are required to make the diagnosis because the patient fails to produce sputum and biopsy specimens are not readily obtainable. IgM serum titers against *Coccidioides immitis* are usually positive within the first week of disease. A serum latex agglutinin test is highly sensitive but may yield false-positives. An immunodiffusion agar test is the preferred method for detecting IgM antibody in serum, cerebrospinal fluid, serous effusions, and synovial fluid. An enzyme-linked immunoassay is also available that detects both IgM and IgG. IgG levels are most commonly tested by complement fixation or immunodiffusion. IgG levels increase after IgM and often persist for years. There is a correlation between IgG serum titer and the severity of disease. A rising titer of ≥1:32 may signal disseminated disease, while a falling titer indicates a favorable prognosis. Patients with no detectable lesions can have titers of ≤1:8 for many years after exposure.

KEY POINTS
The Diagnosis of Coccidioidomycosis

1. Spherules may be seen on induced sputum or following bronchoscopy.
2. Readily cultured on routine bacterial and mycology culture plates.
3. Histopathology: Noncaseating and caseating granulomas; silver stain best, not seen on Gram stain.
4. Multiple serological tests available to measure IgG and IgM antibody titers:
   a. IgM titer elevated in acute disease,
   b. IgG often persists for years, rising titer ≥ 1:32 signals dissemination, falling titer indicative of a favorable prognosis.

TREATMENT

The majority of infections spontaneously resolve. Treatment is reserved for patients with disseminated disease and patients with persistent or progressive coccidioidal pneumonia with hypoxia. Treatment needs to be considered also in patients with pulmonary disease who are at increased risk for dissemination: blacks, Filipinos, pregnant women, diabetics, and im-

munosuppressed patients, including those with AIDS.

Amphotericin B remains the preferred treatment as initial therapy of life-threatening disseminated disease or severe pulmonary disease until the infection is under control. High doses of amphotericin B are recommended: 0.7–1 mg/kg/day. In less severe disease fluconazole (400–800 mg QD) or itraconazole (200 mg BID) is recommended. These agents are preferred because of their low levels of toxicity and the ability to administer them for prolonged periods. Therapy should be continued until the symptoms and signs of infection have resolved. A minimum of six months of therapy is recommended. Complement fixation IgG serum titers are helpful in guiding therapy. An undetectable complement fixation IgG titer or reduction to a stable low titer is associated with a low likelihood of relapse. In patients with meningeal involvement triazole therapy should be continued indefinitely. Surgical debridement of large purulent collections is recommended. Resection of rapidly expanding pulmonary cavities should be performed to prevent rupture into the pleural space. Surgical resection is also recommended to prevent bronchopleural fistula formation and to correct life-threatening pulmonary hemorrhage.

KEY POINTS
The Treatment of Coccidioidomycosis

1. Treatment is usually reserved for disseminated disease.
2. Amphotericin B for severe disease.
3. Fluconazole or itraconazole for less severe disease.
4. Treatment for a minimum of six months.
5. Complement fixation IgG titers should decrease to a stable low titer.
6. For meningitis triazole therapy should be continued indefinitely.
7. Surgical resection for expanding lung lesions.

Additional Reading

General

Baik, I., Curhan, G.C., Rimm, E.B., Bendich, A., Willett, W.C., and Fawzi, W.W. A prospective study of age and lifestyle factors in relation to community-acquired pneumonia in US men and women. *Arch Intern Med* 160:3082–3088, 2000.

Bartlett, J.G., Breiman, R.F., Mandell, L.A., and File, T.M., Jr. Community-acquired pneumonia in adults: guidelines for management. The Infectious Diseases Society of America. *Clin Infect Dis* 26:811–838, 1998.

Ben-David, D., and Rubinstein, E. Appropriate use of antibiotics for respiratory infections: review of recent statements and position papers. *Curr Opin Infect Dis* 15:151, 2002.

Fine, M.J., Stone, R.A., Singer, D.E., et al. Processes and outcomes of care for patients with community-acquired pneumonia: results from the Pneumonia Patient Outcomes Research Team (PORT) cohort study. *Arch Intern Med* 159:970–980, 1999.

Gilbert, K., Gleason, P.P., Singer, D.E., et al. Variations in antimicrobial use and cost in more than 2,000 patients with community-acquired pneumonia. *Am J Med* 104:17–27, 1998.

Guthrie, R. Community-acquired lower respiratory tract infections: etiology and treatment. *Chest* 120:2021–2034, 2001.

Mortensen, E.M., Coley, C.M., Singer, D.E., et al. Causes of death for patients with community-acquired pneumonia: results from the Pneumonia Patient Outcomes Research Team cohort study. *Arch Intern Med* 162:1059–1064, 2002.

Roson, B., Carratala, J., Verdaguer, R., Dorca, J., Manresa, F., and Gudiol, F. Prospective study of the usefulness of sputum Gram stain in the initial approach to community-acquired pneumonia requiring hospitalization. *Clin Infect Dis* 31:869–874, 2000.

Pneumococcal Pneumonia

Bauer, T., Ewig, S., Marcos, M.A., Schultze-Werninghaus, G., and Torres, A. *Streptococcus pneumoniae* in community-acquired pneumonia. How important is drug resistance? *Med Clin North Am* 85:1367–1379, 2001.

Marrie, T.J. Pneumococcal pneumonia: epidemiology and clinical features. *Semin Respir Infect* 14:227–236, 1999.

Musher, D.M., Alexandraki, I., Graviss, E.A., et al. Bacteremic and nonbacteremic pneumococcal pneumonia. A prospective study. *Medicine* (Baltimore) 79:210–221, 2000.

Haemophilus influenzae Pneumonia

Sarangi, J., Cartwright, K., Stuart, J., Brookes, S., Morris, R., and Slack, M. Invasive *Haemophilus influenzae* disease in adults. *Epidemiol Infect* 124:441–447, 2000.

Aspiration Pneumonia

Marik, P.E. Aspiration pneumonitis and aspiration pneumonia. *N Engl J Med* 344:665–671, 2001.

Legionnaires' Pneumonia

Akbas, E., and Yu, V.L. Legionnaires' disease and pneumonia. Beware of the temptation to underestimate this "exotic" cause of infection. *Postgrad Med* 109:135–138, 141–142, 147, 2001.

Waterer, G.W., Baselski, V.S., and Wunderink, R.G. Legionella and community-acquired pneumonia: a review of current diagnostic tests from a clinician's viewpoint. *Am J Med* 110:41–48, 2001.

Atypical Pneumonia

Marrie, T.J., Peeling, R.W., Fine, M.J., Singer, D.E., Coley, C.M., and Kapoor, W.N. Ambulatory patients with community-acquired pneumonia: the frequency of atypical agents and clinical course. *Am J Med* 101:508–515, 1996.

Actinomycosis and Nocardiosis

Heffner, J.E. Pleuropulmonary manifestations of actinomycosis and nocardiosis. *Semin Respir Infect* 3:352–361, 1988.

Tuberculosis

Packham, S. Tuberculosis in the elderly. *Gerontology* 47:175–179, 2001.

Small, P.M., Fujiwara, P.I. Management of tuberculosis in the United States. *N Engl J Med* 345:189–200, 2001.

Histoplasmosis

Gurney, J.W., and Conces, D.J. Pulmonary histoplasmosis. *Radiology* 199:297–306, 1996.

Coccidioidomycosis

Standaert, S.M., Schaffner, W., Galgiani, J.N., et al. Coccidiomycosis among visitors to a *Coccidioides immitis*-endemic area: an outbreak in a military reserve unit. *J Infect Dis* 171:1672–1675, 1995.

Chapter

5

Eye, Ear, Nose, and Throat Infections

Recommended Time to Complete: 1 day

Guiding Questions

1. What is the most common cause of conjunctivitis?
2. What is the greatest risk factor for the development of keratitis?
3. What infection is associated with unsterilized tap water?
4. What is the most likely diagnosis in the patient with a recurrent history of a red eye?
5. What are the three most common ways in which patients develop endophthalmitis?

Eye Infections

Many eye infections are managed by the ophthalmologist, who has the specialized equipment and skills that are required for optimal diagnosis and treatment. However, infectious disease consultants and primary care physicians need to be familiar with these forms of infection to initiate preliminary empiric therapy pending referral.

Conjunctivitis

Potential Severity: Usually responds rapidly to therapy and does not threaten vision.

PREDISPOSING FACTORS

The conjunctiva is a mucous membrane that covers the globe of the eye up to the cornea as well as the lids of the eye. The surface of this transparent membrane is normally protected from infection by tears, which contain numerous antibacterial agents including lysozyme, IgA, and IgG. Patients with decreased tear production (for example, patients with rheumatoid arthritis with infiltration of the lacrimal gland) often suffer from recurrent conjunctivitis as well as keratitis.

CLINICAL MANIFESTATIONS AND ETIOLOGY

Inflammation of the conjunctiva is called conjunctivitis and is accompanied by dilatation of vessels within this membrane and causes the underlying white sclera to appear red. In addition to redness conjunctivitis is accompanied by the formation of pus. Purulent discharge may be associated with swelling of the eyelids as well as pain and/or itching. Dried exudate has often glued the eyelid shut when the patient awakens in the morning. Vision is usually unimpaired, and the cornea and pupil appear normal. Bacteria, viruses, chlamydia, fungi, and parasites can all cause conjunctivitis. Allergic reactions and toxic substances can also result in inflammation of the conjunctiva. The specific findings on eye exam vary and depend on the etiology:

◆ **Bacterial**. *Staphylococcus aureus, Streptococcus pneumoniae, Haemophilus influenzae,* and *Moraxella catarrhalis* are the most common causes of bacterial conjunctivitis. This infection is highly contagious, particularly among children. Copious quantities of pus usually exude from the eye, and when pus is removed, it is quickly replaced by new exudate. The discharge is usually thick and globular. In *S. pneumoniae* or *H. influenzae* conjunctivitis the vessels in the conjunctiva can be damaged, resulting in petechial hemorrhages. *Neisseria gonorrhoeae* and *N. meningitidis* are less common but cause a particularly severe, extremely purulent conjunctivitis that can also involve the cornea. *N. gonorrhoeae* is usually sexually transmitted. This

organism can also infect the conjunctiva of neonates as they pass through an infected birth canal. In chronic care facilities *Serratia marcescens, Pseudomonas aeruginosa,* and Moraxella species may be encountered.

◆ **Viral**. Viral infection is the most common cause of conjunctivitis, representing approximately 14% of diagnosed cases. The exudate in viral infection is less purulent and more serous. In viral, chlamydia, and toxic conjunctivitis the lymphatic tissue in the conjunctiva can become hypertrophied, forming small, smooth bumps called follicles. Viral conjunctivitis is highly contagious, and the second eye commonly becomes involved within 24–48 hours; however, unilateral involvement does not exclude the diagnosis. Adenovirus and enterovirus are most commonly identified. Rarer causes include herpes simplex, varicella-zoster, and measles. The infection is self-limited, resolving over one to three weeks.

◆ **Chlamydial**. *Chlamydia trachomatis* conjunctivitis is a leading cause of blindness worldwide. In the United States this infection is most commonly seen in indigent Native Americans. Another form of *C. trachomatis* infection, inclusion conjunctivitis, is transmitted to adults by genital secretions from an infected sexual partner. As in viral conjunctivitis a follicular inflammatory response is usually encountered. This form of conjunctivitis is also common in neonates who pass through an infected birth canal.

◆ **Fungal**. This form of conjunctivitis is rare. Candida conjunctivitis is usually associated with prolonged use of corticosteroid eye drops. Blastomycosis and *Sporothrix schenckii* are less common etiologies.

◆ **Parasites**. *Trichinella spiralis, Taenia solium, Schisotosoma haematobium, Onchocerca volvulus,* and *Loa loa* (see Chapter 13) infections have all been associated with conjunctivitis.

◆ **Allergic and toxic**. Pollens can induce allergic conjunctivitis that usually involves both eyes and is accompanied by itching of the eyes. In addition to pollens almost any topical solution applied to the eye can result in an allergic conjunctivitis. Hard and soft contact lenses are also frequent offenders, as are cosmetics. Inadvertent splashing of acidic or other toxic solutions into the eye can result in severe irritation and should be quickly followed by extensive irrigation with sterile normal saline.

♦ **Other**. Other clinical conditions in which conjunctivitis is a component of the disease include Reiter's syndrome, keratoconjunctivitis sicca, graft-versus-host disease, and mucous membrane pemphigoid.

DIAGNOSIS

Cultures are not usually obtained in routine cases of conjunctivitis. In more severe cases conjunctival scrapings are obtained for culture and Gram stain. An abundance of polymorphonuclear leukocytes (PMNs) is found in bacterial and chlamydial conjunctivitis. Viral conjunctivitis usually results in a mononuclear cell exudate, and allergic conjunctivitis is associated with a predominance of eosinophils. An exudate containing PMNs combined with follicular inflammation strongly suggests Chlamydia infection.

TREATMENT

In severe bacterial conjunctivitis and Chlamydia conjunctivitis, systemic treatment is recommended. For milder forms, topical antimicrobial agents usually are sufficient. Eye drop preparations include gentamicin or tobramycin for Gram-negative infections and polymyxin B/bacitracin, neomycin/polymyxin, polymyxin B-trimethoprim, or erythromycin for Gram-positive infections. Topical fluoroquinolones effectively cover most Gram-positive and Gram-negative pathogens and are frequently used as initial therapy.

KEY POINTS

Conjunctivitis

1. Tears contain antibacterial agents that protect against conjunctivitis.
2. Bacterial conjunctivitis causes a thick, purulent discharge. The most common causes are *Staphylococcus aureus*, *Streptococcus pneumoniae*, *Haemophilus influenzae*, and Moraxella. *Neisseria gonorrhoeae* causes a very severe conjunctivitis that can progress to keratitis. Topical antibiotics are usually recommended.
3. Viruses are the most common cause. Bilateral involvement is the rule. Result in serous exudate and follicle formation. The disease is self-limited.
4. Allergic conjunctivitis is usually bilateral and accompanied by itching.

Corneal Infections

Potential Severity: Can cause blindness and requires rapid treatment. Often requires management by an experienced ophthalmologist.

Corneal infections cause inflammation of the cornea, also termed keratitis. Any corneal inflammation must be considered sight-threatening and should be promptly treated. Corneal perforation can lead to blindness. Because of the potential subtleties of diagnosis and treatment and the potential consequences of misdiagnosis, all patients with significant corneal lesions should be referred to an ophthalmologist experienced in the management of keratitis.

PREDISPOSING FACTORS

A small break in the cornea is usually required for bacteria and fungi to gain entry into the cornea. Trauma to the eye, contact lens abrasions, eye surgery, and defective tear production all can result in damage to corneal epithelium. Comatose patients receiving respiratory support with incomplete eye closure are at increased risk for keratitis. Immunosuppression and diabetes mellitus also increase the risk of keratitis.

◆ CASE 5.1

A 28-year-old white male had been spending long hours at work and was somewhat sleep deprived. Three days earlier he had gone to the beach for the afternoon. The night prior to seeing the doctor he noted a foreign body sensation in his left eye. Every time he blinked he noted pain. When he awoke the next morning, his left eye was glued shut with yellow exudate. On prying the lid open, he noted that the eye was extremely red and sensitive to light. His vision in that eye was blurred, and images were outlined by halos. In the ophthalmologist's office later that day, slit lamp exam revealed a large dendritic lesion that stained with fluorescein indicative of herpes simplex keratitis (Figure 5.1).

CLINICAL MANIFESTATIONS AND ETIOLOGY

The primary symptom of keratitis is eye pain. The rich enervation of the corneal surface transmits pain sensation each time the eyelid migrates across the corneal ulcer. As described in Case 5.1, patients often complain of a foreign body sensation in their eye. Unlike conjunctivi-

tis, vision is usually impaired as a consequence of corneal haze. Photophobia and reflex tearing are also common. Slit lamp examination allows identification of the corneal break as well as the degree of inflammation. Loss of corneal substance may be apparent and can lead to perforation or corneal scar formation. Intraocular inflammation is commonly seen. Severe inflammation can lead to the collection of inflammatory cells in the anterior chamber that settle by gravity to the bottom of the chamber, forming a hypopyon (see Figure 5.2).

The clinical manifestations including the eye findings vary depending on the etiology:

◆ **Bacterial**. Bacterial infection is the leading cause of keratitis, accounting for 65–90% of cases. Several bacteria produce toxins and enzymes that allow them to penetrate intact corneal epithelium: *Neisseria gonorrhoeae, N. meningitidis, Corynebacterium diphtheriae*, and Listeria and Shigella species. Most other bacteria require a break in the epithelial lining to invade the cornea. Gram-positive or-

Figure 5.2

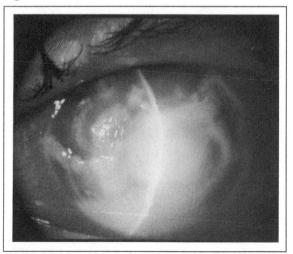

Pseudomonas aeruginosa keratitis. Note the large hypopyon in addition to severe corneal opacification in this patient who used tap water to wash his hard contact lenses. (Courtesy of Dr. William Driebe, University of Florida College of Medicine.) See also on Color Plate 1.

Figure 5.1

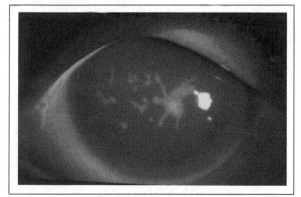

Herpes keratitis. Fluorescein stain showing a typical herpes simplex dendritic lesion. (Courtesy of Dr. William Driebe, University of Florida College of Medicine.) See also on Color Plate 1.

ganisms are most frequently cultured, *Staphylococcus aureus* being the most common pathogen in this group. *Streptococcus pneumoniae* produces a well-circumscribed ulcer that has sharp margins and a gray base, leaving the surrounding cornea clear. The ulcer develops quickly within 24–48 hours of inoculation, and a hypopyon is seen early in the course of the infection. Other Gram-positive cocci that cause keratitis include *Staphylococcus epidermidis*, *Streptococcus viridans*, *Streptococcus pyogenes*, enterococcus, and Peptostreptococcus. In addition to *Corynebacterium diphtheriae*, a number of other Gram-positive bacilli can cause this disease, including Bacillus and Clostridia. One of the most destructive bacteria is *Pseudomonas aeruginosa*. Infection with this Gram-negative rod is commonly associated with hard contact lenses. Pain is severe, and the corneal ulcer spreads rapidly as a consequence of production of bacterial proteases. Development of a large hypopyon is the rule (see Figure 5.2). Perforation can occur quickly. The exudate is often greenish, and the infiltrate appears soupy. Other Gram-negative rods also result in a soupy infiltrate. *Proteus mirabilis*, *Klebsiella pneumoniae*, *Serratia marcescens*, *Escherichia coli*, and *Aeromonas hydrophila* all have been reported to cause keratitis. In addition to Neisseria, other Gram-negative coccobacilli that cause bacterial keratitis include *Pasteurella multocida*, Acinetobacter species, and Moraxella species. *Moraxella liquefaciens* and *M. nonliquefaciens* cause slowly progressive ulcers in debilitated patients, particularly alcoholics and diabetics.

♦ **Viral**. Patients with a history of a recurrent red eye most commonly have recurrent herpes simplex virus keratitis. Latent virus in the fifth cranial nerve reactivates and migrates down the nerve to the corneal surface. Ultraviolet light exposure, menstruation, fever, and other acute stresses can induce viral reactivation. In the hospitalized patient with a unilateral red eye, herpes simplex keratitis should always be considered. Corneal anesthesia may develop initially, minimizing pain. A foreign body sensation is frequently noted that is associated with tearing, and erythema is often present. A classic dendritic lesion that stains with fluorescein dye is readily seen on slit lamp exam (see Figure 5.1). Other forms of viral keratitis include herpes zoster involving the ophthalmic branch of the trigeminal nerve, measles, and Epstein-Barr virus.

♦ **Fungal**. Corneal ulcers caused by hyphal-forming fungi such as Fusarium and Aspergillus most commonly follow an eye injury from organic material such as a tree branch. Use of chronic glucocorticoid eye drops also increases the risk of fungal keratitis. Ulcers tend to be superficial and are often elevated above the corneal surface. The infiltrate tends to be irregular, and an immune ring is often apparent. Smaller satellite lesions are commonly seen surrounding the main infiltrate. A severe anterior chamber reaction associated with a hypopyon is commonly observed. Yeastlike fungi such as Candida can also cause corneal ulcers. They tend to be more indolent but can have all the characteristics described for hyphae-forming fungi.

♦ **Protozoal**. Protozoa are a rare but a very serious cause of corneal ulcers. Acanthamoeba species most commonly develop in contact lens wearers, particularly those who use unsterilized tap water in their cleaning solutions. Acanthamoeba ulcers are painful, are slowly progressive, and fail to respond to topical antibiotics.

DIAGNOSIS AND TREATMENT

Slit lamp examination is helpful in identifying potential causes. If a bacterial or fungal etiology is suspected, corneal scrapings for culture, Gram stain, Giemsa stain, and methenamine silver stain should be performed. A surgical blade is gently scraped across the surface of the ulcer, and the resulting samples are inoculated onto solid media. Aerobic bacteria grow readily on standard media within 48 hours. Special processing is required if Acanthamoeba, fungi, mycobacteria, or Chlamydia are the suspected pathogens. Viral keratitis can usually be diagnosed by appearance and generally does not require culturing.

Treatment must be instituted emergently. Because of the potential risk of perforation and visual loss, patients with bacterial keratitis and significant ulceration are often hospitalized for close observation. Initially, therapy can be based on Gram stain in 75% of patients. In cases in which an etiology is not clearly identified or if the patient has received prior antibiotic therapy, broader antibiotic coverage is warranted. Antibiotics are commonly given topically and in some instances also subconjunctivally. Systemic therapy in addition to topical therapy is recommended for patients with imminent perforation. Topical regimens include bacitracin (5000 U/ml) and gentamicin (13 mg/ml) for *Streptococcus pneumoniae*, cephalothin (50 mg/ml) plus bacitracin for other Gram-positive cocci such as *Staphylococcus aureus*, tobramycin (13.6–15 mg/ml) or gentamicin for Pseudomonas species, gentamicin for other Gram-negative bacilli, amphotericin B (1.5–3 mg/ml) plus flucytosine (1%) for yeast-like fungi, natamycin (5%) for hyphal fungi, and neomycin (5–8 mg/ml) plus pentamidine isethionate (0.15%) for Acanthamoeba species. Topical fluoroquinolones are also efficacious and have been recommended as empiric therapy for non–sight-threatening bacterial keratitis; 0.3% ofloxacin is effective and the least toxic regimen. This fluoroquinolone is often combined with topical cephalothin. Eye drops need to be administered every half hour during the day and hourly during sleep for 7–10 days. Subconjunctival injections should be repeated every 12–24 hours for a total of three to six doses. For herpes simplex keratitis, trifluoridine ophthalmic solution or topical acyclovir is recommended for 7–10 days. Oral acyclovir 400 mg po BID is often given for several months, or in some cases for years, to prevent recurrence.

KEY POINTS

Keratitis (Corneal Infection)

1. Needs to be treated quickly to prevent blindness.
2. Is usually preceded by a break in the cornea (exceptions: Neisseria, *Corynebacteria diphtheriae*, Listera, and Shigella).
3. *Streptococcus pneumoniae* causes a well-circumscribed ulcer with sharp margins.
4. *Pseudomonas aeruginosa* is associated with contact lenses, very destructive and causes severe eye pain.
5. Herpes simplex causes distinct dendritic lesions that take up fluorescein. Consider in the hospitalized patient who develops a unilateral red eye.
6. Fusarium or Aspergillus usually follows eye injury with organic matter (e.g., a tree branch).
7. Acanthamoeba occurs in contact lens wearers who use tap water in their cleaning solutions.

Endophthalmitis

Potential Severity: An ocular emergency. A very serious infection that often leads to permanent visual impairment or blindness.

Endophthalmitis is an inflammatory disease involving the ocular chamber and adjacent structures. When the inflammation involves all the ocular tissue layers and chambers, the disease is called panophthalmitis.

PREDISPOSING FACTORS AND ETIOLOGIES

There are six major causes of endophthalmitis. Each is associated with distinctive pathogens. They are listed in order of frequency:

1. **Acute postoperative endophthalmitis**. These infections generally originate from en-

dogenous flora in the eye. They most frequently develop within one week after surgery but can develop earlier postoperatively. The most common pathogens are Gram-positive cocci, *Staphylococcus epidermidis* being most common, followed by *S. aureus* and streptococcal species. Gram-negative bacilli occur less frequently, and fungal infection is the least common.

2. **Posttraumatic endophthalmitis**. Mixed infections are common. *Staphylococcus epidermidis* and *S. aureus*, Streptococcus species, and Bacillus species are most frequently cultured. Although *Bacillus cereus* is usually a minimally invasive organism, when it gains entry into the eye, this bacteria causes rapidly progressive panophthalmitis. Fungi are encountered in penetrating injuries caused by organic matter. The likelihood of infection is increased when a foreign body is retained in the eye.

3. **Hematogenous endophthalmitis**. Any source of bacteremia can result in seeding of the choroid followed by spread to the retina and vitreous humor. Two thirds of blood-borne infections arise in the right eye, and one quarter of cases involve both eyes. The most common blood-borne pathogens to cause endophthalmitis are fungi, in particular *Candida albicans*. *Bacillus cereus* is the most common cause of hematogenous endophthalmitis in intravenous drug abusers. Patients with bacterial meningitis due to *Streptococcus pneumoniae*, *Neisseria meningitidis*, and *Haemophilus influenzae* may also develop endophthalmitis. In the neonate group B streptococcus is most common; in the elderly group G streptococcus is most common. In the immunocompromised host with pulmonary infiltrates, *Nocardia asteroides* can gain entry into the eye as well as the cerebral cortex. If the primary source of bacteremia is not apparent, subacute bacterial endocarditis should be considered.

4. **Delayed postoperative endophthalmitis**. These infections usually arise weeks to months after surgery and are caused by opportunistic pathogens, including *Proprionobacterium acnes*, Corynebacteria species, Actinomyces species, atypical mycobacteria, and *Torulopsis glabrata*.

5. **Endophthalmitis associated with a filtering bleb**. This surgical procedure allows bacteria to gain entry into the chambers of the eye and is frequently preceded by conjunctivitis. Streptococcus and Haemophilus species are most commonly encountered.

6. **Endophthalmitis in association with uncontrolled bacterial or fungal keratitis**.

CLINICAL MANIFESTATIONS

Eye pain, photophobia, reduced vision, and redness are the primary symptoms of bacterial endophthalmitis. In cases of hematogenous spread, sudden onset of blurred vision without pain, photophobia, or redness is the most common complaint. On exam eyelid edema, chemosis of conjunctiva, and moderate to severe anterior chamber inflammation with a hypopyon are often seen. Loss of the red reflex, retinal hemorrhages, and venous sheathing are noted on retinal exam. In fungal endophthalmitis the symptoms and signs tend to be less severe. The patient often complains only of blurry vision or spots in the visual field. In the comatose patient Candida endophthalmitis is commonly missed unless frequent funduscopic examinations are performed. Monitoring of the fundi is recommended in all patients who have developed candidemia. Findings of focal areas of inflammation, particularly gray-white fluffy exudates in the retina, chorioretina, or inferior vitreous, strongly suggest Candida endophthalmitis. (Figure 5.3).

DIAGNOSIS AND TREATMENT

Cultures and smears must be obtained promptly from the aqueous and vitreous humors, the vitreous giving the highest positive yield. Specimens of exudate from the conjunctiva are often

Figure 5.3

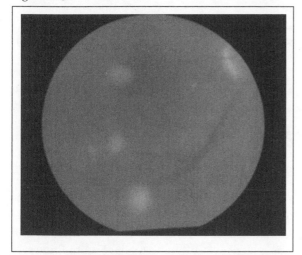

Candida retinitis. Retinal image showing typical fluffy cotton wool exudates caused by seeding from the bloodstream. (Courtesy of Dr. William Driebe, University of Florida College of Medicine.) See also Color Plate 1.

misleading. Cultures of the site of foreign body penetration should be obtained in cases of traumatic endophthalmitis. In patients who are suspected of hematogenous endophthalmitis, blood, urine, and CSF cultures often reveal the etiologic agent. In patients with vision that is better than light perception, vitreous sampling should be followed by intravitreal antibiotic injection. In patients with only light perception, vision is improved by immediate vitrectomy, followed by intravitreal antimicrobials. Initially, broad-spectrum antibiotic treatment is recommended (for example, vancomycin 0.1 cc of a 10 mg/ml solution plus ceftazidime 0.1 cc of a 22.5 mg/ml solution). Systemic therapy must be instituted in cases of hematogenous endophthalmitis but is not of benefit in other forms of endophthalmitis. For Candida endophthalmitis intravenous amphotericin B is recommended, and in more severe cases intravitreous amphotericin B (5–10 µg) is also administered. About half of patients with endophthalmitis retain visual acuity of 20/400 or better. One out of ten patients requires enucleation.

KEY POINTS

Endophthalmitis

1. An ocular emergency; 1 in 10 requires enucleation.
2. Acute postoperative caused by endogenous flora, S*taphylococcus epidermidis*, *S. aureus*, streptococcal species.
3. Posttraumatic results in mixed infections. *Bacillus cereus* very aggressive. Fungal infections after injuries with organic material.
4. Hematogenous form more commonly involves the right eye. Candida most common etiology, *B. cereus* in IV drug abusers.
5. Intravitreal antibiotics required. If light perception only, vitrectomy is recommended.

Throat Infections

Guiding Questions

1. What is the most common cause of pharyngitis?
2. What disease is suggested by the presence of a gray pseudomembrane?
3. What complication is suggested by unilateral tonsillar swelling?
4. What infection should be considered in the patient with inspiratory stridor and sore throat?

Pharyngitis

Potential Severity: Usually a self-limited disease with the exception of the rare, life-threatening complication of peritonsillar abscess.

ETIOLOGY

Pharyngitis is one of the most common infectious diseases that presents to the primary physician's office. There are many causes of pharyngitis. Viruses are most common and include rhinoviruses and coronaviruses (common cold viruses), adenovirus, herpes simplex, parainfluenza, influenza, coxsackievirus A, Epstein-Barr virus, cytomegalovirus, and HIV. The most common bacterial cause is Group A streptococci, which account for over 50% of all cases of pharyngitis in children and about 15% in adults. Other forms of streptococci, groups B and C, have also been associated with pharyngitis in adults. Mixed anaerobic flora can cause a severe form of pharyngitis that extends under the tongue and into the neck, called Vincent's angina. In recent decades *Corynebacterium diphtheriae* has become a rare cause of pharyngitis in the United States. With the waning immunity of the elderly population there is now an increased risk of recrudescence of this dangerous infection. Classically, a grayish pseudomembrane develops that tightly adheres to the pharyngeal wall. This finding should alert the clinician to the possibility of diphtheria. *Neisseria gonorrhoeae* and *Treponema pallidum* are two rarer causes of pharyngitis that need to be included as part of the differential diagnosis in sexually promiscuous patients. Finally, when pharyngitis is accompanied by pneumonia, mycoplasma and chlamydia are the most likely etiologies.

CLINICAL MANIFESTATIONS, DIAGNOSIS, AND TREATMENT

The presence of pharyngeal exudates and tender adenopathy are suggestive of a bacterial etiology but are not entirely specific. Rapid antigen tests now allow the rapid diagnosis of *Streptococcus pyogenes* and have a >90% specificity, but variable sensitivity, 60–95%. If the antigen test is negative and the physical findings are consistent with bacterial pharyngitis, a throat culture should be performed by inoculating a pharyngeal swab onto a sheep blood agar plate.

The possibility of a peritonsillar abscess must always be considered; however, in the antibiotic era this complication has become rare. Medial displacement of one or both tonsils should suggest this possibility. Neck CT with contrast is the diagnostic procedure of choice and allows clear delineation of the location and size of the abscess. Delay in appropriate surgical intervention can result in spread of infection to the retropharyngeal and pretracheal spaces. Entry into the retropharyngeal area can result in spread to the danger space, which extends to the posterior mediastinum, and can result in the development of potentially fatal purulent pericarditis (see Chapter 7).

Treatment depends on the etiology (see Table 5.1). Too often the primary care physician administers antibiotics for viral pharyngitis, and this practice is thought to have contributed to the increasing incidence of penicillin-resistant *Streptococcus pneumoniae* infections (see Chapters 4 and 6). Antibiotics should not be administered to the patient who has a negative rapid antigen test and physical findings suggestive of viral pharyngitis (i.e., lack of pharyngeal exudate and mild lymphadenopathy). In cases of proven *S. pyogenes* the treatment of choice continues to be penicillin: for adults, oral penicillin VK or a single injection of long-acting benzathine penicillin (1.2 million units IM). For penicillin-allergic patients, a 10-day course of erythromycin is recommended. Although antibiotic treatment of *S. pyogenes* shortens the symptomatic period by only 48 hours, eradication of the organism from the pharynx markedly reduces the incidence of poststreptococcal glomerulonephritis and rheumatic heart disease.

KEY POINTS

Pharyngitis

1. Viruses are the most common cause.
2. *Streptococcus pyogenes* is also common (50% in children, 15% in adults).
3. A grayish pseudomembrane should suggest *Corynebacterium diphtheriae*.

4. Keep in mind *Neisseria gonorrhoeae* in the sexually promiscuous patient.
5. If there is asymmetric tonsillar swelling, consider a peritonsillar abscess.
6. Pharyngeal exudate and tender adenopathy suggest but do not prove a bacterial etiology.
7. The rapid antigen test for *S. pyogenes* is specific but varies in sensitivity.
8. Avoid antibiotics in viral pharyngitis; penicillin remains the drug of choice for *S. pyogenes* and reduces the risk of poststreptococcal glomerulonephritis and rheumatic heart disease.

Epiglottitis

Potential Severity: An infectious disease emergency because of the risk of a fatal respiratory arrest.

In the past epiglottitis most commonly occurred in children, but with the advent of the *Haemophilus influenzae* vaccine a higher proportion of cases are now seen in adults. Patients present with a sore throat that subsequently results in difficulty swallowing and drooling, fol-

Table 5-1

Antibiotic Therapy for Ear, Nose, and Throat Infections

DRUG	DOSE	RELATIVE EFFICACY	COMMENTS
PHARYNGITIS			
Viral most frequent	Avoid antibiotics		
Penicillin V-K	500 mg po QID × 10 days	First line	Administer only if proven *Strep-*
Benzathine penicillin	1.2 million units im × 1		*tococcus pyogenes* infection
Erythromycin	500 mg QID × 10 days		For PCN-allergic patients
EPIGLOTTITIS			
Ceftriaxone (or)	1 gm iv or im QD	First line	Intubation recommended for
Cefotaxime	1 gm iv Q8H		children
MALIGNANT OTITIS EXTERNA			
Ciprofloxacin	500 mg iv Q12H	First line	Prolonged therapy × 6 weeks
Ceftazidime	2 gm iv Q8H		
Cefepime	2 gm iv Q12H		
OTITIS MEDIA			
Amoxicillin (or)	500 mg po TID	First line	Amoxicillin more cost-effective,
Amoxicillin-clavulanate	875/125 mg po GID		if no improvement switch to amoxicillin-clavulanate
2nd generation cephalosporin	500 mg po BID	First line	If failure to improve on amoxicillin, also can use one of
Cefuroxime	400 mg po BID		these regimens
Cefpodoxime	500 mg po BID		
Cefprozil			

(continued)

Table 5-1

Antibiotic Therapy for Ear, Nose, and Throat Infections (continued)

DRUG	DOSE	RELATIVE EFFICACY	COMMENTS
MASTOIDITIS (ACUTE)			
Ceftriaxone (or)	1 gm iv or im QD	First line	Therapy × 4–6 weeks
Cefotaxime	1 gm iv Q8H		
MASTOIDITIS (CHRONIC)			
Piperacillin-tazobactam	3/0.375 gm iv Q6H		Polymicrobial including anaer-
Ticarcillin-clavulanate	3.1 gm iv Q4–6H		obes. Intraoperative cultures
Imipenem	500 gm iv Q6H		helpful.
SINUSITIS (OUTPATIENT)			
Amoxicillin-clavulanate	875/125 mg po BID	First line	
Cefuroxime	400 mg po BID	First line	
Gatifloxacin	400 mg po QD	Second line	Danger of selecting for resistant
Levofloxacin	500 mg po QD		*Staphylococcus pneumoniae,*
Moxifloxacin	400 mg po QD		use for the PCN-allergic
SINUSITIS (INPATIENT)			
Ceftriaxone (or)	1 gm iv or im QD	First line	
Cefotaxime (+)	1 gm iv Q8H		
Metronidazole (+)	500 mg iv Q8H		
Nafcillin or Oxacillin	2 gm iv Q4H		

lowed by difficulty breathing. Respiration is often tentative, and inspiratory stridor may be noted. Indirect laryngoscopy reveals a swollen, cherry-red epiglottis, and swelling at this site can be confirmed by lateral neck X-rays. There is high risk of respiratory arrest secondary to airway obstruction, and in children this event is associated with an 80% mortality. For this reason elective endotracheal intubation is recommended in pediatric cases. Adult patients can be closely observed in an intensive-care setting until respiratory distress resolves, and an endotracheal tube should be placed at the bedside. The primary etiology of this infection is *H. influenzae.* However, less commonly *Streptococcus pneumonia*, other streptococcal species, and *Staphylococcus aureus* have been reported in adults. Treatment with intravenous cefotaxime or ceftriaxone for 7–10 days is recommended (see Table 5.1).

KEY POINTS

Epiglottitis

1. Usually a disease of children but increasingly common in adults.
2. Sore throat combined with drooling and inspiratory stridor suggests the diagnosis.
3. Indirect laryngoscopy demonstrates a cherry-red epiglottis.
4. Respiratory arrest is a danger, and pediatric patients should be electively intubated.

5. *Haemophilus influenzae* is the most common cause.
6. Ceftriaxone or cefotaxime is the treatment of choice.

Ear Infections

Guiding Questions

1. What organisms are responsible for malignant otitis externa?

2. Why do children develop otitis media more commonly than adults do?

3. What are the two most common pathogens to cause otitis media?

4. What two complications can result from untreated mastoiditis?

Otitis Externa

Potential Severity: In the normal host, usually an annoying but not serious disease; however, in the diabetic or immunocompromised host, can be life-threatening.

This infection is also called swimmer's ear, and it results from water being trapped in the external auditory canal, resulting in irritation, maceration, and infection. Symptoms include local itching and pain. Physical findings may include redness and swelling of the external canal. Tenderness of the pinna is often noted. Gram-negative bacilli are most commonly cultured, *Pseudomonas aeruginosa* being the major pathogen. Polymyxin drops combined with hydrocortisone (corticosporin otic drops) or an oral fluoroquinolone (ciprofloxacin 500 mg BID)

combined with topical hydrocortisone is the treatment of choice.

A more invasive form of otitis externa called malignant otitis externa can develop in diabetics and immunocompromised patients. This necrotizing infection can spread to the cartilage, blood vessels, and bone. Infection can involve the base of the skull, meninges, and brain, resulting in death. Multiple cranial nerves can be damaged, including cranial nerves VII, IX, X, and XII. *Pseudomonas aeruginosa* is almost always the cause. Systemic therapy for Pseudomonas (ciprofloxacin, ceftazidime, or cefepime) must be instituted for a minimum of six weeks, and necrotic tissue should be surgically debrided.

KEY POINTS

Otitis Externa

1. Due to water trapped in the external ear.
2. Caused by Gram-negative bacilli, *Pseudomonas aeruginosa* most common.
3. Malignant otitis externa:
   a. Occurs in diabetics and immunocompromised patients,
   b. Can infect the base of the skull,
   c. Can be fatal,
   d. Requires prolonged antipseudomonal antibiotic therapy.

Otitis Media

Potential Severity: Rapid treatment and close follow-up reduce the risk of serious complications. Delay in therapy can lead to potentially fatal complications.

Otitis media most commonly occurs in childhood, and by age 3, two thirds of children have had at least one attack. Otitis media with effusion is the consequence of obstruction of the eustachian tube. Loss of drainage results in the accumulation of serous fluid and resorption of air in the middle ear. In younger children the eustachian tube tends to be smaller and more susceptible to obstruction. The initial precipitating event is usually a viral upper respiratory infection. Five to ten days later the sterile fluid collection becomes infected with mouth flora, resulting in ear pain, ear drainage, and occasionally hearing loss. Fever, vertigo, nystagmus, and tinnitus are other associated symptoms. In infants other accompanying symptoms include irritability and loose stools. The finding of redness of the tympanic membrane is consistent with, but not proof of, otitis media and can be the result of diffuse inflammation of the upper respiratory tract. Presence of fluid in the middle ear should be determined by pneumatic otoscopy. More recently, acoustic reflectometry has become available as a method for monitoring ear effusions.

Diagnosis can be made by needle aspiration of the tympanic membrane. Culture of the nasopharynx is not helpful in predicting the bacterial flora in the middle ear. The primary pathogens that cause otitis media are *Streptococcus pneumoniae*, *Haemophilus influenzae* (usually nontypable strains that are not covered by *H. influenzae* B vaccine), *Moraxella catarrhalis*, and, less commonly, *S. pyogenes* and *Staphylococcus aureus*. Amoxicillin is inexpensive and covers the majority of cases of bacterial otitis media. Many experts recommend beginning with amoxicillin, recognizing that patients with β-lactamase-producing organisms (some strains of *H. influenzae* and *M. catarrhalis)* will not respond. If improvement is not seen within 72 hours, the patient should be switched to amoxicillin-clavulanate or cefuroxime. Treatment for 10 days is recommended.

KEY POINTS

Otitis Media

1. Due to obstruction of the eustachian tube in association with a viral upper respiratory infection. More common in children, who have narrow eustachian tubes.

2. Infants may present with irritability and diarrhea.
3. Diagnosis is made by demonstrating the presence of fluid behind the tympanic membrane.
4. *Streptococcus pneumoniae, Haemophilus influenzae,* and *Moraxella catarrhalis* are the most common causes.
5. Amoxicillin to start followed by amoxicillin-clavulanate or cefuroxime if no response within 72 hours.

Mastoiditis

Potential Severity: A rare consequence of otitis media that can lead to fatal complications.

◆ CASE 5.2

A 44-year-old white male began noting purulent drainage from his right ear five months before admission. Drainage was associated with fever and a shaking chill. He received no medical treatment at that time, and symptoms spontaneously resolved. Three weeks prior to admission he again noted increased purulent drainage from the same ear associated with earache and dizziness. One week before admission he developed a severe right-sided headache and experienced difficulty walking because of dizziness. Dizziness was accompanied by nausea and vomiting.

Past medical history: History of chronic right otitis media since age 13 years.

Physical examination: Temperature 38.9°C, foul-smelling purulent discharge from his right perforated tympanic membrane. Tenderness behind right ear with localized erythema and swelling.

Laboratory findings: WBC: 8,900 (68% PMN). Lumbar puncture: 950 WBC (92% mononuclear cells), protein 275 mg/dl, glucose 45 mg/dl. Culture negative. Mastoid films: extensive destruction of the right mastoid air cells as well as the attic and additus. Mastoidectomy was performed, and infection of the temporal bone, epidural space, and mastoid was noted. Intra-operative culture: *Proteus mirabilis*.

With the advent of antibiotics, mastoiditis is now a rare complication of otitis media. However, as described in Case 5.2, rarely infection can spread to the mastoid air cells. Swelling, redness, and tenderness can develop directly behind the ear in the area of the mastoid bone. Chronic mastoid disease can spread to the temporal bone and cause temporal lobe brain abscess. The infection can also spread by epiploic veins to the lateral and sigmoid venous sinuses and cause septic thrombosis. As is seen in Case 5.2, X-rays of the mastoid area may show increased density with soft tissue swelling, loss of mastoid trabeculae, bony sclerosis, lytic lesions of the temporal and parietal bones and contrast enhancement (see Figure 5.4). Treatment is similar to that for otitis media; however, therapy must be prolonged for three to four weeks. Chronic mastoid infections can be associated with Gram-negative aerobic bacteria (as in Case 5.2). If an abscess has formed within the mastoid or if temporal lobe abscess or septic lateral sinus thrombosis has developed, surgical drainage and mastoidectomy need to be per-

Figure 5.4

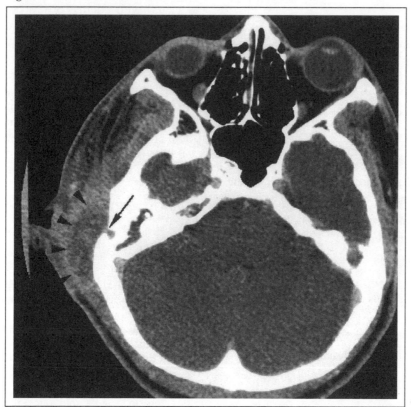

Mastoiditis. CT scan with contrast: axial view showing marked soft tissue swelling in the area of the mastoids surrounded by an enhancing ring (arrowheads). The arrow points to the otic canal. (Courtesy of Dr. Ilona Schamalfus, University of Florida College of Medicine.)

formed. Case 5.2 had headache and severe destruction demonstrated by mastoid X-rays, warranting mastoidectomy and surgical exploration of the temporal region.

KEY POINTS

Mastoiditis

> 1. A rare complication of otitis media.
> 2. Readily diagnosed by mastoid X-rays.
> 3. Requires prolonged antibiotic therapy for three to four weeks.
> 4. Can lead to:
>   a. Brain abscess,
>   b. Septic lateral sinus thrombosis.

Sinus Infections

Guiding Questions

1. Infection of which air sinus is most difficult to evaluate by physical exam?

2. Which physical findings are helpful in evaluating bacterial sinusitis?

3. What is the most common complication associated with ethmoid sinusitis?

4. What complications are associated with frontal sinusitis?

5. What complications are associated with sphenoid sinusitis?

6. How can orbital cellulitis be differentiated from septic cavernous sinus thrombosis?

Potential Severity: Delays in therapy can result in spread of infection outside of the air sinus and lead to fatal complications.

Predisposing Factors

Viral upper respiratory infections caused by rhinoviruses, influenza, parainfluenza, and adenoviruses cause inflammation of the sinuses and the production of serous exudate. An estimated 0.5–1% of viral upper respiratory infections progress to bacterial sinusitis. Anatomic obstruction increases the likelihood of bacterial sinusitis. Causes of obstruction include septal deformities, nasal polyps, foreign bodies, chronic adenoiditis, intranasal neoplasms, and indwelling nasal tubes. Patients undergoing nasotracheal intubation or who have a large-bore nasogastric tube are at increased risk for developing bacterial sinusitis. These tubes interfere with normal drainage of the sinus ostia. Nasal allergies are associated with edema, obstruction, and the accumulation of serous fluid and are another predisposing factor for bacterial sinusitis. Dental abscesses of the upper teeth can spread to the maxillary sinuses and can result in recurrent bacterial sinusitis. Two genetic disorders, cystic fibrosis (associated with abnormal viscous mucous) and Kartagener's syndrome (causing defective mucous cell ciliary function), are rarer predisposing factors for bacterial sinusitis.

Clinical Manifestations

◆ CASE 5.3

A 15-year-old white female developed an upper respiratory infection three weeks before admission. Nasal discharge was clear, but after 10 days she developed a severe left retro-orbital and left occipital headache, associated with left eye tearing. She saw her physician 3 days later complaining of persistent headache and nausea. Tenderness over the left maxillary sinus was noted. She was treated with Neo-Synephrine nose drops and Gantrisin (a sulfa antibiotic). She failed to improve and 2 days later developed swelling of both eyes. Tetracycline was begun, but she became confused and uncooperative.

Physical examination: Temperature 103°F, pulse 140, respiratory rate 40. Toxic, disoriented, lethargic.

HENT: Nose: dry, crusted purulent secretions left middle turbinate. Left eye: proptosis and chemosis and complete ocular paralysis. Right eye: less severe proptosis and chemosis, lateral gaze palsy (sixth nerve deficit). Fundi: left disc blurred margin indicating papilledema. Tenderness over left maxillary and frontal sinuses. Decreased sensation left side of the face in ophthalmic and maxillary branches of the fifth nerve. Neck was very stiff. Remainder of her exam unremarkable.

Laboratory findings: WBC 18.7K (78% PMNs, 10% bands), CSF: 18,000, WBC, 95% PMNs, protein 400 mg/dl, glucose 25 mg/dl. Sinus X-rays: opacification of the left frontal, ethmoid, maxillary, and sphenoid sinuses. Six days after admission she expired. Autopsy revealed pansinusitis, including the left sphenoid sinus, bilateral cavernous sinus thrombosis, and bacterial meningitis. Culture of meninges: group H streptococci.

Although Case 5.3 is unusually severe, this case does illustrate many of the potential clinical manifestations of sinusitis. The most common initial symptom associated with sinusitis is a pressure sensation over the involved sinus or sinuses. Subsequently, pressure progresses to pain in the area of the infected sinus. Infection of the sphenoid sinusitis, because of its deep location within the skull, does not cause an easily recognizable pain syndrome. As described in Case 5.3, sphenoid sinusitis is associated with retro-orbital pain and/or severe pain extending to the frontal, temporal, and occipital regions. Pain is frequently unilateral, severe, interfering with sleep, and not relieved by aspirin. Often sphenoid sinus pain is misdiagnosed as a migraine headache, resulting in delayed diagnosis and treatment. In addition to pain, patients usually experience nasal blockage and often note the drainage of thick, discolored purulent material. However, some deny nasal drainage, complaining of a foul taste or smell. As a conse-quence of chronic postnasal drainage, recurrent coughing is a frequent complaint, particularly at night when the patient is lying in a recumbent position. Surprisingly, despite extensive inflammation in the sinuses a minority of adults experience fever, which develops more commonly in children with sinus infection.

On physical exam, as noted in Case 5.3, localized sinus tenderness over the maxillary and frontal sinuses can be readily elicited. In maxillary sinus infection there may be tooth tenderness. Because of its deeper location within the cranium, infection of the sphenoid sinus is not associated with tenderness. Transillumination can be performed in a darkened room using a flashlight tightly sealed to the skin. Marked reduction in light transmission correlates with fluid accumulation in maxillary sinusitis and also may be helpful for diagnosing frontal sinusitis. Examination of the nose reveals edema and erythema of the nasal mucosa, and if the ostia are not completely obstructed, a purulent discharge may be seen in the nasal passage and posterior pharynx. Inflammation of the fifth cranial nerve is often associated with sphenoid sinusitis, posterior ethmoid sinus infection, cavernous sinus thrombosis, and, less commonly, maxillary sinusitis. Hypoesthesia or hyperesthesia in the regions enervated by the ophthalmic and maxillary branches may be detected on sensory exam. This finding was noted in Case 5.3 and, in combination with oculomotor paralysis, proptosis, papilledema of the left eye, and meningitis, indicated that her bacterial sinusitis was complicated by cavernous sinus thrombosis (see "Complications" below).

KEY POINTS

Clinical Manifestations of Sinusitis

1. Pressure sensation and headache.
2. Retro-orbital and hemicranial headache suggests sphenoid sinusitis.

3. Purulent foul-smelling, bad-tasting drainage.
4. Fever is rare in adults.
5. Sinus tenderness elicited in maxillary and frontal but not sphenoid sinusitis.
6. Transillumination helpful for maxillary and frontal sinusitis.
7. Look for purulent drainage from the ostia and posterior nasopharynx.
8. Hypoesthesia or hyperesthesia of the ophthalmic and maxillary branches of the fifth cranial nerve found in maxillary, ethmoid, and sphenoid disease.

Diagnosis

Despite extensive inflammation of the sinuses, the peripheral white blood cell count is often within normal limits. Case 5.3 had meningitis, explaining her peripheral leukocytosis. Cultures of the nasopharynx correlate poorly with intrasinus cultures and are not recommended. Direct sampling of the infected sinus is required for accurate microbiologic assessment. Fiber-optic cannulation can be performed, but such cultures are often contaminated by normal mouth flora. In children needle aspiration of the infected

Figure 5.5

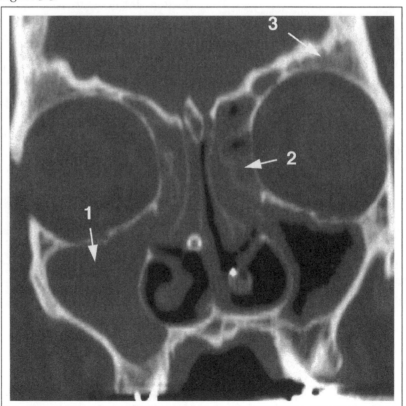

Pansinusitis. CT scan, coronal view of the air sinuses. 1. Maxillary sinus 2. Ethmoid sinus 3. Frontal sinus. Note the marked opacification of the right maxillary (left side of figure) and marked mucosal thickening of the left maxillary sinus. Both ethmoid sinuses are opaque as are the frontal sinuses. (Courtesy of Dr. Ilona Schamalfus, University of Florida College of Medicine.)

maxillary sinuses has allowed accurate sampling. However, this procedure is not recommended in routine cases.

Sinus X-rays are helpful for assessing frontal, ethmoid, and maxillary sinusitis and should include a Water's view. If sphenoid sinusitis is being considered, an overpenetrated lateral sinus film should be ordered, or the diagnosis may be missed. Positive radiographic findings include sinus opacification, air fluid levels, and/or mucosal thickening (≥8 mm). CT scan is the diagnostic study of choice for assessing sinus infections, and a limited CT scan of the sinuses is a cost-effective alternative to conventional sinus films (see Figure 5.5). CT scan allows a more detailed assessment of the integrity of the bony sinus walls. This study can readily detect extension of infection from the ethmoid sinuses to the orbit, as well as the development of an orbital abscess (see Figure 5.6). CT scan is also useful for assessing extension of frontal sinus infection to the epidural or subdural space and for diagnosing frontal brain

abscess, a rare complication of frontal sinusitis. In sphenoid sinusitis, CT with contrast injection is the study of choice for detecting early extension to the cavernous sinuses. This study can also readily detect the development of sinus mucocele.

KEY POINTS
Diagnosis of Sinusitis

1. Nasopharyngeal cultures are not helpful.
2. A limited CT scan of the sinuses is preferred over routine sinus X-rays in sphenoid, ethmoid, and frontal sinusitis.
3. CT allows assessment of bone erosions and extension beyond the sinuses.

Complications

Distinct complications are associated with ethmoid, frontal, and sphenoid sinusitis. To per-

Figure 5.6

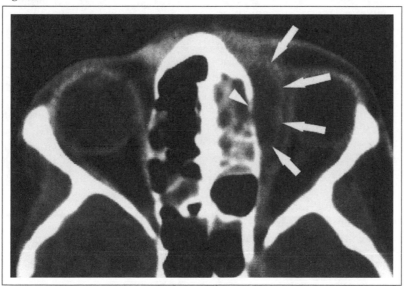

Orbital cellulitis with accompanying orbital abscess. CT scan with contrast: axial view showing the break in the ethmoid sinus wall (arrowhead) and the ring enhancing the orbital abscess (arrows) that is pushing the eye laterally. (Courtesy of Dr. Ilona Schamalfus, University of Florida College of Medicine.)

form the proper diagnostic evaluation and begin prompt therapy, the primary care physician as well as the infectious disease specialist must be able to recognize the early clinical manifestations associated with spread of infection beyond the sinuses. Complicated air sinus infection can be life-threatening and frequently leads to permanent neurologic deficits.

ETHMOID SINUSITIS

The ethmoid sinus is separated from the orbit by the lamina papyracea. This thin layer can be easily breached by infection, particularly in children. Infection in the ethmoid sinus can also spread to the orbit via ethmoid veins. The extent of orbital involvement varies and can cause four different syndromes:

1. **Periorbital cellulitis**. Infection of the skin in the periorbital area results in swollen eyelids; however, eye movements are normal, and there is no displacement of the eye.
2. **Orbital cellulitis**. When infection spreads to the orbital tissue, in addition to swollen eyelids, the eye becomes tender to palpation. Ophthalmoplegia with reduction of all eye movements occurs as a consequence of inflammation of the extraocular muscles. Chemosis (marked swelling and erythema of the conjunctiva) develops and is a reflection of the intense inflammation within the orbit. Finally, proptosis (outward displacement of the eye) is usually seen as a consequence of edematous tissue within the orbit, pushing the eye out of its socket. This infection is usually unilateral.
3. **Orbital abscess**. A discrete abscess can develop in the periosteum or soft tissue of the orbit. This complication cannot be detected by exam, the diagnosis being made by CT scan of the orbit (see Figure 5.6). Abscess formation usually warrants surgical drainage.
4. **Cavernous sinus thrombosis and meningitis**. Orbital infection can spread via the superior ophthalmic veins to the cavernous sinus. Because the cavernous sinuses are connected by the intercavernous sinuses and these veins have no valves, infection usually spreads quickly from one cavernous sinus to the other. As a consequence, bilateral eye involvement is the rule. The finding of bilateral eye involvement makes orbital cellulitis less likely. Other findings that favor the diagnosis of cavernous sinus thrombosis are abnormal fifth nerve sensation, development of papilledema, and inflammatory cells in the CSF. High-resolution CT scan with contrast is now the diagnostic study of choice.

Surgical intervention should be considered if there is progression on antibiotics, loss of visual acuity below 20/60, proptosis, or ophthalmoplegia. The ethmoid sinuses should be drained, further debridement being guided by CT scan findings.

KEY POINTS

Complications of Ethmoid Sinusitis

1. Can easily spread medially through the lamina papyracea to cause:
   a. Preorbital cellulitis,
   b. Orbital cellulitis,
   c. Orbital abscess,
   d. Septic cavernous sinus thrombosis (rare).
2. Orbital cellulitis is usually unilateral, cavernous sinus thrombosis bilateral. Papilledema, fifth nerve deficits, and CSF pleocytosis are also found with septic cavernous sinus thrombosis.
3. Orbital CT scan with contrast delineates the extent of infection.
4. Surgical drainage of the sinus is recommended if there is loss of visual acuity, proptosis, or ophthalmoplegia.

FRONTAL SINUSITIS

Frontal sinusitis can also be life threatening if not managed properly. Infection can spread anteriorly into the frontal bone, causing a subperiosteal abscess that can result in pitting edema of the forehead. The complication has been termed Pott's puffy tumor. Infection can also spread posteriorly. Particularly in teenage males the posterior wall of the frontal sinus may be thin, allowing infection to spread to the epidural or subdural space. Infection can also reach the cerebral cortex, forming a brain abscess. These complications are usually associated with a severe frontal headache that interferes with sleep and is not relieved by aspirin. In some cases seizures may develop, but in most instances frontal brain abscess is neurologically silent. Abscess formation in the subdural or epidural space and brain abscess are readily diagnosed by contrast enhanced CT scan.

KEY POINTS

Complications of Frontal Sinusitis

> 1. Infection can spread anteriorly and cause Pott's puffy tumor.
> 2. Infection can spread posteriorly and cause epidural, subdural, or brain abscess.
> 3. Posterior spread leads to severe headache, but frontal cerebral cortex lesions are usually neurologically silent.
> 4. Contrast enhanced CT scan is recommended in cases of severe frontal sinusitis.

SPHENOID SINUSITIS

Sphenoid sinusitis is the most dangerous sinus infection. If the patient with sphenoid sinusitis does not respond rapidly to oral antibiotics and decongestants, intravenous antibiotics should be initiated. Nafcillin and a third-generation cephalosporin are generally adequate coverage (see below). There should be a low threshold for surgical drainage. This sinus lies deep in the skull. Its walls are adjacent to the pituitary gland, optic canals, dura mater, and cavernous sinuses. The thickness of the lateral walls of the sphenoid sinuses varies. If infection extends beyond these walls, patients can present with the following:

1. Cavernous sinus infection that causes impairment of function of nerves III, IV, and VI causing ophthalmoplegia, fifth nerve dysfunction, and involvement of the ophthalmic and maxillary branches (hypoesthesia or hyperesthesia), as well as proptosis and chemosis. Case 5.3 had all of these characteristics and had sphenoid sinusitis and septic cavernous sinus thrombosis. The intracavernous sinuses allow infection to spread from one sinus to the other, usually within 24 hours. Diagnosis is made most readily by contrast-enhanced CT scan. The early venous phase following administration of contrast demonstrates regions of decreased or irregular enhancement, thickening of the lateral walls, and bulging of the sinus. Anticoagulation with heparin in the very early stages of infection may be helpful, although intravenous antibiotics (covering *Staphylococcus aureus* and other Gram-positive and Gram-negative organisms) are the mainstay of treatment.
2. Bacterial meningitis develops in a significant percentage of cases with cavernous sinus thrombosis, and lumbar puncture can be helpful in differentiating orbital cellulitis from cavernous sinus infection.
3. Infection can spread from the cavernous sinus to the pituitary gland, resulting in the formation of a pituitary abscess.

KEY POINTS

Complications of Sphenoid Sinusitis

> 1. The most dangerous form of sinusitis.
> 2. Most patients require hospitalization and intravenous antibiotics.
> 3. Close to many vital neurologic structures.
> 4. Complications:
>   a. Septic cavernous sinus thrombosis (a leading cause),

b. Bacterial meningitis,
c. Pituitary abscess formation.
5. CT scan with contrast defines the sites of involvement, including cavernous sinus thrombosis.
6. Surgical drainage of the sphenoid sinus is often required to prevent spread outside the sinus walls.

Microbiology

The major pathogens associated with bacterial sinusitis are as follows:

1. *Streptococcus pneumoniae* and *Haemophilus influenzae* are the most common (50–70% in maxillary).
2. Other Gram-positive aerobic mouth flora are also seen (*S. pyogenes, S. viridans*).
3. Other Gram-negative aerobic mouth flora are rare (*Moraxella catarrhalis*).
4. *Staphylococcus aureus* is more frequently seen in ethmoid and sphenoid disease.
5. Anaerobic mouth flora (*Bacteroides melanogenicus* and anaerobic streptococci) are found more frequently in adults and in patients with chronic sinusitis.
6. Gram-negative organisms are rare in the normal host, most frequently being found in chronic sinusitis. In AIDS patients *Pseudomonas aeruginosa* is a frequent pathogen.
7. Fungal sinusitis, particularly Aspergillus, is becoming an increasing problem in the immunocompromised patient, being most frequently associated with neutropenia.

KEY POINTS

Microbiology and Treatment of Sinusitis

1. *Streptococcus pneumoniae* and *Haemophilus influenzae* are most common; anaerobes are seen in adults and in chronic dis-

ease, *Staphylococcus aureus* in sphenoid disease.
2. Gram-negatives (*Pseudomonas aeruginosa*) in AIDS patients.
3. Fungi (Aspergillus) in neutropenic patients.
4. The threshold for antibiotic treatment must be low:
a. Amoxicillin-clavulanate,
b. Cefuroxime axetil,
c. Fluoroquinolones (concerns about resistance),
d. Azithromycin, no better than amoxicillin,
e. Amoxicillin no longer recommended for initial therapy.
5. Patients with frontal, ethmoid, or sphenoid sinus infection often require hospitalization and intravenous antibiotics (oxacillin + third-generation cephalosporin + metronidazole).

Treatment

Nasal decongestants are helpful for preventing sinus obstruction during acute viral upper respiratory tract infections. Neo-Synephrine nose drops, 1/4–1/2%, Q4H are effective, but treatment for longer than 3–4 days results in tachyphylaxis or rebound nasal congestion. Pseudoephedrine may also be used, but concern has been raised that this treatment may unduly dry out the nasal passages and increase the viscosity of the nasal discharge. Theoretically, inhalation of steam should improve nasal drainage by clearing the ostia; however, no studies are available that support this treatment.

The threshold for treatment with antibiotics should be low because patients with acute bacterial sinusitis may become asymptomatic despite the persistence of pus and active infection. Persistent infection may result in irreversible mucosal damage of the sinus wall and chronic sinusitis. The timing of antibiotic therapy remains controversial. A reasonable guideline is to institute antibiotics if symptoms of sinusitis persist for 7–10 days after the initial onset of a viral upper respiratory infection. The presence of purulent, foul-smelling exudate should also encourage the initiation of antibiotics. No single antibiotic will treat all possible pathogens. Treatment should be continued for a minimum of 10 days. Recommended oral regimens are the following:

1. Augmentin (amoxicillin and clavulanic acid) is probably the drug of choice. Covers *Streptococcus pneumoniae*, *Haemophilus influenzae* including ampicillin-resistant strains, *Moraxella catarrhalis*, and *Staphylococcus aureus*.
2. Cefuroxime axetil, a second-generation cephalosporin, has a spectrum of activity similar to that of Augmentin. Several other third-generation oral cephalosporins have also been recommended.
3. The fluoroquinolones levofloxacin, gatifloxacin, and moxifloxacin cover all of the major pathogens that cause acute bacterial sinusitis. The development of fluoroquinolone-resistant *Streptococcus pneumoniae* is a major concern; therefore these antibiotics should be reserved for the penicillin-allergic patient.
4. Amoxicillin is a cheaper alternative but is not as broad in spectrum. This antibiotic was previously considered the drug of choice for initial therapy. However, more recent bacteriologic studies reveal a high percentage of β-lactamase-producing organisms capable of degrading amoxicillin.
5. Azithromycin is no more efficacious than amoxicillin but is more costly.

Patients suffering with frontal, ethmoid, and sphenoid sinusitis frequently require hospitalization and intravenous antibiotic therapy to prevent the spread of infection to vital organs beyond the sinus walls. High-dose intravenous antibiotics should be instituted emergently and directed at the probable organisms (see "Microbiology" above). Empiric therapy should include a penicillinase-resistant penicillin, either nafcillin or oxacillin, at maximal doses plus a third-generation cephalosporin, either ceftriaxone or cefotaxime. Anaerobic coverage should also be instituted with intravenous metronidazole.

Additional Reading

Eye Infections
Benson, W.H., and Lanier, J.D. Current diagnosis and treatment of corneal ulcers. *Curr Opin Ophthalmol* 9:45–49, 1998.

Callegan, M.C., Engelbert, M., Parke, D.W., 2nd, Jett, B.D., and Gilmore, M.S. Bacterial endophthalmitis: epidemiology, therapeutics, and bacterium-host interactions. *Clin Microbiol Rev* 15:111–124, 2002.

Durand, M.L., and Heier, J.S. Endophthalmitis. *Curr Clin Top Infect Dis* 20:271–297, 2000.

Sheikh, A., and Hurwitz, B. Topical antibiotics for acute bacterial conjunctivitis: a systematic review. *Br J Gen Pract* 51:473–477, 2001.

Shields, S.R. Managing eye disease in primary care. Part 2. How to recognize and treat common eye problems. *Postgrad Med* 108:83–86, 91–96, 2000.

Pharyngitis
Ebell, M.H., Smith, M.A., Barry, H.C., Ives, K., and Carey, M. The rational clinical examination. Does this patient have strep throat? *JAMA* 284:2912–2918, 2000.

Hayes, C.S., and Williamson, H., Jr. Management of Group A beta-hemolytic streptococcal pharyngitis. *Am Fam Physician* 63:1557–1564, 2001.

Otitis Media
Schwartz, L.E., Brown, R.B. Purulent otitis media in adults. *Arch Intern Med* 152:2301–2304, 1992.

Stool, S., Carlson, L.H., and Johnson, C.E. Otitis media: diagnosis, management, and judicious use of antibiotics. *Curr Allergy Asthma Rep* 2:297–300, 2002.

Sinusitis
Chow, A.W. Acute sinusitis: current status of etiologies, diagnosis, and treatment. *Curr Clin Top Infect Dis* 21:31–63, 2001.

Conrad, D.A., and Jenson, H.B. Management of acute bacterial rhinosinusitis. *Curr Opin Pediatr* 14:86–90, 2002.

Erkan, M., Aslan,T., Ozcan, M., and Koc, N. Bacteriology of antrum in adults with chronic maxillary sinusitis. *Laryngoscope* 104:321–324, 1994.

Lew, D., Southwick, F.S., Montgomery, W.W., Weber, A.L., Baker, A.S. Sphenoid sinusitis. *N Engl J Med* 309:1149–1154, 1983.

Tami, T.A. The management of sinusitis in patients infected with the human immunodeficiency virus (HIV). *Ear Nose Throat J* 74:360–363, 1995.

Wald, E.R., Milmoe, G.J., Bowen, A., Ledesma-Medina, J., Salamon, N., Bluestone, C.D. Acute maxillary sinusitis in children. *N Engl J Med* 304:749–754, 1981.

Complications of ENT Infections

Ramsey, P.G., and Weymuller, E.A. Complications of bacterial infection of the ears, paranasal sinuses, and oropharynx in adults. *Emerg Med Clin North Am* 3(1):143–160, 1985.

Southwick, F.S. Septic thrombophlebitis of major dural venous sinuses. *Curr Clin Topic Infect Dis* 15:179–203, 1995.

Central Nervous System Infections

Recommended Time to Complete: 2 days

Guiding Questions

1. What layers of the brain make up the meninges?
2. Where is the subdural space?
3. What is the blood-brain barrier and why is it important to consider when treating CNS infections?

Introduction

Potential Severity: Often life-threatening illnesses. Infections of the central nervous system are infectious disease emergencies and require immediate treatment.

Fortunately, central nervous system infections are rare, but they are extremely serious. The cerebral cortex and spinal cord are confined within the restricted boundaries of the skull and bony spinal canal. Therefore inflammation and edema have devastating consequences, often leading to tissue infarction that in turn results in permanent neurologic sequelae or death.

To understand the pathogenesis and clinical consequences of central nervous system infections, it is important to have a working knowledge of basic neuroanatomy and neurophysiology. The cerebral cortex and spinal cord are suspended and bathed by cerebrospinal fluid (CSF) that is produced by the choroid plexus

Figure 6.1

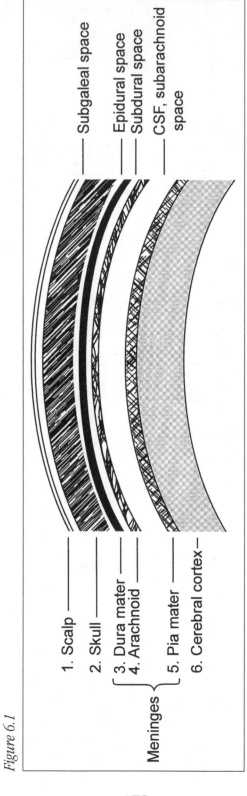

Schematic depiction of the epidural, subdural, and subarachnoid spaces in the CNS.

lining the walls of the cerebral ventricles and resorbed by arachnoid villi, which drain into a large midline vein, the superior sagittal sinus. The cortex and spinal cord are surrounded by three layers called the meninges. The two layers closest to the cortex are called the pia mater (directly overlying the cerebral cortex) and the arachnoid. These layers make up the leptomeninges, and the third layer, the dura mater or pachymeninges, serves as the outer layer (see Figure 6.1). The CSF flows between the pia mater and arachnoid in the subarachnoid space. Central nervous system infections are classified by the site of infection. Infection of the cerebral cortex is called encephalitis, and infection of meninges is called meningitis. Abscesses usually form in three locations within the central nervous system: the cerebral cortex, termed a brain abscess; between the dura and arachnoid, called a subdural abscess; or immediately outside the dura, forming an epidural abscess.

The capillaries of the brain and spinal cord differ from those in other regions of the body. The tight junctions linking the endothelial cells of the vessels in this region are less permeable than vessels in other parts of the body. The limited permeability of central nervous system vessels forms a physiologic barrier that is commonly termed the blood-brain barrier. This barrier protects the central nervous system from invading pathogens and toxic substances. However, in addition to its protective effect, the impermeability of the CNS capillaries prevents the entry of immunoglobulins, complement, and antibiotics. Therefore if a pathogen breaches the blood-brain barrier, the host's initial defense mechanisms are impaired, partly explaining the rapid progression and serious consequences of CNS infections. Antibiotics that are used to treat central nervous system infections must be capable of penetrating this barrier, and because penetration of all antibiotics is impeded, maximal doses (sometimes termed "meningeal doses") are required to cure CNS infections.

Bacterial Meningitis

Guiding Questions

1. When should a lumbar puncture be performed?

2. A patient has meningeal symptoms and signs but is noted to have a focal neurologic deficit. What tests should you perform? Is there any therapeutic intervention you would begin before sending the patient for tests?

3. A college student arrives in the emergency room with a generalized headache and stiff neck. The lumbar puncture reveals CSF with a white blood cell count (WBC) of 50 (100% lymphocytes), protein 75 mg%, and glucose 80 mg%. What is the most likely diagnosis and how would you treat the patient?

4. A previously healthy 30-year-old man arrives in the emergency room complaining of a severe generalized headache and fevers. After lumbar puncture his CSF is found to have 500 WBC (95% PMNs), protein 300 mg%, and a glucose of 25 with serum glucose of 75 mg%. What is the most likely diagnosis and how would you treat this patient?

Bacterial meningitis remains one of the most feared and dangerous infectious diseases a physician can encounter. This form of meningitis constitutes a true infectious disease emergency. It is important that the physician quickly make the appropriate diagnosis and initiate antibiotic therapy. Minutes can make the difference between life and death in bacterial meningitis. Because of the rapid progression of the disease there is no time to look through textbooks to decide on appropriate management. To ensure the best outcome, every clinician needs to have a basic understanding of bacterial meningitis and its management.

Epidemiology and Etiology

With the advent of the *Haemophilus influenzae* B vaccine the incidence of bacterial meningitis in children has declined dramatically in the United States, and this is now primarily an adult disease. The wider use of pneumococcal vaccine in patients age ≥65 years and in patients with chronic underlying diseases also promises to reduce the incidence in adults. Because bacterial meningitis is not a reportable disease in the United States, an exact incidence is not available but has been estimated to be about 3–4 per 100,000. In underdeveloped countries the incidence is at least tenfold higher, reflecting crowded conditions and the lack of vaccination programs or other public health preventive measures.

Four pathogens have been the major causes of community acquired bacterial meningitis in children and adults (see Table 6.1):

1. **Streptococcus pneumoniae**. This is the most common cause of community-acquired meningitis in the United States. In other parts of the world, *Neisseria meningitidis* predominates. *S. pneumoniae* first causes infection of the ear, sinuses, or lungs and then spreads to

the bloodstream, where it seeds the meninges. *S. pneumoniae* is also the most common cause of recurrent meningitis in patients with a CSF leak following head trauma.

2. **Neisseria meningitidis**. This pathogen can cause isolated sporadic infection or cause an epidemic. *N. meningitidis* first infects the nasopharynx, causing sore throat. In individuals lacking antimeningococcal antibodies, nasopharyngeal carriage may be followed by bacteremia and seeding of the meninges. Crowded environments such as college dormitories or military training facilities increase the risk of contracting *N. meningitidis*. Epidemics usually occur in the winter months, when person-to-person spread by respiratory secretions is most frequent. Patients with defects in the terminal complement components are also at increased risk of contracting sporadic meningococcal infection.

3. **Listeria monocytogenes**. This organism primarily infects individuals with depressed cell-mediated immunity, including pregnant woman, neonates, patients on immunosuppressives, and individuals infected with HIV. Finally, individuals over the age of 50 may have an increased risk of developing Listeria. This form of meningitis is contracted by ingesting contaminated foods. Heavy contamination with Listeria can occur when foods are stored for prolonged periods at 4°C, because this organism can grow in a cool environment. Listeria can contaminate unpasteurized soft cheeses as well as other improperly processed dairy products. High counts of this organism have also been found in defectively processed hot dogs and fish. When Listeria enters the gastrointestinal (GI) tract, it is able to silently invade the GI lining, enter the bloodstream, and infect the meninges.

4. **Haemophilus influenzae**. Prior to the administration of the *H. influenzae* B vaccine, *H. influenzae* meningitis was the most common pathogen to cause meningitis in chil-

Table 6.1

Bacterial Etiologies of Meningitis in Adults

	COMMUNITY	NOSOCOMIAL
Streptococcus pneumoniae	38%	8%
Gram-negative bacilli	4%	38%
Neisseria meningitidis	14%	1%
Listeria	11%	3%
Streptococci	7%	12%
Staphylococcus aureus	5%	9%
Haemophilus influenzae	4%	4%

dren; however, meningitis due to this organism is now rare.

The causes of bacterial meningitis in neonates reflect the organisms they contact during passage through the birth canal. *Escherichia coli* is the most common cause of neonatal meningitis, followed by Group B streptococci.

Nosocomial bacterial meningitis has increased in frequency over the past two decades. This increased incidence can be explained by the increased numbers of patients undergoing neurosurgical procedures and having hardware placed in their cerebral ventricles. The bacteriology of nosocomial meningitis is very different from that of community-acquired disease. Gram-negative rods predominate, *E. coli* and *Klebsiella* being the most common. *Staphylococcus aureus* is another frequent pathogen (see Table 6.1). Patients undergoing ventricular shunt placement can develop meningitis due to contamination of the plastic shunt tubing. *S. epidermidis, S. aureus,* enterococci, *Bacillus subtilis,* and corynebacteria (previously called diptheroids) are most commonly encountered.

KEY POINTS

The Epidemiology and Etiologies of Bacterial Meningitis

1. Primarily a disease of adults.
2. Four major pathogens are associated with community-acquired disease:
   a. *Streptococcus pneumoniae* is most common and follows bacteremia from ear, sinus, or lung infection. Also associated with chronic CSF leaks.
   b. *Neisseria meningitidis* begins with colonization of the nasopharynx. Sporadic cases often associated with terminal complement defects. Epidemics occur in crowded environments such as dormitories and military training camps.
   c. *Listeria monocytogenes* occurs in neonates, pregnant women, and immunocompromised patients. Contracted by eating contaminated refrigerated foods.
   d. *Haemophilus influenzae* was the most common form of meningitis in children. Now is rare following widespread administration of *H. influenzae* B vaccine.
3. Neonates develop Gram-negative and group B streptococcus meningitis.
4. Nosocomial meningitis is usually associated with neurosurgery and/or placement of a ventriculostomy tube and is caused by Gram-negative rods, *Staphylococcus aureus,* enterococci, *S. epidermidis, Bacillus subtilis,* and corynebacteria.

Pathogenesis

Bacterial meningitis is most commonly blood borne. Primary infections of the ears, sinuses, throat, lungs, heart, and gastrointestinal tract can all lead to bacteremia, and on rare occasion blood-borne bacteria gain entry into the subarachnoid space (see Figure 6.2). Blood-borne bacteria may gain entry through the large venous sinuses in the brain. Bacteria can settle along these slow-flowing venous channels, then escape and penetrate the dura and arachnoid, infecting the CSF. Less commonly, bacteria can enter the CSF through a break in the cribriform plate or defect in the base of the skull following basilar skull fracture. Patients suffering head trauma can develop CSF leakage at these sites, and bacteria from the nasopharynx or middle ear, primary *Streptococcus pneumoniae,* can track up through the leak into the subarachnoid space. Finally, patients who develop brain abscesses secondary to otitis media and mastoiditis or bacterial sinusitis on rare occasion can develop meningitis due to direct spread of bacteria from the abscess to the subarachnoid space.

Figure 6.2

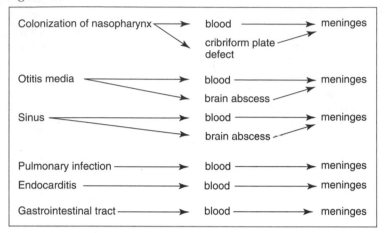

Routes for bacterial invasion of the meninges.

Because the blood-brain barrier blocks entry of immunoglobulins and complement, in the early phases of infection bacteria are able to grow unimpeded by the host's immune system. As the number of organisms increases, polymorphonuclear leukocytes (PMNs) are attracted to the site. As they attempt to kill organisms, PMNs often lyse, releasing toxic oxygen products, proteolytic enzymes, and inflammatory cytokines. These products lead to necrosis and edema of the surrounding tissue. The marked inflammatory response in the subarachnoid space damages the cerebral microvasculature, increasing the permeability of the blood-brain barrier. Leakage of serum from the damaged vessels results in an increase in the CSF protein level. Inflammation at the surface of the cerebral cortex can induce vasculitis and occlusion of both small arteries and cortical veins, causing cerebral infarction. Inflammation of the arachnoid and pia mater alters glucose transport into this region, lowering CSF glucose levels. Inflammation of the subarachnoid space may impair CSF flow and cause hydrocephalus. Finally, inflammation damages neural cells in the cerebral cortex and causes cerebral edema. The ultimate consequences of intense inflammation and bacterial invasion of the meninges are increased intracranial pressure, decreased cerebral blood flow, and cerebral cortex hypoxia, leading to irreversible ischemic damage.

KEY POINTS

The Pathogenesis of Bacterial Meningitis

1. Gain entry to the subarachnoid space and CSF:
   a. Most commonly by bacteremia, gain entry via large venous channels,
   b. By nasopharyngeal spread through a CSF leak caused by a cribriform plate defect or basilar skull fracture,
   c. Direct spread from a brain abscess or air sinus infection.
2. Rapid growth in the CSF because the blood-brain barrier blocks entry of immunoglobulins and complement.
3. Inflammation damages the blood-brain barrier, increasing permeability, allowing entry of serum protein, and impairing glucose transport.
4. Progressive cerebral edema, increased CSF pressure, and decreased cerebral blood flow lead to irreversible ischemic damage.

Clinical Manifestations of Bacterial Meningitis

◆ CASE 6.1

A 47-year-old sales manager and father of two arrived in the emergency room in deep coma. Mr. H. T. had a history of recurrent ear infections since age 12. Three days prior to admission, Mr. T. complained of a severe left earache. He took ear drops prescribed by his local physician, and the pain disappeared during the night. The evening prior to admission, he began complaining of headache and felt "sort of disoriented." An hour after the onset of headache he began vomiting, vomiting five times during the night. The morning of admission his wife reported that he appeared drowsy. He stayed home from work, sleeping most of the morning. About noon he awoke but did not recognize his wife and began speaking incoherent sentences and became very restless. By 4 P.M. he failed to respond when his wife called his name, and he was brought to the emergency room.

Physical examination: Temperature 104°F, blood pressure 140/100, pulse 140, respiratory rate 20.
Very ill-appearing man who did not respond to his name, moving all limbs only in response to deep pain. Ears bilaterally blocked with cerumen. Eyes: Pupils were dilated 8 mm but reacted to light. Optic disc margins were flat. Neck: Very stiff, both Kernig's and Brudzinski's signs were present. Lungs: Coarse diffuse rhonchi throughout all lung fields.
Skin: No lesions seen.
Neurologic exam: No cranial nerve abnormalities. Symmetric reflexes. Moved all limbs.
Laboratory findings: Peripheral WBC 19,500 (39% polymorphonuclear leukocytes, 50% band forms, 6% lymphocytes, 5% monocytes). Hct 35.5. Chest X-ray: no infiltrates.
Lumbar puncture performed in the emergency room: Opening CSF pressure: 560 mm H_2O (normal 70–180 mm); CSF WBC: 9,500 WBCs (95% PMNs); CSF protein: 970 mg% (normal 14–45 mg%), CSF glucose: 25 mg% , with simultaneous serum glucose of 210 (normal 50–75 mg%, generally 2/3 of serum glucose); CSF Gram stain: Gram-positive lancet-shaped diplococci. CSF and blood cultures grew *Streptococcus pneumoniae*.

Understanding that meningitis is usually the consequence of hematogenous spread from a primary infection, the clinician needs to inquire about antecedent symptoms of ear, nose, and throat infections as well as symptoms of pneumonia. Meningitis in Case 6.1 was preceded by otitis media.

Case 6.1 had many of the typical symptoms of meningitis. Classically, patients with bacterial meningitis have symptoms of an upper respiratory tract or ear infection that is abruptly interrupted by worsening fever accompanied by one or more "meningeal" symptoms:

1. Headache is usually severe and unremitting, often being reported as the most severe headache ever experienced. Generalized pain is the rule, reflecting diffuse inflammation of the meninges. Pain may radiate down the neck. Aspirin and other over-the-counter pain medications are usually ineffective.
2. Neck stiffness is frequently noted and is a consequence of meningeal inflammation precipitating muscle spasms of the back of the neck.
3. Vomiting is a frequent symptom, as experienced in Case 6.1. The cause of vomiting is unclear, but it may be secondary to brain stem irritation and/or elevated intracerebral pressure.
4. Altered consciousness usually develops within hours of the onset of headache. As noted in Case 6.1, the patient may become difficult to arouse and often becomes confused and disoriented. It is surprising how long family members wait before becoming concerned enough to bring the patient to the hospital. Unfortunately, such delays dramatically worsen the prognosis of bacterial meningitis. In more severe cases loss of consciousness may be accompanied by grand mal or focal seizures.

Physical examination usually demonstrates high fever as well as neck stiffness. Two maneuvers are commonly used to test for meningeal inflammation. Brudzinski's nape of the neck sign is elicited by flexing the neck forward. This movement stretches the meninges and is resisted by the patient with meningeal inflammation because this maneuver causes severe pain. Kernig's sign requires that the hip be flexed at a 90° angle and the knee be bent at a 45° angle as the patient lies on his or her back. As the knee is straightened, the patient with meningeal irritation will resist straightening, complaining of lower back and hamstring pain.

A careful ear, nose, and throat examination should be performed. Findings of otitis media (dull tympanic membrane, fluid behind the eardrum) may be discovered in cases of *Streptococcus pneumoniae* and *Haemophilus influenzae,* or pharyngeal erythema maybe noted in cases of *Neisseria meningitidis.* The nose should be carefully examined looking for a clear nasal discharge suggestive' of a CSF leak. However, usually at the time of presentation meningeal inflammation temporarily closes the CSF leak, and leakage becomes apparent only after the patient has recovered. The nasal passage and posterior pharynx may also reveal a purulent discharge suggestive of sinusitis, a less common infection that can predispose to meningitis. Auscultation of the heart may reveal a diastolic murmur suggesting aortic insufficiency and would strongly suggest bacterial endocarditis as the primary infection leading to meningitis. Most cases of endocarditis complicated by meningitis are due to *Staphylococcus aureus.* Lung exam may reveal findings of pneumonia (asymmetric lung expansion, bronchovesicular breath sounds, rales, egophony, and dullness to percussion) and would make *S. pneumoniae* the most likely etiology. A chest X-ray should also be performed in all patients with meningitis to exclude pneumonia. A thorough examination of the skin needs to be performed looking for purpuric lesions. Petechiae and purpura are most commonly encountered in patients with meningococcemia but also may be found in *S. aureus* endocarditis, Echo 9 virus, and rickettsial infections (see Chapter 13, "Zoonotic Infections"). In patients who are asplenic, pneumococcal or *H. influenzae* sepsis is commonly associated with disseminated intravascular coagulation and petechial lesions. The finding of petechiae or purpura is usually a bad prognostic sign.

Finally and most important, a neurologic exam must be performed. First the mental status must be carefully described. The exact level of neurologic function should be documented. For example, does the patient respond to voice or only to a deep sternal rub? The level of consciousness on admission is a very useful prognostic indicator. Patients who are unresponsive to deep pain have a much higher mortality rate than do patients who respond to voice. The cranial nerves should be assessed. Lateral gaze palsy due to sixth nerve dysfunction can result from increased intracranial pressure. Focal findings such as hemiparesis, asymmetric pupillary response to light, or other unilateral cranial nerve deficits are uncommon in bacterial meningitis and raise the possibility of a space-occupying lesion such as a brain abscess or tumor. The finding of papilledema on funduscopic exam is rare in meningitis and usually indicates the presence of a space-occupying lesion.

It is important to keep in mind that meningitis in the very young and the very old does not present with these classic symptoms and signs. In the elderly the onset of meningitis is often more insidious. The earliest symptoms usually are fever and alterations in mental status. Meningeal signs are less commonly reported, and many elderly patients have neck stiffness as a consequence of osteoarthritis, an old cerebrovascular accident, or Parkinson's disease. The physician must have a high index of suspicion and must aggressively exclude the possibility of bacterial meningitis in the elderly patient with fever and confusion. In the very young, neonatal and infant meningitis simply presents as fever and irritability. No history is obtainable, and as a consequence lumbar puncture should be included in the fever workup of the very young patient.

KEY POINTS

The Clinical Manifestations in Bacterial Meningitis

1. Upper respiratory or ear infection interrupted by the abrupt onset of meningeal symptoms:
   a. Generalized, severe headache,
   b. Neck stiffness,
   c. Vomiting,
   d. Depression of mental status.
2. Physical findings:
   a. Brudzinski's (neck flexion) and Kernig's (straight leg raise) signs,
   b. Abnormal ear exam (*Streptococcus pneumoniae* or *Haemophilus influenzae*), pharyngeal erythema (*Neisseria meningitidis*), clear nasal discharge due to CSF leak (*S. pneumoniae*),
   c. Petechial or purpuric skin lesions most common with *N. meningitidis*, also seen with rickettsial infection, echovirus, *Staphylococcus aureus*, and asplenic sepsis,
   d. Neurologic exam, look for focal findings (suggests a space-occupying lesion) and assess mental status (important prognostic factor).

Diagnosis

The critical test for making the diagnosis of meningitis is the lumbar puncture. If the clinician has included meningitis as part of his or her differential diagnosis, a lumbar puncture needs to be performed. If no focal neurologic deficits are apparent and papilledema is not seen on funduscopic examination, a lumbar puncture can be safely performed (see Figure 6.3). Too often the clinician orders a CT scan before performing the lumbar puncture, needlessly delaying the appropriate diagnostic study. The one major exception to this rule is patients with AIDS, who have a high frequency of cortical space-occupying lesions.

At the time of lumbar puncture, CSF pressure should be documented by manometry. In cases of bacterial meningitis, CSF pressure is almost always elevated, and high elevation suggests severe cerebral edema and/or defective CSF resorption. Cellular and biochemical analysis of the CSF is very helpful in deciding on the most likely etiology of meningitis (see Table 6.2). Patients with bacterial meningitis who have not received prior antibiotics have increased numbers of WBC in their CSF with more than 90% PMNs. Patients with *Listeria monocytogenes* can have a lower percentage of PMNs. This organism grows and survives within the cytoplasm of host cells, a condition that can stimulate a monocytic CSF response in some patients. Patients who have received antibiotic therapy prior to lumbar puncture may also have a reduced percentage of PMNs. Because bacterial meningitis causes marked inflammation of the meninges, glucose transport is impaired, and CSF glucose is usually low (termed hypoglycorrachia). Normally, the CSF glucose concentration is two thirds of the serum glucose; therefore a serum glucose should be drawn at the time of the lumbar puncture to more accurately assess the CSF glucose level. In patients with pneumococcal meningitis a CSF glucose of < 25 mg/dl is associated with worse clinical outcome. As a consequence of inflammatory damage to vessels within the meninges, serum leaks into the cerebrospinal fluid, causing a rise in protein concentration. Concentrations can reach 1000 mg/dl in some cases, and the CSF protein almost always exceeds the normal adult concentration of 50 mg/dl in cases of bacterial meningitis. The combination of PMNs, low glucose, and high protein in the CSF is almost always caused by bacterial meningitis, and the finding of this CSF formula warrants treatment with antibiotics. In addition to a CSF cell count, glucose, and protein, CSF Gram stain and culture need to be obtained. In more than 75% of bacterial meningitis cases the Gram stain is positive. The one exception is *Listeria monocytogenes*. Because this organism

Figure 6.3

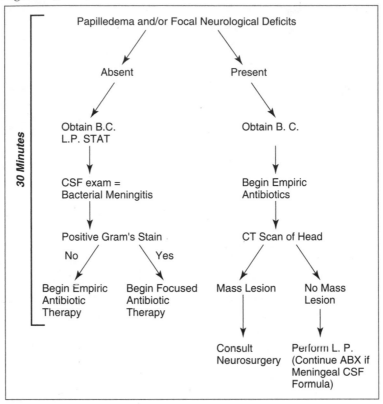

Initial management of suspected bacterial meningitis. (Source: Adapted from Tunkel, A. R., and Sheld, W. M. Acute bacterial meningitis. *Lancet* 346:1675–1680, 1995.)

usually remains intracellular, the Gram stain is positive in only 25% of cases. Latex agglutination tests for *Haemophilus influenzae, Streptococcus pneumoniae,* and *Neisseria meningitidis* are available and may be ordered in patients with negative Gram stain. However, it must be emphasized that the sensitivity of these tests is somewhat variable, and a negative latex agglutination test does not exclude the possibility of bacterial meningitis. The CSF culture should be planted immediately after lumbar puncture and in the absence of prior antibiotics remains the most sensitive test for diagnosis. In addition, a positive culture allows antibiotic sensitivity testing, which is particularly important for guiding

the treatment of *S. pneumoniae* as well as enteric pathogens.

KEY POINTS

The Diagnosis of Bacterial Meningitis

1. If meningitis is a consideration, a lumbar puncture must be performed.
2. Lumbar puncture can be performed before CT scan if there are no focal neurologic deficits and papilledema is not seen.
3. CSF opening pressure should be measured and is often elevated.

Table 6.2

CSF Profiles

TYPE OF INFECTION	WBCs	GLUCOSE (NL 2/3 OF SERUM)	PROTEIN
Untreated bacterial Tuberculosis	Polys	Low (often < 25 mg%)	Elevated (150–1000 mg%)
Fungi Treated bacterial	Lymphs	Low	Moderately elevated (80–500 mg%)
Viral	Lymphs	Normal (low in early mumps)	Mildly elevated (usually <150 mg%)
Parameningeal infection (brain abscess)	Polys or lymphs	Normal	Normal or slight elevation

4. CSF formula is very helpful in deciding whether or not the patient has bacterial meningitis. Bacterial meningitis has:
   a. >90% PMNs (exception: Listeria),
   b. Elevated CSF protein (usually 150–1000 mg/dl),
   c. Low CSF glucose, <2/3 the serum value (<25 mg/dl: poor prognosis).
5. CSF Gram stain positive in >75% of cases (exception: Listeria, 25%).
6. Blood and CSF cultures allow antibiotic sensitivity testing.

Treatment

Evaluation and institution of antibiotic therapy should occur within 30 minutes if a diagnosis of bacterial meningitis is being strongly considered. In cases in which a focal neurologic deficit is evident or papilledema is found, empiric antibiotic therapy should be instituted prior to sending the patient to CT scan (see Figure 6.3). Blood cultures should be drawn before antibiotics are begun and often subsequently yield the etiology.

Empiric antibiotic treatment is also required if the CSF Gram stain proves to be negative and the CSF formula indicates bacterial meningitis. Empiric therapy depends on the age and immune status of the patient and whether infection is nosocomial or community acquired (see Table 6.1). For community-acquired meningitis in patients ages 3 months to 50 years, maximal doses of a third-generation cephalosporin (ceftriaxone or cefotaxime) is recommended (for doses, see Table 6.3). If the patient is severely ill, vancomycin should be added to this regimen to cover for the possibility of penicillin-resistant *Streptococcus pneumoniae* (see Chapter 4, "Pulmonary Infections," for a full discussion of penicillin-resistant *S. pneumoniae*). In the patient with an immediate hypersensitivity reaction to penicillin or a history of allergy to cephalosporins, vancomycin is recommended. In patients over the age of 50 maximal doses of ampicillin are added to the third-generation cephalosporin to cover for *Listeria monocytogenes*. This organism is not sensitive to cephalosporins, and penicillin or ampicillin is the treatment of choice. For the immunocompromised host a third-generation cephalosporin, ampicillin, and vancomycin are recommended for empiric

Table 6.3

Antibiotic Treatment for Bacterial Meningitis

ORGANISM	ANTIBIOTIC	DOSE	ALTERNATIVE
Streptococcus pneumoniae (PCN MIC < 0.1 µg/ml)	Penicillin	20–24 million units/day (divided Q4H)	Chloramphenicol 4–6 g/day (divided Q6H)
	Ceftriaxone	2–4 g/day (divided Q12H)	
	Cefotaxime	12 g/day (divided Q6H)	
S. pneumoniae (MIC ≥ 0.1 µg/ml	Vancomycin ± rifampin	2 g/day (divided Q12H)	Chloramphenicol
Neisseria meningitidis	Penicillin	20–24 million units/day (divided Q4H)	Ceftriaxone Cefotaxime
Listeria monocytogenes	Ampicillin ± gentamicin	12 g/day (divided Q4H) 4–8 mg intrathecal 5 mg/kg/day systemic	Trimethoprim-sulfamethoxazole 15–20 mg/day (trimethroprim) (divided Q6H)
Haemophilus influenzae	Ceftriaxone Cefotaxime	2–4 g/day (divided Q12H) 12 g/day (divided Q6H)	Chloramphenicol
Enterobacteriaceae	Ceftriaxone ± gentamicin	2–4 g/day (divided Q12H) 4–8 mg intrathecal 5 mg/kg/day systemic	Aztreonam 6–8 g/day (divided Q6H) Trimethoprim-sulfa
	Cefotaxim ± gentamicin	12 g/day (divided Q6H)	
Pseudomonas aeruginosa	Ceftazidime + gentamicin	6–12 g/day (divided Q8H) 4–8 mg intrathecal 5 mg/kg/day systemic	Antipseudomonal penicillin 18–24 g/day (divided Q4H) + intrathecal gentamicin
Staphylococcus aureus (methicillin-sensitive)	Nafcillin or oxacillin ± rifampin	9–12 g/day (divided Q4H) 9–12 g/day (divided Q4H) 1200 mg/day (divided Q12H)	Vancomycin + rifampin Trimethoprim-sulfamethoxazole + rifampin
S. aureus (methicillin-resistant)	Vancomycin + rifampin	2 g/day (divided Q12H) 1200 mg/day (divided Q12H)	
S. epidermidis	Vancomycin + rifampin	2 g/day (divided Q12H) 1200 mg/day (divided Q12H)	

therapy. In patients who are post neurosurgery or have a cerebrospinal fluid shunt, vancomycin and ceftriaxone or cefepime are recommended.

Once a specific bacterium has been identified, the regimen can be focused. Table 6.3 outlines the recommended regimens for each major pathogen. Penicillin-resistant *Streptococcus pneumoniae* is a particular concern, given the high prevalence of these strains and the poor penetra-

tion of antibiotics across the blood-brain barrier. Intermediately resistant stains (penicillin MIC 0.1–1 µg/ml) may initially improve on penicillin therapy; however, as the integrity of the blood-brain barrier improves, the patient may relapse as a consequence of reduced levels of penicillin in the CSF. For this reason vancomycin is recommended for intermediately penicillin-resistant *S. pneumoniae* meningitis. For infections with high-level penicillin-resistant *S. pneumoniae* (penicillin MIC > 2 μg/ml) vancomycin is also the treatment of choice. Vancomycin penetrates the intact blood-brain barrier poorly, and in some patients therapeutic CSF levels might not be achieved without intrathecal administration. Rifampin combined with vancomycin may also be effective for the treatment of highly resistant *S. pneumoniae*. This regimen has been recommended for patients receiving high-dose dexamethasone because corticosteroid therapy reduces meningeal inflammation and improves the integrity of the blood-brain barrier, decreasing vancomycin CSF levels (see below). The antibiotic response should be monitored in patients who are infected with highly penicillin-resistant pneumococcus. In these patients the lumbar puncture should be repeated 24–36 hours after the initiation of therapy. Aminoglycosides, erythromycin, clindamycin, tetracyclines, and first-generation cephalosporins should not be used to treat meningitis because these drugs do not cross the blood-brain barrier.

Neurologic damage is primarily the consequence of an excessive inflammatory response. Corticosteroids reduce inflammation, and in children with *Haemophilus influenzae* bacterial meningitis, dexamethasone (0.15 mg/kg Q6H × 4 days) has been shown to reduce CSF pressure, CSF PMNs, and protein; increase CSF glucose; and improve cerebral blood perfusion. Dexamethasone also significantly reduces the incidence of deafness. The efficacy of dexamethasone in adults has not been clearly proven. However, in patients with severe mental status changes or markedly elevated CSF pressure, dexamethasone 10 mg Q6H for 2–3 days is recommended. Dexamethasone should be given just before or simultaneously with antibiotics because inflammatory mediators are released in response to the lysis of bacteria induced by antibiotic treatment. Given the lack of proven efficacy in adults, dexamethasone treatment should probably be avoided in adults infected with highly penicillin-resistant *Streptococcus pneumoniae* (MIC ≥ 2 μg/ml) because the resulting reduction in inflammation improves the integrity

of the blood-brain barrier and reduces vancomycin CSF levels. Other inhibitors of inflammation, such as a monoclonal antibody directed against the adherence receptors of leukocytes, are potentially promising but remain experimental at this time.

Additional therapeutic measures are primarily directed at reducing cerebral edema and controlling seizures. Administration of hypotonic solutions should be avoided. The airway must be protected, and hypoventilation with associated hypercarbia should be avoided because elevated pCO_2 levels cause cerebral vessel dilation and may increase intracranial pressure. Hyperventilation can also be harmful for the opposite reason: Reductions in pCO_2 may reduce cerebral perfusion and increase the risk of infarction. When the intracranial pressure is documented to be markedly elevated by lumbar puncture, intravenous 20% mannitol can be administered to remove free water from the cerebral cortex and quickly reduce cerebral edema. Oral glycerol may also reduce cerebral edema, and its efficacy is currently being investigated. Seizures develop in 20–30% of patients with meningitis; however, antiseizure medications (dilantin and diazepam are most commonly used) are not recommended for prophylaxis but are administered after the first seizure.

KEY POINTS
Treatment of Bacterial Meningitis

1. Antibiotics should be given within 30 minutes if bacterial meningitis suspected.
2. Blood cultures should be drawn and antibiotics given **prior** to CT scan.
3. Maximal doses of antibiotics must given because of limited passage through the blood-brain barrier.
4. Empiric therapy:
   a. Community-acquired, age 3 months to 50 years: ceftriaxone or cefotaxime; if se-

verely ill, add vancomycin. More than 50
years old or immunocompromised: ceftriaxone or cefotaxime and ampicillin and
vancomycin.
   b. Nosocomial: vancomycin and ceftazidime
      or cefepime.
5. Dexamethasone: Give 30 minutes before antibiotics:
   a. Children: Shown to be efficacious in
      Haemophilus influenzae.
   b. Adults: Possibly helpful, give in patients
      with coma or increased CSF pressure.
6. Maintain ventilation, prevent increased
   pCO_2 or decreased pO_2.
7. Avoid hypotonic solutions, consider mannitol or glycerol for increased CSF pressure.
8. Antiseizure medications after first seizure.

Complications

Mortality rates remain high in patients with bacterial meningitis. *Listeria monocytogenes* is associated with the highest mortality rate, 26%, followed by *Streptococcus pneumoniae*, 19%, and
Neisseria meningitidis, 13%. *Haemophilus influenzae* meningitis tends to be less severe and
is now associated with an average mortality rate
of 3%. Mortality rates are higher in the very
young and the elderly. Neurologic sequelae in
surviving patients are common. The young patient, whose brain is developing, often suffers
mental retardation, hearing loss, seizure disorders, or cerebral palsy. Older patients may develop hydrocephalus, cerebellar dysfunction,
paresis, a seizure disorder, and hearing loss.

Prevention

Given the high mortality rates and high incidence of permanent neurologic sequelae associated with bacterial meningitis, the medical community must strive to reduce the incidence of
these devastating infections.

VACCINES

Because three of the primary pathogens that
causing community-acquired bacterial meningitis are encapsulated organisms, opsonins (IgG
and complement) play a critical role in allowing
the host macrophages and PMNs to ingest these
pathogens and clear them from the bloodstream. Reduced time in the bloodstream reduces the likelihood of seeding the meninges.
The remarkable reduction in invasive *Haemophilus influenzae* type B following the widespread
administration of the *H. influenzae* B (HIB) vaccine illustrates the power of this preventive
measure. Protective levels of immunoglobulin
are achieved when the PedvaxHIB vaccine is
administered at two and four months of age.
Two other HIB vaccines are also available that
should be administered at two, four, and six
months of age.

A quadravalent meningococcal vaccine directed against serogroups A, C, Y, and W135 is
now available and is recommended for high-risk
groups, including military recruits, college students, asplenic patients, and patients with terminal complement deficiencies. The vaccine is also
useful for controlling epidemics and should be
administered to travelers going to areas where
the prevalence of meningococcal disease is high
(see *www.CDC.gov* for current recommendations for travelers). A major problem with the
present vaccine is the lack of a suitable im-
munogen against serogroup B. This serogroup
and serogroup C are the serogroups that are primarily responsible for meningococcal meningitis
in the United States. The second problem with
the meningococcal vaccine is the fact that immunity tends to be short lived, antibody titers
decreasing after three years following a single
dose of the vaccine. The incidence of meningococcal disease remains low in the United States
(approximately 1 per 100,000); therefore this
vaccine is not recommended for routine immunization.

A safe, inexpensive, efficacious 23-valent
pneumococcal vaccine is available and has been

underutilized. The mortality rate attributable to pneumococcal infection is higher than that for any other vaccine-preventable infection (approximately 40,000 per year in the United States), and about half of these deaths could be prevented by vaccination. Individuals 65 years of age or older are at higher risk for developing invasive pneumococcal infection, including meningitis, and should be vaccinated. Other groups that warrant vaccination include patients with chronic cardiovascular, pulmonary, or liver disease, diabetes mellitus, or sickle-cell disease and other patients with functional asplenia and those who have had a splenectomy. A single intramuscular or subcutaneous injection is protective for five to ten years. For most patients revaccination is not recommended. Exceptions are the immunocompromised host and patients over age 65 years, who often develop a more rapid decline in protective antibody levels. Revaccination may be considered more than five years after the initial vaccination. A 7-valent conjugated vaccine is now available that is immunogenic in children under 2 years of age. The vaccine is given in four doses at ages 2, 4, 6, and 12–15 months.

CHEMOPROPHYLAXIS

Brief antibiotic treatment has been used to prevent secondary cases of *Haemophilus influenzae* and *Neisseria meningitidis*. Secondary cases generally occur within 6 days of the index case of *H. influenzae* and within 5 days of the index case of *N. meningitidis* meningitis. Both organisms are carried in the nasopharynx, and in the person lacking specific humoral immunity these organisms can become invasive. Which individuals should be targeted for prophylaxis has been carefully delineated by epidemiologic data; however, fear plays a major role in determining who eventually receives prophylaxis. For *H. influenzae* household contacts with at least one unvaccinated child under the age of two years require prophylaxis. Data on day care exposure remains controversial; however, most experts

agree that children under age two years who may have been exposed in a day care setting should receive chemoprophylaxis. Rifampin 20 mg/kg/day (maximum dose in adults 600 mg QD) for 4 days is recommended. Rifampin prophylaxis is not recommended for pregnant women because of the potential risk of rifampin to the fetus. For *N. meningitidis* a single dose of ciprofloxacin 500 mg is the preferred prophylactic regimen and is recommended for close contacts, including household members, day care contacts, and those who may have been directly exposed to the index patient's oral secretions (e.g., kissing, mouth-to-mouth resuscitation, endotracheal tube intubation). Given the potential severity of this disease and the minimal harm of a single dose of antibiotic, physicians should probably have a low threshold for using prophylaxis. This brief treatment may help to alleviate the extreme anxiety associated with meningococcal disease.

KEY POINTS

The Outcome and Prevention of Bacterial Meningitis

1. Mortality is high: 26% Listeria, 19% *Streptococcus pneumoniae*, 13% *Neisseria meningitidis*, 3% *Haemophilus influenzae*.
2. Permanent sequelae are common:
   a. Children: Mental retardation, hearing loss, seizure disorders, cerebral palsy.
   b. Adults: Hydrocephalus, cerebellar dysfunction, paresis, a seizure disorder, hearing loss.
3. Vaccines efficacious:
   a. *S. pneumoniae*: 23-valent vaccine, safe, inexpensive. Recommended if ≥65 years old; chronic cardiovascular, pulmonary, or liver disease; diabetes mellitus; sickle-cell disease; or asplenia.
   b. *H. influenzae*: PedvaxHIB vaccine at two and four months of age, safe and inexpensive.

c. *N. meningitidis*: Quadravalent meningo-coccal vaccine serogroups A, C, Y, and W135; misses group B. Recommended: military recruits, college students, asplenia, and terminal complement defects.
4. Chemoprophylaxis:
   a. *H. influenzae*: Rifampin within 6 days for household contacts with unvaccinated child under two years old and children under two years old exposed in a day care center.
   b. *N. meningitidis*: Single dose of ciprofloxacin within 5 days for house-hold and day care contacts and those ex-posed to index case's oral secretions.

Other Forms of Meningitis

Viral Meningitis

◆ CASE 6.2

H.W. is a 45-year-old woman who was admitted to the hospital with a chief complaint of severe headache and neck stiffness × 8 days. 10 days prior to admission (PTA) she noted some mild stiffness of the back of her neck associated with fever and mild shivering. 8 days PTA she devel-oped a throbbing, sharp bitemporal headache that radiated to the vertex. Her headache was made worse by sitting up or moving. Bright light both-ered her eyes. She also noted some muscle stiff-ness in other areas, in particular her lower back. She felt very tired and lost her appetite. Although at times she felt lethargic, she never lost touch with reality.

Epidemiology: This fall (several weeks PTA) she administered psychometric admission tests to a large number of students (ages 10–20).

Physical examination: Temperature 100.4°F. Mildly ill-appearing, alert, middle-aged woman sitting in a dark room complaining of severe head-ache. Eyes: mild conjunctival erythema; fundi: normal discs. Neck: mildly stiff, negative Ker-nig's and Brudzinki's signs. Remainder of exam within normal limits including ENT and neuro-logic exams.

Laboratory findings: Hct 40, WBC 6,000 (45% PMNs, 50% lymphocytes, 5% monocytes). Lumbar puncture: OP 100, CSF WBC: 180/mm^3 (50% PMNs, 48% lymphocytes, 2% monocytes), CSF protein 59, glucose 61 with simultaneous serum glucose 84. CSF Gram stain: negative for organ-isms. A repeat lumbar puncture 8 hours later revealed OP 100; cell count 170 (2% PMNs, 95% lymphocytes, 3% monocytes), protein 58, glucose 61 (no serum glucose drawn). Gram stain: negative. CSF bacterial cultures: negative.

Hospital course: Her headache persisted, as did her low-grade fever. She remained alert and continued to have photophobia and a mildly stiff neck. She was discharged on the third hos-pital day, and her symptoms resolved over the next week.

Viral meningitis is the most common form of meningitis and is primarily caused by the non-polio enteroviruses, echoviruses, and coxsack-ieviruses. In temperate climates infections usu-ally occur during the warmer months of the year, generally during the summer and early fall. In tropical climates this infection occurs year-round. Enteroviruses are spread via the fecal-oral route, and small epidemics are frequently reported. Other viruses less commonly cause aseptic meningitis. In the nonimmune patient mumps virus is often associated with aseptic meningitis. Meningitis can occur in the absence of salivary gland swelling. The peak incidence of this virus is age five to nine years. During pri-mary genital infection with herpes simplex virus type 2, aseptic meningitis can develop. Herpes simplex type 1 less commonly causes meningi-tis. Recurrent Mollaret's aseptic meningitis has been associated with both herpes simplex types 1 and 2, as well as with Epstein-Barr virus. Acute aseptic meningitis can also be caused by varicella-zoster virus in the presence or absence of skin lesions. Epstein-Barr virus and cytomegalovirus mononucleosis syndromes can be accompanied by meningitis. Lymphocytic choriomeningitis virus was previously thought to be a common cause of aseptic meningitis, but recent studies have found this virus to be rare. The virus is transmitted in the urine of rodents, and this diagnosis should be considered in individuals who have had potential contact with rodents or rodent excreta. This infection occurs most commonly in the winter, when rodents are more likely to take up residence in human dwellings. Finally, at the time of initial human immunodeficiency virus infection 5–10% of patients may experience symptoms of aseptic meningitis, and in some of these cases HIV has been isolated from the CSF (see Chapter 17, "HIV Infection").

As is illustrated in Case 6.2, severe headache is the most common complaint. Headache is usually generalized but may localize bilaterally to the frontal, temporal, or occipital regions. Photophobia is another very common complaint, and patients usually request that their room remain darkened. Neck stiffness and diffuse myalgias are also common. On physical examination the skin should be carefully examined for maculopapular rashes (found in some strains of echovirus). Eye exam may reveal conjunctivitis, which is frequently associated with enteroviral infections. Significant nuchal rigidity is found in over half of cases with aseptic meningitis. Patients may be slightly lethargic; however, unlike patients with bacterial and fungal meningitis, patients with viral meningitis rarely exhibit significant depression in mental status. Focal neurologic findings should not be observed in this disease.

Lumbar puncture usually reveals a predominance of lymphocytes, a normal glucose, and a mildly elevated CSF protein (see Table 6.2). The CSF leukocyte count usually ranges from 100 to 1000 cells/mm^3. In some forms of viral meningitis (mumps and lymphocytic choriomeningitis) the CSF glucose may be lowered early in the disease. Also early in the disease, PMNs may predominate in the CSF, and bacterial meningitis

cannot be safely excluded. Therefore these patients should not be sent home but should be covered with empiric antibiotics pending CSF culture, blood cultures, and follow-up lumbar puncture. In most cases a repeat lumbar puncture 6–24 hours later reveals a predominance of lymphocytes, and the patient can be discharged. However, in some patients PMNs may persist for up to 48 hours, necessitating continued observation in the hospital and antibiotic administration. A negative CSF culture after 48 hours greatly reduces the probability of bacterial meningitis. However, the threshold for antibiotic coverage must be low to prevent inadvertent delays in the treatment of bacterial meningitis. PCR diagnosis of enterovirus in the CSF is highly sensitive and specific but is not yet commercially available. Proof of enterovirus CSF infection would allow the patient to be discharged home because with the exception of patients with severe immunoglobulin deficiency, viral meningitis is a self-limiting disease that usually resolves spontaneously within 7–10 days. In patients with agammaglobulinemia a chronic enteroviral viral meningitis or meningoencephalitis can develop that continues for years and is often fatal. Treatment with systemic and intraventricular pooled IgG preparations has been successful in some of these patients.

KEY POINTS
Viral Meningitis

> 1. The most common form of meningitis:
>   a. Enteroviruses, echovirus, and coxsackievirus most frequent, summer and early fall,
>   b. Mumps in the nonimmune, may be no parotid gland swelling, ages 5–9 years,
>   c. Herpes simplex type 2 primary disease, also cause of Mollaret's recurrent meningitis,
>   d. Epstein-Barr virus and cytomegalovirus, rare,

e. Lymphocytic choriomeningitis excreted in rodent urine, rare,
    f. Can be the initial presentation of HIV infection.
2. Primary clinical manifestations:
    a. Headache and photophobia, stiff neck,
    b. No loss of consciousness,
    c. Conjunctivitis, maculopapular, and rarely petechial rashes with echovirus.
3. CSF: Predominance of lymphs, rarely PMNs early, normal glucose, mild protein increase.
4. Diagnosis: PCR not commercially available, often presumptive.
5. Treatment: Observation, antibiotics if PMNs in CSF, self-limited disease lasting 7–10 days.

Tuberculous Meningitis

This disease most commonly arises in association with miliary tuberculosis. Meningitis can also develop if a tubercle ruptures into the subarachnoid space. The symptoms and signs of tuberculous meningitis vary and can mimic other forms of acute bacterial meningitis. This disease can also be indolent and present with a mild headache and malaise. Because tuberculous meningitis primarily involves the basilar meninges, inflammation often involves the pons and optic chiasm, leading to third, fourth, and sixth cranial nerve dysfunction, causing abnormalities in extraocular movements as well as the pupillary response. Mental status changes need to be carefully documented, and outcome closely correlates with the neurologic findings. Patients who are stuporous or have hemiplegia have nearly a 50% risk of dying or suffering severe neurologic sequelae.

Chest X-ray demonstrates changes consistent with tuberculosis in most children but in only 50% of adults. Tuberculin skin test is helpful and is usually positive. However, a negative PPD does not exclude the diagnosis. Lumbar puncture is the key to diagnosis and usually obeys the "500 rule"; that is, the leukocyte count is usu-

ally ≤500 cells mm³ (usual range: 100–500 cells/mm³), and the protein is usually ≤500 mg/dl (range: 100–500 mg/dl). In addition a moderate depression in CSF glucose is usually encountered (≤45 mg/dl); however, in a significant number of cases the CSF glucose may exceed this value. A predominance of mononuclear leukocytes is the usual cellular response; however, early in tuberculous meningitis PMNs may predominate in up to one quarter of patients. The CSF AFB smear is positive in slightly over one third of cases, but repeat examination of multiple samples that have been centrifuged increases the sensitivity. Large volumes of CSF should be collected for culture and increase the culture yield. PCR amplification tests for tuberculosis are now available that are highly specific; however, their sensitivity has not yet matched that of culture. CT or MRI with contrast may reveal rounded densities that are indicative of tuberculomas, basilar arachnoid inflammation, and hydrocephalus. Flow of CSF may be impaired as a consequence of basilar inflammation that blocks flow through the aqueduct of Sylvius.

After appropriate cultures are obtained, treatment should be initiated immediately. Untreated tuberculous meningitis is fatal within five to eight weeks of the onset of symptoms. Prognosis is worse in patients under five years or over 50 years of age. A three-drug regimen consisting of INH, rifampin, and pyrazinamide is recommended. Ethambutol can be added if infection with a resistant organism is suspected. In addition to antituberculous agents, a glucocorticoid (60 mg prednisone QD in adults and 1–3 mg/kg in children) is recommended in patients with hydrocephalus to reduce basilar inflammation.

KEY POINTS
Tuberculous Meningitis

1. Usually develops during miliary tuberculosis.
2. No pulmonary disease is evident in 50%.

3. Clinically similar to other forms of meningitis:
   a. A basilar process involving the pons and optic chiasm,
   b. Third, fourth, and sixth cranial nerve deficits,
   c. Can cause noncommunicating hydrocephalus,
   d. Development of coma is a bad prognostic sign.
4. CSF obeys the 500 rule: < 500 WBC, usually lymphocytes, protein < 500 mg/dl, glucose often < 45 mg/dl.
5. Culture large volumes of CSF, AFB smear positive in one third, PCR sensitive.
6. Fatal if not treated within 5–8 weeks.
7. Treatment with INH, rifampin, and pyrazinamide.

Cryptococcal Meningoencephalitis

Cryptococcus neoformans is found predominantly in pigeon droppings. High concentrations of this yeastlike fungus are found in pigeon nesting areas and on ledges where pigeons perch. The organism is inhaled and subsequently gains entry into the bloodstream and seeds the brain and meninges, causing a meningoencephalitis. Cryptococcus contains a thick capsule made up of negatively charged polysaccharides that are immunosuppressive, blocking cell-mediated immune responses as well as leukocyte migration. These effects explain the minimal inflammatory response elicited by invading cryptococci. Strains that produce melanin demonstrate increased virulence, and this cell wall product is thought to provide protection against oxidants. The high concentrations of dopamine in the CNS serve as a substrate for melanin production. Cryptococcus also produces mannitol, a product that may induce cerebral edema and inhibit phagocyte function.

This organism most commonly infects immunocompromised hosts; however, infections in normal hosts are also reported. This is the most common form of meningitis in AIDS patients (see Chapter 17, "HIV Infection"). In the non–HIV-infected patient, cryptococcal CNS infection usually has a slowly progressive, waxing and waning course characterized by severe intermittent headache followed by mild confusion and personality changes that can progress to stupor and coma. The subacute onset and nonspecific nature of this illness often delay the diagnosis. On average, the diagnosis is determined one month after the onset of symptoms. The progression of this illness tends to be more rapid in HIV-infected patients, and the larger burden of organisms results in marked inhibition of the inflammatory response (see Chapter 17, "HIV Infection"). Like *Mycobacterium tuberculosis*, cryptococcus produces a basilar meningitis that can cause oculomotor palsies due to third, fourth, and sixth cranial nerve dysfunction, hearing loss, and hydrocephalus. Patients may experience decreased visual acuity and diplopia. Neck stiffness is often minimal, and the possibility of meningoencephalitis might not be considered. Papilledema is noted in up to one third of cases. Focal motor deficits and seizures are rare.

The diagnosis is made by lumbar puncture. CSF pressure is often elevated above 200 mm H_2O, reflecting disturbances in CSF flow and resorption. The CSF formula typically has 20–200 WBC/mm^3 with a predominance of mononuclear cells, mildly elevated protein, and moderately decreased glucose. The CSF can be mixed 1:1 with India ink, and this preparation reveals encapsulated, rounded particles in 25–50% of infected non-HIV patients. Lymphocytes and starch granules can be mistaken for yeast forms. True cryptococcal forms have a double refractile wall, a distinctly outlined capsule, and refractile inclusions within their cytoplasm (see Figure 6.4). The most useful finding is a budding yeast form, and when this is encountered, it provides strong proof of a true cryptococcal infection. Cryptococcal polysaccharide antigen latex agglutination is highly sensitive and specific. The CSF antigen titer is determined by serially dilut-

Figure 6.4

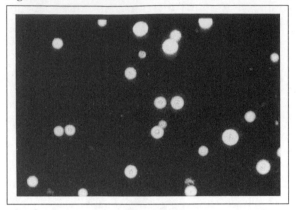

India ink preparation of CSF in cryptococcal meningitis. Two examples of budding yeast are seen, and this finding is highly specific for a true positive test.

ing the CSF. In most cases of cryptococcal meningitis, cryptococcal antigen can also be detected in the serum. The CSF culture is positive in 90% of patients, and culturing large volumes of CSF (10–15 ml) can increase the yield. The organism usually grows within 5–7 days on standard media, and use of birdseed agar can enhance growth. In addition to CSF analysis, brain CT scan or MRI with contrast is recommended to assess the degree of hydrocephalus and the extent of cerebral edema and to look for the presence of discrete, ring-enhancing masses, termed cryptococcomas.

In the non-AIDS patient the goal of therapy is to eradicate the infection. Amphotericin B (0.5–0.7 mg/kg/day) and flucytosine (100–150 mg/kg/day given in four divided doses) are recommended for a minimum of two weeks (see Chapter 1, "Anti-Infective Agents," for a description of toxicities). If the patient has improved clinically, therapy can be switched to oral fluconazole (400 mg QD), and consolidation therapy is then continued for three to six months. In patients who respond poorly to therapy, a lumbar puncture should be repeated at two weeks. Amphotericin B and flucytosine should be continued until CSF cultures are sterile.

The mortality rate for cryptococcal meningitis is 25–30% in non-AIDS patients. Poor prognostic factors include a positive CSF India ink preparation, CSF cryptococcal antigen titer of > 1:32, CSF WBC < 20/mm^3, elevated CSF opening pressure, and extraneural infection.

KEY POINTS
Cryptococcal Meningoencephalitis

1. Transmitted by pigeon excreta.
2. Inhaled, infects the lung, enters the bloodstream, and seeds the meninges and brain.
3. Yeastlike fungus with a thick, negatively charged polysaccharide capsule that is immunosuppressive. Also produces melanin and mannitol.
4. Waxing and waning symptoms, and diagnosis often delayed for ≥ 1 month.
   a. Headache most common,
   b. Personality change, confusion,
   c. Stiff neck uncommon,
   d. Cranial nerve deficits: III, IV, VI, and VIII.
5. Lumbar puncture required for diagnosis:
   a. 20–200 WBC/mm^3, predominance of mononuclear cells,
   b. Mildly elevated protein,
   c. Moderately depressed glucose,
   d. Positive India ink preparation 25–50%,
   e. Positive cryptococcal antigen,
   f. Culture usually positive in 5–7 days.
6. CT scan or MRI with contrast may show:
   a. Hydrocephalus,
   b. Cerebral edema,
   c. Ring-enhancing lesions (cryptococcomas).
7. Treatment with amphotericin B and flucytosine × 2 weeks, fluconazole for 3–6 months.
8. Mortality 25–30%, worse prognosis if CSF: + India Ink prep, antigen > 1:32, WBC < 20/mm^3, or increased opening pressure or if there is also an extraneural infection.

Viral Encephalitis

Potential Severity: An acute and severe illness associated with a high mortality.

◆ CASE 6.3

A 74-year-old white male with a history of chronic steroid (10 mg prednisone QD) use and stage I chronic lymphocytic leukemia (CLL) came to the emergency room with confusion and fever. Four days prior to admission (PTA) he complained of being increasingly tired. Two days PTA he became lethargic and was found sleeping on the floor. His wife had difficulty arousing him, and she noted that he was no longer interested in any activity. The morning of admission he displayed bizarre behavior (example: putting underwear on top of his pajama bottoms). He also became unsteady, requiring help from his wife to walk. His temperature at home was 102°F.

Epidemiology: Lives in Florida with his wife. His wife reported that he spent considerable time outside and was bitten by multiple mosquitoes.

Physical examination: Temperature 103.6°F. On arrival to the emergency room, he was mildly lethargic but was talking and answering simple questions. ENT: no lesions in mouth, sclera without erythema. Neck: some increased muscle tone, without Kernig's or Brudzinski's signs. Lungs: few rhonchi. Heart: no murmurs or rubs. Abdomen: unremarkable. Skin: no lesions noted. Neurologic exam: ataxic gait, moving all extremities, diffuse hyperreflexia, generalized increased muscle tone.

By hospital day 2 his mental status had deteriorated. He only groaned and winced with painful stimuli.

Laboratory studies: Head CT and MRI were within normal limits. Lumbar puncture: CSF WBC 100 cells/mm^3 (40% PMNs, 47% lymphocytes, 13% monocytes), protein 106 mg/dl, glucose 68 mg/dl. Serum IgM for West Nile virus: markedly elevated.

The recent outbreaks of West Nile viral encephalitis have raised the public's awareness and concern about viral encephalitis. There are two major groups of encephalitides: those that are arthropod borne and those that are caused by viruses spread from person to person. Mosquito-borne disease is caused by arboviruses, which include the alphaviruses, flaviviruses, and bunyaviruses. These infections occur in the summer months when mosquitoes are active. In addition to humans these viruses often infect birds and horses. In the case of West Nile virus crows are particularly susceptible, and the finding of a dead crow warrants increased surveillance. Public health officials frequently set out sentinel chickens in areas that are heavily infested with mosquitoes to document disease activity. The different arboviruses tend to be associated with outbreaks in specific areas of the country and have somewhat different host preferences (see Table 6.4). Prevention is best accomplished by avoiding mosquito bites. Long-sleeved shirts and long pants should be worn when outdoors. During times of increased viral encephalitis activity people should avoid the outdoors in the early evening, when mosquitoes prefer to feed. Insect repellants are also an important protective measure. Viruses that are spread from person to person and cause encephalitis include mumps, measles, varicella-zoster virus, and the most common form of sporadic encephalitis: herpes simplex type I. These forms of viral encephalitis can occur any time during the year. Other, rarer causes of viral encephalitis include cytomegalovirus, Epstein-Barr virus, and enteroviruses. Finally, a particularly deadly form of encephalitis, rabies, caused by the rabies virus, is spread by animal bites, most commonly those of bats.

With the exception of rabies, these viruses all present with similar symptoms and signs and cannot be differentiated clinically. The clinical manifestations of encephalitis differ from those of meningitis. The virus directly invades the cerebral cortex and causes abnormalities in upper cortical function. Patients may experience

Table 6.4

Encephalitis Caused by Arboviruses

DISEASE	VIRUS	LOCATION	HOSTS	CLINICAL
Eastern equine encephalitis	Alphavirus	Eastern U.S., Canada, Central and South America, Caribbean, Guyana	Birds, horses	Severe disease, high mortality
Western equine encephalitis	Alphavirus	U.S., Canada, Central and South America, Guyana	Birds, small mammals, snakes, horses	Mild disease, primarily in children
Venezuelan equine encephalitis	Alphavirus	Northern South America, Central America, Florida, Texas	Horses, rodents, birds	Febrile illness, encephalitis uncommon
St. Louis encephalitis	Flavivirus	Western, central, and southern U.S., Central and South America, Caribbean	Birds	Attacks those over 50
West Nile encephalitis	Flavivirus	Throughout the U.S. (New York, Louisiana, Georgia, Florida)	Birds	Usually mild disease, in elderly severe disease
Japanese encephalitis	Flavivirus	Japan, Siberia, Korea, China, Southeast Asia, India	Birds, pigs horses	Can cause severe encephalitis
California group encephalitis	Bunyavirus	U.S., Canada	Small mammals	School-age children, permanent behavior changes

visual or auditory hallucinations. As described in Case 6.3, patients may perform peculiar higher motor functions such as unbuttoning and buttoning a shirt or placing underwear over their pants. Patients with encephalitis frequently develop seizures that are either grand mal or focal in character. They may also develop motor or sensory deficits such as ataxia. These symptoms and signs are usually accompanied by severe headache. As the disease progresses and cerebral edema occurs, the patient may become comatose. Development of coma is associated with a poor prognosis. In herpes encephalitis the typical vesicular herpetic lesions on the lip or face are usually not seen because reactivated virus migrates up cranial nerves toward the central nervous system rather than to the periphery.

Patients who contract rabies encephalitis often suffer the acute onset of hydrophobia. When they attempt to drink water, their pharynx spasms. Spasms spread from the pharynx to the respiratory muscles, causing shallow, quick respirations. These abnormalities are thought to be the result of brain stem involvement and damage to the nucleus ambiguus found in the upper medulla. Hyperactivity, seizures, and coma usually follow. Pituitary dysfunction is often evident and can result in diabetes insipidus (which causes loss of free water) or inappropriate antidiuretic hormone secretion (which causes hyponatremia). Cardiac arrhythmias and autonomic dysfunction are also common. Patients usually die within one to two weeks after the onset of coma. Less commonly, patients present with ascending paralysis resembling Guillain-Barré syndrome and subsequently develop coma.

Diagnostic studies usually include CT scan or MRI with contrast. MRI is more sensitive and detects smaller lesions and early areas of edematous cerebral cortex. In herpes simplex encephalitis involvement of the temporal lobes is the rule. In other forms of encephalitis diffuse cerebral edema may be found in severe cases; however, as seen in Case 6.3, these imaging studies are often normal. EEG is particularly helpful in herpes simplex encephalitis, frequently demonstrating electrical spikes in the region of the infected temporal lobe. Lumbar puncture usually reveals fewer than 500 WBC/mm^3 in the CSF with a predominance of mononuclear cells. However, in early infection PMNs may be noted, and this finding warrants a follow-up lumbar puncture to document a shift to lymphocytes. The CSF protein is usually normal or mildly elevated, and the CSF glucose is usually normal, although a low glucose may be seen in herpes. Also in herpes simplex type I encephalitis increased numbers of red blood cells may be found in the CSF.

With the exception of rabies a specific diagnosis is usually difficult to determine. Acute and convalescent serum IgM and IgG titers for the viral causes of encephalitis should be sent. CSF samples should be cultured for virus in addition to bacteria and fungi. Throat swabs for viral culture are also recommended. The yield for viral cultures is highest early in the illness. CSF PCR for herpes simplex is both sensitive and specific and is the diagnostic test of choice where available. In the absence of this test, brain biopsy of the affected temporal lobe remains the diagnostic procedure of choice for herpes simplex encephalitis. Herpes immunofluorescence stain of cortical tissue has an 80% yield. Viral culture of the brain should also be obtained and takes 1–5 days to grow. In herpes encephalitis, histopathology classically reveals Cowdry Type A intranuclear inclusions. Other stains, including AFB smear and fungal stains, should also be performed.

With the exception of herpes simplex I there is no specific treatment for the most common causes of viral encephalitis. One approach to the treatment of viral encephalitis is to initiate acyclovir therapy (10 mg/kg Q8H iv) while awaiting diagnostic tests, recognizing that a delay in therapy for herpes encephalitis worsens the prognosis. If temporal lobe abnormalities are found and the patient has failed to improve on acyclovir, a brain biopsy should be strongly considered. In other forms of encephalitis in which no focal cortical abnormalities are noted, the usefulness of brain biopsy remains to be determined.

The prognosis of viral encephalitis varies depending on the agent. Untreated herpes simplex type I has a mortality of 50–60% and a high frequency of neurologic sequelae. Early treatment reduces mortality (15%). The mortality for rabies is nearly 100%, justifying vaccination of anyone who might have been exposed to the rabies virus. The prognosis for the arboviruses depends on the patient's age, the extent of cortical involvement, and the specific agent. Eastern equine encephalitis tends to be the most virulent, having a 70% mortality rate, while western equine encephalitis is usually mild and often subclinical, primarily infecting young children. West Nile virus infection often is subclinical or causes mild disease; however, in some patients, particularly the elderly, this infection can be fatal. Venezuelan equine encephalitis is usually mild, and Japanese encephalitis varies in severity.

The management of rabies exposure is complex, and specific guidelines have been published by the Advisory Committee on Immunization Practices (*Morbidity and Mortality Weekly Report,* 48(RR-1):1–21, 1999; *http://www.cdc.gov/mmwr/PDF/RR/RR4801.pdf.* Bite wounds should be washed with a 20% soap solution and irrigated with a virucidal agent such as povidone-iodine solution. Rabies immune globulin (20 IU/kg) should be injected around the wound and given intramuscularly. Several safe and effective antirabies vaccines are available. The vaccine should be given on days 0, 3, 7, 14, and 28.

KEY POINTS
Viral Encephalitis

1. Three major categories:
   a. Mosquito borne: Arboviruses,
   b. Animal to human: Rabies virus,
   c. Human to human: Herpes simplex type I, mumps, measles, varicella-zoster; less commonly Epstein-Barr virus, cytomegalovirus, and enteroviruses.
2. Symptoms of cortical dysfunction are evident:
   a. Hallucinations, repetitive higher motor activity such as dressing and undressing,
   b. Seizures,
   c. Severe headache,
   d. Ataxia.
3. Rabies causes distinct syndromes:
   a. Hydrophobia,
   b. Rapid, short respirations,
   c. Hyperactivity and autonomic dysfunction,
   d. Less commonly ascending paralysis.
4. Diagnosis often presumptive, requires acute and convalescent serum:
   a. Lumbar puncture CSF < 500 WBC/mm³, mild increase protein, RBCs in herpes simplex I,
   b. CSF PCR for herpes simplex, culture rarely positive,
   c. MRI/CT scan: Temporal lobe abnormalities in herpes simplex I,
   d. EEG: Localized temporal lobe abnormalities in herpes,
   e. Brain biopsy if temporal lobe abnormalities and no improvement on acyclovir.
5. Treatment: Acyclovir for possible herpes simplex I.
6. Prevention: Avoid mosquito bites during epidemics. For rabies, wash wound, immune globulin and rabies vaccine.

Brain Abscess

Potential Severity: Often subacute in onset but may be life-threatening if improperly managed. Early neurosurgical consultation is of critical importance.

◆ CASE 6.4

A 19-year-old white male noted the gradual onset of severe left frontal headache. His headache was sharp and constant, interfered with sleep, and was not relieved by aspirin. Two weeks after the onset of headache he was noted to have a grand mal seizure associated with urinary incontinence that lasted 15 minutes. On admission to the hospital he was afebrile, alert, but somewhat confused. He was oriented to person but not to time or place. HENT examination: Teeth in poor repair with evidence of several cavities and gingivitis. Funduscopic examination revealed sharp disc margins. Mild left-sided weakness was noted on neurologic exam. CT scan with contrast demonstrated a 3-cm, ring-enhancing lesion in the right frontal cortex. No evidence of sinusitis.

Prevalence and Pathogenesis

Brain abscess is an uncommon disease, found in about 1 out of 10,000 general hospital admissions. Infection of the cerebral cortex can result from the direct spread of bacteria from another focus of infection (accounts for 20–60% of cases) or through hematogenous seeding.

DIRECT SPREAD

The direct spread of microorganisms from a contiguous site usually causes a single brain abscess. Primary infections that can directly spread to the cerebral cortex include the following:

1. Subacute and chronic otitis media and mastoiditis (spread to the inferior temporal lobe and cerebellum)
2. Infection of the frontal or ethmoid sinuses (spreads to the frontal lobes)
3. Dental infection (usually spreads to the frontal lobes)

In Case 5.4 it is likely that his brain abscess spread from a dental focus. Brain abscess as a complication of ear infections has decreased in frequency, especially in developed countries. By contrast, brain abscess arising from a sinus infection remains an important consideration in both adults and children. Bullet wounds to the brain devitalize tissue and may leave fragments of metal that can serve as a focus for infection. Other foreign bodies that have been associated with brain abscesses are a pencil tip lodged in the orbit and a lawn dart. In these cases brain abscess may develop many years after the injury. Brain abscess can occasionally result from facial trauma or as a complication of a neurosurgical procedure. The development of brain abscess after neurosurgery may be delayed, symptomatic infection occurring 3–15 months after surgery.

HEMATOGENOUS SPREAD

Abscesses associated with bacteremia are usually multiple and are located in the distribution of the middle cerebral artery. Initially, they tend to be located at the gray-white matter junction where brain capillary blood flow is slow and septic emboli are more likely to lodge. Microinfarction causes damage to the blood-brain barrier, allowing bacteria to invade the cerebral cortex. Primary infections that lead to hematogenous seeding the brain include the following:

1. Chronic pulmonary infections, such as lung abscess and empyema, often in hosts with bronchiectasis or cystic fibrosis
2. Skin infections

3. Pelvic infection
4. Intra-abdominal infection
5. Esophageal dilation and endoscopic sclerosis of esophageal varices
6. Bacterial endocarditis (2–4% of cases)
7. Cyanotic congenital heart diseases (most common in children)

No primary site or underlying condition can be identified in 20–40% of patients with brain abscess.

The location of a brain abscess reflects the site of the primary infection. The most common locations of abscesses in order of decreasing frequency are frontal or temporal lobes, frontoparietal, parietal, cerebellar, and occipital. The histologic changes in the brain depend on the age of the infection. The early lesion (in the first one to two weeks) is poorly demarcated and is associated with localized edema. There is evidence of acute inflammation but no tissue necrosis. This early stage is commonly called cerebritis. After two to three weeks necrosis and liquefaction occur, and the lesion becomes surrounded by a fibrotic capsule.

KEY POINTS

The Pathogenesis of Brain Abscess

1. Two major causes:
   a. Direct spread from middle ear, frontal sinus, or dental infection,
   b. Hematogenous spread from chronic pulmonary, skin, pelvic, and intra-abdominal infection. Also endocarditis, bacteremia after esophageal dilatation, cyanotic heart disease. Abscess at the gray-white matter junction.
2. Location: Frontal or temporal > fronto-parietal > parietal > cerebellar > occipital.
3. Cerebritis (acute inflammation and edema) progresses to necrosis followed by fibrotic capsule formation.

Microbiology

The bacterial etiology of brain abscess is highly variable. The pathogens that are involved differ depending on the site of the primary infection, the age of the patient (microorganisms often differ in children and adults), and the immune status of the host. The organism(s) that are recovered from a brain abscess frequently provide a clue about the primary site of infection and any potential undiagnosed underlying conditions in the host.

Anaerobic bacteria are common constituents of brain abscesses, generally originating as part of the normal mouth flora. However, intra-abdominal or pelvic infections can occasionally lead to bacteremia with an anaerobic organism that seeds the cerebral cortex. The anaerobes in such cases usually reflect colonic or female genital tract flora. The most frequent anaerobes that are cultured from brain abscess include anaerobic streptococci, Bacteroides species (including *B. fragilis*), *Prevotella melaninogenica,* Propionibacterium, Fusobacterium, Eubacterium, Veillonella, and Actinomyces.

Aerobic Gram-positive cocci are also frequently encountered and include viridans streptococci, *Streptococcus milleri,* microaerophilic streptococci, *S. pneumoniae* (rare), and *Staphylococcus aureus. S. aureus* is a more frequent pathogen in brain abscess following trauma or a neurosurgical procedure. *Streptococcus milleri* is particularly common, and this organism possesses proteolytic enzymes that predispose to necrosis of tissue and the formation of abscesses.

Aerobic Gram-negative rods are not usually recovered in brain abscess except following neurosurgery or head trauma. When Gram-negative rods are isolated, Pseudomonas species, *Haemophilus aphrophilus, Actinobacillus actinomycetemcomitans,* and Klebsiella species are the most common pathogens.

IMMUNOCOMPROMISED HOST

In the immunocompromised patient the range of organisms, particularly opportunistic pathogens, is considerably broader. *Toxoplasma gondii* can reactivate when the cell-mediated immune system becomes compromised. *Nocardia asteroides,* a common soil organism, can enter the bloodstream via the lungs and seed the cerebral cortex. Aspergillus, *Cryptococcus neoformans,* and *Coccidioides immitis* also can enter through the lungs and subsequently invade the cerebral cortex. Other pathogens that cause brain abscess in the immunocompromised host include *Candida albicans,* Mucormycosis (Zygomyces), *Cladosporium trichoides,* and Curvularia species.

Individuals who are infected with the human immunodeficiency virus (HIV) frequently develop infections of the cerebral cortex. *Toxoplasma gondii* is the most common cause of brain abscess in these patients, but more than one CNS infection can occur simultaneously. Tuberculomas, cryptococcoma, early progressive multifocal leukoencephalopathy, *Listeria monocytogenes,* Salmonella, Candida, Histoplasma, and Aspergillus have been reported to cause CNS lesions in association with HIV infection. CNS lymphoma also commonly mimics brain abscess in the patient with the acquired immunodeficiency syndrome (AIDS) (see Chapter 17, "HIV Infection").

IMMIGRANTS

Parasites are the most common etiology of brain abscess in individuals who previously lived outside the United States. Cysticercosis represents 85% of brain infections in Mexico City (see Chapter 12, "Parasitic Infections"). Other parasites that can cause brain abscess include *Entamoeba histolytica, Schistosoma japonicum,* and Paragonimus species.

KEY POINTS
The Etiology of Brain Abscess

> 1. Anaerobes from mouth flora, pelvis, and
>   gastrointestinal tract:
>   a. Bacteroides (may include *B. fragilis*),
>   b. *Prevotella melaninogenica,*

c. Proprionobacterium, Fusobacterium, Eubacterium, Veillonella,
d. Actinomyces.
2. Aerobic Gram-positive cocci:
   a. *Streptococcus milleri* (protease activity,
      predisposition to form abscesses),
   b. Microaerophilic streptococci,
   c. *Staphylococcus aureus* (endocarditis,
      trauma, neurosurgery),
   d. Viridans streptococci.
3. Gram-negative rods rare: Pseudomonas species, *Haemophilus aphrophilus*, *Actinobacillus actinomycetemcomitans*, and Klebsiella.
4. Immunocompromised host:
   a. Toxoplasmosis,
   b. Nocardia,
   c. Fungal: Aspergillus, *Cryptococcus neofor-
      mans*, and *Coccidioides immitis*.
5. Parasites in immigrants: Cysticercosis.

Clinical Symptoms and Signs

The symptoms of brain abscess tend to come on
gradually and are often nonspecific, delaying
the diagnosis. The mean interval between the
first symptom and diagnosis is two weeks. As
observed Case 6.4, headache is the most common symptom and usually localizes to the side
where the abscess is located, but in some cases
headache is generalized. As is observed with
bacterial meningitis, headache is usually severe
and is not relieved by aspirin or other over-the-
counter pain medications. In patients with cyanotic heart disease and unexplained headache,
the diagnosis of brain abscess must always be
excluded. About 15% of patients complain of
neck stiffness, mimicking meningitis. Meningis-
mus is most commonly associated with occipital
lobe brain abscess or with an abscess that has
leaked into a lateral ventricle.

Changes in mental status are common. In patients with frontal abscess subtle disturbances in
judgment and inattentiveness may be the primary symptoms. Lethargy can progress to coma,

and these changes are thought to be primarily
the consequence of cerebral edema and increased intracranial pressure. The development
of coma is associated with a poor prognosis.
Vomiting may also develop as a consequence of
increased intracranial pressure.

The absence of fever does not exclude the diagnosis of brain abscess. A significant percentage of patients with this disease (45–50%) fail to
mount a febrile response. Focal neurologic deficits usually develop days to weeks after the
onset of headache and are observed in half the
patients at the time of admission. The specific
neurologic deficits depend on the location of
the abscess (see Table 6.5). Sixth and third cra-

Table 6.5

Neurologic Manifestations of Brain Abscess

LOCATION	NEUROLOGIC DEFICITS
Temporal	Wernicke's aphasia, homonymous superior quadranopsia, mild contralateral facial muscle weakness
Frontal	Drowsy, inattentive, disturbed judgment, mutism, seizures; + grasp, suck and snout reflexes; contralateral hemiparesis when the abscess is large
Parietal	Impaired position sense, two-point discrimination and stere-ognosis, focal sensory and motor seizures, homonymous hemianopsia, impaired optico-kinetic nystagmus
Cerebellar	Ataxia, nystagmus (coarser on gaze toward the lesion), ipsilat-eral incoordination of arm and leg movements with intention tremor, rapid progression (usu-ally not encapsulated)
Brain stem	Facial weakness and dysphagia, multiple other cranial nerve palsies, contralateral hemiparesis

nial nerve palsies may be seen and are the consequence of increased intracranial pressure. Papilledema is a late manifestation of increased intracranial pressure and is found in 25% of patients. As was observed in Case 6.4, focal or grand mal seizures develop in 25% of patients and are most commonly associated with frontal lobe brain abscess.

KEY POINTS

Clinical Manifestations of Brain Abscess

1. Symptoms are initially nonspecific, and delay in diagnosis is common (2 weeks):
   a. Severe headache is often localized to the site where the abscess has formed,
   b. Neck stiffness is noted in occipital brain abscess or after rupture into the ventricle,
   c. Alterations in mental status, inattentiveness, lethargy, coma (a bad prognostic sign),
   d. Vomiting is associated with increased CSF pressure.
2. Physical findings often minimal:
   a. Fever not present in half of patients,
   b. Focal neurological findings late,
   c. Papilledema, a late manifestation, seen in 25%,
   d. Sixth and third nerve deficits due to increased CSF pressure,
   e. Seizures most common in association with frontal brain abscess.

Diagnosis

Focal symptoms (e.g., unilateral headache) or signs (e.g., unilateral cranial nerve deficits, hemiparesis) and papilledema suggest a space-occupying lesion in the cerebral cortex. In this circumstance a lumbar puncture is contraindicated until this possibility is excluded. The asymmetric cerebral edema associated with brain abscess can cause brain stem herniation in 15–30% of patients if CSF pressure is reduced below the tentorium

by lumbar puncture. CT scan with contrast or MRI should be performed prior to lumbar puncture to exclude a focal cerebral lesion. Blood cultures should be drawn (positive in 15% of cases) and empiric parenteral antibiotic therapy initiated before CT scan or MRI. If the study is negative, a lumbar puncture can then be performed.

COMPUTED TOMOGRAPHIC SCAN

CT scan is not as sensitive as MRI for the diagnosis of brain abscess but can frequently be obtained more easily on an emergent basis. When brain abscess is a serious consideration, this study must be performed with a contrast agent. The lesion has different appearances depending on its age, and these differences reflect the histopathology:

1. **Early cerebritis**. An irregular area of low density that does not enhance following contrast injection.
2. **Later cerebritis**. The lesion enlarges and demonstrates a thick, diffuse ring of enhancement following contrast injection. The ring of contrast enhancement represents breakdown of the blood-brain barrier and the development of an inflammatory capsule (see Figure 6.5).
3. **Late cerebritis**. Necrosis often develops at this stage. Precontrast images reveal a ring of higher density than the surrounding edematous brain. Injection of contrast demonstrates a thin ring that is not of uniform thickness.
4. **Healed abscess**. Once the abscess has healed, the resulting collagen capsule becomes isodense (has the same density as the surrounding tissue), and infusion of contrast no longer results in ring enhancement.

MAGNETIC RESONANCE IMAGING (MRI)

This is the diagnostic study of choice for evaluating brain abscess and should be performed with gadolinium diethylenetriamine peta-acetic acid, which crosses the damaged blood-brain barrier. This agent increases the T1 intensity and causes more prominent enhancement of lesions than CT scan does. Compared to CT scan, MRI:

1. Is more sensitive for detecting early cerebritis
2. Is more sensitive for detecting satellite lesions and is capable of detecting smaller-diameter lesions (1 mm resolution)
3. More accurately estimates the extent of central necrosis, ring enhancement, and cerebral edema
4. Better visualizes the brain stem

LUMBAR PUNCTURE

As was noted earlier, this test is contraindicated in patients with brain abscess because of the danger of herniation. When this test has been performed inadvertently, the cerebrospinal pro-

Figure 6.5

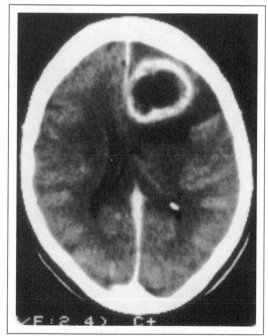

CT scan with contrast of brain abscess. Note the large ring-enhancing lesion in the left frontal cortex associated with the marked edema and obliteration of the lateral ventricle.

file is indicative of a parameningeal abscess, that is, moderate numbers of WBCs (<500), usually with a predominance of mononuclear cells, normal CSF glucose, and normal CSF protein (see Table 6.1). On rare occasion an abscess may rupture into the lateral ventricle, causing frank meningitis resulting in a CSF formula with a predominance of PMNs (up to 160,000/mm^3), low glucose, and high protein.

KEY POINTS
Diagnosis of Brain Abscess

1. Focal symptoms or neurologic signs as well as papilledema = possible space-occupying lesion; lumbar puncture is contraindicated.
2. After blood cultures and empiric antibiotics, perform CT scan or MRI with contrast.
3. MRI is preferred over CT scan (detects early cerebritis and smaller lesions and visualizes the brain stem).
4. Four stages detected on imaging:
   a. Early cerebritis (edema, no ring enhancement),
   b. Later cerebritis (ring enhancement with early capsule, edema),
   c. Late cerebritis (necrosis, ring seen without contrast, thin, nonuniform contrast-enhancing ring),
   d. Healed abscess (no longer ring enhancing, lesion becomes isodense).

Treatment

The goals of therapy are to sterilize the abscess or abscesses and reduce the mass effect caused by necrosis and cerebral edema. Because surgical drainage of the brain abscess is usually necessary, a neurosurgeon should be contacted as soon as the diagnosis is made.

ANTIBIOTICS

Prolonged antibiotic therapy (six to eight weeks) is required to cure brain abscess. A number of drugs can be chosen depending on the probable pathogen(s) involved. Once the etiologic organisms have been isolated and susceptibility testing has been performed, the drug regimen can be modified. High-dose penicillin remains the mainstay of therapy and covers all mouth flora, including both aerobic and anaerobic streptococci. Metronidazole is also recommended for most patients because this antibiotic readily penetrates brain abscesses, intralesional concentrations reaching 40 µg/ml. This drug has excellent cidal activity against all anaerobes but is not active against aerobic organisms. In most patients a third-generation cephalosporin should also be included in the regimen to cover Enterobacteriaciae that may be present, particularly in patients with a brain abscess associated with a chronic ear infection. High-dose ceftriaxone and cefotaxime are equally effective and should be used unless *Pseudomonas aeruginosa* is strongly suspected. When *P. aeruginosa* is cultured or when a brain abscess develops after a neurosurgical procedure, maximum doses of ceftazidime or cefepime should be used. In patients who develop brain abscess following penetrating head trauma or craniotomy and in the patient with *Staphylococcus aureus* bacteremia, high-dose oxacillin or nafcillin needs to be included. Aminoglycosides, erythromycin, tetracyclines, and first-generation cephalosporins should not be used to treat brain abscess because these drugs do not cross the blood-brain barrier.

Surgery

Surgical drainage generally is required for both diagnosis and treatment. Needle aspiration is preferred in most cases because this procedure reduces the extent of neurologic damage. In patients with a traumatic brain abscess an open procedure is preferred to remove bone chips and foreign material. Surgical removal of the entire capsule greatly increases the likelihood of cure in fungal brain abscesses. Surgery can be delayed or avoided in patients with early cerebritis without evidence of cerebral necrosis

and in patients with abscesses located in vital regions of the brain that are inaccessible to aspiration. When the decision is made not to drain immediately, careful follow-up with sequential CT or MRI is critical. Following the initiation of empiric antibiotics for an established brain abscess, indications for surgical intervention include lack of clinical improvement within a week, depressed sensorium, signs of increased intracranial pressure, and progressive increase in the ring diameter of the abscess. Contrast enhancement at the site of the abscess may persist for several months. Therefore this finding is not helpful for deciding on surgical intervention or continued antibiotic therapy.

Glucocorticoids

Glucocorticoids should be given only to patients who have evidence of mass effect and a depressed mental status. Dexamethasone should be administered at a loading dose of 10 mg iv followed by 4 mg Q6H; the drug should be discontinued as soon as possible. The addition of glucocorticoids has several disadvantages. They reduce contrast enhancement on CT scan, making monitoring of changes in abscess size more difficult. Second, glucocorticoids slow capsule formation, increasing the risk of ventricular rupture. Finally, they decrease antibiotic penetration into the abscess by improving the integrity of the blood-brain barrier.

Key Points

Treatment and Outcome of Brain Abscess

1. Antibiotic therapy must be prolonged (6–8 weeks) and use high doses of:
   a. Penicillin: Covers mouth flora,
   b. Metronidazole: Concentrates in abscesses and kills all anaerobes,
   c. Ceftriaxone or cefotaxime: Covers Gram-positive and Gram-negative aerobes; if

Pseudomonas is possible, replace with ceftazidime or cefepime,

   d. Nafcillin or oxacillin for abscess following head trauma, neurosurgery, or *Staphylococcus aureus* bacteremia.

2. Neurosurgery usually required for culture and drainage. Always consult neurosurgery.

   a. Needle aspiration is usually preferred (less collateral damage),

   b. Open resection is recommended after head trauma and with fungal abscess,

   c. Observation in cases of early cerebritis with frequent follow-up MRI or CT scan,

3. Dexamethasone used when there is mass effect and depressed mental status. Avoid when possible:

   a. Reduces contrast enhancement during imaging,

   b. Slows capsule formation and increases the risk of ventricular rupture,

   c. Reduces antibiotic penetration into the abscess.

4. Mortality ranges from 0% to 30%. Poor prognosis is associated with:

   a. Rapid progression in the hospital,

   b. Coma on admission,

   c. Rupture into the ventricle.

Prognosis and Outcome

Mortality rates from brain abscess currently range from 0% to 30%. CT and/or MRI have improved outcome by allowing earlier diagnosis and more accurate monitoring of the response to therapy. Poor prognostic factors for recovery from a brain abscess include rapid progression of the infection before hospitalization, stupor or coma on admission (60–100% mortality), and rupture of the abscess into the ventricle (80–100% mortality). In surviving patients there is a high incidence of neurologic sequelae (30–60%), recurrent seizures being most common. This persistent problem most frequently follows frontal brain abscess.

Intracranial Epidural and Subdural Abscess

Potential Severity: Subdural abscess spreads rapidly. Emergency surgical drainage is life-saving.

These abscesses are rare and usually result from spread of infection from a nidus of osteomyelitis following neurosurgery, an infected sinus (in particular the frontal sinus), or, less commonly, an infected middle ear or mastoid. In infants subdural effusions may complicate bacterial meningitis; however, unlike the adult form, they rarely require drainage. The bacteria causing these closed space infections reflect the primary sites of infection. *Staphylococcus aureus* is most common, followed by aerobic streptococci. Other pathogens include *Streptococcus pneumoniae, Haemophilus influenzae,* and Gram-negative organisms. Anaerobes such as anaerobic streptococci and *Bacillus fragilis* can also be associated with this infection. Patients with sinusitis and chronic mastoiditis often have polymicrobial abscesses.

Epidural abscesses form between the skull and dura (see Figure 6.1). Because the dura is normally tightly adherent to the skull, this infection usually remains localized and spreads slowly, mimicking brain abscess in its clinical presentation. On exam localized erythema, swelling, and tenderness of the subgaleal region may be seen. Subdural empyema in the cranial region progresses much more rapidly than epidural abscess, usually spreading rapidly throughout the cranium. Patients appear acutely ill and septic. They complain of severe headache that is localized to the site of infection, and nuchal rigidity commonly develops, suggesting the diagnosis of meningitis. Within 24–48 hours focal neurologic deficits are noted, and half of the patients develop seizures. Lumbar puncture is contraindicated because of the high risk of brain stem herniation. CT scan with contrast should be performed and in most instances demonstrates the abscess as well as overlying osteomyelitis, sinus infection, or mastoiditis. In early epidural or subdural abscess MRI is capable of detecting early cortical edema and smaller collections of inflammatory fluid. MRI should be performed in patients who are suspected of having early disease and who have a negative CT scan.

Subdural empyema is a neurosurgical emergency. Immediate drainage is required to prevent death from cerebral herniation. Exploratory burr holes and blind drainage have been life-saving in rapidly progressing cases. Antibiotic therapy should be instituted immediately. The same regimens that are recommended for brain abscess are used. The mortality rate from subdural empyema remains high, 14–18%, the prognosis being especially poor in patients who are comatose. Epidural abscess is less dangerous but also requires surgical drainage. Mortality is low; however, if left untreated, this infection can spread to the subdural space.

KEY POINTS

Epidural and Subdural Intracranial Abscesses

1. Associated with frontal sinusitis, mastoiditis, and neurosurgery.
2. *Staphylococcus aureus* common; otherwise, the microbiology is similar to that of brain abscess.
3. Epidural abscess progresses slowly, requires surgical drainage.
4. Subdural abscess spreads quickly:
   a. Often mimics meningitis,
   b. Lumbar puncture contraindicated, CT scan or MRI emergently,
   c. Requires immediate drainage,
   d. Mortality 14–18%.

Spinal Epidural Abscess

Potential Severity: Often subacute in onset. Development of motor weakness indicates imminent spinal cord infarction and requires emergency surgical drainage.

After the dura passes below the foramen magnum, it no longer tightly adheres to the bone surrounding the spinal cord. Both an anterior and a posterior space are present that contain fat and blood vessels. Infection can spread to the epidural space from vertebral osteomyelitis or disk space infection. Infection of the epidural space following epidural catheter placement is increasingly common, as is postoperative infection following other surgical procedures in spinal cord area. Skin and soft tissue infections and urinary tract infections as well as intravenous drug abuse can lead to bacteremia and seeding of the epidural space. In approximately one third of patients no primary cause is identified.

The inflammatory mass associated with infection can compress the nerve roots as they exit the spinal canal, causing radicular pain and findings consistent with lower motor neuron dysfunction (decreased reflexes, loss of light touch and pain sensation in specific dermatomes). In addition to radicular pain patients complain of localized back pain. These symptoms often are accompanied by malaise and fever. As the epidural mass expands, the spinal cord is compressed, resulting in upper motor neuron findings such as a positive Babinski's reflex, hyperreflexia, loss of motor function, and bladder dysfunction. Usually within 24 hours of the onset of paralysis the spinal cord's vascular supply becomes irreversibly compromised, leading to infarction and permanent paraplegia. To prevent this devastating outcome, clinicians need to consider spinal epidural abscess in their differential diagnosis for back pain. In the patient with back pain and fever, spinal epidural abscess must be strongly considered. Another helpful clue can be derived from the physical examination. In posterior epidural abscesses severe, localized tenderness over the infected area is encountered. However, in anterior epidural abscess, a rarer event, infection is deep seated, and tenderness cannot be elicited. Epidural abscess formation can be readily visualized by MRI (see Figure 6.6). CT scan with contrast is a less effective method for diagnosis.

The bacteriology of epidural abscess reflects the primary site of infection. *Staphylococcus aureus* is cultured from over half of cases. Gram-negative aerobes are the second most frequent cause, followed by aerobic streptococci, *S. epidermidis,* and anaerobes. *Mycobacterium tuberculosis* is another important etiology, most commonly being associated with tuberculous infection of the thoracic vertebrae.

Because of the unpredictability of neurologic complications surgical decompression is recommended in all cases with any neurologic com-

Figure 6.6

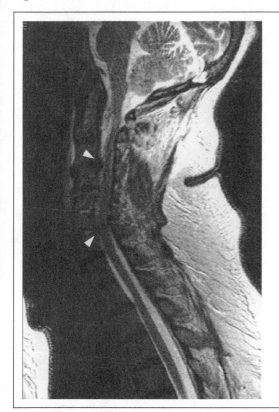
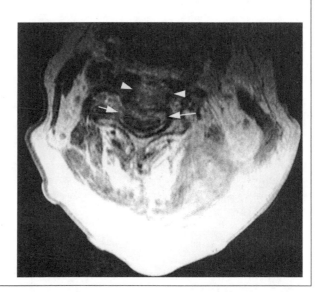

MRI of spinal epidural abscess. (Left) Sagittal view. Anterior mass can be seen compressing the spinal cord. Diffuse enhancement can be seen indicating extensive inflammation. The area of spinal canal narrowing is demarcated by the arrowheads. (Right) Axial view. An anterior epidural abscess is seen in the spinal canal (arrowheads) compressing the spinal cord (arrows) against the posterior wall of the canal. (Courtesy of Dr. Ron Quisling, University of Florida College of Medicine.)

promise or evidence of significant cord compression on MRI. Drainage is combined with prolonged antibiotic treatment (four to six weeks). High doses of nafcillin or oxacillin, ceftriaxone, and metronidazole are recommended as empiric therapy pending culture results.

KEY POINTS

Spinal Epidural Abscess

1. The spinal canal contains both an anterior and a posterior epidural space containing fat and small vessels.
2. The spinal epidural space can become infected by:
   a. Spread of infection from osteomyelitis or disk space infection,
   b. Spinal surgery or epidural catheter placement,
   c. Hematogenous spread following skin or urinary tract infection, as well as IV drug abuse.
3. Symptoms and signs include:
   a. Low back pain and fever,
   b. Radicular pain accompanied by lower motor neuron deficits,
   c. Later, signs of cord compression (Babinski's reflex, hyperreflexia, loss of motor function, bladder dysfunction). Within 24 hours of onset, irreversible paraplegia may occur,
   d. Localized spinous process tenderness in posterior epidural abscesses.
4. In the patient with back pain and fever, always consider spinal epidural abscess.
5. MRI with contrast is the diagnostic study of choice.
6. Treatment:
   a. Emergency surgical drainage if signs of cord compression or significant compression on MRI,
   b. Prolonged antibiotic therapy (four to six weeks) with nafcillin or oxacillin, metronidazole, and ceftriaxone.

Additional Reading

Bacterial Meningitis

Choi, C. Bacterial meningitis in aging adults. *Clin Infect Dis* 33:1380-1385, 2001.

Durand, M.L. Calderwood, S.B., Weber, D.J., Miller, S.I., Southwick, F.S., Caviness, V.S., Swartz, M.N. Acute bacterial meningitis in adults: A review of 493 episodes. *N Engl J Med* 328:21-28, 1993.

Hussein, A.S., and Shafran, S.D. Acute bacterial meningitis in adults. A 12-year review. *Medicine* (Baltimore) 79:360-368, 2000.

Odio, C.M. et al. The beneficial effects of early dexamethasone administration in infants and children with bacterial meningitis. *N Engl J Med* 324:1525, 1531, 1991.

Swartz, M.N., and Dodge, P.R. Bacterial meningitis. A review of selected aspects. N Engl J Med 272:725, 779, 842, 898, 954, 1,003, 1965.

Viral Meningitis

Wynants, H., Taelman, H., Martin, J.J., and Van den Ende, J. Recurring aseptic meningitis after travel to the tropics: a case of Mollaret's meningitis? Case report with review of the literature. *Clin Neurol Neurosurg* 102:113-115, 2000.

Tuberculous Meningitis

Berger, J.R. Tuberculous meningitis. *Curr Opin Neurol* 7:191-200, 1994.

Offenbacher, H., Fazekas, F., Schmidt, R., et al. MRI in tuberculous meningoencephalitis: Report of four cases and review of the neuroimaging literature. *J Neurol* 238:340-344.

Cryptococcal Meningitis

Ely, E.W., Peacock, J.E., Jr., Haponik, E.F., and Washburn, R.G. Cryptococcal pneumonia complicating pregnancy. *Medicine* (Baltimore) 77:153-167, 1998.

Mitchell, D.H., Sorrell, T.C., Allworth, A.M., et al. Cryptococcal disease of the CNS in immunocompetent hosts: Influence of cryptococcal variety on clinical manifestations and outcome. *Clin Infect Dis* 20:611-616, 1995.

Rex, J.H., Larsen, R.A., Dismukes, W.E., Cloud, G.A., and Bennett, J.E. Catastrophic visual loss due to *Cryptococcus neoformans* meningitis. *Medicine* (Baltimore) 72:207-224, 1993.

Brain Abscess

Samson, D.S., Clark, K. A current review of brain abscess. *Am J Med* 54.201-210, 1973.

Corson, M.A., Postlethwaite, K.P., and Seymour, R.A. Are dental infections a cause of brain abscess? Case report and review of the literature. *Oral Dis* 7:61-65, 2001.

Seydoux, C., and Francioli, P. Bacterial brain abscesses: Factors influencing mortality and sequelae. *Clin Infect Dis* 15:394-401, 1992.

Carpenter, J.L. Brain stem abscesses: Cure with medical therapy, case report, and review. *Clin Infect Dis* 18:219-226, 1994.

Subdural and Epidural Abscess

Dill, S.R., Cobbs, C.G., and McDonald, C.K. Subdural empyema: analysis of 32 cases and review. *Clin Infect Dis* 20:372-386, 1995.

Mackenzie, A.R., Laing, R.B., Smith, C.C., Kaar, G.F., and Smith, F.W. Spinal epidural abscess: The importance of early diagnosis and treatment. *J Neurol Neurosurg Psychiatry* 65:209-212, 1998.

Nussbaum, E.S., Rigamonti, D., Standiford, H., Numaguchi, Y., Wolf, A.L., and Robinson, W.L. Spinal epidural abscess: A report of 40 cases and review. *Surg Neurol* 38:225-231, 1992.

Rich, P.M., Deasy, N.P., and Jarosz, J.M. Intracranial dural empyema. *Br J Radiol* 73:1329-1336, 2000.

Cardiovascular
Infections

Recommended Time to Complete: 1 day

Guiding Questions

1. What cardiac lesions predispose to bacterial endocarditis?

2. If the physician is going to administer antibiotic prophylaxis, when should the antibiotic be given?

3. What symptoms are most common in subacute bacterial endocarditis?

4. What skin lesions should be searched for when you suspect bacterial endocarditis and how often are they seen?

5. How should blood cultures be drawn if the clinician suspects bacterial endocarditis?

6. Are bacteriostatic antibiotics effective in the treatment of bacterial endocarditis?

7. In the patient with *Staphylococcus aureus* line-related bacteremia how long should antibiotics be administered?

8. What key physical finding is most helpful for detecting cardiac tamponade?

Infective Endocarditis

Potential Severity: Acute endocarditis is life threatening and often requires surgical intervention. Subacute endocarditis is an indolent disease that can continue for months.

Epidemiology

Infective endocarditis remains a serious but relatively uncommon problem. The incidence varies from series to series and is estimated to be as high as 11 per 100,000 and as low as 0.6 per 100,000. The exact incidence is difficult to ascertain because the definitions for endocarditis differ in many surveys. A reasonable estimate is probably 2 per 100,000. This means that during a primary care physician's lifetime he or she will encounter only one or two cases. Endocarditis is more common in males than in females, and the disease is increasingly becoming a disease of the elderly. In recent series over half of the patients with endocarditis were over the age of 50 years. With the rapid treatment of group A streptococcal infections the incidence of rheumatic heart disease has declined, eliminating this important risk factor for endocarditis in the young. With increasing life expectancies worldwide the percentage of elderly will continue to rise, and we can expect an increasing number of elderly patients with infective endocarditis in the future.

KEY POINTS

The Epidemiology of Infective Endocarditis

1. A rare disease, each primary physician is likely to see one to two cases in a career.
2. More common in males.
3. Increasingly a disease of the elderly.

HOST FACTORS

Infective endocarditis is usually preceded by the formation of a predisposing cardiac lesion. Preexisting endocardial damage leads to the accumulation of platelets and fibrin, producing nonbacterial thrombotic endocarditis (NBTE). This sterile lesion serves as an ideal site to trap bacteria as they pass through the bloodstream. Cardiac lesions that result in endocardial damage and predispose to the formation of NBTE include rheumatic heart disease, congenital heart disease (bicuspid aortic valve, ventricular septal defect, coarctation of the aorta, and tetralogy of Fallot), mitral valve prolapse, degenerative heart disease (calcific aortic valve disease), and prosthetic valve placement. Risk factors for endocarditis reflect the pathogenesis of the disease. Patients with congenital heart disease or rheumatic heart disease, those with an audible murmur associated with mitral valve prolapse, and elderly patients with calcific aortic stenosis are all at increased risk. The higher the pressure gradient in aortic stenosis, the greater is the risk of developing endocarditis. Intravenous drug abusers are at high risk of developing endocarditis as a consequence of injecting bacterially contaminated solutions intravenously.

Platelets and bacteria tend to accumulate in specific areas of the heart on the basis of the Venturi effect. When a fluid or gas passes at high pressure through a narrow orifice, an area of low pressure is created directly downstream of the orifice. The Venturi effect is most easily appreciated by examining a rapidly flowing, rock-filled river. When the flow of water is confined to a narrower channel by large rocks, the velocity of water flow increases. As a consequence of the Venturi effect, twigs and other debris can be seen to accumulate on the downstream side of the obstructing rocks, in the area of lowest pressure. Similarly, vegetations form on the downstream or low-pressure side of a valvular lesion. In aortic stenosis vegetations tend to form in the aortic coronary cusps on the downstream side of the obstructing lesion. In mitral regurgitation vegetations are most commonly seen in the atrium, the low-pressure side of regurgitant flow. On attaching to the endocardium, pathogenic bacteria induce platelet aggregation, and the resulting dense platelet-fibrin complex provides a protective environment. Phagocytes are incapable of entering this site, so an important host defense is eliminated. Colony counts in vegetations are usually 10^9–10^{11} bacteria/gm of tissue, and bacteria within the vegetations periodically lapse into a metabolically inactive, dormant phase.

The frequency with which the four valves become infected reflects the likelihood of endocardial damage. Shear stress would be expected to be highest in the valves that are exposed to high pressure, and the majority of cases of bacterial endocarditis involve the valves of the left side of the heart. The closed mitral valve is subjected to the highest pressures and is most commonly infected, followed in frequency by the aortic valve. With the exception of intravenous drug abusers, right-sided endocarditis is uncommon, and when it does occur, it most commonly involves the tricuspid valve. The closed pulmonic valve is subjected to the lowest pressure, and infection of this valve is rare.

Patients with prosthetic valves must be particularly alert to the symptoms and signs of endocarditis because the artificial material serves as an excellent site for bacterial adherence. Finally, patients who have recovered from infective endocarditis are at increased risk of developing a second episode.

KEY POINTS

Host Factors in the Pathogenesis of Infective Endocarditis

1. Nonbacterial thrombotic endocarditis (NBTE) due to valve damage followed by platelet and fibrin deposition.
2. NBTE results from:
   a. Rheumatic heart disease,
   b. Congenital heart disease (bicuspid valve and VSD),
   c. Mitral valve prolapse,
   d. Degenerative valve disease (calcific aortic valve disease),
   e. Prosthetic valve.
3. Venturi effect results in vegetation formation on the low-pressure side of high-flow valvular lesions.
4. Mitral valve > aortic valve > tricuspid valve (usually iv drug abusers).

BACTERIAL FACTORS

The organisms that are responsible for infective endocarditis are sticky. They more readily adhere to inert surfaces and to the endocardium. Streptococci that express dextran on their cell wall surface adhere more tightly to dental enamel and to other inert surfaces. Streptococci that produce higher levels of dextran demonstrate an increased ability to cause dental caries and to cause bacterial endocarditis. Viridans streptococci, named for their ability to cause green or alpha hemolysis on blood agar plates, often have a high dextran content and are a leading cause of dental caries and bacterial endocarditis. *Streptococcus mutans* and *S. sanguis* are the most common species in this group to cause endocarditis. One group D streptococcus, *S. bovis*, has high levels of dextran and demonstrates an increased propensity to cause endocarditis. This bacterium often enters the bloodstream via the gastrointestinal tract as a consequence of a colonic carcinoma. Viridans streptococci also express the surface adhesin Fim A, and this protein is expressed in strains that cause endocarditis. *Candida albicans* readily adheres to NBTE in vitro and causes endocarditis, particularly in intravenous drug abusers and patients with prosthetic valves. *C. krusei* is nonadherent and rarely causes infective endocarditis. Adherence to specific constituents in the NBTE also may be important virulence characteristics. For example, pathogenic strains of *S. sanguis* are able to bind to platelet receptors, and endocarditis-causing strains of *Staphy-*

lococcus aureus demonstrate increased binding to fibronectin.

KEY POINTS

Bacterial Factors in the Pathogenesis of Infective Endocarditis and Causes of Bacteremia

1. Bacteria with high dextran content stick to NBTE more readily and also cause dental caries.
   a. *Streptococcus viridans* is the leading cause of subacute bacterial endocarditis,
   b. *S. bovis* also has high dextran content, associated with colonic carcinoma.
2. *Candida albicans* adheres well to NBTE, *C. krusei* adheres poorly.
3. Causes of bacteremia that lead to infective endocarditis:
   a. Dental manipulations (extraction and periodontal surgery), water picks,
   b. Tonsillectomy,
   c. Urology procedures (urethral dilatation, cystoscopy, and prostatectomy),
   d. Pulmonary procedures (rigid bronchoscopy, intubation),
   e. Gastrointestinal procedures (upper GI endoscopy, sigmoidoscopy, colonoscopy).

CAUSES OF BACTEREMIA LEADING TO ENDOCARDITIS

For bacteria to adhere to NBTE, they must gain entry into the bloodstream. Whenever a mucosal surface that is heavily colonized with bacterial flora is traumatized, small numbers of bacteria enter the bloodstream and are quickly cleared by the spleen and liver. As outlined in Table 7.1, dental manipulations frequently precipitate transient bacteremia. Patients undergoing dental extraction or periodontal surgery are at particularly high risk. However, gum chewing and tooth brushing can also lead to bacteremia. Oral irrigation devices such as water picks should be avoided by patients with known valvular heart disease or prosthetic valves because these devices precipitate bacteremia more frequently than simple tooth brushing does. Other manipulations that can cause significant transient bacteremia include tonsillectomy, urethral dilatation, transurethral prostatic resection, and cystoscopy. Pulmonary and gastrointestinal procedures cause bacteremia in a low percentage of patients (see Table 7.1).

Etiologies of Infective Endocarditis

The organisms that are most frequently associated with infective endocarditis are able to colonize the mucosa, enter the bloodstream, and adhere to NBTE or native endocardium (see Table 7.2). In native valve endocarditis, Streptococcus species are the most common cause, representing more than half of the cases. *S. viridans* species are most frequent, followed by *S. bovis* and enterococcus (*S. faecalis* and *S. faecium*). Staphylococcus species are second in frequency. *Staphylococcus aureus* predominates; coagulase-negative staphylococcus plays a minor role. Other, rarer organisms include Gram-negative aerobic bacteria and the HACEK group. The HACEK group includes *Haemophilus aphrophilus, Actinobacillus actinomycetemcomitans, Cardiobacterium hominis, Eikenella corrodens,* and *Kingella kingae*. These slow-growing organisms are found in the mouth and require CO_2 for optimal growth. They might not be detected on routine blood cultures that are discarded after 7 days. Anaerobes, *Coxiella burnetti* (Q fever endocarditis), and Chlamydia species are exceedingly rare etiologies. In about 3–5% of cases cultures are repeatedly negative.

In intravenous drug abusers the microbiology differs, *Staphylococcus aureus* and Gram-negative organisms predominating (see Table 7.2). In certain areas of the country, such as Detroit, Michigan, methicillin-resistant *Staphylococcus aureus* is the predominant pathogen. *Pseudomonas*

Table 7.1

Causes of Bacteremia Leading to Potential Endocarditis

PROCEDURE OR MANIPULATION	PERCENT POSITIVE BLOOD CULTURES
Dental	
Dental extraction	18–85
Periodontal surgery	32–88
Chewing gum	15–51
Tooth brushing	0–26
Oral irrigation device	27–50
Upper airway	
Bronchoscopy (rigid scope)	15
Intubation/nasotracheal suction	16
Gastrointestinal	
Upper GI endoscopy	8–12
Sigmoidoscopy/colonoscopy	0–9.5
Barium enema	11
Liver biopsy, percutaneous	3–13
Urologic	
Urethral dilatation	18–33
Urethral catheter	8
Cystoscopy	0–17
Transurethral prostatectomy	12–46

Source: Everett, E.D., and Hirschmann, J.V., *Medicine*, 56:61, 1977.

aeruginosa, found in tap water, is the most common Gram-negative. Streptococci also are common, particularly enterococcus and *Streptococcus viridans* species. Fungi, primarily *Candida albicans*, are another important cause of endocarditis in this population. Polymicrobial disease is also more frequent.

The causes of prosthetic valve endocarditis depend on the timing of the infection (see Table 7.2). The development of endocarditis within the first two months of surgery, early prosthetic valve endocarditis, is primarily caused by nosocomial pathogens. Staphylococcal species, both coagulase-positive and coagulase-negative strains, Gram-negative aerobic bacilli, and fungi predominate. In late prosthetic valve endocarditis, developing more than two months after surgery, organisms originating from the mouth and skin

flora predominate: *Streptococcus viridans* species, *Staphylococcus aureus,* and coagulase-negative Staphylococcus species being most common. Gram-negative aerobic bacilli and fungi are less common but important pathogens as well.

KEY POINTS

Etiologies of Infective Endocarditis

1. Native valve endocarditis:
   a. Most commonly caused by streptococci: *S. viridans* most common, *S. faecalis* (enterococcus), *S. bovis* (associated with colonic cancer),
   b. *Staphylococcus aureus* second most common,

Table 7.2

Microorganisms Causing Infective Endocarditis

Organism	% Native	IV drug user	Early PVE	Late PVE
Streptococcal species	60–80	15	<10	35
Viridans	30–40	5	<5	25
S. bovis	10	<5	<5	<5
S. faecalis (GpD)	5–18	8	<5	<5
Other	<5	<5	<5	<5
Staphylococcus species	20–35	50	50	30
Coagulase-positive	10–27	50	20	10
Coagulase-negative	1–3	<5	30	20
Gram-negative bacilli	<5	15	20	20
Miscellaneous bacteria	<5	5	5	5
HACEK group	<5	<1	<1	<5
Corynebacteria and Propionibacteria	<1	<5	<5	<5
Anaerobes	<1	<1	<1	<1
Fungi	<5	5	5	5
Coxiella burnetii	<1	<1	<1	<1
Polymicrobial	<1	<5	<5	<5
Culture negative	3–5	3–5	<5	<5

Source: Adapted from Schlant, R.C., Alexander, R.W., O'Rourke, R.A., and Soonneblick, E.H. (Eds.) *Hurst's The Heart,* 8th edition. New York, McGraw Hill, pp. 1681–1709, 1994.)

c. HACEK group uncommon, consider in culture-negative cases (hold blood culture > 7 days).

2. In intravenous drug users:
   a. Most commonly caused by *S. aureus,*
   b. Gram-negative aerobic bacilli second most common, *Pseudomonas aeruginosa,*
   c. Fungi,
   d. Polymicrobial.

3. In prosthetic valve:
   a. Early, nosocomial pathogens: *Staphylococcus aureus,* coagulase-negative staphylococci, Gram-negative bacilli, and fungi,
   b. Late (> 2 months postoperative), mouth and skin flora: *Streptococcus viridans,* coagulase-negative staphylococci, *Staphylococcus aureus,* Gram-negative bacilli, and fungi.

Clinical Manifestations

◆ CASE 7.1

A 78-year-old retired advertising executive was admitted to the hospital with a chief complaint of increasing shortness of breath and ankle swelling. He had some dental work done 3½ months prior to admission. He felt well until three months prior to admission, when he began experiencing shortness of breath following any physical exertion. He also noted increasing fatigue and night sweats as well as intermittent low-grade fever. A diastolic murmur, II/VI, was noted along the left sternal border maximal at the third intercostal space. He was treated as an outpatient with diuretics for left-sided congestive heart failure. One day prior to admission, he began experiencing increasingly severe shortness of breath. He also began coughing frothy pink phlegm and arrived in the emergency room gasping for air.

Physical examination: Temperature 39°C, blood pressure 106/66, pulse 85 regular, respiratory rate 36/min. He appeared lethargic and had rapid, shallow respirations. His teeth were in good repair. Fundi: No hemorrhages or exudates. Neck: sitting up at a 30° angle, his jugular veins were distended to the level of his jaw. Lungs: diffuse wheezes and rales lower 2/3rds both lung fields. Heart: loud S3 gallop, II/VI nearly holosystolic murmur heard loudest in the left 3rd intercostal space radiating to the apex, and a II/VI diastolic murmur heard best along left sternal border. Abdomen: liver and spleen were not palpable. Extremities: 2+ pitting edema of the ankles extending midway up the thighs. Nail beds without splinter hemorrhages. Pulses: 2+ bilaterally.

Laboratory findings: WBC 11,700 (69 PMNs 4% band forms, 22% lymphocytes, and 3% mononuclear cells). Hct 30, normochromic, normocytic. Urinalysis: 1+ protein, 10–20 red blood cells, 5–10 white blood cells. Erythrocyte sedimentation rate 67. EKG: normal sinus rhythm, PR interval prolonged, left bundle branch block. Chest X-ray: extensive diffuse perihilar infiltration bilaterally. Four of four blood cultures were positive for *Streptococcus viridans*.

When the event leading to bacteremia can be identified, the usual incubation period required before symptoms develop is less than two weeks. In Case 7.1 the onset of symptoms occurred 15 days after dental work. Because the symptoms are usually nonspecific, on average there is a delay of five weeks between the onset of symptoms and diagnosis. In Case 7.1 the delay was three months. As observed in this patient, the most common symptom is low-grade fever. Body temperature is usually only mildly elevated in the 38°C range and, with the exception of acute endocarditis, rarely rises above 40°C. Fever is frequently accompanied by chills and less commonly by night sweats. Fatigue, anorexia, weakness, and malaise are common complaints, and the patient often experiences weight loss. Myalgias and arthralgias are also common complaints. Patients are often mistakenly suspected of having a malignancy, connective tissue disease, or other chronic infection such as tuberculosis. Another prominent complaint in a smaller percentage of patients is low back pain. Debilitating back pain that limits movement can be the presenting complaint, and health care personnel should always consider infective endocarditis as one possible cause of low back pain and fever. Systemic emboli can result in sudden hemiparesis or sudden limb pain as a consequence of tissue ischemia. In all patients who suffer a sudden cerebrovascular accident consistent with an embolic stoke, infective endocarditis should be excluded.

In addition to a subacute onset, some patients can present with rapid onset (hours to days) of symptoms and signs. Acute infective endocarditis is most commonly associated with *Staphylococcus aureus* or enterococcus and rarely with *Streptococcus pneumoniae*. Fever is often high, 40°C, accompanied by rigors. These patients are usually brought to the emergency room acutely ill. The likelihood of serious cardiac and extravascular complications is higher, particularly with acute *S. aureus* endocarditis. Rapid diagnosis and treatment are mandatory to reduce valvular destruction and embolic complications.

KEY POINTS

The History in Infective Endocarditis

1. Symptoms usually begin 2 weeks after initial bacteremia and are nonspecific.

2. Diagnosis takes an average of 5 weeks from onset of symptoms.
3. Low-grade fever most common; may be accompanied by night sweats.
4. Symptoms include fatigue, malaise, generalized weakness, anorexia, and weight loss; mimics cancer.
5. Myalgias and arthralgias may suggest a connective tissue disease.
6. Low back pain can be the initial primary complaint. Consider endocarditis as well as epidural abscess and osteomyelitis when back pain is accompanied by fever.
7. Infective endocarditis must be excluded in all cases of embolic cerebrovascular accidents, particularly in younger patients.
8. In acute endocarditis, fever is high and the patient appears acutely ill.

The classic physical findings of infective endocarditis should be carefully searched for. Fever is the rule and is detected in 95% of patients. A heart murmur is almost always appreciated. The absence of an audible murmur should call into question the diagnosis of endocarditis, except in cases of right-sided endocarditis or infection of a mural thrombus (rare). Although the murmur is classically described as a changing murmur, its character usually does not change significantly over time unless a valve leaflet is destroyed (which most commonly occurs with *Staphylococcus aureus*) or a chordae tendineae ruptures. Detection of a new aortic regurgitant murmur is a bad prognostic sign and is commonly associated with the development of congestive heart failure, as described in Case 7.1. The most common cause of acute aortic regurgitation is infective endocarditis; therefore if a high-pitched diastolic murmur radiating along the left sternal border is heard, the initial work-up should always include blood cultures. In Case 7.1 the diagnosis was delayed because his outpatient physician did not exclude infective endocarditis as the cause of his new diastolic murmur.

Careful attention must be paid to the fundi, skin, nail beds, and peripheral pulses because manifestations attributable to emboli are noted in over half of infective endocarditis cases. Funduscopic exam may reveal classic Roth spots, retinal hemorrhages with pale centers, or, more commonly, flame-shaped hemorrhages. One of the most common locations to detect petechial hemorrhages is the conjunctiva (see Figure 7.1A); however, this finding is not specific for endocarditis and is also seen in patients following cardiac surgery and in patients with thrombocytopenia. Clusters of petechiae can be seen on any part of the body. Other common locations are the buccal mucosa, palate, and extremities. Their presence alone should be considered a nonspecific finding. Splinter hemorrhages, linear red or brownish streaks, develop under the nail beds of the hands and feet and are caused by emboli lodging in distal capillaries (Figure 7.1B). These lesions can also be caused by trauma to the fingers or toes. Osler nodes are small, pea-sized subcutaneous, painful erythematous nodules that arise in the pads of the fingers and toes as well as the thenar eminence (Figure 7.1C). They are usually present only for a brief period, disappearing within hours to days. Janeway lesions are most commonly seen in association with *Staphylococcus aureus* (Figure 7.1D). These painless hemorrhagic plaques usually develop on the palms and soles. Bacteria can sometimes be visualized on a skin biopsy of the lesion (Figure 7.1D). It must be kept in mind that, as observed in Case 7.1, about half of patients with infective endocarditis fail to demonstrate any physical evidence of peripheral emboli. Therefore the absence of embolic phenomena does not exclude this diagnosis.

Other findings can include clubbing of the fingers and toes. This manifestation is less common than it was in the past as a consequence of earlier diagnosis and treatment, but it may be found in patients with prolonged symptoms. Another commonly reported finding is splenomegaly. Some patients experience left upper quadrant pain and tenderness as result of splenic infarction, caused by septic emboli. Joint ef-

Figure 7.1

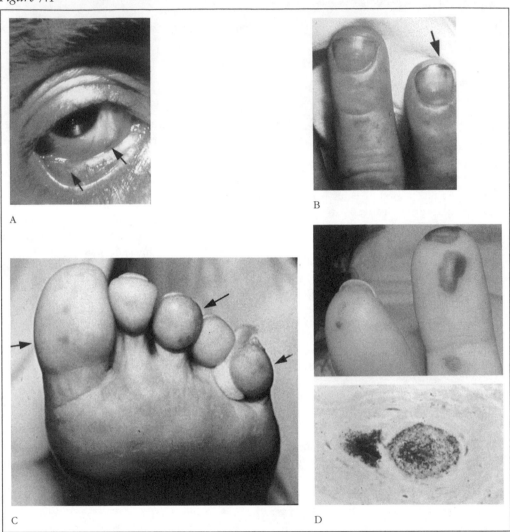

Embolic lesions in infective endocarditis. (A) Conjunctival hemorrhages: Arrows point to two discrete linear hemorrhages. (B) Nail bed splinter hemorrhage: Multiple petechiae are seen on both fingers. Arrow points to a splinter hemorrhage underlying the nail bed. (C) Osler nodes: Arrows point to subtle discolorations of the pads of the toes. These sites were raised and tender to palpation. (D) Janeway lesions: Top: Painless hemorrhagic lesions are seen. Bottom: Biopsy of a typical lesion shows thrombosis and intravascular gram-positive cocci. Culture was positive for *S. aureus*. See also Color Plate 2.

fusions are uncommon; however, diffuse arthralgias and joint stiffness are frequently encountered. Finally, all pulses should be checked periodically, and the sudden loss of a peripheral pulse accompanied by limb pain warrants immediate arteriography to identify and extract occluding emboli. A thorough neurologic exam must also be performed. Confusion, severe headache, or focal neurologic deficits should be further investigated by head CT scan or MRI with contrast looking for embolic infarction, intracerebral hemorrhage, or brain abscess.

KEY POINTS

Physical Findings in Infective Endocarditis

1. A cardiac murmur is heard in nearly all patients:
   a. Absence of a murmur should call into question the diagnosis of infective endocarditis,
   b. Classic changing murmur is rare, may occur with rupture of chordae tendineae,
   c. New aortic regurgitation is due to infective endocarditis until proven otherwise.
2. Embolic phenomena are found in over 50% of cases:
   a. Petechiae: Most common in conjunctiva, clusters can be found anywhere,
   b. Splinter hemorrhages: Linear streaks found under nails,
   c. Osler nodes: Painful raised lesion in the pads of the fingers or toes, evanescent,
   d. Janeway lesions: Painless, red macules, persistent, most common in acute endocarditis due to *Staphylococcus aureus*,
   e. Roth spots, retinal hemorrhage with a clear center.
3. Splenomegaly can be found, left upper quadrant tenderness can occur with embolic infarction.
4. Check all pulses as a baseline because of the risk of obstructive emboli.
5. Perform a thorough neurologic exam; a sudden embolic stroke can develop.

Laboratory abnormalities are nonspecific in nature. Case 7.1 had many of the typical laboratory findings of infective endocarditis. Anemia of chronic disease is noted in 70–90% of subacute cases. A normocytic normochromic red cell morphology, low serum iron, and low iron-binding capacity characterize this form of anemia. The peripheral leukocyte count is usually normal. The finding of an elevated peripheral white blood count should raise the possibility of a myocardial abscess or other extravascular focus of infection. Leukocytosis is also often found in patients with acute bacterial endocarditis. The erythrocyte sedimentation rate, a measure of chronic inflammation, is almost always elevated. With the exception of patients with hemoglobinopathies that falsely lower the rate of red blood cell sedimentation, the finding of a normal erythrocyte sedimentation rate (ESR) virtually excludes the diagnosis of infective endocarditis. C-reactive protein, another inflammatory marker, is also elevated in nearly all cases. A positive rheumatoid factor is detected in half of patients, and elevated serum globulins are found in 20–30% of cases. Cryoglobulins, depressed complement levels, positive tests for immune complexes, and a false positive serology for syphilis are other nonspecific findings that may accompany infective endocarditis. The urinalysis is frequently abnormal, proteinuria being found in 50–65% of cases and hematuria in 30–50%. These abnormalities are the consequence of embolic injury and/or deposition of immune complexes causing glomerulonephritis.

Finally, a chest X-ray should be performed in all patients with suspected endocarditis. In patients with right-sided disease, distinct round, cannonball-like infiltrates may be detected and represent pulmonary emboli. In cases of acute mitral regurgitation or decompensated left-sided failure due to aortic regurgitation diffuse alveolar fluid may be detected, indicating pulmonary edema. Finally the EKG should be closely monitored. The finding of a conduction defect raises concern that infection has spread to the conduction system and in some cases may progress to complete heart block. In Case 7.1 the PR interval was prolonged, and this patient subsequently developed complete heart block. Findings consistent with myocardial infarct may be detected when emboli are released from vegetations in the coronary cusps into the coronary arteries.

KEY POINTS

Laboratory Findings in Infective Endocarditis

1. Anemia of chronic disease found in most patients.
2. Normal peripheral WBC, unless myocardial abscess or acute disease.
3. Manifestations of chronic antigenemia, mimics a connective tissue disorder:
   a. Elevated ESR and C-reactive protein,
   b. Positive rheumatoid factor,
   c. Elevated immunoglobulins, cryoglobulins, and immune complexes,
   d. Decreased complement,
   e. Hematuria and proteinuria.
4. Chest X-ray may be abnormal:
   a. Circular, cannonball-like lesions in embolic right-sided endocarditis,
   b. Pulmonary edema pattern secondary to left-sided CHF.
5. EKG: Monitor closely, conduction defects can progress to complete heart block.

Diagnosis

BLOOD CULTURES

Blood cultures are the critical test for making the diagnosis of infective endocarditis. Compared to most tissue infections, such as pneumonia and pyelonephritis, that result in the intermittent release of large numbers of bacteria into the blood, infective endocarditis is associated with a constant low-level bacteremia (see Figure 7.2). The vegetation is like a time-release tablet, with bacteria being constantly released in small numbers into the bloodstream. It is this constant antigenic stimulus that accounts for the rheumatic complaints and multiple abnormal serum markers associated with infective endocarditis. To document the presence of a constant bacteremia, blood cultures should be drawn at least 15 minutes apart. In patients with suspected subacute infective endocarditis, three blood cultures are recommended over the first 24 hours. In these patients antibiotics should be withheld

Figure 7.2

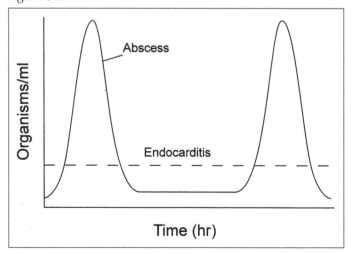

Concentration of bacteria in the blood stream over time in infective endocarditis versus bacteremia caused by other infections.

until the blood cultures are confirmed to be positive, because administration of even a single dose of antibiotics can lower the number of bacteria in the bloodstream to undetectable levels and prevent identification of the pathogen. However, if the patient is acutely ill, three blood cultures should be drawn over 45 minutes, and empiric therapy should be immediately begun. Because the number of bacteria in the blood is usually low, approximately 100 bacteria/ml, a minimum of 10 ml of blood should be inoculated into each blood culture flask. Lower volumes decrease the yield and may account for many culture-negative cases. Routinely, blood cultures are held in the microbiology laboratory for 7 days and discarded if negative. However, if a member of the slow-growing HACEK group is suspected, the laboratory must be alerted to hold the blood cultures for four weeks and to subculture the samples on chocolate agar in 5% CO_2. If nutritionally deficient streptococci are suspected, specific nutrients need to be added to the blood culture media. The sensitivity of blood cultures is excellent, yields being estimated to be 85–95% on the first blood culture and improving to 95–100% with a second blood culture. The third blood culture is drawn primarily to document the constancy of the bacteremia and does not significantly improve overall sensitivity. The administration of antibiotics within two weeks of blood cultures lowers the sensitivity, and patients who have received antibiotics often require multiple blood cultures spaced over days to weeks to identify the etiology.

ECHOCARDIOGRAPHY

Echocardiography is the other essential test that needs to be performed in all patients with suspected infective endocarditis. Transthoracic echocardiography (TTE) is relatively insensitive for detecting vegetations (44–63% sensitivity) compared to transesophageal echocardiography (TEE) (94–100% sensitivity), which can detect vegetations smaller than 3 mm. Compared to TTE, TEE more readily detects extravalvular extension of infection (87% versus 28% sensitivity) and more accurately visualizes valve perforations (95% versus 45% sensitivity). TEE is also preferred for investigating prosthetic valve endocarditis. When accompanied by Doppler color flow analysis, echocardiography allows assessment of valve function, myocardial contractility, and chamber volume; vital information for deciding on surgical intervention.

The Modified Duke Criteria

The definitive diagnosis of infective endocarditis in the absence of valve tissue histopathology or culture is often difficult, and many investigations of this disease have been plagued by differences in the clinical definition of infective endocarditis. Clinical criteria have been established that allow the classification of cases as definite and possible (see Table 7.3). Findings of two major criteria, one major and three minor criteria, or five minor criteria are classified by the modified Duke criteria as a definite cases of infective endocarditis. Possible infective endocarditis is defined as having one major criterion and one minor criterion or three minor criteria.

KEY POINTS
Diagnosis of Infective Endocarditis

1. Blood cultures documenting constant bacteremia with endocarditis-associated pathogen:
   a. Blood cultures need to be spaced at least 15 minutes apart, three over 24 hours for subacute bacterial endocarditis,
   b. Large volumes (at least 10 ml) of blood need to be added to blood cultures,
   c. Blood cultures are usually negative for at least 7 days after an antibiotic is given.
2. Documentation of endocardial involvement (TEE is more sensitive than TTE), TEE

always preferred in prosthetic valve endocarditis.

3. Duke criteria are helpful for making the
   clinical diagnosis of infective endocarditis in
   the absence of pathologic tissue.

Table 7.3

Modified Duke Criteria for Infective Endocarditis

Major Criteria

1. (+) Blood cultures with typical endocarditis-
   associated organisms including *Staphylococcus aureus:*

   2 separate (+) blood cultures

   (OR)

   Persistent (+) blood culture (2 positive over
   12 hours apart or 3 or the majority of >4
   blood cultures positive, first and last drawn
   at least 1 hour apart)

2. Evidence of endocardial involvement:

   (+) echo (in patients with possible IE, a TEE
   is recommended.)

   (OR)

   New regurgitant murmur

3. + Q fever serology (antiphase I IgG > 1:800)
   or single blood culture + *Coxiella burnetii*

Minor Criteria

1. Predisposing heart condition
2. Fever ≥ 38°C
3. Vascular phenomena
4. Immunologic phenomena
5. Single positive blood culture with typical
   organism
6. The previous minor criteria of suspicious lesion on TTE eliminated

Definite Infective Endocarditis

2 major

1 major and 3 minor

5 minor

Possible Infective Endocarditis

1 major and 1 minor

3 minor

Source: Li, J.S., et al. *Clin Infect Dis*, 30:633–638, 2000.

Complications

In the modern antibiotic era complications associated with infective endocarditis remain common: Approximately 60% of patients suffer one
complication, 25% suffer two complications, and
8% suffer three or more complications.

CARDIAC COMPLICATIONS

Complications involving the heart are most frequent and occur in one third to one half of patients. Congestive heart failure is the most common
complication that leads to surgical intervention.
Destruction of the valve leaflets results in regurgitation. Less commonly, vegetations become large
enough to obstruct the outflow tract and cause
stenosis. Perivalvular extension of infection also
requires surgical intervention. This complication
is more common with aortic valve disease, and
spread from the aortic valvular ring to the adjacent conduction system can lead to heart block.
This complication should be suspected in the infective endocarditis patient with peripheral leukocytosis, persistent fever while on appropriate antibiotics, or an abnormal conduction time on
EKG. Transesophageal echo detects the majority
of cases, and this test should be performed in all
cases of aortic valve endocarditis. Less common
complications include pericarditis and mycocar-
dial infarction.

SYSTEMIC EMBOLI

Pieces of the vegetation consisting of a friable
collection of platelets, fibrin, and bacteria frequently break off and become lodged in arteries
and arterioles throughout the body. It is likely
that small emboli are released in all cases of endocarditis; however, they are symptomatic in one
sixth to one third of patients. Because the right
brachiocephalic trunk (innominate artery) is the
first vessel that branches from the ascending aortic arch, emboli have a higher likelihood of passing through this vessel and into the right internal
carotid artery. The second branch coming off the

aortic arch is the left common carotid artery, and there is also a higher likelihood of emboli entering this vessel. These anatomic considerations probably account for the observation that two thirds of left-sided systemic emboli from the heart lodge in the central nervous system. In addition to sudden neurologic deficits, patients can suffer with ischemic limbs as well as splenic and renal infarction. Patients with right-sided endocarditis frequently develop recurrent pulmonary emboli. Symptomatic emboli more commonly occur in patients with fungal endocarditis and patients infected with slow-growing organisms such as the HACEK group. Antibiotic therapy is associated with fibrotic changes in the vegetation and reduces the risk of emboli.

MYCOTIC ANEURYSMS

Infectious emboli can become lodged at arterial bifurcations, where they occlude the vasa vasorum or the entire vessel lumen, damaging the muscular layer of the vessel. The systemic arterial pressure causes ballooning of the weakened vessel wall and formation of an aneurysm. Aneurysms are most commonly encountered in the middle cerebral artery, abdominal aorta, and mesenteric arteries. On occasion these aneurysms can burst, resulting in intracerebral or intra-abdominal hemorrhage. Because of the increased risk of hemorrhage, anticoagulation should be avoided in patients with infective endocarditis. Mycotic aneurysms are most commonly encountered in *Staphylococcus aureus* endocarditis.

NEUROLOGIC COMPLICATIONS

Complications arising in the central nervous system are second only to cardiac complications in frequency and are seen in 25–35% of patients. In addition to embolic strokes and intracerebral hemorrhage, patients can develop encephalopathy, meningitis, meningoencephalitis, and brain abscess. The development of a neurologic deficit in the past was considered a contraindication to cardiac surgery. More recent experience indicates that surgery within a week of the neuro-

logic event is not accompanied by worsening neurologic deficits.

RENAL COMPLICATIONS

Significant renal failure (serum creatinine ≥ 2 mg/dl) can develop in up to one third of patients and is more likely in the elderly and patients with thrombocytopenia. Renal dysfunction can be caused by immune complex glomerulonephritis, renal emboli, and drug-induced interstitial nephritis. Glomerulonephritis results from immune complex deposition in the basement membranes of the glomeruli and results in the microscopic changes of membranoproliferative disease. The urinalysis reveals hematuria and mild proteinuria. Red cell casts are observed in glomerulonephritis but not in interstitial nephritis. Glomerulonephritis usually rapidly improves with antibiotic therapy.

KEY POINTS

Complications Associated with Infective Endocarditis

1. Cardiac complications occur in up to half of patients:
   a. Congestive heart failure,
   b. Myocardial abscess (aortic disease associated with conduction defects),
   c. Myocardial infarction a rare complication of aortic disease.
2. Systemic emboli: Two thirds go to the cerebral cortex.
3. Neurological complications:
   a. Embolic stroke (most common with fungi and HACEK group),
   b. Mycotic aneurysms (most common in *Staphylococcus aureus*),
   c. Encephalopathy, meningitis, and brain abscess.
4. Renal complications:
   a. Membranoproliferative glomerulonephritis due to immune complex deposition,
   b. Interstitial nephritis,
   c. Embolic damage.

Treatment

ANTIBIOTICS

Whenever possible, the antibiotic therapy of subacute infective endocarditis should be based on the antibiotic sensitivities of the offending organism. Because bacteria are protected from neutrophil ingestion by the dense coating of fibrin found in the vegetation, bactericidal antibiotics are required to cure this infection. To design the most effective regimen, minimal bactericidal levels should be determined for multiple antibiotics, and combinations of antibiotics should be tested for synergy (see Chapter 1). The goal is to achieve serum cidal levels of 1:8–1:32, this level of cidal activity being associated with cure. A second important principle of antibiotic therapy is the requirement for prolonged antibiotic therapy. The concentrations of bacteria in the vegetation are high, and a significant percentage of the bacteria slow their metabolism and stop actively dividing for significant periods. These conditions prevent immediate sterilization by cidal antibiotics that require active bacterial growth such as penicillins, cephalosporins, and glycopeptide antibiotics. Most curative regimens are continued for four to six weeks to prevent relapse. One exception to this rule is uncomplicated subacute bacterial endocarditis caused by *Streptococcus viridans* species. The combination of penicillin G (12–18 million units QD given iv Q4H) and gentamicin (1 mg/kg iv Q8H) is synergistic and is associated with more rapid killing of bacteria in vegetations. Two weeks of combination therapy results in cure rates similar to those for penicillin alone for four weeks. A two-week course of ceftriaxone (2 gm iv QD) and gentamicin achieves comparable results. The gentamicin dose should be adjusted to maintain peak serum levels of 3 µg/ml, the concentration that is required to achieve synergy.

In acute bacterial endocarditis, intravenous empiric antibiotic therapy should be initiated immediately after drawing of three blood cultures. A combination of vancomycin 1 g Q12H, ampicillin 2 g Q4H, and gentamicin 1 mg/kg Q8H is recommended to cover the most likely pathogens, *Staphylococcus aureus*, including MRSA, and enterococcus, pending culture results. Empiric therapy for culture-negative subacute bacterial endocarditis should include ampicillin and gentamicin to cover for enterococcus, the HACEK group, and nutritional deficient streptococci.

The regimens for specific bacterial causes of endocarditis are outlined in Table 7.4. Whenever possible, a synergistic regimen consisting of a β-lactam antibiotic and an aminoglycoside is preferred. One exception to this rule is *Staphylococcus aureus*. Combination therapy of nafcillin or oxacillin and gentamicin may shorten the duration of positive blood cultures but has not been shown to improve mortality or overall cure rates, and therefore dual-antibiotic therapy is not recommended. With the exception of ceftazidime, MIC values for cephalosporins correlate well with therapeutic response and are often therapeutically equivalent to the semisynthetic penicillins. β-lactam antibiotics are preferred over vancomycin because vancomycin is less rapidly cidal, and failure rates of up to 40% have been reported when *S. aureus* endocarditis is treated with vancomycin. In the penicillin-allergic patient with *S. aureus* endocarditis, β-lactam desensitization should be strongly considered. In patients with enterococcal endocarditis, cephalosporins are ineffective and should not be used. Maximal doses of intravenous penicillin (18–30 million units QD in Q4H doses) or ampicillin (12 gm QD in Q4H doses) combined with gentamicin (1 mg/kg Q8H) is preferred, and this combination should be continued for the full course of therapy. Vancomycin (1 gm Q12H) combined with gentamicin is a suitable alternative in the penicillin-allergic patient. With the exception of uncomplicated *Streptococcus viridans* species, antibiotic treatment should be continued for four to six weeks.

Antibiotic therapy for prosthetic valve endocarditis presents a particularly difficult challenge.

Table 7.4

Antibiotic Therapy for Infective Endocarditis

DRUG	DOSE	RELATIVE EFFICACY	COMMENTS
Acute, empiric	Duration 4–6 weeks unless otherwise noted		
Vancomycin (+)	1 gm iv Q12H		Vancomycin more slowly
Ampicillin (+)	2 gm iv Q4H		cidal. Whenever possible,
Gentamicin	1 mg/kg iv Q8H		use an alternative.
Culture negative			
Ampicillin (+)	2 gm iv Q4H		
Gentamicin	1 mg/kg iv Q8H		
Prosthetic, empiric			
Vancomycin (+)	1 gm iv Q12H		
Gentamicin (+)	1 mg/kg iv Q8H		
Rifampin	600 mg po QD		
Streptococcus viridans			
Penicillin G (or)	2–3 million units iv Q4H	First line	Short course if uncompli-
ampicillin (+)	2 gm iv Q4H		cated. Use sensitivity
Gentamicin	1 mg/kg iv Q8H × 2 weeks		testing to determine
			best regimen.
Ceftriaxone (+)	1 gm iv QD	Alternative	Short course if uncompli-
Gentamicin	1 mg/kg iv Q8H × 4 weeks		cated
Vancomycin	1 gm iv Q12H × 4 weeks	Alternative	For PCN-allergic patient
Enterococcus			
Ampicillin (or)	2 gm iv Q4H	First line	Relapse is common in the
penicillin G (+)	2–3 million units iv Q4H		absence of gentamicin.
Gentamicin	1 mg/kg iv Q8H		Use sensitivity testing
			to determine best regi-
			men.
Staphylococcus aureus **MSSA**			
Nafcillin or oxacillin (+)	2 gm iv Q4H	First line	Addition of gentamicin may
Gentamicin	1 mg/kg iv Q8H for 3–5 days		shorten bacteremia but has no effect on final outcome
S. aureus MRSA			
Vancomycin	1 gm iv Q12H	First line	
S. aureus (tricuspid)		First line	
Nafcillin or oxacillin (+)	2 gm iv Q4H	First line	Short course effective if no
Gentamicin	1 mg/kg iv Q8H × 2 weeks		metastatic lesions and MSSA
Ciprofloxacin (+)	750 mg po BID	Second line	May be effective in MSSA
Rifampin	300 mg po BID × 4 weeks		

The deposition of biofilm on the prosthetic material makes cure with antibiotics alone difficult, and the valve often has to be replaced. Some patients with late-onset prosthetic valve endocarditis caused by very antibiotic-sensitive organisms can be cured by antibiotic treatment alone. In patients with coagulase-negative Staphylococcus a combination of intravenous vancomycin (1 gm Q12H) and rifampin (300 mg Q8H) for six weeks or more plus gentamicin (1 mg/kg Q8H) for two weeks is the preferred treatment for methicillin-resistant strains. For methicillin-sensitive strains nafcillin or oxacillin (2 gm Q4H) should be substituted for vancomycin.

Intravenous drug abusers with uncomplicated tricuspid valve *Staphylococcus aureus* endocarditis can be treated with two weeks of intravenous nafcillin or oxacillin (2 gm Q4H) combined with tobramycin (1 mg/kg Q8H). This abbreviated regimen is not recommended in HIV-positive patients. An oral regimen of ciprofloxacin (750 mg BID) and rifampin (300 mg BID) for four weeks has also proved effective, provided that the *S. aureus* strain is sensitive to ciprofloxacin.

KEY POINTS

Antibiotic Therapy of Infective Endocarditis

1. Cidal antibiotics must be used, and therapy must be prolonged.
   a. Therapy four to six weeks, except for uncomplicated *Streptococcus viridans* in which penicillin or ceftriaxone combined with low-dose gentamicin can be used; two weeks effective,
   b. Therapy must be guided by MIC values and synergy testing,
   c. Synergistic therapy not shown to be of benefit for *S. aureus*.
2. β-lactam antibiotics are preferred over vancomycin whenever possible.
3. Antibiotics alone rarely sterilize prosthetic valves. Some success with coagulase-nega-

tive Staphylococcus using vancomycin, gentamicin, and rifampin.
4. Tricuspid endocarditis:
   a. Nafcillin or oxacillin plus tobramycin × two weeks effective except for HIV-infected patients,
   b. Oral ciprofloxacin plus rifampin × four weeks also may be effective.

SURGERY

Medical therapy alone often is not curative, particularly in prosthetic valve endocarditis. In a significant percentage of patients surgical removal of the infected valve or debridement of vegetations greatly increases the likelihood of survival. As a consequence, in recent years the threshold for surgery has lowered. In almost all cases of infective endocarditis the cardiologist and cardiac surgeon should be consulted early in the course of illness. The decision to operate is often complex, and appropriate timing of surgery must balance the risk of progressive complications with the risk of intraoperative and postoperative morbidity and mortality. Indications for surgery include the following:

1. **Moderate to severe congestive heart failure (CHF)**. This is the most frequent indication for surgery. A delay in surgery often results in a fatal outcome due to irreversible left ventricular dysfunction. In patients with CHF, death can be very sudden.
2. **More than one systemic embolus**. The ability to predict the likelihood of recurrent emboli by echocardiography is questionable. In some studies, large vegetations, >10 mm in diameter, were found to have a higher probability of embolizing; however, more recent studies have not confirmed this finding.
3. **Uncontrolled infection**. *Staphylococcus aureus* is one of the most common pathogens to cause persistently positive blood cultures. Extravascular foci of infection should always be excluded before surgical intervention is considered.

4. **Resistant organisms or fungal infection**. The mortality in fungal endocarditis approaches 90%, and with the exception of a rare case of *Candida albicans* cures have not been achieved by medical therapy alone.

5. **Perivalvular/myocardial abscess**. With the exception of very small abscesses these lesions usually enlarge on medical therapy and require surgical debridement and repair.

As was discussed above (see "Neurologic Complications"), a focal neurologic deficit is not an absolute contraindication for surgery. Whenever possible, surgery should be delayed until blood cultures are negative to reduce the risk of septic intraoperative complications. However, even in the setting of ongoing positive blood cultures, infection of the new valve is uncommon, particularly if the surgeon thoroughly debrides the infected site.

be associated with a 50% mortality in patients over age 50 years. Fungal infections and infections with Gram-negative aerobic bacilli are also associated with poor outcomes. Development of CHF or onset of neurologic deficits is associated with a worse prognosis. Patients with early prosthetic valve endocarditis often do poorly despite valve replacement, cure rates ranging from 30% to 50%. Late prosthetic valve endocarditis has a better outcome. In patients with late prosthetic valve infection with *Streptococcus viridans* species, cure rates of 90% have been achieved when antibiotic therapy is accompanied by surgery and 80% with antibiotic treatment alone. Patients with *Staphylococcus epidermidis* late prosthetic valve endocarditis have been cured 60% of the time medically and have a 70% cure rate when medical treatment is combined with valve replacement.

KEY POINTS

Surgery for Infective Endocarditis

---
1. The threshold for surgery should be low and increases the likelihood of cure.
2. The cardiologist and cardiac surgeon should be consulted early.
3. Indications for surgery include:
   a. Moderate to severe CHF. Early surgery lowers intraoperative and postoperative mortality,
   b. More than one systemic embolus,
   c. Uncontrolled infection,
   d. Resistant bacteria or a fungal pathogen,
   e. Perivalvular leak or myocardial abscess.
4. Neurologic deficits are not an absolute contraindication for surgery.

KEY POINTS

The Prognosis in Infective Endocarditis

---
1. Outcome strongly correlates with the organism and valve infected:
   a. *Staphylococcus aureus* has 50% mortality in patients > 50 years of age,
   b. Fungal infections are difficult to cure,
   c. Gram-negative bacilli are associated with a poor outcome.
2. CHF or neurological deficits = worse prognosis.
3. Prosthetic valve endocarditis associated with a poorer outcome:
   a. Early prosthetic endocarditis, cure rates only 30–50%,
   b. Late disease has higher cure rates, particularly *Staphylococcus epidermidis* and *Streptococcus viridans*.

Prognosis

Cure rates depend on the organism involved and the valve infected. *Staphylococcus aureus* remains a particularly virulent pathogen and continues to

Prevention

The efficacy of prophylaxis has never been proven for native valve endocarditis. As documented in Table 7.1, individuals probably experience multiple episodes of transient bacteremia each day, and this cumulative exposure is hundreds of times greater than that of a single exposure. Despite these concerns, the standard of care is to provide antibiotic prophylaxis during invasive procedures for high- and moderate-risk patients. High-risk patients are defined as patients with prosthetic valves (including bioprosthetic and homograft valves), patients with a past history of endocarditis, patients with complex cyanotic congenital heart disease, and patients with surgically constructed systemic pulmonary shunts. Moderate-risk patients are defined as those with rheumatic and other acquired valvular dysfunction, patients with hypertrophic cardiomyopathy, and patients with mitral valve prolapse with valve regurgitation. Invasive procedures that warrant prophylaxis include the following:

1. Dental procedures: periodontal procedures, tooth cleaning if bleeding is anticipated, initial placement of orthodontic bands, intraligamentary local anesthetic injections. These recommendations have been questioned, and some authorities recommend prophylaxis only with dental extractions and gingival surgery in patients with prosthetic valves or previous endocarditis (*Annals of Internal Medicine*, 129:829, 1998).
2. Tonsillectomy and adenoidectomy
3. Surgical procedures that involve intestinal or respiratory mucosa
4. Sclerotherapy of esophageal varices or esophageal dilation in high-risk patients
5. Endoscopic retrograde cholangiography with biliary obstruction
6. Gallbladder surgery in high-risk patients
7. Cystoscopy, urethral dilation, or prostate surgery

The timing of antibiotics is important. The antibiotic should be administered before the procedure and timed so that peak serum levels are achieved at the time of the procedure. For dental, oral, and upper respiratory procedures:

◆ Amoxicillin 2 gm po should be administered 1 hour before the procedure; alternatively, penicillin V, 2 gm po can be given 1 hour before and 1 gm 6 hours after the first dose.
◆ Clindamycin, 600 mg po; cephalexin or cefadroxil, 2 gm po; azithromycin or clarithromycin, 500 mg po can be given 1 hour before the procedure in the penicillin-allergic patient.
◆ If parenteral therapy is required, ampicillin, 2 gm im or iv ampicillin or, in the penicillin-allergic patient, clindamycin; 600 mg iv or cefazolin, 1 gm im or iv can be given 30 minutes before the procedure.

For genitourinary or gastrointestinal procedures:

◆ **High-risk patient**. Ampicillin 2 gm im or iv plus gentamicin 1.5 mg/kg 30 minutes or less before the procedure and ampicillin, 1 gm iv or amoxicillin po 6 hours later.
◆ **High-risk patient with penicillin allergy**. Vancomycin, 1 gm iv over 1–2 hours plus gentamicin, 1.5 mg/kg iv or im; complete infusion within 30 minutes of starting the procedure.
◆ **Moderate-risk patient**. Amoxicillin, 2 gm po 1 hour before the procedure or ampicillin, 2 gm im or iv 30 minutes before the procedure.
◆ **Moderate-risk patient with penicillin allergy**. Vancomycin, 1 gm iv over 1–2 hours; complete the infusion within 30 minutes of starting the procedure.

KEY POINTS
Prophylaxis in Infective Endocarditis

1. The efficacy of prophylaxis has not been proven; however, it is considered the standard of care.
2. Give to high-risk patients (prosthetic valves, previous endocarditis, cyanotic heart disease, and surgical shunts) and moderate-risk patients (rheumatic and other acquired valvular

dysfunction, hypertrophic cardiomyopathy, mitral valve prolapse with regurgitation).
3. Give just prior to the procedure to achieve peak antibiotic levels at the time of the invasive procedure.

Intravascular Catheter-Related Infections

Potential Severity: Can be life-threatening. Often prolong a hospital stay and can be complicated by metastatic lesions and bacterial endocarditis.

◆ CASE 7.2

A 53-year-old white female was admitted to the hospital with complaints of severe shaking during the infusion of her hyperalimentation solution. She had been receiving intravenous hyperalimentation for 16 years for a severe dumping syndrome that prevented eating by mouth. She had had multiple complications from her intravenous lines, including venous occlusions and line-associated bacteremia, requiring replacement of 24 lines. She was last admitted 6 months earlier with infection of her intravascular catheter with *Enterobacter cloacae*, requiring line removal and intravenous cefepime. A tunneled catheter was placed at that time in her left subclavian vein, and she did well until the evening prior to admission. As she was infusing her solution, she developed rigors, and her temperature rose to 102.6°F. She continued to experience chills and developed a headache.

Physical examination: Temperature 38°C, blood pressure 136/50, nontoxic appearing. Heart: A II/VI systolic ejection murmur along the left sternal border (present for years). The site of the catheter was not erythematous or tender. Two blood cultures were positive for *E. coli*. The culture drawn from the catheter became positive 6 hours after being drawn, while a simultaneous peripheral blood culture became positive 5 hours later (11 hours after being drawn).

Epidemiology, Pathogenesis, and Etiology

More than 200,000 nosocomial bloodstream infections occur annually in the United States. A major percentage of these infections are related to intravascular devices. Bacteria most commonly infect catheters by tracking subcutaneously along the outside of the catheter into the fibrin sheath that surrounds the intravascular segment of the catheter. Bacteria can also be inadvertently introduced into the hub and lumen of the catheter from the skin of a caregiver or as a consequence of a contaminated infusate. Less commonly, catheters can be infected by hematogenous spread caused by a primary infection at another site. Once bacteria invade the fibrin sheath surrounding the catheter, they generate a biofilm that protects them from attack by neutrophils. This condition makes sterilization by antibiotics alone difficult. The risk of infection is greater for some devices than others:

1. Femoral vein > internal jugular vein > subclavian vein catheters
2. Nontunneled > tunneled catheters
3. Tunneled > totally implanted devices
4. Conventional catheter tips > silver-impregnated catheter tips
5. Centrally inserted central venous catheters > peripherally inserted central catheters
6. Hemodialysis > other catheters
7. Hyperalimentation > standard infusion ports

Regular exchange of central venous catheters over guide wires does not reduce the incidence of infection. In fact reinsertion of a catheter through an infected soft tissue site can precipitate bacteremia.

The organisms that are most commonly associated with intravascular device infection are skin flora. Gram-positive cocci predominate, coagulase-negative Staphylococcus being most common, followed by *S. aureus*. Coagulase-negative Staphylococcus produces a glycocalyx that enhances its adherence to synthetic materials such as catheter tips. Enterococci and corynebacteria are other common Gram-positive pathogens. Gram-negative bacilli account for up to one third of infections, *Klebsiella pneumoniae*, Enterobacter species, *E. coli*, Pseudomonas species, Acinetobacter species, and Serratia species being most common. Positive blood cultures for *Klebsiella*, *Citrobacter*, and non-aeruginosa strains of Pseudomonas suggest a contaminated infusate. Fungi now account for 20% of central venous catheter infections, *Candida albicans* predominating. Like coagulase-negative Staphylococcus, *C. albicans* is able to form a glycocalyx that enhances adherence to catheters. Patients receiving high-glucose solutions for hyperalimentation are at particularly high risk for this infection.

KEY POINTS

Epidemiology, Pathogenesis, and Etiology of Intravascular Catheter-Related Infections

1. Bacteria infect catheters in three ways:
   a. Skin flora migrates along the catheter track,
   b. Bacteria are injected into the port,
   c. Hematogenous spread.
2. Catheter location and type affect the risk of infection.
3. Regular exchange of central venous catheters over guide wires does not reduce the incidence of infection; not recommended, can precipitate bacteremia.
4. Gram-positive cocci predominate:
   a. Coagulase-negative Staphylococcus most common, adheres to catheters by a glycocalyx,
   b. *S. aureus*,
   c. Enterococci,
   d. Corynebacteria.
5. Gram-negatives account for one third:
   a. Enterobacter species, *E. coli,* Acinetobacter species, Pseudomonas species, and Serratia species,
   b. Contaminated infusate associated with Klebsiella species, Citrobacter, or non-aeruginosa strains of Pseudomonas.
6. *Candida albicans:* Also forms an adherent glycocalyx, associated with high-glucose solutions.

Clinical Manifestations and Diagnosis

The clinical presentation of intravascular device-related infection is nonspecific, generally being accompanied by fever, chills, and malaise. The finding of purulence around the intravascular device is helpful, but it is not always present. The absence of an alternative source for bacteremia should always raise the possibility of intravascular device infection. As observed in Case 7.2, the abrupt onset of chills and/or hypotension during the infusion of a solution through the device strongly suggests catheter-associated infection or contamination of the infusate. The rapid resolution of symptoms following removal of the device, and positive blood cultures for coagulase-negative Staphylococcus, Corynebacterium, or a fungus are other findings that suggest an infected intravascular device. The absence of these findings, however, does not exclude the diagnosis.

Rapid diagnosis can be achieved by drawing 100 µl of blood from the catheter while it is still in place, subjecting the sample to cytospin, and performing both Gram stain and acridine orange stain. This method, however, is less sensitive than cultures of the removed catheter tip. Two methods are recommended. The roll method (the catheter is rolled across the culture plate) is semiquantitative (positive ≥ 15 cfu), and the vortex or sonication method (releases bacteria into liquid media) is quantitative (positive ≥ 100 cfu). The roll method detects bacteria on the outer surface of the catheter, while the vortex/sonication method also detects bacteria from the inner lumen. The sonication method is more sensitive but more difficult to perform than the roll method. With the use of antibiotic- and silver-impregnated catheters these methods may yield false negative results. Cultures of removed catheter tips should be performed only when a catheter-related bloodstream infection is suspected. Routine surveillance culturing of removed catheter tips is not recommended.

When an intravascular device infection is suspected, at least two blood cultures should be drawn: one set from the intravenous catheter and one set from a peripheral vein. A negative blood culture drawn from the intravenous line is very helpful in excluding the diagnosis of catheter-related bloodstream infection. A positive culture requires clinical interpretation. As in Case 7.2, when removal of the catheter is not desirable, quantitative blood culturing has been recommended. The finding of fivefold to tenfold higher colony counts in the catheter sample compared to the peripheral samples suggests catheter-related infection. A more practical approach (used in Case 7.2) takes advantage of automated colorimetric, continuous monitoring of blood cultures now available in most clinical microbiology laboratories. The time required to detect bacteria in the catheter sample is compared to the time required for the peripheral sample. Detection of bacteria 2 hours or more earlier in the catheter sample as compared to the peripheral sample suggests a catheter-associated infection. In Case 7.2 the history of rigors during intravenous infusion combined with the earlier detection of bacteria in the catheter culture as compared to the peripheral culture provided strong evidence that the infection originated in the intravascular device.

KEY POINTS

Clinical Manifestations and Diagnosis of Intravascular Catheter-Related Infections

1. Symptoms are nonspecific. Suggestive historical facts include:
   a. Rigors or chills associated with infusion,
   b. Resolution of symptoms on removal of the intravenous catheter,
   c. Blood cultures positive for *Staphylococcus epidermidis*, *Corynebacteria*, or *Candida albicans*.
2. Purulence around the catheter site provides strong evidence but is absent in many cases.
3. Cytospin Gram stain or acridine orange stain of catheter sample for rapid diagnosis.
4. Roll and sonication methods for quantitating bacteria on catheter tip. Surveillance cultures not recommended.
5. Simultaneous blood cultures should be drawn from the catheter and a peripheral vein:
   a. Quantitative cultures: Catheter sample 5–10× > peripheral sample = catheter infection,
   b. Measurement of the time interval required for detection: catheter positive > 2 hours earlier than peripheral sample = catheter infection.

Treatment

Empiric antibiotic therapy should be initiated after appropriate cultures have been obtained. Vancomycin is usually recommended to cover for MRSA as well as methicillin-resistant coagulase-negative Staphylococcus. In the severely ill or immunocompromised patient additional coverage for Gram-negative bacilli is recommended with an anti-pseudomonal third- (cefazidime) or fourth-generation cephalosporin (cefepime). In the severely ill patient the catheter should be immediately removed. The catheter should also be removed if fever persists and blood cultures continue to be positive for 48 hours or more and if the patient is infected with virulent, difficult-to-treat pathogens such as *S. aureus*; Gram-negative bacilli, particularly *Pseudomonas aeruginosa;* and fungi. Polymicrobial bacteremia suggests heavy contamination of the line and usually warrants catheter removal. Other indications for removal include neutropenia, tunnel or pocket infection, valvular heart disease or endo-carditis, septic thrombophlebitis, and the presence of metastatic abscesses.

The duration of therapy has not been examined in carefully controlled trials. Therapy is usually continued for two weeks in uncomplicated infection. For patients with coagulase-negative staphylococcus, treatment for 5–7 days is sufficient if the catheter is removed but should be continued for a minimum of two weeks if the catheter is left in place. In complicated infections in which bacteremia continues despite removal of the catheter, treatment must be continued for four to six weeks. On average most catheter-associated infections are treated for three weeks. Because of the high incidence of relapse, follow-up blood cultures are important if the line was kept in place.

The salvage rate for tunnel catheters can be improved by filling the catheter lumen with pharmacologic concentrations of antibiotic, termed antibiotic lock therapy. Vancomycin (25 mg in 5 ml of solution) is usually recommended for Gram-positive infections, and gentamicin (5 mg in 5 ml of solution) for Gram-negative bacilli. This treatment exposes the bacteria to very high concentrations of antibiotic and is more likely to kill bacteria protected by biofilm. Antibiotic lock therapy is particularly helpful in tunnel-catheter infections because infections associated with this catheter type usually develop within the lumen. Cure rates from 60% to 80% have been achieved.

Because of the ability of *Staphylococcus aureus* to attach to and destroy normal heart valves (70% of *S. aureus* endocarditis cases occur on previously normal heart valves), this pathogen poses a unique challenge. The duration of therapy after prompt catheter removal is best guided by transesophageal echo (TEE). The presence of valvular vegetations on TEE warrants four weeks of therapy, while the absence of vegetations on this test allows treatment for two weeks without significant risk of relapse. Short-course therapy should be considered only in patients who promptly defervesce on antibi-

otic therapy and who do not have valvular heart disease or an extravascular focus of infection.

In patients with Candida species the intravenous catheter must be removed. Removal must be accompanied by antifungal therapy because of the high risk of Candida endophthalmitis (10–15%) in untreated patients. In uncomplicated *C. albicans* infection fluconazole (400 mg/day for ≥14 days) is as effective as amphotericin B and is accompanied by minimal toxicity. For fungemia due to other, more resistant strains such as *C. kruzei*, prolonged positive blood cultures, severe systemic complaints, or the presence of neutropenia warrants therapy with systemic amphotericin B (0.3–1 mg/kg/day).

KEY POINTS

Treatment of Intravascular Catheter-Related Infections

1. The catheter should be removed if:
   a. The patient is severely ill,
   b. Fever and positive blood cultures persist for >48 hours,
   c. Infected with a virulent organism,
   d. Polymicrobial bacteremia,
   e. Tunnel infection, neutropenia, endocarditis, metastatic infection, septic thrombophlebitis.
2. Empiric therapy: Vancomycin and antipseudomonal third- or fourth-generation cephalosporin.
3. Duration of therapy not studied:
   a. Average duration three weeks,
   b. One week for coagulase-negative Staphylococcus if line is removed and two weeks if line is kept in place,
   c. Four to six weeks for complicated infections.
4. Antibiotic lock therapy improves cure rate for tunnel catheters (vancomycin, gentamicin).
5. *S. aureus*: High risk of endocarditis, TEE helpful in determining the length of therapy.

6. *Candida albicans*: Always remove the line, treat for two weeks to prevent endophthalmitis:
   a. Fluconazole for uncomplicated catheter-related infection,
   b. Amphotericin B for severely ill, neutropenia, or infection with a resistant fungus.

Myocarditis

Potential Severity: Fulminant myocarditis can be fatal or lead to chronic congestive heart failure. Most cases are self-limited and are followed by full recovery.

The true incidence of myocarditis or inflammation of the heart is unknown because the majority of cases are asymptomatic. In systemic viral illnesses it has been estimated that 1–5% of cases have myocardial involvement. Young males are at higher risk for serious myocarditis, as are pregnant women, neonates, and immunocompromised patients.

Etiology and Pathogenesis

Viruses are a major cause of myocarditis. Enteroviruses are the most frequent viruses associated with myocarditis and have been detected by PCR in 25% of patients with myocarditis. Coxsackieviruses B are the major strains implicated. Echoviruses have also been detected. Adenovirus is another common viral cause, particularly in adults. However, many other viruses have been implicated, including cytomegalovirus and Epstein-Barr virus, varicella-zoster, and mumps. Patients with asymptomatic HIV infection have a high incidence of myocarditis (1.6% per year). Many bacteria have also been implicated as

causes of myocarditis, including Legionella and Chlamydia species. Spirochetes can invade the heart, and patients with Lyme disease may present with cardiac arrhythmias (see Chapter 13). Severe disseminated fungal infections due to Aspergillus, Candida, and Cryptococcus species can result in myocarditis. Parasites are also implicated; *Trypanosoma cruzi* attacks the heart in 30% of patients with Chagas' disease, and heavy infestation with Trichinella can cause fatal myocarditis (see Chapter 12).

Viruses can directly invade myocytes and can cause direct damage to the infected cells. The immune response to infection also causes cytotoxicity. Myocyte infiltration by T cells predominates, accompanied by macrophages and B cells. Circulating autoantibodies directed against mitochondria and contractile proteins are frequently detected. Cytokines and oxygen free radicals have also been implicated as contributors to myocyte damage. Forced exercise, pregnancy, use of steroids or nonsteroidal anti-inflammatory agents, use of ethanol, and nutritional deficiencies have all been implicated as factors that predispose to symptomatic myocarditis.

Clinical Manifestations, Diagnosis, and Treatment

The pace of illness and symptoms varies greatly from patient to patient. Some patients experience a flulike illness that can be accompanied by chest pain when the pericardium is involved. Other patients present with arrhythmias or symptoms of right- and left-sided congestive heart failure. On physical exam the presence of an S_3 gallop indicates significant left-sided congestive heart failure. Left ventricular dilatation can lead to expansion of the mitral valve ring and a mitral regurgitant murmur. In patients with pericardial involvement a pericardial friction rub may be present.

Cardiac enzymes are elevated in the minority of cases. CK-MB levels are elevated in only 5%

of cases, and cardiac troponin I in 34%. Elevations are most commonly detected within the first month of symptoms and suggest ongoing myocyte necrosis. Acute and convalescent viral titers may be drawn and will detect recent viral infections, but this test should not be considered proof of etiology. Electrocardiogram may demonstrate nonspecific ST and T wave changes, ventricular or atrial arrhythmias, and conduction defects. Chest X-ray will detect pulmonary edema and cardiac dilatation. Echocardiography is very helpful for assessing cardiac contractility, chamber size, valve function, and wall thickness. Contrast-enhanced MRI allows detection of the extent and degree of inflammation, parameters that correlate with left ventricular function and clinical status. Definitive diagnosis requires endomyocardial biopsy. Timing of biopsy and interpretation by an experienced pathologist are critical. PCR analysis of biopsy tissue remains experimental, and the specificity and sensitivity of these assays remain to be determined.

No specific treatment for viral myocarditis is available. A randomized trial of immunosuppressive agents failed to improve outcome. Administration of immunoglobulins may be of benefit; however, a randomized trial has not been performed. Exercise restriction limits the work required by the inflamed heart and has been shown to be beneficial in a mouse model of viral myocarditis. In-hospital cardiac monitoring may be required during the acute phase of myocarditis to prevent potentially life-threatening arrhythmias. Antiarrhythmic drugs must be used cautiously because of their negative inotropic effects. Warfarin anticoagulation should be considered in patients with ejection fractions below 20% to reduce the risk of mural thrombi and systemic emboli. The majority of cases of viral myocarditis recover completely; however, patients with fulminant disease may die. Severe cardiac damage can lead to refractory congestive heart failure that can be corrected only by cardiac transplantation.

KEY POINTS

Myocarditis

1. Primarily caused by enteroviruses (coxsackievirus most frequent).
2. Asymptomatic HIV, incidence of mycocarditis 1.6% per year.
3. Risk factors for symptomatic disease: Forced exercise, pregnancy, steroids or nonsteroidal anti-inflammatory agents, alcohol, and nutritional deficiencies.
4. Many patients are asymptomatic; others develop:
   a. Flulike illness, chest pain,
   b. Arrhythmias,
   c. CHF.
5. Physical exam: S_3 gallop = left-sided CHF, mitral regurgitation due to ring dilatation.
6. Cardiac enzymes elevated in the minority of cases.
7. Cardiac echocardiogram very helpful; MRI allows assessment of extent of inflammation.
8. Endomyocardial biopsy combined with PCR experimental.
9. Treatment: Bed rest, drugs for CHF and arrhythmias, anticoagulation.
10. Usually full recovery; however, fulminant cases may require heart transplant.

Pericarditis

Potential Severity: Viral pericarditis usually has a self-limited benign course. However, patients with purulent pericarditis have a high mortality rate and require emergent care.

Etiology and Pathogenesis

Inflammation of the pericardium has multiple infectious and noninfectious causes. Of cases in which an etiology can be determined, a viral cause is most common. The same viruses that invade the myocardium also attack the pericardium. Coxsackievirus A and B and echovirus are most common. Bacteria can also cause pericarditis, resulting in purulent pericarditis. This disease is now rare in the antibiotic era. *Staphylococcus aureus, Streptococcus pneumoniae,* and other streptococci are the leading etiologies, although virtually any bacterium can cause purulent pericarditis. The pericardium can become infected as a result of hematogenous spread (the most common route in the antibiotic era) or by spread from a pulmonary, myocardial, or subdiaphragmatic focus. Finally, purulent pericarditis can be a delayed complication of a penetrating injury or cardiac surgery. Postoperative infections are most commonly caused by *Staphylococcus aureus,* Gram-negative aerobic rods, and Candida species.

Tuberculous pericarditis results from hematogenous spread during primary disease or can spread to the pericardium by lymphatics draining from the respiratory tract or via direct spread from the lung or pleura. Initially, infection causes fibrin deposition and granulomas containing viable mycobacteria, followed by the gradual accumulation of pericardial fluid, initially containing PMNs followed by lymphocytes, monocytes, and plasma cells. Finally, the effusion is absorbed, and the pericardium thickens, becomes fibrotic, and calcifies. Over time the pericardial space shrinks, causing constrictive pericarditis.

KEY POINTS

Etiology, Pathogenesis, and Clinical Manifestations of Pericarditis

1. Three forms of pericarditis:
   a. Viral: Enteroviruses most common (coxsackievirus and echovirus),
   b. Purulent pericarditis usually hematogenous (multiple organisms, including *Staphylococcus aureus*),
   c. Tuberculous pericarditis: Usually seeded during primary disease but can spread from a pulmonary focus.
2. Symptoms: Substernal chest pain, relieved by sitting forward. Less common in purulent pericarditis, gradual onset in tuberculous disease.
3. Physical exam:
   a. Three-component friction rub early, later disappears with increased pericardial fluid,
   b. Pulsus paradoxicus > 10 mm abnormal,
   c. Jugular venous distension with depressed y descent.

Clinical Manifestations

Clinical manifestations vary depending on the etiology. Viral pericarditis and idiopathic pericarditis usually present with substernal chest pain that is usually sharp and made worse by inspiration. Pain is also worsened by lying supine; the patient prefers to sit up and lean forward. In acute bacterial pericarditis the patient suddenly develops fever and dyspnea, and only one third of patients complain of chest pain. Because of the lack of specific symptoms the diagnosis of purulent pericarditis is often not considered, and the diagnosis is made only at autopsy. Tuberculous pericarditis is more insidious in clinical onset. Vague, dull chest pain; weight loss; night sweats; cough; and dyspnea are most commonly reported.

The classic physical findings of pericarditis include a scratchy three-component friction rub due to rubbing of the moving heart against the abnormal pericardium during atrial systole, early ventricular filling, and ventricular systole. When the pericardial effusion increases in volume, the friction rub usually disappears. The hemodynamic consequences of the pericardial effusion can be assessed by checking for pulsus paradoxicus. The blood pressure cuff is inflated above systole and then slowly released until the first Korotkoff sound is heard during expiration. The cuff is again released slowly until the blood pressure sounds are heard with each systolic beat. The difference between the pressure at which the first sounds related to respiration and that at which all systolic sounds are detected is the paradoxic pulse pressure and is abnormal if greater than 10 mm Hg. The accentuated drop in blood pressure during inspiration is caused by pericardial fluid limiting the ability of the heart to expand. Inspiration increases right ventricular filling, causing this chamber to balloon into the left ventricle, reducing left ventricular filling volume, thus reducing the volume of blood that can be ejected into the systemic circulation. A second hemodynamic consequence of pericardial tamponade is a rise in right ventricular filling pressure. High right-sided pressures cause an increase in jugular venous distention as well as abnormal jugular venous pulsations with a loss of y descent. The patient often has a rapid respiratory rate and complains of dyspnea. However, because of the equalization of right- and left-sided cardiac pressures, pulmonary edema does not develop, and the lung fields are clear on auscultation.

Diagnosis and Treatment

The EKG is abnormal in 90% of patients and may show diffuse ST segment elevation, depression of the PR segment, and, when the effusion is large, decreased QRS voltage and electrical alternans. The EKG findings are usually not specific, and when pericarditis is being considered, echocardiography is the critical test that needs to be ordered. The echocardiogram readily detects pericardial thickening and pericardial fluid accumulation. In life-threatening tamponade, echocardiography can be used to guide pericardiocentesis. Determining the etiology of pericarditis is often difficult. Viral etiologies can be determined only retrospectively by acute and convalescent antibody titers. In young patients viral or idiopathic pericarditis is most likely. In the absence of hemodynamic compromise, pericardiocentesis is not recommended because of the low diagnostic yield and the moderate risk of the procedure. However, in patients with significant pericardial tamponade, pericardial fluid yields a diagnosis in one quarter of cases, and pericardial biopsy in half of patients. Pericardial fluid drainage and pericardial biopsy can be performed surgically. In an emergency, echocardiography-guided catheter pericardiocentesis can be performed. In patients with a thickened pericardium a percutaneous pericardial biopsy can be performed safely.

KEY POINTS
Diagnosis and Treatment of Pericarditis

1. Echocardiography should be performed immediately:
   a. Allows assessment of pericardial thickness, pericardial fluid, and tamponade,
   b. Can be used to guide emergency pericardiocentesis.
2. EKG: Diffuse ST and T changes, depressed PR interval, decreased QRS voltage, electrical alternans.
3. Pericardiocentesis only for those with tamponade or suspected of having purulent pericarditis. Pericardial biopsy improves the diagnostic yield.
4. Viral or idiopathic pericarditis self-limited:
   a. Nonsteroidals only if no myocarditis,
   b. Colchicine.
5. Purulent pericarditis: Emergency surgical drainage and systemic antibiotics (mortality: 30%).
6. Tuberculous pericarditis:
   a. Four-drug antituberculous regimen,

> b. Prednisone to prevent constriction
>   (20–50% incidence during treatment),
> c. Calcific form requires pericardectomy.

Viral and idiopathic pericarditis are usually benign, self-limited disorders that can be treated with bed rest. Nonsteroidal anti-inflammatory agents are helpful for reducing chest pain but probably should be avoided in patients with accompanying myocarditis. Colchicine (1 mg/day) may also be helpful for reducing symptoms in cases of idiopathic disease. In patients with purulent pericarditis, surgical drainage of the pericardium should be performed emergently and be accompanied by systemic antibiotic therapy. This disease continues to be accompanied by a 30% mortality rate. Tuberculous pericarditis should receive four-drug antituberculous therapy. However, during treatment 20–50% of patients progress to constrictive pericarditis. This complication can be prevented by simultaneously administering oral prednisone (60 mg × 4 weeks, 30 mg × 4 weeks, 15 mg × 2 weeks, and 5 mg × 1 week). Patients who have developed calcific tuberculous pericarditis at the time of diagnosis require pericardiectomy for relief of symptoms.

Additional Reading

Infective Endocarditis

Andrews, M.M., and von Reyn, C.F. Patient selection criteria and management guidelines for outpatient parenteral antibiotic therapy for native valve infective endocarditis. *Clin Infect Dis* 33:203-209, 2001.

Dhawan, V.K. Infective endocarditis in elderly patients. *Clin Infect Dis* 34:806-812, 2002.

McKay, G., Bunton, R., Galvin, I., Shaw, D., and Singh, H. Infective endocarditis—a twelve year surgical outcome series. *N Z Med J* 115:124-126, 2002.

Mylonakis, E., and Calderwood, S.B. Infective endocarditis in adults. *N Engl J Med* 345:1318-1330, 2001.

Piper, C., Korfer, R., and Horstkotte, D. Prosthetic valve endocarditis. *Heart* 85:590-593, 2001.

Ryan, E.W., and Bolger, A.F. Transesophageal echocardiography (TEE) in the evaluation of infective endocarditis. *Cardiol Clin* 18:773-787, 2000.

Catheter-Associated Infections

Bouza, E., Burillo, A., and Munoz, P. Catheter-related infections: diagnosis and intravascular treatment. *Clin Microbiol Infect* 8:265-274, 2002.

Mermel, L.A., Farr, B.M., Sherertz, R.J., et al. Guidelines for the management of intravascular catheter-related infections. *Clin Infect Dis* 32:1249-1272, 2001.

Raad, I.I., and Hanna, H.A. Intravascular catheter-related infections: new horizons and recent advances. *Arch Intern Med* 162:871-878, 2002.

Myocarditis

Feldman, A.M., and McNamara, D. Myocarditis. *N Engl J Med* 343:1388-1398, 2000.

Haas, G.J. Etiology, evaluation, and management of acute myocarditis. *Cardiol Rev* 9:88-95, 2001.

Lewis, W. Cardiomyopathy in AIDS: a pathophysiological perspective. *Prog Cardiovasc Dis* 43:151-170, 2000.

Pericarditis

Adler, Y., Finkelstein, Y., Guindo, J., et al. Colchicine treatment for recurrent pericarditis. A decade of experience. *Circulation* 97:2183-2185, 1998.

Aikat, S., and Ghaffari, S. A review of pericardial diseases: clinical, ECG and hemodynamic features and management. *Cleve Clin J Med* 67:903-914, 2000.

Maisch, B. Pericardial diseases, with a focus on etiology, pathogenesis, pathophysiology, new diagnostic imaging methods, and treatment. *Curr Opin Cardiol* 9:379-388, 1994.

Trautner, B.W., and Darouiche, R.O. Tuberculous pericarditis: optimal diagnosis and management. *Clin Infect Dis* 33:954-961, 2001.

Gastrointestinal and Hepatobiliary Infections

Recommended Time to Complete: 3 days

Guiding Questions

1. What are the three most common bacterial causes of infectious diarrhea and how are these infections contracted?

2. What test is useful for differentiating viral diarrhea from bacterial diarrhea?

3. How does *Clostridium difficile* cause diarrhea and how is pseudomembranous colitis diagnosed?

4. What findings suggest the development of spontaneous peritonitis?

5. How do abdominal abscesses usually form and how are they best managed?

6. What pathogen most commonly causes peptic ulcer disease?

7. How do hepatic abscesses usually develop and which bacteria are most commonly cultured?

8. What are the three most common forms of viral hepatitis and how are they contracted?

9. What are the major complications of viral hepatitis?

Infectious Diarrhea

Potential Severity Can be life-threatening in infants, young children, and the elderly. In most patients this illness can be managed on an outpatient basis.

Diarrheal illness is one the leading causes of death worldwide, accounting for nearly 2.5 million deaths annually. These diseases are most commonly encountered in developing countries and are a less serious problem in the United States. With appropriate medical care these infections are rarely fatal. Pathogens causing diarrhea can be transmitted in three ways: in food, in water, or by person-to-person spread. These differences in modes of transmission reflect differences in the ability of each pathogen to survive in the environment and reflect the inoculum size required for each pathogen to cause disease.

Bacterial Diarrhea

The three most common bacterial causes of acute infectious diarrhea are Salmonella, Shigella, and Campylobacter. Each of these pathogens has a unique life cycle and unique virulence characteristics. Other important bacterial pathogens include *Escherichia coli, Yersinia enterocolitica, Vibrio cholerae,* and *V. parahaemolyticus.* The various causes of bacterial diarrhea are usually not distinguishable clinically, and diagnosis requires isolation of the organism on stool culture.

◆ CASE 8.1

A 52-year-old black female with rheumatoid arthritis for 24 years was admitted to the hospital with complaints of fever and diarrhea × 24 hours. One month earlier she was hospitalized for neck surgery and received a 10-day course of broad-spectrum antibiotics (ceftazidime). Antibiotic treatment was completed the day of discharge (18 days prior to her second admission). She was doing well in a rehabilitation hospital until 3 days prior to admission, when she was noted to have fever to 102°F (38.9°C) associated with shaking chills and severe watery diarrhea (25–30 bowel movements/day), which persisted. One day before admission she developed abdominal cramps, nausea, vomiting, and anorexia. The rehabilitation nurse found her blood pressure to be 70/50 and referred her to the emergency room.

Medications: Aspirin, large quantities of antacids.
Epidemiology: Her son brought her an egg-salad sandwich from Famous Deli, which they shared 16 hours prior to the onset of the illness. Her son also had severe diarrhea.
Physical examination: Temperature 102.2°F, blood pressure 70/50, pulse 120, respiratory rate 20. She was moderately ill-appearing. She had dry mucous membranes and a dry, fissured tongue. Abdomen: hyperactive bowel sounds, mild diffuse tenderness. Skin: no lesions seen.
Laboratory findings: WBC 7,100 (10% PMNs, 63% bands, 19% lymphocytes), BUN 63, serum creatinine 2.1. Methylene blue smear of stool: few PMNs, few mononuclear cells. Gram stain: mixed flora. Stool culture: *Salmonella enteritidis.*

MICROBIOLOGY, PATHOGENESIS, AND EPIDEMIOLOGY

SALMONELLA This aerobic Gram-negative bacillus can grow readily on simple culture media. It is motile, and most strains do not ferment lactose. There are three major species: *Salmonella typhi, S. choleraesuis,* and *S. enteritidis. S. typhi* is adapted to humans and rarely infects other animals; however, the other Salmonella species readily infect both wild and domestic animals. These organisms attach to epithelial cells in the small intestine and colon. Once attached, they inject specific proteins into host cells that cause the formation of large ruffles that surround the bacteria and internale them into large vacuoles. Here Salmonella are able to replicate and eventually lyse the infected cell, escaping into the extracellular environment and in some cases gaining entry to the bloodstream to cause bacteremia. *S. typhi* is particularly adept at surviving within cells and often causes little intestinal epithelial damage and little diarrhea, primarily entering mesenteric lymph nodes and the bloodstream to cause classic enteric fever. *S. choleraesuis* is also adept at invading the bloodstream and is the most common cause of nontyphoidal Salmonella bacteremia. The ingestion of large numbers of bacteria (10^4–10^8 organisms) is generally required to produce symptomatic disease. Stomach acidity kills many of the organisms before they enter the more hospitable intestinal tract. The use of antacids (as in Case 8.1) or gastrectomy markedly reduces the number of organisms required to cause disease. The critical inoculum size is also affected by the normal bowel flora. Reduction in the flora caused by prior antibiotic treatment reduces competition for nutrients (as in Case 8.1) and allows Salmonella to more readily multiply within the bowel lumen. Depressed immune function increases the risk of salmonellosis, AIDS patients and patients with lymphoma and other neoplasms being at higher risk. Patients with sickle-cell disease have an increased incidence of Salmonella bacteremia that is often complicated by osteomyelitis.

Salmonella requires large numbers of organisms to cause disease, and as a consequence gastroenteritis is almost always associated with the ingestion of heavily contaminated food. In Case 8.1 it is likely that the sandwich from the delicatessen had become contaminated. Because chickens often excrete Salmonella in their stools, eggs, egg products, and undercooked chicken are the most common foods associated with this disease. Contamination of processed foods has occurred resulting in large outbreaks of salmonellosis. Processed foods causing outbreaks have included ice cream, unpasteurized goat's cheese, paprika-powdered potato chips, and white fish. Salmonella-infected human or animal feces can contaminate fruits and vegetables. Pet turtles, iguanas, and birds can carry large numbers of organisms and can infect humans, particularly young children. Contamination of the water supply with sewage also can lead to gastrointestinal infection. *S. typhi* is frequently contracted from contaminated water, and typhoid fever is most commonly found in developing countries where sanitation is poor. Salmonella infections are more common in the summer months, when the warmer temperatures allow the organism to multiply more rapidly on contaminated foods.

KEY POINTS
Salmonella Gastroenteritis

1. Gram-negative bacillus, does not ferment lactose, motile.
2. Attaches to intestinal and colonic cells and injects proteins that stimulate internalization.
3. Spread to mesenteric nodes; *S. choleraesuis* and *S. typhi* often enter the bloodstream.
4. The organism is acid-sensitive. Large numbers of organisms are required to induce infection. Risk factors for disease include:
   a. Antacid use (acid-sensitive),
   b. Prior antibiotics (reduces competition by normal flora),
   c. Depressed immune function (AIDS and transplant patients, sickle-cell disease).
5. Contracted from contaminated foods (more common in the summer months):
   a. Chicken products: eggs, undercooked meat,
   b. Contaminated processed foods: ice cream, unpasteurized goat's cheese, white fish, contaminated fruits and vegetables,
   c. Infected pet turtles, iguanas, birds,
   d. Contaminated water supply: *S. typhi*.

SHIGELLA   This Gram-negative bacillus is nonmotile and does not ferment lactose. It grows readily on standard media. There are four major serological groups: A–D. Group A, *S. dysenteriae,* and Group D, *S. boydii,* are rarely found in the United States. The most common species encountered in the United States are Group B, *S. flexneri,* and Group D, *S. sonnei.*

Shigella contains a series of surface proteins that induce intestinal epithelial cells and M cells to ingest it. Like Salmonella this organism injects proteins into host cells, stimulating ruffling. Unlike Salmonella, once phagocytosed, Shigella possesses a surface hemolysin that allows it to lyse the phagosome membrane and escape into the cytoplasm. Here the bacterium induces the assembly of actin rocket tails that propel it through the cytoplasm. When the bacterium reaches the cell periphery, it pushes outward to form membrane projections that can be ingested by adjacent cells, allowing efficient spread from cell to cell. Shigella produces a cytotoxic Shiga toxin and also induces premature cell death. As a consequence of efficient cell-to-cell spread combined with host cell destruction, Shigella produces superficial ulcers in the bowel mucosa and induces an extensive acute inflammatory response that usually prevents entry into the bloodstream.

Shigella is relatively resistant to acid and can survive in the gastric juices of the stomach for several hours. This characteristic explains why ingestion of as few as 200 bacteria can cause disease. The organism first takes up residence in the small intestine, and after several days, the organism is cleared by the small intestine; however, the pathogen then invades the colon, where it causes an intense inflammatory response, forming microabscesses and mucosal ulcerations.

Because such a low inoculum is required to cause disease, the epidemiology of Shigella is different from that of Salmonella. Shigella has no intermediate animal hosts; the bacteria reside only in the intestinal tract of humans. The primary mode of spread is from person to person by anal-oral transmission. Food-borne and water-borne outbreaks may also occur as a consequence of fecal contamination and are most commonly reported in developing countries where public health standards are poor. Toilet seats can become heavily contaminated by Shigella, and this condition may account for some cases in the United States. Children in day care centers have a high incidence of infection, as do institutionalized individuals, particularly mentally challenged children. On U.S. Indian reservations, high numbers of Shigella dysentery cases have been reported. In tropical areas, spread of Shigella has been attributed to flies, and epidemics of shigellosis have been reported to correlate with heavy fly infestation.

KEY POINTS

Shigella Dysentery

1. Shigella is a Gram-negative rod, does not ferment lactose, nonmotile.
2. Induces ruffling of host cells, once internalized it escapes to the cytoplasm:
   a. Moves through the cytoplasm and spreads from cell to cell by polymerizing actin,
   b. Accelerates cell death, forming plaques of necrotic cells,
   c. Induces marked inflammation and rarely invades the bloodstream.
3. Resistance to gastric acid allows small numbers of organisms (200 bacteria) to cause disease.
4. Initially grows in the small intestine and then spreads to the colon.
5. Spreads from person to person. Day care centers, toilet seats, contaminated water. Can be spread by flies. Less commonly food-borne.

CAMPYLOBACTER These organisms are comma-shaped Gram-negative rods. On microscopic examination they have a distinctive seagull shape.

Campylobacter are microaerophilic and, with the exception of *Campylobacter fetus,* are unable to grow at 25°C. Ideal growth conditions for *C. jejuni,* the most common strain causing diarrhea, are 42°C, 6% oxygen, and 5–10% carbon dioxide. Other bowel flora often overgrow on routine MacConkey's media and selective Campy BAP medium (10% sheep blood in brucella agar containing amphotericin B, cephalothin, vancomycin, polymyxin B, and trimethoprim) is recommended.

The life cycle of Campylobacter is not as well defined as those of Salmonella and Shigella. This pathogen can be ingested by monocytes, where it can survive within cells for 6–7 days. Endocytosis by intestinal epithelial cells and M cells is also likely to occur. Once it becomes intracellular, this pathogen induces cell death and tissue necrosis, leading to ulceration of the bowel wall and intense acute inflammation. Possibly as a consequence of transport by monocytes, Campylobacter can gain entry into the bloodstream. *Campylobacter fetus,* subspecies *fetus,* is particularly adept at causing bacteremia and often causes little or no diarrhea. This strain's resistance to the bactericidal activity of serum may explain its ability to produce persistent bacteremia leading to vascular infections, soft tissue abscesses, and meningitis.

Like Salmonella, Campylobacter is sensitive to acid; therefore large numbers of organisms (>10^4 organisms) are required to cause disease. The epidemiology of Campylobacter is similar to that of Salmonella. *C. jejuni* is the primary species that causes diarrhea. This species frequently contaminates poultry, and its high carriage rate may be partly explained by the bird's high body temperature, a condition that would be expected to enhance growth of *C. jejuni.* This organism is 10 times more frequently cultured from commercial chicken carcasses than is Salmonella (approximately 30% versus 3%). *C. jejuni* can also be carried in water, raw milk, sheep, cattle, swine, and reptiles. As is observed with Salmonella, infections are more common in the summer months.

KEY POINTS

Campylobacter Gastroenteritis

1. Campylobacter is a comma-shaped rod, microaerophilic.
2. Grows best at 42°C, requires Campy BAP selective media or other bowel flora overgrowth. Only *C. fetus* can grow at 25°C.
3. Internalized by and lives in monocytes and intestinal epithelial cells, induces cell death, bowel ulceration, and intense inflammation.
4. *C. fetus* is carried by monocytes to the bloodstream, resists serum bactericidal activity, and causes persistent bacteremia.
5. Like Salmonella, sensitive to gastric acid and requires a high inoculum (>10^4 bacteria).
6. Epidemiology is similar to that of Salmonella. *C. jejuni* primarily responsible for diarrhea.
   a. Survives well in chickens because of their high body temperature (30% of carcasses +),
   b. Carried in water, raw milk, sheep, cattle, swine, and reptiles.

ESCHERICHIA COLI   There are multiple strains of *Escherichia coli* that can cause diarrheal illness. These strains cannot be easily distinguished from nonpathogenic strains of *E. coli* that normally colonize the bowel. Serotyping methods are available on an experimental basis that can identify specific lipopolysaccharide antigens (O antigens) and flagellar antigens (H antigens) associated with specific pathogenic characteristics. For example, *E. coli* 0157:H7 strain is a member of the EHEC group and causes hemorrhagic colitis and hemolytic uremic syndrome. Diarrhea-causing *E. coli* strains are generally classified into five major classes on the basis of their mechanisms of virulence:

1. Enterotoxigenic (ETEC) strains colonize the small bowel and produce a choleralike toxin or heat-stable toxin that stimulates secretion of chloride, causing watery diarrhea. These

organisms are most commonly encountered in developing countries and are contracted from human sewage–contaminated water.

2. Enteropathogenic (EPEC) strains adhere to the small bowel and induce the polymerization of actin filaments to form a pedestal directly beneath the site of bacterial attachment. This process is associated with mild inflammation and usually causes watery diarrhea. These strains are transmitted by contaminated food and water and by person-to-person spread in nurseries. This is primarily a disease of children under three years of age and is more common in developing countries.

3. Enterohemorrhagic (EHEC) strains produce verotoxins or Shiga-like cytotoxins that inhibit protein synthesis and causes cell death. In certain strains the toxin damages vascular endothelium in the bowel and glomeruli, causing hemorrhagic colitis and hemolytic uremic syndrome. O157:H7 is the most common strain associated with these complications. Cattle appear to be the primary reservoir, and disease is most commonly associated with ingestion of undercooked contaminated ground beef. Less commonly, cases have developed after the drinking of unpasteurized milk or contaminated apple cider or the ingesting of contaminated commercial mayonnaise. Person-to-person spread can occur in day care centers and nursing homes. This is primarily an infection of industrialized nations and usually occurs during the summer months.

4. Enteroinvasive (EIEC) strains invade colonic epithelial cells by the same mechanisms as are used by Shigella. These strains do not produce toxins but cause an inflammatory colitis that is indistinguishable from that caused by Shigella. These strains require ingestion of a large inoculum (10^8 organisms) to cause disease. Outbreaks are rare and are usually associated with contaminated foods in developing countries.

5. Enteroaggregative (EaggEC) strains adhere in large aggregates to human colonic mucosa and produce a low-molecular-weight entero-

toxin that causes watery diarrhea. Diarrhea is often prolonged. These strains are contracted by ingesting contaminated water or food. Enteroaggregative *E. coli* strains are reported in developing countries and are an important cause of travelers' diarrhea.

KEY POINTS

E. Coli Gastroenteritis

1. Serotyping identifies specific O (lipopolysaccharide) and H (flagellar proteins) antigens.
2. There are five pathogenic classes:
   a. Enterotoxigenic (ETEC) produce a choleralike toxin. Spread by human sewage–contaminated water in developing countries,
   b. Enteropathogenic (EPEC) induce pedestals that cause mild inflammation. Watery diarrhea primarily in children < 3 years old, person-to-person spread in developing countries,
   c. Enterohemorrhagic (EHEC) produce verotoxins or Shiga-like cytotoxin, damage vessels. O157:H7 causes hemolytic-uremic syndrome. Cattle primary reservoir, undercooked hamburger, unpasteurized milk, contaminated apple cider, and mayonnaise,
   d. Enteroinvasive (EIEC) similar to Shigella. Requires large inoculum, found in developing countries,
   e. Enteroaggregative (EaggEC) adhere as large aggregates, enterotoxin produces watery diarrhea. A major cause of traveler's diarrhea.

YERSINIA   *Yersinia enterocolitica* is a Gram-negative bacillus that grows aerobically on standard media. Large numbers of organisms need to be ingested to cause disease (as high as 10^9 organisms). The organism primarily invades the mucosa of the terminal ileum and causes painful enlargement of the mesenteric nodes. As a consequence of right-sided abdominal pain, Yersinia enterocolitis can be mistaken for appendicitis. This infection is rare in the United States, being more commonly reported in northern Europe, South America, Africa, and Asia. The disease usually occurs in children. *Y. enterocolitica* is generally contracted from contaminated meat products, and because this bacterium can grow at 4°C, refrigerated meats are a particular concern. Contamination of pasteurized milk has been associated with several outbreaks in the United States. As compared to other forms of bacterial diarrhea, which peak during the summer months, most cases of *Y. enterocolitica* occur during the winter months.

KEY POINTS

Yersinia Gastroenteritis

1. Aerobic Gram-negative bacillus, requires large inoculum (10^9).
2. Infects terminal ileum, mesenteric node inflammation mimics appendicitis.
3. Common in northern Europe, South America, Africa, and Asia; rare in the U.S.
4. Contaminated meat products and milk, grows at 4°C.
5. Most common in children, more frequent during winter months.

VIBRIO   The two primary strains associated with diarrhea are *Vibrio cholerae* and *V. parahaemolyticus*. This small, slightly curved Gram-negative rod has a single flagellum at one end that causes the bacterium to move erratically under the microscope. The organism can be isolated from the stool using thiosulfate, citrate, bile salt, sucrose agar, or tellurite taurocholate gelatin agar.

V. cholerae   This strain gains entry to the small bowel by ingestion of contaminated water (requires 10^3–10^6 organisms to cause disease) or food (requires 10^2–10^4 organisms). Neutralization of stomach acid lowers the inoculum required to cause disease. The organism attaches

to the small intestine, where it produces cholera toxin. This exotoxin binds to a specific receptor in the bowel mucosa that activates adenylate cyclase, causing an increase in cyclic adenosine monophosphate (cyclic AMP). Elevated cyclic AMP in turn promotes secretion of chloride and water, causing voluminous, watery diarrhea.

Vibrio cholerae is able to grow and survive in aquatic environments, particularly in estuaries, where it attaches to algae, plankton, and shellfish. During periods when the environment is unfavorable for growth, the organism can convert to a dormant state that can no longer be cultured. The bacteria can also form a rugose, an aggregate of bacteria that is surrounded by a protective biofilm that blocks killing by chlorine and other disinfectants. These characteristics allow *V. cholerae* to persist in water and shellfish. Oysters harvested during the summer months off the Gulf Coast of the United States are frequently positive for *V. cholerae*. Fortunately, these strains do not produce cholera toxin and produce only occasional cases of gastroenteritis. Cholera toxin–producing strains are usually found in areas of poor sanitation where fecal contamination of food and water are common. This organism is capable of producing large epidemics or pandemics; major outbreaks frequently take place in India and Bangladesh. Epidemics have also been reported in Asia, Africa, and Europe. In 1991 there was a large outbreak in Peru, and cholera has been reported in other regions of South America and in Central America. Epidemics usually begin during the hot seasons of the year.

KEY POINTS

Vibrio cholerae Diarrhea

1. Vibrio is a slightly curved Gram-negative bacillus with a single flagellum. Requires special culture media (tellurite taurocholate gelatin).
2. Spread by contaminated water (10^3–10^6 organisms) or food (10^2–10^4 organisms).

3. Attaches to small intestine and produces cholera toxin which binds to a receptor that increases cyclic AMP, promoting chloride and water secretion.
4. Survives in algae, plankton, and shellfish. Can convert to dormant state or form aggregates surrounded by biofilm (rugose).
5. Noncholera toxin strains in Gulf of Mexico.
6. Cholera toxin strains spread by contaminated water in India, Bangladesh, Asia, Africa, Europe, South America (Peru), and Central America. Occur in the hot seasons of the year.

V. parahaemolyticus This strain is halophilic, or salt loving, and grows in estuaries and marine environments, attaching to plankton and shellfish. Little is known about its pathogenesis other than the close correlation between hemolysis and the ability to cause disease. Nonhemolytic strains are almost always avirulent. This organism produces an enterotoxin and causes moderate bowel inflammation, resulting in mild to moderately severe diarrhea. Clams and oysters that filter large volumes of water become heavily contaminated with V. parahaemolyticus, and the ingestion of raw or undercooked shellfish is the primary cause of human disease. Other forms of inadequately cooked seafood can harbor small numbers of Vibrio, and the tradition of eating uncooked seafood (sushi) explains the high incidence of V. parahaemolyticus diarrhea in Japan. The increasing popularity of sushi in the United States is likely to be accompanied by an increasing incidence of V. parahaemolyticus diarrhea in this country.

KEY POINTS

Vibrio parahaemolyticus Diarrhea

1. Thrives in salt water, concentrates in shellfish.
2. Nonhemolytic strains are nonpathogenic.

3. Produces an enterotoxin causing moderate inflammation and watery diarrhea.
4. Very common in Japan, being contracted from sushi.
5. Incidence may increase in the U.S. as sushi becomes more popular.

CLINICAL MANIFESTATIONS

With the exception of certain strains of *E. coli* and *Vibrio parahaemolyticus* most cases of bacterial diarrhea present with enterocolitis. As illustrated in Case 8.1, after ingestion of Salmonella-contaminated food, the incubation period is usually 8–24 hours (Shigella: 36–72 hours, EHEC: 4 days). Enterocolitis is characterized by diarrhea and abdominal pain. Stools may be frequent but small, or as in Case 8.1, diarrhea may be voluminous. In some patients stool may be watery as a consequence of increased secretion of fluids into the bowel. Watery diarrhea is most commonly encountered in enterotoxigenic (ETEC), enteropathogenic (EPEC), and enteroaggregative (EaggEC) *E. coli*, as well as Vibrio. Other patients have purulent, mucusy stools. This form of diarrhea is most commonly encountered in Shigella dysentery, reflecting the exuberant acute inflammatory response of the bowel. Finally, stools may be bloody as a result of bowel ulceration and tissue necrosis. Bloody stools are most commonly encountered in Shigella, Campylobacter, enterotoxigenic (ETEC), and enteroinvasive (EIEC) *E. coli*. In patients with significant colonic involvement, tenesmus and marked pain on attempting to defecate are common complaints. On physical exam a significant percentage of patients have fever, usually in the 38–39°C range. Abdominal exam reveals hyperactive bowel sounds, reflecting increased peristalsis. Diffuse tenderness is typical, usually not accompanied by guarding or rebound. However, in some cases severe tenderness with rebound may be present, suggesting the diagnosis of acute appendicitis or cholecystitis. The peripheral leukocyte count is often normal; however, some patients develop moderate leukocytosis. Fluid loss can be profound, leading to hypotension and electrolyte abnormalities. Positive blood cultures can accompany Salmonella enterocolitis but are rare in Shigella or *C. jejuni* infections.

KEY POINTS

The Clinical Presentation of Bacterial Diarrhea

1. Incubation period: 8–24 hours for Salmonella, 36–72 hours for Shigella, 4 days for EHEC.
2. Diarrhea varies in volume and consistency:
   a. Watery with EPEC, ETEC, EaggEC, and Vibrio,
   b. Mucusy with Shigella,
   c. Bloody with Shigella, Campylobacter, EHEC, and EIEC.
3. Abdominal pain associated with hyperactive bowel sounds and diffuse tenderness, in some cases severe, mimicking appendicitis or cholecystitis.
4. Tenesmus and pain on defecating when the colon involved. Most common with Shigella.

ENTERIC FEVER

Enteric fever is most commonly associated with *Salmonella typhi* and *S. paratyphi*. The incubation for typhoid fever is usually 8–14 days, being longer with a lower inoculum. Fever is the first manifestation, and the infection usually mimics an influenzalike illness, characterized by continuous frontal headache, generalized aches, malaise, anorexia, and lethargy. A large percentage of patients also have a nonproductive cough. Most patients complain of mild abdominal discomfort and constipation that is often followed by bloody diarrhea during the second week of the illness. Fever increases to 40°C during the second week, and the patient often becomes severely ill. Abdominal pain and distention worsen, and mental status dulls. In the absence of antibiotic treatment, by the third

week a significant percentage of patients recover, while 10% die of septic shock or bowel perforation. On physical exam the pulse may be inappropriately slow despite high fever (temperature-pulse dissociation). The abdomen is often markedly distended and tender during the later phases of the disease, and splenomegaly is noted in a significant percentage of patients. Small rose-colored, 2- to 5-mm maculopapular lesions that blanch on pressure develop on the upper abdomen and chest regions in 80% of patients by the second to third week. The rose spots usually persist for 2–4 days. Normochromic normocytic anemia and moderate peripheral leukopenia (WBC 2,500/mm³ range) are common. Other patients may have mild elevations in their peripheral leukocyte count. Blood cultures are positive in 90% of patients during the first week and in 50% during the second week. Stool cultures remain positive for many weeks. *Campylobacter fetus* and *Yersinia enterocolitica* can produce a syndrome that is clinically indistinguishable from typhoid fever.

KEY POINTS

Enteric Fever

1. Caused by *Salmonella typhi, S. paratyphi, C. fetus,* and *Yersinia enterocolitica.*
2. Incubation period 8–14 days, longer with lower inocula.
3. Influenzalike syndrome: headache, muscle aches, malaise, lethargy, nonproductive cough.
4. Mild abdominal discomfort that worsens, constipation or minimal bloody diarrhea.
5. Progresses to high fever (40°C) and slow pulse, septic shock and bowel perforation.
6. Skin: Small, rose-colored macules = rose spots.
7. Normochromic, normocytic anemia, leukopenia.
8. Positive blood cultures: 90% first week.

DIAGNOSIS

Direct examination of the stool using a methylene blue stain should be performed in all patients to assess the cellular response. The presence of polymorphonuclear leukocytes (PMNs) on stool smear strongly suggests acute bacterial enterocolitis but may also be seen in amoebic dysentery and in antibiotic-associated pseudomembranous colitis. An abundant PMN response is seen in Shigella, Campylobacter, and enteroinvasive E. coli (EIEC). Cases of Salmonella enterocolitis tend to have a less vigorous PMN response in the stool, and patients with S. typhi may demonstrate increased numbers of fecal monocytes. The finding of seagull-shaped Gram-negative forms on stool Gram stain is highly suggestive of Campylobacter. The stool culture should be immediately planted on the appropriate media to maximize sensitivity. In the case of Campylobacter, special selective media and microaerophilic conditions must be used (see above). Pathogenic strains of E. coli cannot be readily identified by culture; immunologic and molecular biology methods are required. Slide agglutination using specific antiserum against O antigens has been performed in several epidemics. PCR primers and DNA hybridization probes are also available for investigative purposes.

KEY POINTS

Diagnosis of Bacterial Diarrhea

> 1. Direct examination of the stool using methylene blue stain to assess PMN response:
>   a. Abundant PMN seen in Shigella, Campylobacter, and EIEC,
>   b. Salmonella: Moderate PMNs, with S. typhi may see monocytes,
>   c. PMNs also seen with amoebic dysentery and C. difficile toxin–associated diarrhea.

> 2. Gram stain showing seagull-shaped Gram-negative forms = Campylobacter.
> 3. Stool culture with standard media and Campylobacter-selective media.
> 4. E. coli strains are identified by slide agglutination tests using specific O antisera.

TREATMENT AND OUTCOME

The majority of cases of bacterial enterocolitis are self-limited, usually lasting 3–7 days, and may not require antibiotic therapy. Fluid and electrolyte replacement is generally the most important supportive measure. Agents that slow peristalsis are contraindicated in patients with bacterial enterocolitis. These drugs may prolong fever, increase the risk of bacteremia, and prolong fecal excretion of the pathogen. Antibiotic therapy for Salmonella enterocolitis prolongs carriage in the stool and has not been shown to shorten the duration of gastroenteritis. Patients with typhoid fever warrant immediate antibiotic treatment. Chloramphenicol (500 mg iv Q6H × 14–28 days) was the treatment of choice until recently. However, relapses have occurred with this regimen, and increasing numbers of S. typhi strains have become resistant to chloramphenicol. A floroquinolone (ciprofloxacin, standard dose for 10 days) or a third-generation cephalosporin (ceftriaxone, standard dose × 10–14 days) is now the recommended first-line regimen. To prevent potential complications associated with bacteremia, nontyphoidal Salmonella should also be treated with antibiotics when this disease develops in neonates, persons over age 50 years, immunocompromised patients, and patients with prosthetic valves or vascular grafts. Antibiotic therapy should be continued for only 48–72 hours or until the patient no longer has a fever. An oral fluoroquinolone, amoxicillin, or trimethoprim-sulfamethoxazole is generally recommended. To prevent person-to-person spread and shorten the course of the illness of shigellosis, trimethoprim-sulfamethoxazole (1 DS po BID × 3–5 days) or ciprofloxacin (standard dose × 3–5 days) is usually administered. Although antibiotic treatment of *Campylobacter jejuni* diarrhea has not been proven to shorten the course of the illness, it has been shown to shorten the carrier state. Useful regimens include erythromycin (250 mg po QID × 5–7 days), azithromycin (standard dose × 5 days), or ciprofloxacin (standard dose × 5–7 days). *Yersinia enterocolitica* is usually not treated; however, in severe cases trimethoprim-sulfamethoxazole, a fluoroquinolone, or a third-generation cephalosporin may be administered. *Vibrio parahaemolyticus* can be treated with tetracycline or ciprofloxacin. Finally, the course of travelers' diarrhea can be shortened from 3–5 days to 1.5 days by a brief course of ciprofloxacin.

KEY POINTS
Treatment of Bacterial Diarrhea

1. Self-limited diseases and often do not require antibiotic treatment.
2. Fluid and electrolyte replacement most important.
3. Avoid agents the slow peristalsis, increase the risk of bacteremia, or prolong fever and carrier state.
4. Antibiotic treatment of Salmonella gastroenteritis prolongs the carrier state. However, to prevent complications associated with bacteremia, treat (ciprofloxacin, amoxicillin, or trimethoprim-sulfa):
   a. Neonates,
   b. Persons > 50 years,
   c. Immunocompromised or prosthetic valve or synthetic vascular grafts.
5. Treat enteric fever emergently with ciprofloxacin or ceftriaxone.
6. Shigella: Trimethoprim-sulfamethoxazole or ciprofloxacin reduces person-to-person spread.
7. *Campylobacter jejuni*: Erythromycin, azithromycin, or ciprofloxacin shortens the carrier state.

8. Yersinia: Usually not treated, severe cases use trimethoprim-sulfamethoxazole, ciprofloxacin, or ceftriaxone.
9. *Vibrio parahemolyticus* I: Treat with tetracycline or ciprofloxacin.
10. Travelers' diarrhea: Ciprofloxacin × 3–5 days shortens the course of illness.

PREVENTION

Public health measures are the most efficient and cost-effective way of reducing these diseases. Understanding the epidemiology of each pathogen allows the public health investigator to track down the source of bacterial contamination and prevent additional cases. After symptomatic disease, Salmonella fecal carriage may be prolonged, particularly if the patient received antibiotics. The carrier state can usually be eradicated by prolonged therapy with amoxicillin (standard dose × 4–6 weeks) or a fluoroquinolone (ciprofloxacin: standard dose × 4–6 weeks). In patients with gallstones the carrier state often cannot be eliminated.

KEY POINTS
Prevention of Bacterial Diarrhea

1. Investigation of sources of contamination is a cost-effective preventive measure.
2. Salmonella fecal carriage can be prolonged:
   a. Carrier state can often be eradicated by prolonged therapy (4–6 weeks) with amoxicillin or ciprofloxacin,
   b. Carrier state often cannot be eliminated in patients with gallstones.

Viral Diarrhea

This is the most common form of diarrhea, usually causing mild self-limited watery diarrhea. The most common viruses to be associated with viral diarrhea are Norwalk virus, rotaviruses, enteric adenoviruses, and astroviruses.

VIROLOGY, PATHOGENESIS, AND EPIDEMIOLOGY

NORWALK VIRUS This single-stranded RNA virus is a calicivirus, a viral group that derives its name from the distinct cup or chalicelike indentations of the viral capsid seen on electron microscopy. Because there is no convenient method for propagating the virus and no animal model of Norwalk virus gastroenteritis, little is known about its pathogenesis. Histopathology from infected human volunteers has revealed that the virus causes blunting of villi as well as PMN infiltration of the lamina propria in the jejunum. Diarrhea is associated with a mild malabsorption of nutrients and decreased production of brush border enzymes. The virus is shed in the stool for 24–48 hours after the onset of illness. Infection is transmitted by contaminated water and foods and by person-to-person spread. In addition to contaminated drinking water, swimming pools and lakes can transmit the disease. Norwalk virus is relatively resistant to chlorine. Shellfish are a leading food source, and because the virus is relatively heat resistant, cooking contaminated shellfish does not completely eliminate the risk of infection. Infected food handlers can contaminate food, resulting in large outbreaks. Large outbreaks have also been reported in closed environments such as ships, military installations, hospitals, and nursing homes. Norwalk virus is most commonly associated with outbreaks in adults; however, infants and children may be infected by this virus or another member of the calicivirus group.

ROTAVIRUS The name (from the Latin *rota,* meaning "wheel") of this double-stranded RNA virus is derived from the wheellike appearance of the viral capsid on electron micrographs. The capsid contains short, spokelike structures that radiate from a central hub toward a rim structure. It is a member of the reovirus family. Rotaviruses are able to replicate in mature villous epithelial cells in the small intestine. The viral capsid attaches, penetrates the host cell peripheral membrane, and enters the cytoplasm. Diarrhea is thought to be caused by loss of absorption by epithelial villi, lactase deficiency, and a decrease in the intestinal concentrations of other disaccharidases. The virus may also increase chloride secretion. Rotavirus is the most common cause of infant diarrhea, and by age 3 years over 90% of children acquire antibodies to rotaviruses. Repeated infections may occur, indicating minimal cross-protection between strains. Adults may also contract the infection, most commonly from infected children as a consequence of fecal-oral transmission. The virus is resistant to hand washing and to many commonly used disinfectants but is inactivated by chlorine. It is able to survive on surfaces, in water, and on the hands for prolonged periods. In developed countries infections most commonly occur during the winter months.

ENTERIC ADENOVIRUSES Two serotypes of this double-stranded DNA virus have been designated as enteric forms. They are found primarily in the diarrheal stools and are resistant to serum. They are the second most frequent cause of nonbacterial gastroenteritis in infants and young children. Infections occur most commonly during the summer months.

ASTROVIRUSES These single-stranded RNA viruses have the appearance of a five- or six-pointed star on electron micrographs. Astroviruses have been associated with outbreaks of gastroenteritis in children on pediatric wards and in elderly patients in nursing homes. The prevalence of this type of virus is currently being determined.

CLINICAL MANIFESTATIONS, DIAGNOSIS, AND TREATMENT

◆ CASE 8.2

A young physician arrived in Tuba City, Arizona, to work in an Indian Health Service clinic. Three days later, he became ill with mild midabdominal cramps and watery diarrhea, but he denied fever. He continued working, added additional salt and fluid to his diet, and was inconvenienced but not incapacitated by his illness. On the third day of symptoms a stool smear revealed no PMNs, and bacterial culture grew no pathogens.

The clinical manifestations vary. At one end of the clinical spectrum patients experience mild, watery diarrhea with minimal symptoms as described in Case 8.2, and at the other extreme the patient may develop severe nausea, vomiting, abdominal cramps, headache, myalgias, and fevers to 39°C. Stool smear reveals no leukocytes, and cultures are negative for bacterial pathogens. Identification of the specific viral agent is usually not possible. Most agents are most readily identified by their appearance on electron microscopy. Commercial ELISA assays for rotavirus are available and provide satisfactory results. These diseases are self-limited, lasting 2–6 days depending on the agent. Maintaining hydration is the primary goal of therapy.

KEY POINTS

Viral Diarrhea

1. The most common form of infectious diarrhea.
2. Caused primarily by four viral groups:
   a. Norwalk virus: A calicivirus, blunts intestinal villi, causes mild malabsorption, resistant to chlorine, spread by contaminated water, including swimming pools, primarily infects adults,
   b. Rotavirus: Causes lactase deficiency, primarily infects infants, resists hand washing, peaks in winter,
   c. Enteric adenovirus: Infects infants and young children, peaks in summer months,
   d. Astroviruses: Infect children in pediatric wards and the elderly in nursing homes.
3. Clinical spectrum: Mild, watery diarrhea to severe nausea, vomiting, and fever. No

PMNs in the stool. Commercial ELISA available for rotavirus.
4. Self-limited diseases; supportive care with hydration.

Parasitic Infections

Amebiasis can mimic bacterial enterocolitis, while other parasites such as *Giardia lamblia,* Cryptosporidium, *Isospora belli,* and Microsporida often present with complaints that mimic viral gastroenteritis. However, in most instances these parasitic infections are not self-limited and persist for prolonged periods.

Amebiasis

LIFE CYCLE AND EPIDEMIOLOGY

Amebiasis is caused by *Entamoeba histolytica.* Other amoebic species found in the feces of humans, including *Entamoeba coli, E. hartmanni, E. polecki, Endolimax nana,* and *Iodamoeba buetschlii,* do not cause disease in humans. *E. histolytica* can be distinguished from other amoebas because it is the only species that ingests erythrocytes. Trophozoites are large, 10–60 μm in diameter, and contain a lucent cytoplasm, a single nucleus, and multiple intracellular granules. They crawl by chemotaxis, using an actin-based mechanism that is similar to human macrophages and neutrophils. Trophozoites attach to specific galactose receptors on host cells and, following contact, rapidly kill the host cells by a calcium-dependent mechanism. The amoeba also releases numerous proteolytic enzymes that break down the anchoring host cell matrix. Flask-shaped mucosal ulcers may be found in the colon at sites of trophozoite invasion. Ulcers can extend into the submucosa and result in invasion of the bloodstream. Amoebas can also travel up the portal vein and form abscesses in the liver. Because *E. histolytica* can lyse host neutrophils, acute inflammatory cells are rarely seen in the regions of active infection. Immunity against amoebas is primarily cell-mediated, and patients with depressed cell-mediated immunity are at greater risk for disseminated disease.

In addition to the trophozoite form, under unfavorable environmental conditions *E. histolytica* forms dormant cysts. The cyst has a distinctive morphology consisting of a rounded structure with three or four distinct nuclei (see Figure 8.1). These hardy cysts can remain viable for months outside the host in moist, warm environments. Trophozoites are very sensitive to the acid pH of the stomach; however, cysts readily survive the gastric environment, and ingestion of cysts accounts for fecal-oral spread of the infection. Cysts can also contaminate food and water. In developing countries a high percentage of the population become infected with *E. histolytica* and usually carry the parasite in their stool for 12 months. In the United States institutionalized patients, particularly the mentally challenged, have a high incidence of stool carriage and disease. An increased incidence has also been observed in sexually promiscuous homosexual males. The risk of amebiasis is increased by travel to a developing country and is

particularly high in individuals who reside in the endemic area for over one month.

KEY POINTS

Life Cycle and Epidemiology of Amebiasis

1. Caused by *Entamoeba histolytica*, contains ingested red blood cells, 10–60 µm in diameter.
2. Bind to galactose receptors on host cells and kill host cells, causes flasklike ulcers.
3. Able to invade portal vein and form abscesses in the liver.
4. Able to lyse host PMNs, acute inflammatory cells rarely seen in areas of infection, protection by cell-mediated immunity.
5. Forms dormant cysts that can survive for months in moist, warm environments.
6. Cysts can contaminate food and water.
7. Very common in developing countries.
8. In U.S. found in institutionalized patients, homosexuals, and tourists.

CLINICAL MANIFESTATIONS

Symptoms depend on the degree of bowel invasion. Superficial bowel infection is associated with watery diarrhea and nonspecific gastrointestinal complaints. Invasive intestinal disease

Figure 8.1

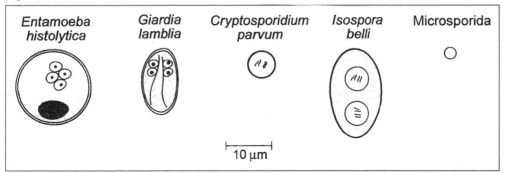

Parasites that cause diarrhea. Each pathogen is schematically drawn to scale and represents the form most commonly detected on stool smears.

presents with the gradual onset (one to three weeks) of abdominal pain and bloody diarrhea associated with tenesmus and abdominal tenderness. Fever is noted in the minority of patients. Amebiasis can be mistaken for ulcerative colitis, and administration of corticosteroids can dramatically worsen the disease and lead to toxic megacolon. Amoebic liver abscess can develop in conjunction with colitis. Patients complain of right upper quadrant pain and can also experience pain referred to the right shoulder. Hepatomegaly is noted in half of cases.

DIAGNOSIS AND TREATMENT

Stool smears usually demonstrate PMNs. However, because the amoebic trophozoites destroy human PMNs, the numbers are often reduced in comparison to patients with shigellosis. The stools are always heme-positive, reflecting trophozoite invasion and destruction of bowel mucosa. The alkaline phosphatase and erythrocyte sedimentation rate are usually elevated when there is hepatic involvement.

The diagnosis is made by identifying trophozoites or cysts in the stool. Specimens that are obtained during endoscopy should be immediately examined looking for motile trophozoites. Because cysts are only intermittently released, at least three stools should be examined to safely exclude amebiasis. The serum antiamoebic antibody is positive in most patients who have had symptomatic disease for over one week. DNA probes and PCR may be available for stool analysis in the future. Abdominal CT scan should be performed in patients with symptoms consistent with hepatic disease and readily identifies abscesses. Serum antiamoebic antibodies are elevated in 99% of patients with hepatic amebic abscess. Aspiration of the abscess yields sterile, odorless, brownish liquid without PMNs. Amoebas are generally not seen and only rarely are cultured because the parasite concentrates in the walls of the abscess.

Invasive enterocolitis and hepatic abscess should be treated with metronidazole (750 mg

po TID × 10 days) or tinidazole (2 gm po QD divided in TID doses × 3–5 days, not available in the United States). For asymptomatic cyst excretors, iodoquinol (650 mg po TID × 20 days) or paromomycin (25–35 mg/kg/day po in TID doses × 7 days) is recommended. Diloxanide fuoroate (500 mg po TID × 10 days) can be used as an alternative therapy.

KEY POINTS

Clinical Manifestations, Diagnosis, and Treatment of Amebiasis

1. Clinical presentation depends on the degree of invasion:
   a. Watery diarrhea associated with superficial infection,
   b. Bloody diarrhea, tenesmus, abdominal pain, and tenderness associated with more invasive disease,
   c. Misdiagnosed as ulcerative colitis; corticosteroids can lead to toxic megacolon,
   d. Right upper quadrant pain, right shoulder pain, and hepatomegaly seen with liver abscess.
2. Diagnosis:
   a. Stool smears: PMNs < shigellosis, trophozoites destroy PMNs,
   b. Stools always heme-positive,
   c. Alkaline phosphatase and ESR usually elevated in hepatic abscess,
   d. Three stool examinations usually reveal trophozoites or cysts,
   e. Serum antiamoebic antibody is positive in most patients after 1 week of symptoms,
   f. Liver abscess aspirates brownish sterile liquid without PMNs, parasite not seen.
3. Treatment: Metronidazole; for carrier state, iodoquinol or paromomycin.

Giardia lamblia

LIFE CYCLE AND EPIDEMIOLOGY

This enteric flagellated protozoa, like amoeba, has two stages: the free-living trophozoite and the dormant cyst. The trophozoite consists of a dorsal convex surface and a flat, disk-shaped ventral surface made up of microtubules and microribbons, two nuclei, and four pairs of flagella. On stained preparations it has the appearance of a bearded human face (see Figure 8.1). Trophozoites adhere to GI endothelial cells, disrupt the brush border, cause disaccharidase deficiency, and induce inflammation. All these mechanisms are thought to account for watery diarrhea and malabsorption. Both cell-mediated and humoral immunity play roles in host defense. Patients with X-linked agammaglobulinemia have an increased risk of contracting severe prolonged disease, emphasizing the contribution of humoral immunity. Under unfavorable environmental conditions Giardia can form dormant cysts that are excreted in the stool and account for spread of disease. Giardiasis is found throughout the world and is a common infection in the United States. Giardia cysts most commonly are spread by contaminated water, and multiple water-borne outbreaks have occurred in mountainous regions of the Northeast, Northwest, and Rocky Mountain States, as well as British Columbia. Campers must aggressively sterilize drinking water from mountain streams to prevent this common infection. Food-borne outbreaks are increasingly being recognized. Giardia can also be transmitted from person to person in day care centers and other confining institutions. This pathogen also has been spread from person to person by sexually active homosexuals.

1. Giardia exists as trophozoites and dormant cysts.
2. Trophozoites attach to GI endothelial cells, cause malabsorption and inflammation.
3. Giardia cysts spread by contaminated water, person to person, less commonly by food.
4. Worldwide infection; common in mountainous regions of the U.S.
5. A disease of campers (sterilization of water is critical for prevention), day care centers, and sexually active homosexuals.

CLINICAL MANIFESTATIONS, DIAGNOSIS, AND TREATMENT

This parasite usually causes mild symptoms or is asymptomatic. Adults may complain of abdominal cramps, bloating, diarrhea, anorexia, nausea, and malaise. Belching is also a common complaint. Children most often develop watery diarrhea. Symptoms usually resolve spontaneously in four to six weeks. Chronic disease is less common and results in malabsorption, chronic diarrhea, and weight loss.

The diagnosis of giardiasis should be considered in all patients with prolonged diarrhea. Stool smears reveal no PMNs. Examination for cysts using concentration techniques have a 90% yield after three stool samples. ELISA or immunofluorescence antigen tests are now available, have high sensitivity (up to 98%) and specificity (90–100%), and are now the test of choice. Endoscopy and duodenal biopsy or duodenal aspiration is no longer necessary in most cases. Metronidazole (250 mg po TID × 5–7 days) is the treatment of choice.

KEY POINTS

Clinical Manifestations, Diagnosis, and Treatment of Giardiasis

1. Clinical manifestations are usually mild; self-limited, lasting 4–6 weeks:
   a. Adults: symptoms mild: abdominal cramps, anorexia, watery diarrhea, nausea, and belching,
   b. Children: more severe watery diarrhea,
   c. Can cause a chronic malabsorption syndrome, primarily with immunoglobulin deficiency.

2. Diagnosis:
  a. Stool smear: no PMNs, cysts seen in 90% after three stool exams,
  b. ELISA or immunofluorescence antigen tests are the tests of choice,
  c. Endoscopy is no longer necessary.
3. Treat with metronidazole.

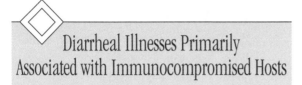

Diarrheal Illnesses Primarily Associated with Immunocompromised Hosts

Cryptosporidium

This intestinal protozoon survives and replicates within the intestinal microvilli, eventually generating oocysts that are excreted in the stool and are responsible for the spread of infection (see Figure 8.1). Autoinfection can also occur, explaining how ingestion of small numbers of oocytes can cause severe persistent infection in the immunocompromised host. Loss of cell-mediated immunity increases the risk of infection and explains the higher incidence of cryptosporidium intestinal disease in AIDS patients. Cryptosporidium is classified as an intestinal coccidium and is related to malarial organisms. The mechanisms by which cryptosporidium causes diarrhea are not completely understood. The pathogen affects intestinal ion transport and causes inflammatory damage of the intestinal microvilli, resulting in malabsorption. This parasite is carried in the intestinal tract of many animals and is also found in water. The oocyst is resistant to chlorination, and large outbreaks due to contaminated drinking water supplies have been reported. Ingestion of 130 oocysts can causes diarrheal disease in 50% of volunteers. Person-to-person spread has also been reported and can occur in households as well as in institutional settings such as day care centers

and hospitals. Animal-to-person spread can take place following exposure to infected farm animals.

Isospora belli

This intestinal coccidium is found most frequently in tropical environments but has been identified as a cause of watery diarrhea in AIDS patients in the United States. A characteristic oocyst is excreted in the stool (see Figure 8.1).

Microsporida

This obligate intracellular parasite is very small in comparison to the other parasites that cause diarrhea (see Figure 8.1). It was known to be a common pathogen in insects and fish; however, in 1985 intestinal microsporidiosis was first described in an AIDS patient. This parasite causes significant diarrhea only in immunocompromised hosts. It infects mucosal epithelial cells, causing villous atrophy, and may ascend into the biliary tract to cause cholangitis. Diagnosis is made by demonstrating the organisms in stool or after intestinal biopsy. Giemsa, Ziehl-Neelsen, or Gram stain may be used to identify the organism.

Clinical Manifestations, Diagnosis, and Treatment

Cryptosporidia, Isospora belli, and Microsporida all present with chronic watery diarrhea that is often associated with abdominal cramps. The majority of cases occur in immunocompromised hosts, most frequently AIDS patients. Minimal findings are noted on physical examination. Patients may appear malnourished and be dehydrated. Diagnosis is made by stool smear. In addition to iodine, stool samples should be stained with modified Kinyoun acid-fast stain and concentrated. Cryptosporidium cysts are acid-fast. *Isospora belli* sporocysts are transparent and can be easily overlooked. They demonstrate blue autofluorescence when observed under a fluorescence microscope with a 330- to 380-nm UV filter. A modified trichrome stain is recommended for the diagnosis of microsporidium; it stains the cysts reddish pink. A number of fluorescence stains are commercially available and are sensitive and specific (for example, Calcofluor white stain, Sigma).

There is no reliable treatment for cryptosporidiosis. Nonspecific antidiarrheal agents may be used to provide temporary relief. *Isospora belli* can be effectively treated with trimethoprim-sulfamethoxazole (1 DS QID × 10 days). In sulfa-allergic patients pyrimethamine (75 mg/kg/day) combined with folinic acid (10–25 mg/day) has proved to be a successful alternative. Treatment of Microsporidia with albendazole (400 mg po BID × 3 weeks) leads to clinical improvement; however, most patients relapse when the medication is discontinued. Fumagillin (20 mg TID × 2 weeks), an antibiotic derived from *Aspergillus fumigatus*, results in clearance of spores, and relapse occurs in a minority of patients. Fumagillin is toxic to the bone marrow and may result in reversible neutropenia and/or thrombocytopenia.

KEY POINTS

Cryptosporidia, *Isospora belli*, and Microsporida

1. Survive and multiply on or in the mucosal epithelial cells of the intestine.
2. Cryptosporidium can spread via contamination of the water supply, oocysts resist chlorination. Small numbers of oocysts can cause disease (130 oocysts).
3. Primarily infect AIDS patients with severely depressed cell-mediated immunity.
4. Cause watery diarrhea and abdominal cramps, dehydration, and malnutrition.
5. Diagnosis by stool smear:

    a. Cryptosporidium cysts modified Kinyoun acid-fast,

    b. *Isospora belli* sporocysts transparent, fluoresce with UV light,

    c. Microsporidium: Modified trichrome and fluorescence stains sensitive and specific.

6. Treatment:

    a. No therapy available for Cryptosporidia,

    b. Trimethoprim-sulfa for *Isospora belli*,

    c. Fumagillin effective for microsporidia.

Antibiotic-Associated Diarrhea

Potential Severity: Undiagnosed *Clostridium difficile* can progress to severe colitis that may require colectomy or result in bowel perforation and death.

Antibiotic-associated diarrhea develops in up to 30% of hospitalized patients. Systemic antibiotics reduce the normal flora and interfere with the bacterial breakdown of carbohydrates. The increased concentrations of undigested carbohydrate increase the intraluminal osmotic load, preventing water resorption and causing watery diarrhea. Antibiotic-induced reductions in the normal bowel flora also allow resistant bacteria to overgrow. Overgrowth of *Staphylococcus aureus* was once thought to cause diarrhea; however, in recent studies, this bacterium has rarely been found in the feces of patients with antibiotic-associated diarrhea. Overgrowth of Candida species has also been implicated, and some patients have improved following administration of oral nystatin; however, others with heavy colonization with Candida fail to develop diarrhea. *Clostridium difficile* is the only pathogen that has been definitively proven to cause antibiotic-associated diarrhea. This organism has been implicated in 20–30% of patients with antibiotic-associated diarrhea and 50–75% of those who develop antibiotic-associated colitis.

Microbiology, Pathogenesis, and Epidemiology

Clostridium difficile is an obligate anaerobic, spore-forming, Gram-positive rod. The organism's name reflects the difficulty of isolating the pathogen on routine media. A cycloserine, cefoxitin, fructose agar with an egg-yolk base (CCFA medium) is capable of selecting this organism from total fecal flora. When the bowel flora is exposed to broad-spectrum antibiotics, *C. difficile* overgrows and releases two high-molecular-weight exotoxins, Toxin A and Toxin B, which bind to and kill cells in the bowel wall. Their mechanisms of action include stimulation of mitogen-activated protein kinases (MAP-kinases) and inactivation of small GTP-binding Rho proteins that regulate actin filament assembly. Exposure of tissue-cultured cells to filtrate from *C. difficile*–infected feces results in dramatic cytopathic changes. Exposure of the human colon to these cytotoxins results in depolymerization of actin filaments, the rounding up and detachment of cells, and the formation of shallow ulcers. Acute inflammation with pus and mucus forms pseudomembranes that are readily seen by colonoscopy. Early lesions are superficial; however, as the disease progresses and as the levels of toxin increase, inflammation can extend through the full thickness of the bowel.

This disease develops in 10% of patients who are hospitalized for over 2 days. *Clostridium difficile* diarrhea is rarely encountered in outpatients. The incidence of disease is higher in the elderly and in those who have severe underlying diseases or have undergone gastrointestinal surgery. An increased incidence is also associated with broad-spectrum antibiotics (clindamycin, ampicillin, amoxicillin, and cephalosporins are associated with the highest incidence), anticancer chemotherapy (methotrexate, 5-Fu, doxorubicin, and

cyclophosphamide), bowel enemas or stimulants, enteral feedings, and close proximity to another patient with *C. difficile* diarrhea. This infection is spread from patient to patient, primarily by hospital personnel. Spores can be readily carried on the hands, clothes, and stethoscopes. Numerous hospital outbreaks have been reported and occur more commonly on wards where clindamycin is frequently administered.

KEY POINTS

Microbiology, Pathogenesis, and Epidemiology of *Clostridium difficile*

1. Obligate anaerobic, spore-forming, Gram-positive rod.
2. Produces two cytotoxins, Toxin A and Toxin B, that bind to and kill host cells.
3. Bowel wall necrosis leads to acute inflammation.
4. A disease of hospitalized patients. Risk factors for disease:
   a. Broad-spectrum antibiotic administration reduces competing normal flora. Clindamycin associated with highest incidence followed by ampicillin/amoxicillin,
   b. Cancer chemotherapy,
   c. Bowel enemas or stimulants, enteral feedings,
   d. Elderly, patients with underlying disease, and after GI surgery,
   e. Spread from patient to patient by hospital personnel, spores carried on hands.

Clinical Manifestations

Clostridium difficile causes a spectrum of disease manifestations, ranging from an asymptomatic carrier state to fulminant colitis. The severity of symptoms does not appear to relate to the amount of toxin released into the stool and may relate to the number of toxin receptors in the host's bowel. High titers of IgG directed against

Toxin A appear to be protective and are often high in the asymptomatic carrier. The most common form of symptomatic disease is diarrhea without colitis. Diarrhea usually begins 5–10 days after the initiation of antibiotics. However, diarrhea can develop up to ten weeks after the completion of antibiotic therapy. Diarrhea is usually watery, consisting of 5–15 bowel movements per day. Crampy bilateral lower quadrant pain that decreases after a bowel movement, low-grade fever, and mild peripheral blood leukocytosis are common characteristics. Pseudomembranous colitis presents with the same symptoms, and findings except pseudomembranes are seen on colonoscopy, and marked thickened of the colonic bowel wall is seen on CT scan. These forms of *C. difficile*–induced diarrhea can be difficult to differentiate clinically from the most common form of antibiotic-associated diarrhea: osmotic diarrhea. Lack of fever or leukocytosis, absence of PMNs in the stool,

and improvement when oral intake is reduced favor osmotic diarrhea.

Fulminant colitis develops in 2–3% of patients infected with *Clostridium difficile*. This disease is associated with severe morbidity and a high mortality. Diarrhea is usually present; however, some patients develop constipation. Abdominal pain is usually diffuse and severe and can be associated with hypoactive bowel sounds, abdominal distention, and guarding. Findings of peritonitis can develop and usually indicate bowel perforation. Toxic megacolon (bowel loops dilated > 7 cm) is a feared complication. Full-thickness involvement of the bowel wall leads to bowel distention and air fluid levels seen on abdominal CT scan or KUB. Thumbprinting is often seen, reflecting submucosal edema, and can mimic bowel ischemia (see Figure 8.2). Sigmoidoscopy must be performed cautiously under these conditions because of the high risk of perforation. Marked elevation in the peripheral white blood count (25,000–35,000

Figure 8.2

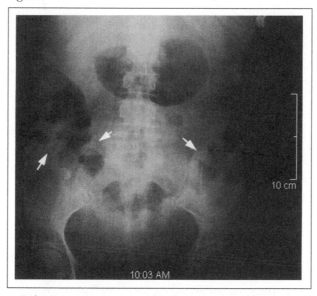

KUB demonstrating prominent thumbprinting. Arrows point to the thickened folds of the large intestine indicative of marked bowel edema. These changes are seen in bowel ishemia and with *C. difficile* colitis. (Courtesy of Dr. Pat Abbitt, University of Florida College of Medicine.)

cells/mm^3) is common. The development of lactic acidosis usually indicates impending bowel perforation and irreversible bowel damage that requires immediate surgical intervention.

KEY POINTS
Clinical Manifestations of *Clostridium difficile* Diarrhea

1. Symptoms do not correlate with the level of toxin production.
2. Mild to moderate disease:
   a. Watery diarrhea and crampy abdominal pain,
   b. Low-grade fever and mild leukocytosis common,
   c. Patients with colitis same symptoms + pseudomembranes seen on colonoscopy.
3. Severe disease has a high fatality rate:
   a. Diarrhea or constipation,
   b. Diffuse abdominal pain and tenderness, signs of peritonitis = impending perforation,
   c. CT scan: Toxic megacolon > 7 cm bowel dilatation, air fluid levels, bowel wall thickening, and thumbprinting (can mimic ischemic bowel),
   d. Marked leukocytosis (25,000–35,000/mm^3), lactic acidosis = impending perforation.

Diagnosis

Stool smear demonstrates PMNs in half of cases and may be heme-positive. Stool culture for *Clostridium difficile* is not recommended because this organism is difficult and expensive to isolate and because culture yields many false positive results. Therefore diagnostic laboratories have focused on toxin detection. The original cytotoxicity assay remains the gold standard. Stool filtrate is overlaid onto fibroblasts. If the toxin is present, the cells round up and eventually detach from the monolayer. Specificity is confirmed if these effects are blocked by preincubating the filtrate with toxin-neutralizing antibody. The assay is sensitive (94–100%) and specific (99%) when performed by experienced personnel but is expensive and requires 2–3 days to perform. Enzyme-linked immunosorbent assay (ELISA) kits that detect toxin A and B are now preferred as the initial screening test. They are rapid and less expensive, but they have a lower sensitivity (70–90%), though comparable specificity. Many assays detect only Toxin A and fail to detect a small percentage of *C. difficile* strains that exclusively produce Toxin B. In cases in which the diagnosis is strongly suspected, a negative ELISA assay should be confirmed by the cytotoxic assay. Sigmoidoscopy is usually not required because patients with positive findings almost always have a positive toxin test. Endoscopy can be performed with caution in the patient who requires immediate diagnosis or is unable to produce stool or if other colonic disorders are also being considered. A significant percentage of patients will have negative findings; however, the presence of pseudomembranes is considered diagnostic.

Treatment, Outcome, and Prevention

Whenever possible, the first step should be to discontinue the offending antibiotic or antibiotics. In many cases patients will fully recover without further intervention. This approach is preferred when symptoms are mild because it allows the bowel to recolonize with competing normal flora and prevents relapse. This contrasts with the 10–25% relapse rate associated with the administration of metronidazole or vancomycin. As in other forms of diarrhea, fluids and electrolytes need to be replaced. Diarrhea serves to protect the mucosa by flushing away *Clostridium difficile* toxins; therefore antiperistaltic agents must be avoided. Their use increases the risk of full-blown colitis and toxic megacolon. If these measurers are not effective or not practical, specific therapy with oral metronidazole (250 mg QID × 10 days) should be initiated. Asymptomatic patients colonized with *C. difficile* should not be treated. Recurrent disease is common as a consequence of residual spores in the stool that are not killed by the antibiotic. First-time recurrences should be treated with the same regimen that is used to treat the initial episode. Oral vancomycin should be avoided whenever possible because of the increased risk of selecting for vancomycin-resistant enterococci (VRE). Nearly all strains of *C. difficile* are killed by metronidazole, and bactericidal levels are readily achieved in the bowel of symptomatic patients. Cure rates of 95% have been reported with the use of this agent.

Oral vancomycin (125 mg QID × 10 days) should be reserved for patients with severe disease. The bowel does not absorb vancomycin, and stool levels of vancomycin reach concentrations that are 1,000–3,000 times the MIC for *Clostridium difficile*. In contrast to metronidazole, in which stool concentrations decrease as the integrity of the bowel mucosa improves, levels of vancomycin remain high throughout the course of the disease. Response rates and relapse rates for oral vancomycin are comparable to those for oral metronidazole. In the patient who is unable to take oral medications, intravenous metronidazole (500 mg Q8H) should be administered. Intravenous metronidazole is excreted in the biliary tract, and therapeutic levels of the antibiotic are achieved in the stool. Intravenous vancomycin fails to achieve significant intraluminal bowel concentrations and is not recommended.

The most feared complications of pseudomembranous colitis are the development of toxic megacolon and bowel perforation. These complications arise in a low percentage of patients (0.4–4%) but are associated with a high mortality rate (30–50%). Persistent fever, marked elevation of the peripheral white blood cell count, lack of response to antibiotics, and marked bowel thickening on CT scan are worrisome findings and warrant consultation with a general surgeon. When these complications arise, bowel resection and ileostomy are recommended.

Standard infection control measures must be scrupulously followed to prevent hospital personnel from spreading *Clostridium difficile* spores from patient to patient. Thorough hand washing can never be overemphasized. Prolonged use of broad-spectrum antibiotics should be avoided whenever possible. Limiting the use of clindamycin has proved effective in reducing the attack rate in several hospital outbreaks.

KEY POINTS

Diagnosis, Treatment, and Prevention of *Clostridium difficile* Diarrhea

1. Diagnosis:
   a. Stool smear: 50% have PMNs in stool,
   b. ELISA assay for Toxins A and B are the preferred assays. Many assays detect only Toxin A and can miss *C. difficile* that produces only Toxin B,
   c. The cytotoxicity assay remains the gold standard; it is expensive and takes several days,
   d. Endoscopy usually is not required. Can cause perforation.
2. Treatment:
   a. Oral metronidazole the treatment of choice,
   b. Oral vancomycin only for severe illness because of the risk of VRE superinfection,
   c. Relapse is common because of residual spores, retreat with metronidazole,
   d. Intravenous metronidazole usually effective, excreted in the bile,
   e. Severe disease may require bowel resection, mortality rate 30–50%.
3. Prevention: Hand washing by hospital personnel is critical. Limiting clindamycin use may reduce the attack rate.

Intra-abdominal Infections

The overall incidence of intra-abdominal infections is difficult to ascertain, but certainly this group of diseases accounts for a significant number of admissions through the emergency room. Intra-abdominal infections often fall between the interface of internal medicine and surgery. In many cases the infectious disease specialist, gastroenterologist, radiologist, and general surgeon need to coordinate their care to ensure the most favorable outcome.

Primary or Spontaneous Peritonitis

Potential Severity: A frequently fatal infection that requires immediate paracentesis and empiric antibiotic therapy.

MICROBIOLOGY AND PATHOGENESIS

In adults spontaneous or primary peritonitis develops in patients with severe cirrhosis and ascites. Ascites caused by congestive heart failure, malignancy, and lymphedema have also led to this infection. Bacteria may enter the peritoneal space by hematogenous spread, lymphatic spread, or migration through the bowel wall. In patients with severe cirrhosis the reticuloendothelial system of the liver is often bypassed secondary to shunting, increasing the risk of prolonged bacteremia. Bowel motility is also slowed in these patients, resulting in bacterial overgrowth. The most common pathogens are enteric bowel flora, *E. coli* being most common, followed by *Klebsiella pneumoniae*. *Streptococcus pneumoniae* and other streptococci, including enterococci, may also be cultured. *Staphylococcus aureus* and anaerobes are infrequently encountered.

CLINICAL MANIFESTATIONS

The initial symptoms and signs may be subtle, and physicians need to maintain a low threshold for diagnostic and therapeutic intervention. Fever is the most common manifestation and often initially is low-grade (38°C range). Abdominal pain is usually diffuse and constant and differs from the usual sensation of tightness experienced with tense ascites. A third common manifestation is a deterioration of mental status. Infection is well known to exacerbate hepatic encephalopathy, and spontaneous peritonitis should be excluded as part of any mental status workup of a patient with end-stage liver disease. Diarrhea may precede other symptoms and signs and is usually precipitated by overgrowth of the bowel flora. Abdominal tenderness is diffuse and is not associated with guarding because the ascites separates the visceral and parietal peritoneum, preventing severe inflammatory irritation of the abdominal wall muscles. In the late stages of infection, rebound tenderness may be elicited. If hypotension and hypothermia develop prior to the initiation of antibiotics, the prognosis is grave.

KEY POINTS

Microbiology, Pathogenesis, and Clinical Manifestations of Primary Peritonitis

1. Most commonly associated with end-stage liver disease and portal hypertension.
2. Organisms infect the ascitic fluid by hematogenous spread, lymphatic spread, and bowel leakage.
3. Infecting organisms:
   a. Enteric Gram-negatives most common: *E. coli* and *Klebsiella pneumoniae*,
   b. *Streptococcus pneumoniae* and enterococci,
   c. Anaerobes and *Staphylococcus aureus* are uncommon.

4. Clinical presentation may be subtle:
   a. Low-grade fever (38°C),
   b. Constant, diffuse abdominal pain without guarding,
   c. Worsening mental status.

DIAGNOSIS

The diagnosis of spontaneous peritonitis can be made only by obtaining a sample of ascitic fluid. Needle aspiration of peritoneal fluid is a simple and safe procedure. Significant bleeding requiring transfusion occurs in fewer than 1% of patients despite abnormally elevated prothrombin times in a high percentage of patients. Paracentesis is a minimally traumatic procedure and does not require prophylactic plasma transfusions. Proper handling of the samples is critical for making an accurate diagnosis. A minimum of 10 ml of ascitic fluid should be inoculated into a blood culture flask. Care must be taken to exchange the needle used to penetrate the skin for a new sterile needle prior to puncturing the blood culture flask. Second, a sample should be inoculated into a tube containing anticoagulant for cell counts. If this precaution is not taken, the ascites fluid may clot, preventing accurate cytological analysis. Third, a tube should be sent to measure total protein, albumin, lactic dehydrogenase (LDH), glucose, and amylase levels. Finally, a separate syringe or tube should be sent for Gram stain. The leukocyte count in the ascitic fluid of patients with spontaneous peritonitis is almost always >300 cells/mm^3 with predominance of PMNs. The diagnosis is strongly suggested by an absolute PMN count of $\geq$250 cells/mm^3. Gram stain is positive in 20–40% of cases and is helpful in guiding antibiotic therapy. Other ascites fluid values help to differentiate primary from secondary peritonitis. A high ascites fluid total protein, LDH, and amylase and a low fluid glucose are more commonly found in secondary peritonitis and should raise the possibility of bowel perforation.

TREATMENT AND OUTCOME

Empiric therapy should be initiated emergently. Delays in therapy can result in sepsis, hypotension, lactic acidosis, and death. In the patient with cirrhosis and ascites and who has fever, abdominal pain or tenderness, changes in mental status, and/or $\geq$ 250 mm^3 PMNs in the ascitic fluid, antibiotics should be initiated as soon as blood, urine, and ascites fluid cultures have been obtained. A third-generation cephalosporin (cefotaxime or ceftriaxone) covers the majority of potential pathogens. If secondary peritonitis is suspected, anaerobic coverage with metronidazole should be added. Treatment should be continued for 5–10 days depending on the response to therapy. The mortality rate remains high in this disease (60–70%), reflecting the patients' severe underlying liver disease and the serious nature of this infection. Early diagnosis may reduce mortality to the 40% range. Death is often due to end-stage cirrhosis, spontaneous peritonitis representing a manifestation of this terminal disease. Patients who have had their first bout of spontaneous peritonitis should be strongly considered for liver transplant. Intermittent prophylaxis may be considered in patients at risk for recurrent spontaneous peritonitis. Prophylactic regimens have included trimethoprim-sulfamethoxazole (1 DS po QD 5 out of 7 days) or ciprofloxacin (750 mg po once per week).

KEY POINTS
Diagnosis, Treatment, and Outcome of Spontaneous Peritonitis

1. Paracentesis needs to be performed when this diagnosis is considered:
   a. 10 ml of fluid in a blood culture flask,
   b. Cell count from an anticoagulated sample >250 PMNs/mm^3 or >300 WBCs/mm^3 with predominance of PMNs,
   c. Gram stain positive 20–40%,
   d. Elevated protein, LDH, and amylase and low glucose suggest secondary peritonitis.

2. Empiric antibiotics given emergently as soon as cultures are obtained:
   a. Ceftriaxone or cefotaxime, add metronidazole if suspect secondary peritonitis,
   b. Mortality rate 60–70% reduced to 40% with early treatment.
3. Marker of severe end-stage liver disease. Patients should be considered for liver transplant.
4. Trimethoprim-sulfamethoxazole or ciprofloxacin prophylaxis recommended for patients at risk.

Secondary Peritonitis

Potential Severity: A life-threatening illness that usually requires acute surgical intervention.

MICROBIOLOGY AND PATHOGENESIS

Spillage of the bowel flora into the peritoneal cavity has multiple causes. Perforation of a gastric ulcer, appendicitis with rupture, diverticulitis, bowel neoplasm, gangrenous bowel due to strangulation or mesenteric artery insufficiency, and pancreatitis are some of the most common diseases leading to secondary peritonitis. The types of organisms that are associated with peritonitis depend on the site of mucosal breakdown. Gastric perforation most commonly results in infection with mouth flora including streptococci, Candida, and lactobacilli as well as anaerobes. Perforation in the lower regions of the bowel result in infections with mixed enteric flora. Feces in the colon consist of bacteria concentrations averaging 10^{11} colony-forming units/ml. Anaerobes comprise a major component, *Bacteroides fragilis* being one of the most common species. Aerobic Gram-negative bacteria are abundant, *E. coli* predominating; Klebsiella species, Proteus species, and Enterobacter species are also common. Gram- positive bacteria also are found in the bowel flora; *Streptococcus viridans*, enterococci, and *Clostridia perfringens*

predominate. The peritoneum's response to infection is usually rapid and exuberant. Large amounts of proteinaceous exudate are released into the peritoneum, and there is a massive influx of PMNs and macrophages. The influx of fluid can result in intravascular fluid losses of 300–500 ml/hour. Mechanical clearance via the diaphragmatic lymphatic system can clear large numbers of bacteria quickly. However, once in the lymphatic system, bacteria usually invade the bloodstream. Phagocytic cells ingest large numbers of bacteria and kill them. Finally, the deposition of fibrinous exudate can wall off the infection to form discrete abscesses. When the peritoneal host defenses are overwhelmed, the patient develops metabolic acidosis, tissue hypoxia, irreversible shock, and multiorgan failure and dies.

KEY POINTS

Microbiology and Pathogenesis of Peritonitis

1. Bacteriology depends on the site of perforation:
   a. Gastric perforation: Mouth flora including Candida and anaerobes,
   b. Lower bowel contains 10^{11} bacteria/ml and perforation causes massive soilage. Anaerobes are a major component, *Bacteroides fragilis* common. Aerobic Gram-negative bacteria, *E. coli* predominates; Klebsiella species, Proteus species, and Enterobacter species are also common. Gram-positive *Streptococcus viridans*, enterococci, and *Clostridium perfringens*.
2. Peritoneum exudes 300–500 ml/hour of proteinaceous material, masses of PMNs; bacteria enter the lymphatics and then the bloodstream. Fibrinous material can wall off abscesses.
3. Metabolic acidosis, hypoxia, multiorgan failure, and death may follow.

CLINICAL MANIFESTATIONS

The anterior peritoneum is richly innervated, and the first manifestation of inflammation is abdominal pain that is usually sharp, localized to the initial site of spillage, and aggravated by motion. Pain is almost always accompanied by loss of appetite and nausea. Fever, chills, constipation, and abdominal distention are common. Patients usually lie still in bed, breathing with shallow respirations. Fever, tachycardia, and hypotension develop in the later stages. On abdominal exam the bowel sounds are decreased or absent, and the abdomen is tender to palpation. Guarding and involuntary spasm of the abdominal muscles can result in a boardlike abdomen. If slow compression of the abdomen followed by rapid release of pressure causes severe pain, the patient has rebound tenderness, indicating peritoneal irritation. On rectal exam tenderness can often be elicited. Elderly patients often fail to present with the classic findings of peritonitis. They often have only mild to moderate tenderness and do not exhibit guarding or rebound. A high index of suspicion must be maintained when the elderly patient presents with abdominal pain. These patients are at increased risk for diverticulitis, perforated colonic carcinoma, and bowel ischemia.

KEY POINTS

Clinical Presentation of Peritonitis

1. Abdominal pain is usually sharp and begins at the site of spillage.
2. Any movement or deep breathing worsens the pain.
3. Peritoneal inflammation causes abdominal spasm (guarding) and rebound.
4. Rectal tenderness may be found.
5. Elderly often don't have the typical findings of peritonitis.

DIAGNOSIS AND TREATMENT

Serial abdominal examinations and careful monitoring of vital signs as well as peripheral white blood cell count are helpful in deciding whether or not to perform an exploratory laparotomy. A high peripheral white blood cell count in the range of 17,000–25,000 WBCs/mm^3 with an increased percentage of PMNs and band forms is usually noted. A normal peripheral leukocyte count without a predominance of PMN forms should call into question the diagnosis of secondary peritonitis. Supine and upright abdominal X-rays should be performed to exclude free air under the diaphragm (indicative of bowel or gastric perforation), to assess the bowel gas pattern, and to search for areas of thickened edematous bowel wall. A chest X-ray must always be performed to exclude lower lobe pneumonia, which can cause ileus and upper quadrant tenderness mimicking peritonitis. CT scan of the abdomen and pelvis following oral and intravenous contrast is now considered the initial diagnostic test of choice for patients with suspected intra-abdominal infection. This diagnostic procedure often obviates the need for exploratory laparotomy and allows the accurate diagnosis of appendicitis, localization and needle aspiration of abscesses, and the identification of areas of bowel obstruction.

KEY POINTS

Diagnosis of Secondary Peritonitis

1. Serial abdominal exams should be performed and vital signs closely monitored.
2. Peripheral leukocytosis should be present.
3. KUB X-ray with upright view should be performed looking for free air.
4. Chest X-ray should always be performed to exclude basilar pneumonia.
5. CT scan with oral and intravenous contrast is the diagnostic study of choice.

Antibiotic treatment should be initiated emergently in patients who are suspected of having secondary peritonitis. Broad-spectrum antibiotic coverage is necessary to cover the multiple organisms infecting the peritoneum. A number of regimens have been recommended. Single agents are available that are effective for community-acquired infections of mild to moderate severity and include high doses of cefoxitin, cefotetan, ticarcillin-clavulanate, and piperacillin-tazobactam. Imipenem-cilastatin can be used as a single agent in severe peritonitis, hospital-acquired infection, or resistant infections. Combination therapy may also be used and often is used in severe cases. Potential regimens include the following:

1. Cefoxitin or cefotetan plus gentamicin
2. Metronidazole and a third-generation cephalosporin (ceftriaxone, cefotaxime, ceftizoxime)
3. Metronidazole plus a fluoroquinolone (ciprofloxacin, levofloxacin, gatifloxacin)
4. Clindamycin plus aztreonam

When secondary peritonitis is being considered, a general surgeon should be consulted emergently. Repeated abdominal exam allows the surgeon to follow the progression of findings. If tenderness becomes more diffuse, or if increased guarding and rebound are noted, exploratory laparotomy is often required for diagnosis, drainage, and bowel repair. Peritoneal irrigation is performed intraoperatively, and drains are placed at sites where purulent collections are noted. Multiple operations are often required for the surgical treatment of patients with diffuse purulent peritonitis. Antibiotic coverage should be adjusted based on the cultures and sensitivities of the intraoperative cultures.

KEY POINTS
Treatment of Secondary Peritonitis

1. Empiric antibiotics should be initiated emergently:
   a. Mild to moderately severe disease: Single-drug therapy with cefoxitin, cefotetan, ticarcillin-clavulanate, or piperacillin-tazobactam,
   b. Severe disease: Combination therapy with cefoxitin or cefotetan + gentamicin, metronidazole + third-generation cephalosporin, metronidazole + fluoro-

quinolone (ciprofloxacin, levofloxacin, or gatifloxacin), clindamycin + aztreonam, or a carbapenem alone (imipenem-cilastin).
2. Surgical consultation immediately to follow abdominal exam:
   a. Laparotomy is often required for drainage and bowel repair,
   b. Peritoneal lavage and placement of drains are often required,
   c. Intraoperative cultures help to direct antibiotic coverage.

SECONDARY PERITONITIS ASSOCIATED WITH PERITONEAL DIALYSIS

Bacterial peritonitis is a frequent complication of chronic ambulatory peritoneal dialysis (CAPD) and is the most frequent reason for discontinuation of CAPD. *Staphylococcus epidermidis* and *S. aureus* are the most common bacteria associated with this infection. Gram-negative bacteria more commonly encountered in patients with diverticulitis. Although enteric Gram-negatives may be cultured, *E. coli* is uncommon. *Pseudomonas aeruginosa* grows readily in water and is the etiologic agent in up to 5% of cases. Fungal peritonitis has become increasingly common. Atypical mycobacteria and less commonly *Mycobacterium tuberculosis* have also caused peritonitis in this setting. As is observed in spontaneous peritonitis, fever and diffuse abdominal pain are the most common complaints. The peritoneal dialysis fluid usually becomes cloudy as a consequence of inflammatory cells. Peritoneal fluid white blood cell counts are usually >100 cells/mm^3 with a predominance of PMNs. A predominance of lymphocytes should raise the possibility of fungal or tuberculous infection. Peritoneal fluid culture (two cultures consisting of 10 ml in each blood culture flask) and Gram stain should be obtained. Yield from Gram stain is low; however, properly obtained peritoneal cultures are positive in over 90% of cases. Blood cultures should be obtained if there are systemic symptoms but are rarely positive. After cultures are obtained, antibiotic should be added to the dialysate. Initial empiric therapy should include a first-generation cephalosporin (cefazolin 500 mg/l loading dose followed by 125 mg/l in each bag) and an aminoglycoside (gentamicin or tobramycin 20 mg/l or amikacin 60 mg/l once per day). Once-a-day aminoglycoside therapy rather than constant treatment is now recommended to reduce the risk of ototoxicity. If the patient fails to improve over 48 hours, removal of the dialysis catheter should be considered.

KEY POINTS

Secondary Peritonitis Associated with Peritoneal Dialysis

1. Clinical presentation similar to that of primary peritonitis accompanied by cloudy dialysate.
2. *Staphylococcus epidermidis* and *S. aureus* most common, *Pseudomonas aeruginosa*, fungi, and atypical mycobacteria are also found. *Mycobacterium tuberculosis* is less common.
3. Diagnosis:
   a. WBC in peritoneal fluid > 100/mm^3 with a predominance of PMNs,
   b. Culture 10 ml peritoneal fluid into blood culture flask × 2; blood cultures rarely positive.
4. Treatment with intraperitoneal antibiotics: First-generation cephalosporin + once-per-day aminoglycoside for empiric therapy.

Hepatic Abscess

Potential Severity: Usually presents subacutely. With appropriate drainage and antibiotics prognosis is excellent.

PATHOGENESIS AND MICROBIOLOGY

Spread of pyogenic infection to the liver can occur in multiple ways. Biliary tract infection is most common, followed by portal vein bacteremia associated with intra-abdominal infections, primarily appendicitis, diverticulitis, and inflammatory bowel disease. Direct extension into the liver from a contiguous infection can occur after perforation of the gallbladder or duodenal ulcer and in association with a perinephric, pancreatic, or subphrenic abscess. Penetrating wounds and postoperative complications may result in liver abscess. Bacteremia from any source can seed the liver via the hepatic artery and result in the formation of multiple abscesses. Finally, in approximately one quarter of cases a cause cannot be determined. The bacteriology of this infection reflects the primary site of infection. As in secondary peritonitis this infection is usually polymicrobial. Anaerobes are commonly cultured, including Bacteroides species, Fusobacterium and Peptostreptococcus species, and Actinomyces species. Microaerophilic streptococci (*S. milleri* being most frequent) are found in one quarter of cases. Enteric Gram-negative rods, particularly *E. coli* and Klebsiella species are other important pathogens. Candida can also invade the liver, candidal abscesses being most commonly encountered in leukemia patients following chemotherapy-induced neutropenia. Amebic liver abscess is rare and complicates 3–9% of patients with amoebic colitis.

KEY POINTS

Pathogenesis and Microbiology of Liver Abscess

1. Bacteria seed the liver by multiple routes:
   a. Biliary tract most common,
   b. Portal system in association with intra-abdominal infection,
   c. Direct extension from intra-abdominal infections,
   d. Penetrating wounds and postoperative complications,
   e. Hematogenous.

> 2. Bacteriology usually similar to secondary peritonitis:
>   a. Microaerophilic streptococci frequent, in particular *S. milleri,*
>   b. Candida in leukemia patients following neutropenia.

CLINICAL MANIFESTATIONS

Fever with or without chills is the most common presenting complaint. This may be the only complaint, hepatic abscess being one of the more common infectious causes of fever of undetermined origin. Abdominal pain develops in about half of the patients and is often confined to the right upper quadrant. Pain is usually dull and constant. Weight loss (10 pounds or more during 3 months or less) is another frequent complaint. Physical exam often reveals tenderness over the liver. Jaundice is rare. In patients with abscess in the upper regions of the right hepatic lobe pulmonary exam may reveal decreased breath sounds on that side, owing to atelectasis or a pleural effusion.

DIAGNOSIS, TREATMENT, AND OUTCOME

With the exception of amoebic liver abscess, the peripheral white blood cell count is usually elevated (>20,000 WBCs/mm^3) with increased numbers of immature neutrophils. The serum alkaline phosphatase is also elevated in the majority of cases. Blood cultures are positive in up to half of patients. Abdominal CT scan is the most sensitive test for identifying liver abscesses and demonstrates a discrete area of attenuation at the abscess site (see Figure 12.7). Ultrasound is somewhat less sensitive but also useful. Both CT and ultrasound can be used to guide needle aspiration for culture and drainage. The finding of brownish fluid without a foul odor suggests the possibility of amoebic abscess.

Initial empiric antibiotic therapy should be identical to secondary peritonitis. The antibiotic regimen can be subsequently tailored to the abscess

culture results. Percutaneous drainage in combination with antibiotics is now the treatment of choice. Open surgical drainage should be considered in patients who continue to have fever after two weeks of antibiotic treatment and percutaneous drainage. Open surgery may also be required in patients with biliary obstruction, multiloculated abscesses (other than echinococcus; see Chapter 12), and highly viscous abscesses. Mortality was high in early series, approaching 100% when abscesses were not drained; however, with modern antibiotics and drainage techniques nearly 100% of patients are now cured.

KEY POINTS KEY POINTS
Clinical Manifestations, Diagnosis, and Treatment of Liver Abscess

> 1. May present as fever of unknown origin. Dull right upper quadrant pain associated with right upper quadrant tenderness.
> 2. Leukocytosis and elevated alkaline phosphatase.
> 3. CT scan is the diagnostic study of choice.
> 4. Percutaneous drainage and broad-spectrum coverage using the same regimens as for secondary peritonitis.
> 5. Open drainage for patient with:
>   a. Biliary obstruction,
>   b. Multiloculated abscess other than echinococcus,
>   c. Viscous exudate.

Pancreatic Abscess

Potential Severity: A serious but usually not fatal complication of pancreatitis that presents subacutely.

Pancreatic abscesses usually arise as complication of pancreatitis. Release of pancreatic enzymes leads to tissue necrosis. Subsequently, necrotic tissue can become infected by reflux of contaminated bile or by hematogenous spread. Like other intra-abdominal abscesses, pancreatic abscesses are usually polymicrobial. CT scan and ultrasound arc employed for culture and drainage. Because of the significant quantities of necrotic tissue, open drainage and debridement are usually required in combination with broad-spectrum antibiotics. The same antibiotic regimens that are recommended for secondary peritonitis offer excellent empiric coverage pending cultures and sensitivities. Survival is improved by early surgical drainage. A fatal outcome is more likely in the elderly patient, who more often has accompanying biliary tract disease.

KEY POINTS

Pancreatic Abscess

1. Necrotic tissue can become infected by contaminated bile or hematogenous spread.
2. Abscesses are polymicrobial.
3. CT scan and ultrasound to guide drainage.
4. Open surgical drainage is usually required to debride necrotic tissue.
5. The same broad-spectrum coverage used for secondary peritonitis is recommended.
6. Fatal outcome is more likely in the elderly.

Cholecystitis and Cholangitis

Potential Severity: An acute potentially life-threatening infection that can be complicated by sepsis. Rapid treatment reduces morbidity and mortality.

PATHOGENESIS AND MICROBIOLOGY

Biliary obstruction is most frequently caused by gallstones and results in increased pressure in and distention of the gallbladder. These changes compromise blood flow and interfere with lymphatic drainage, leading to tissue necrosis and inflammation leading to cholecystitis. Although infection is not the primary cause of acute cholecystitis, obstruction prevents the flushing of bacteria from the gallbladder and is associated with infection in over half of the cases. If treatment is delayed, infection can spread from the gallbladder to the hepatic biliary ducts and common bile duct causing cholangitis. The organisms associated with cholecystitis and cholangitis reflect the bowel flora and are similar to the organisms encountered in secondary peritonitis. *E. coli,* Klebsiella species, enterococci, and anaerobes are most frequently cultured from biliary drainage.

CLINICAL MANIFESTATIONS

The acute onset of right upper quadrant pain, high fever, and chills are most common. Jaundice may also be noted, fulfilling Charcot's triad (fever, right upper quadrant pain, and jaundice). On physical exam marked tenderness over the liver is commonly elicited. Hypotension may be present, indicating early Gram-negative sepsis. Elderly patients might not complain of pain, presenting solely with hypotension. Marked peripheral leukocytosis with increased number of PMNs and band forms is the rule. Liver function tests are usually consistent with obstruction, demonstrating an elevated serum alkaline phosphatase and gamma glutamyl transpeptidase (GGT) and bilirubin. On rare occasion the serum amino transferase enzymes, reflecting hepatocellular damage, may also be elevated (up to 1,000 IU) as a result of microabscess formation in the liver. Blood cultures are frequently positive.

DIAGNOSIS AND TREATMENT

Ultrasonography is the preferred diagnostic study, and can usually detect gallstones, dilatation of the gallbladder, and dilatation of the biliary ducts including the common bile duct. Other adjunctive tests may include CT scan or MRI; however, these tests are generally not recommended for initial screening. Endoscopic ret-

rograde cholangiopancreatography (ERCP) is helpful for confirming the diagnosis, dilating the
sphincter of Oddi, stone removal, and placing
stents to maintain biliary flow in fibrotic-con-
stricted biliary channels. This procedure should
be performed under antibiotic coverage and
should be avoided in cases of cholangitis because of the risk of precipitating high-level bacteremia. Broad-spectrum antibiotics should be
initiated immediately. Regimens similar to those
for secondary peritonitis may be used. Many experts prefer ampicillin and gentamicin because
this regimen covers enterococci in addition to
the enteric Gram-negative pathogens. Imipenem
also effectively covers enterococci as well as the
enteric Gram-negative rods and anaerobes. Despite its poor activity against enterococci, ciprofloxacin has also proved effective. Metronidazole
may be added to ciprofloxacin to improve anaerobic coverage. Prompt surgical intervention is required for patients with a gangrenous gallbladder
and gallbladder perforation. In cases of acute
cholecystitis decompression of the gallbladder
and stone removal are now most commonly accomplished by ERCP. The outcome is usually favorable for mild to moderate disease; however,
mortality approaches 50% in those with severe
cholangitis.

KEY POINTS
Cholecystitis and Cholangitis

1. Caused by obstruction of the biliary
   tree leading to necrosis and inflammation.
2. Polymicrobial infection occurs in over half
   of cases; *E. coli*, Klebsiella species, enterococci, and anaerobes are most common.
3. Charcot's triad may be noted: fever, right
   upper quadrant pain, and jaundice. The elderly may present with hypotension and no
   abdominal pain.
4. Diagnosis:

   a. Elevated alkaline phosphatase, GGT, and
      bilirubin. Transaminases can rarely reach
      1,000 IU,
   b. Abdominal ultrasound is the preferred di-
      agnostic screening tool,
   c. ERCP confirms the diagnosis, can dilate
      the sphincter of Oddi, remove stones,
      and place stents to maintain biliary flow.
5. Treatment:
   a. Broad-spectrum antibiotics: Ampicillin +
      gentamicin, imipenem, metronidazole +
      ciprofloxacin,
   b. Biliary drainage and stone removal by
      ERCP, now the treatment of choice,
   c. Surgery for perforated or gangrenous
      gallbladder.
6. Mortality rate in severe cholangitis approaching 50%.

Helicobacter pylori–Associated Peptic Ulcer Disease

Potential Severity: A chronic disease that
causes discomfort but is usually not life threatening.

MICROBIOLOGY AND PATHOGENESIS

Helicobacter pylori is a small, curved, microaerophilic Gram-negative rod that is closely
related to Campylobacter. This organism is able
to survive and multiply within the gastric mucosa. The majority of *H. pylori* live freely in this
environment; however, a small number adhere
exclusively to gastric epithelial cells, forming adherence pedestals similar to those observed with
enteropathogenic *E. coli*. This organism demonstrates corkscrewlike motility, allowing it to migrate within the gastric and duodenal mucosa.
All pathogenic strains express high concentrations of urease, allowing them to generate ammonium ions that buffer the gastric acid. The
mechanism by which ulcers are formed is not

completely understood. In addition to urease activity that induces inflammation, the presence of the *cagA* gene and production of a cytotoxic protein vac A are virulence factors associated with the ability to cause peptic ulcer disease. Colonization with *H. pylori* may be associated with the accumulation of increased numbers of inflammatory cells in the lamina propria of gastric epithelial cells. Production of inflammatory cytokines reduces somatostatin levels and causes an increase in gastrin levels. Chronic inflammation caused by *H. pylori* is thought to produce aplastic changes in the gastric mucosa and may lead to gastric carcinomas.

CLINICAL MANIFESTATIONS, DIAGNOSIS, AND TREATMENT

Patients with *Helicobacter pylori* peptic ulcer disease usually have the classic symptoms of dyspepsia consisting of burning pain several hours after meals, relieved by food and antacids. Belching, indigestion, and heartburn are also frequent complaints. Other than mild midepigastric tenderness the physical examination is usually normal.

Testing for *Helicobacter pylori* is recommended only in symptomatic patients. Diagnosis is most commonly made by endoscopic biopsy. A biopsy specimen should be first tested for urease (Clotest), which has high sensitivity and specificity in patients who are not taking bismuth, H_2 blockers, or proton pump inhibitors. This is the most cost-effective diagnostic method. Biopsy specimens can also be cultured using selective media and microaerophilic conditions. Culture should be performed in patients who have proved refractory to therapy in order to obtain antibiotic sensitivities. *H. pylori* can also be visualized using silver, Gram, or Gicmsa stain as well as by immunofluorescence. Noninvasive studies include the urease breath test, in which the patient ingests ^{13}C- or ^{14}C-labeled urea and the patient's breath is analyzed for ^{13}C or ^{14}C over the next hour. This test requires expensive equipment but is specific and sensitive. Measurement of IgG antibody levels by ELISA assay is now commercially available, inexpensive, and sensitive. However, false-positive results are reported in some patients over age 50 years. Antibody titers drop as the infection is eradicated and is a potentially useful parameter for assessing the response to antibiotic therapy. The urea breath test remains the most accurate method for documenting cure.

Multiple regimens have been used to treat *Helicobacter pylori*, and the ideal regimen has not been determined. Triple therapy with a proton pump inhibitor (lansoprazole 30 mg BID or omeprazole 20 mg BID), amoxicillin (1 g po BID), and clarithromycin (500 mg po BID) for two weeks is associated with a 90% cure rate. In the patient who is penicillin allergic, metronidazole (500 mg po BID) can be substituted for amoxicillin. A proton pump inhibitor can also be combined with bismuth (525 mg QID) and two other oral antibiotics (amoxicillin, clarithromycin, metronidazole, tetracycline).

KEY POINTS

Helicobacter pylori–Associated Peptic Ulcer Disease

1. A small, curved, microaerophilic Gram-negative rod:
   a. Survives on the mucosal surface of the stomach,
   b. Synthesizes high concentrations of urease that produces ammonium ions to neutralize acid.
2. Dyspepsia, belching, and heartburn are the most common symptoms.
3. Diagnosis: Test only symptomatic patients:
   a. Endoscopic biopsy with Clotest for urease preferred,
   b. Culture only for refractory cases,
   c. Urease breath test expensive but accurate,
   d. ELISA antibody test, false positive in those >50 years old, titer decreases with treatment.
4. Treatment:

a. Proton pump inhibitor + amoxicillin + clarithromycin (PCN allergy: replace amoxicillin with metronidazole),

b. Proton pump inhibitor + bismuth + amoxicillin + clarithromycin (or metronidazole or tetracycline).

Viral Hepatitis

Potential Severity: Fulminant hepatitis is rare but usually fatal. Chronic active hepatitis can lead to liver failure and may require liver transplantation.

Acute viral hepatitis is a common disease affecting approximately 700,000 Americans per year. Three viral agents—hepatitis A, hepatitis B, and hepatitis C virus—are primarily responsible for acute hepatitis. Less common causes include hepatitis D or delta agent and hepatitis E. A number of other viral agents affect multiple organs in addition to the liver. Epstein-Barr virus and cytomegalovirus are the most common viruses in this category. Less commonly, herpes simplex viruses, varicella-zoster virus, coxsackievirus B, measles, rubella, rubeola, and adenovirus can infect the liver. Fulminant hepatitis is rare but serious, occurring in approximately 1% of cases with icteric hepatitis. Fulminant disease is most commonly reported with hepatitis B and D but is also reported in pregnant woman with hepatitis E.

Clinical Manifestations of Acute Hepatitis

There are no clinical features that definitively differentiate one form of viral hepatitis from another. Acute viral hepatitis has four stages of illness:

1. **Incubation period**. This period varies from a few weeks to six months depending on the viral agent (see Table 8.1). During this period the patient has no symptoms.

2. **Preicteric stage**. The symptoms during this stage are nonspecific. The most common initial complaint is malaise, patients reporting a general sense of not feeling well. Fatigue may also be a prominent complaint, accompanied by generalized weakness. Anorexia, nausea, and vomiting are other common symptoms. Loss of taste for cigarettes is reported among smokers. Dull right upper quadrant pain is also a frequent complaint. Some patients experience a flulike illness consisting of myalgias, headache, chills, and fever. Finally, a minority develop a serum-sickness syndrome consisting of fever, rash, and arthritis or arthralgias. These symptoms are due to immune-complex (virus plus antibody) deposition. Most of the symptoms associated with viral hepatitis dramatically resolve with the onset of jaundice.

3. **Icteric stage**. This stage begins 4–10 days after the onset of the preicteric stage. Jaundice and dark urine are the classic symptoms. Scleral icterus may be unnoticed and is best visualized in natural rather than artificial light. Pale-colored stools can develop as a consequence of decreased excretion of bile pigments. Immune-complex formation at this stage can result in vasculitis primarily with hepatitis B, and glomerulonephritis can develop in association with hepatitis B or C infection.

4. **Convalescent stage**. The duration of this phase depends on the severity of the attack and the viral etiology.

The most prominent physical finding is icterus that can be detected in the sclera or under the tongue when bilirubin levels reach 2.5–3.0 mg/dl. Slight hepatic enlargement with mild to moderate tenderness is common. Tenderness can be elicited by placing one hand over the liver and pounding this site gently with the fist of the other hand (termed "punch tenderness"). The skin may exhibit scratch marks as a result of severe pruritus. Fulminant hepatitis may be ac-

Table 8.1

Clinical Characteristics of the Different Forms of Viral Hepatitis

VIRUS TYPE	INCUBATION PERIOD	EPIDEMIOLOGY	SEQUELAE
Hepatitis A	4 weeks	Fecal oral route Food-borne Water Sexually transmitted	Self-limited disease Can relapse up to 6 months after primary attack Fulminant hepatitis rare

Hepatitis B	12 weeks	Person to person
		Blood and blood products
		Other body fluids
		Intravenous drug abuse
		Sexually transmitted
			Chronic infection common: 90%
			  neonates, 20–50% children,
			  5–10% adults
			Hepatocellular carcinoma

Hepatitis C	6–10 weeks	Person to person Blood and blood products Intravenous drug abuse Sexual transmission rare Higher risk with HIV infection	Usually a chronic infection Cirrhosis in 25% Requires liver transplant Hepatocellular carcinoma
Hepatitis D + B	12 weeks	Person to person Blood and blood products Other body fluids Intravenous drug abuse Sexually transmitted Household contacts	Same as hepatitis B Hepatic failure more common among IV drug abusers
Hepatitis E	4 weeks	Fecal-oral route Only in developing countries	Self-limited disease Fulminant hepatitis in pregnancy

companied by hepatic encephalopathy, causing depression in mental status and asterixis (irregular flapping of the outstretched hands after forcible dorsiflexion).

Laboratory findings are distinctive in viral hepatitis. Levels of aspartate aminotransferase (AST) and alanine aminotransferase (ALT) often increase to 1,000–2,000 IU, and the ratio of AST/ALT is usually less than 1, while in alcoholic hepatitis this ratio is usually >1.5. Alkaline phosphatase, a reflection of biliary obstruction or cholestasis, is only mildly elevated. LDH also is mildly elevated. Transaminase values usually peak in the early icteric stage. Direct and indirect bilirubin fractions are usually equally elevated. High levels of direct or conjugated bilirubin suggest cholestasis, while high levels of

indirect or unconjugated bilirubin usually indicate red blood cell hemolysis, which can develop in patients with viral hepatitis who have glucose-6-dehydrogenase deficiency or sickle-cell anemia. Significant elevation of the prothrombin time is a bad prognostic sign. A prothrombin time of greater than 100 seconds indicates irreversible hepatic damage, and such patients should be promptly considered for liver transplant. In fulminant hepatitis, disseminated intravascular coagulation can develop, leading to thrombocytopenia. Liver biopsy is generally not required to diagnose acute viral hepatitis. This test should be performed when several causes of hepatitis are possible or when therapy is being considered. Histopathology classically reveals ballooning and hepatocyte necrosis, disarray of liver lobules, mononuclear cell infiltration, and cholestasis.

Chronic hepatitis can follow acute hepatitis B and hepatitis C infections. Particularly in patients with hepatitis C, chronic infection can follow asymptomatic acute infection. The majority of patients experience no symptoms until they progress to liver failure. In most instances of hepatitis C, hepatic failure takes more than 20 years, but it usually occurs more rapidly in hepatitis B virus infection. Elevations of transaminase values are often detected during routine screening. Levels are usually mildly to moderately elevated and do not exceed 7–10 × normal values. Mild fatigue may develop and cause the patient to seek medical attention. Other patients may present with symptoms and signs of cirrhosis. The chronic generation of high antibody levels directed against the virus can result in the production of immune complexes that deposit in the glomeruli and small to medium-sized blood vessels causing membranous glomerulonephritis and vasculitis in a minority of patients with chronic disease. Polyarteritis nodosa is frequently associated with persistent hepatitis B infection.

KEY POINTS
Clinical Manifestations of Acute Viral Hepatitis

1. Four clinical states:
   a. Incubation period: Asymptomatic,
   b. Preicteric stage: Nonspecific symptoms, malaise, fatigue, generalized weakness. Anorexia, nausea and vomiting, loss of taste for cigarettes, minority develop a serum-sickness syndrome,
   c. Icteric stage: Symptoms dramatically resolve with the onset of jaundice, itching may develop, pale stools,
   d. Convalescent stage: Duration varies.
2. Fulminant hepatitis leads to encephalitis with asterixis.
3. LFTs:

   a. Transaminase values 1000-2000 IU AST/ALT < 1 (> 1.5 with alcohol),
   b. High direct bilirubin = cholestasis, high indirect bilirubin = hemolysis,
   c. High PT = bad prognosis >100 s = liver transplant.
4. Complications: Chronic active hepatitis B or C, vasculitis, and glomerulonephritis.

Hepatitis A

VIROLOGY, PATHOGENESIS, AND EPIDEMIOLOGY

Hepatitis A is a small, nonenveloped single-stranded RNA virus. This picornavirus is highly resistant to heating and drying. The virus is inactivated by chlorine and does not survive well in buffered saline; however, in protein solutions such as milk the virus is able to withstand high temperatures for brief periods. In tissue culture the virus is not cytopathic, and replication has to be detected by immunofluorescent antibody staining. Isolation of wild-type virus is often unsuccessful, making tissue culture an ineffective diagnostic tool. Virus enters the host via the gastrointestinal tract, traversing the intestine and infecting the hepatocyte, where it survives and multiplies within the cell cytoplasm. The virus primarily infects hepatocytes and then is released into the bloodstream and excreted into the bile, resulting in high levels of virus in the stool. Hepatocyte damage is caused by the host's cell-mediated immune response. Peak titers of virus in the blood and stool occur just prior to or at the time that liver function tests become abnormal. Virus continues to be excreted in the feces for several weeks.

Hepatitis A causes an estimated 1.4 million cases of acute hepatitis worldwide. This virus is spread by the fecal-oral route and is highly infectious. Spread occurs readily in households. Preschool day care centers are an important source for infection because children under the age of two years develop asymptomatic disease and excrete high concentrations of virus in their stool that can be readily spread to nonimmune parents and caregivers. Sexual transmission of the virus occurs in male homosexuals, and intravenous drug addicts readily spread hepatitis A to each other; however, the virus is rarely spread by blood transfusions. Common-source outbreaks occur as a consequence of contaminated water, milk, and food. Raw or undercooked clams, oysters, and mussels are major sources of food-borne disease. These bivalved shellfish filter large volumes of contaminated water, concentrating the virus. A large food-borne outbreak occurred in Maine and Michigan that was traced to contaminated frozen strawberries that had been shipped to both states. Infected food handlers have caused several outbreaks, and hand washing is an important measure for preventing spread of this disease. Breakdowns in sanitary conditions that occur during natural disasters and war increase the risk of hepatitis A. Inactivation of the virus can be readily accomplished by treating potentially contaminated surfaces with a 1:100 dilution of household bleach.

KEY POINTS

Pathogenesis and Epidemiology of Hepatitis A

> 1. A single-stranded RNA picornovirus that is highly resistant to heating and drying.
> 2. Survives in protein solutions, killed by chlorine.
> 3. Enters via the gastrointestinal tract, penetrates the bowel, infects hepatocytes, multiplies in the cytoplasm, is excreted in the bile, high concentrations in the feces.
> 4. Epidemiology:
>   a. Spread by fecal-oral route in day care centers, children < 2 years old asymptomatic infection,
>   b. Sexual transmission among homosexuals,
>   c. IV drug abusers, not usually spread by blood transfusions,

> d. Food-borne: water, milk, bivalved shellfish, food contaminated by food handlers.

CLINICAL MANIFESTATIONS AND DIAGNOSIS

After a four-week incubation period, patients infected with hepatitis A usually experience the acute onset of a flulike illness. The disease is usually self-limited, resolving within two to three months (see Figure 8.3). However, 10% of hospitalized patients have a relapsing course characterized by improvement followed by a second episode of jaundice that usually develops six to twelve weeks later but can occur up to six months after the first symptomatic attack. Prolonged but benign cholestasis has also been reported. Patients with hepatitis A do not develop chronic hepatitis. Young children who have a less robust immune response to the virus often have few symptoms and do not develop jaundice. Fulminant hepatitis is a rare complication and occurs more frequently in patients who are coinfected with hepatitis C or hepatitis B.

Diagnosis is made by measuring serum anti–hepatitis A IgM antibody titers. Levels are observed at the time of symptomatic disease and usually persist for six months. Anti–hepatitis A IgG antibodies progressively increase, titers being low during early symptomatic disease but continuing to rise, peaking at about four months. IgG titers persist for decades (see Figure 8.3).

KEY POINTS

Clinical Manifestations and Diagnosis of Hepatitis A

> 1. Incubation period 4 weeks.
> 2. Self-limited illness of two to three months' duration.
> 3. Relapse can occur up to six months after the primary attack.
> 4. Chronic hepatitis does not develop.

Figure 8.3

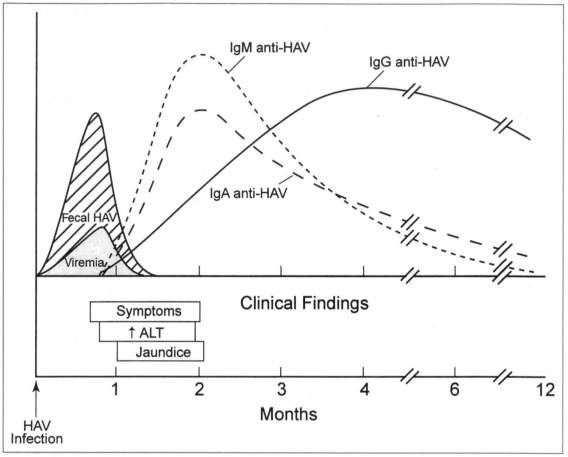

Clinical course of hepatitis A. (Adapted from *Hoeprich Infectious Diseases,* 1994.)

5. Diagnosis: IgM antibody titer detected at the time of symptoms, persists × six months; IgG antibody titer increases later and peaks at four months; persists for decades.

TREATMENT AND PREVENTION

The majority of patients can be managed as outpatients. No therapy is available that will alter the course of infection. Strict bed rest is not warranted, and moderate activity as tolerated is now recommended. In patients with fulminant hepatitis, exchange transfusions and glucocorticoids fail to alter the clinical course, and liver transplantation may be required for survival.

Administration of pooled human immunoglobulin (IG) has been shown to prevent or reduce the symptoms of hepatitis A. Prophylaxis should be given within two weeks of exposure. The duration of protection is dose-dependent; 0.02 ml/kg im affords two months of protection, while 0.06 ml/kg usually protects for five months. IG administration should be considered in U.S. residents who plan to travel in endemic areas if they wish to travel outside of the usual tourist routes. After recognition of the index case, postexposure prophylaxis is recommended for household and sexual contacts; day care center staff and attendees; classroom contacts in school-centered outbreaks; persons residing or working in institutions with crowded living conditions such as prisons, military barracks, and facilities housing the disabled; and hospital personnel who have come into direct contact with feces or body fluids from an infected patient. Prophylaxis is not recommended for casual contacts or in common-source outbreaks.

A safe and effective formalin-killed vaccine is available. The indications for vaccination are currently evolving. Vaccination should be considered for travelers who are planning to travel more than three times to endemic areas over a 10-year period. Passive immunoglobulin therapy is more cost-effective for those who travel less frequently. Significant protective titers take four weeks to develop; therefore if the traveler does not receive the vaccine within this time frame, passive immunization with IG should also be administered. Immunization following exposure is not completely protective. Passive immunization is the preventive measure of choice; however, if the individual is likely to be exposed to hepatitis A repeatedly, IG and vaccine can be administered simultaneously without interfering with the immune response of the vaccine or the protective efficacy of IG.

The vaccine should also be considered for individuals who are at high risk of hepatitis A: homosexual men, illicit drug users, heterosexuals with multiple sexual partners, persons requiring repeated administration of concentrated coagulation factors, and those with an occupational risk of exposure. The vaccine is also recommended for patients with preexisting chronic liver disease. In areas where the incidence of hepatitis A is over 20 per 1,000, vaccination should be considered for children over the age of two years. The dose of vaccine recommended for adults in the United States is 1,440 EL.U (enzyme-linked immunosorbent assay units) given as a 1-ml im injection followed by a booster dose of the same amount at six to twelve months. In children two doses of 720 EL.U in 0.5 ml im given one month apart followed by a booster at six to twelve months is recommended. In other countries a more elaborate immunization protocol is used consisting of three 720 EL.U im doses given at 0, 1, and 6–12 months. The duration of protection has been estimated to be 20–30 years.

KEY POINTS
Treatment and Prevention of Hepatitis A

1. No therapy available.
2. Pooled immunoglobulin (IG) protective if given within 2 weeks of exposure.
3. IG prophylaxis recommended for:
   a. Household and sexual contacts,
   b. Day care center staff and attendees,
   c. Classroom contacts in school-centered outbreaks,
   d. Persons residing or working in institutions with crowded living conditions,
   e. Hospital personnel with direct contact with feces or body fluids from an infected patient,
   f. Travelers to endemic areas,
   g. Not recommended for casual contacts or in common-source outbreaks.
4. Vaccine indications are evolving; recommended for:
   a. Homosexual men and illicit drug users,
   b. Heterosexuals with multiple sexual partners,
   c. Persons requiring repeated administration of concentrated coagulation factors,
   d. Occupational risk of exposure,
   e. Patients with preexisting chronic liver disease,
   f. Children over age of two where high incidence of hepatitis A.

Hepatitis E

This small, single-stranded RNA virus is related to the caliciviruses. The pathogenesis, epidemiology, and clinical manifestations are similar to those of hepatitis A. The average incubation period is similar to that of hepatitis A: 32 days. The virus is secreted in the stool and spread by the fecal-oral route. Outbreaks have been associated with contaminated water in India, Nepal, Southeast Asia, Africa, China, and Mexico. Infection occurs in areas where sanitation is poor and fecal contamination of water is likely. Indigenous cases have not been reported in the United States, Canada, or the developed countries of Europe and Asia. In these countries infection has been reported in tourists who have traveled to endemic areas. As is observed with hepatitis A, the disease is self-limited and does not result in chronic hepatitis. The hepatitis E virus can cause fulminant hepatitis in pregnant women in their third trimester, resulting in mortality rates of 15–25%. Diagnostic tests to identify hepatitis E are not currently commercially available. Immunoglobulin injections have not been proven to protect against hepatitis E, and no vaccine is currently available.

KEY POINTS

Hepatitis E

1. A single-stranded RNA virus related to the caliciviruses.
2. Incubation period: 1 month.
3. Transmitted by the fecal-oral route.
4. Reported in developing countries with poor sanitation, not in U.S. except for travelers.
5. A self-limited disease.
6. Causes fulminant hepatitis in women in their 3rd trimester of pregnancy.
7. No blood test available.
8. Pooled immunoglobulins are not helpful for prevention.

Hepatitis B

VIROLOGY AND PATHOGENESIS

Hepatitis B is a small, enveloped, spherical, partially double-stranded DNA virus and is a hepadnavirus. The outer core contains lipid, as well as the hepatitis B surface antigen (HBsAg) (see Figure 8.4). The host directs viral-neutralizing antibody (anti-HBs) against the HBsAg. In addition to fully competent viral particles, a higher abundance of defective viral particles that form small spheres and filaments are found in the bloodstream of infected patients. These are the most abundant forms of hepatitis B found in the bloodstream. They are noninfectious and are composed of HBsAg and host membrane lipid. The inner DNA-containing core can be released by nonionic detergent treatment of intact virus and contains the hepatitis B core antigen (HBcAg). Infected patients also generate antibody against this antigen (anti-HBc). In addition to viral DNA, the core contains DNA polymerase and protein kinase activities. Treatment of the core with the ionic detergent sodium dodecyl sulfate (SDS) releases a third commonly detected antigen: the hepatitis B e antigen (HBeAg). The presence of this particle in a patient's serum indicates active viral replication, and the generation of antibody to this particle (anti-HBe) signals the end of active viral replication (see Figure 8.5). Mutant hepatitis B viruses have now been reported that do not release the e antigen; therefore the absence of HBeAg does not always indicate cessation of viral replication. These mutant strains are primarily found in Eastern Europe.

The virus has a unique tropism for hepatocytes and has a narrow host range that includes humans, chimpanzees, and a few other higher primates. Hepatitis B virus cannot be reliably maintained in tissue culture cells. It survives in serum for months at 4°C and for years when frozen at −20°C but is killed within 2 minutes when heated to 98°C and when treated with many detergents. Hepatitis B viral DNA can integrate into host cell DNA, and integration may account for the increased incidence of hepatocellular carcinoma in patients who are chronic carriers of hepatitis B virus. These inserts may alter the expression of critical regulatory genes and upregulate host oncogenes.

KEY POINTS

Virology and Pathogenesis of Hepatitis B

1. An enveloped, partially double-stranded DNA hepadnavirus,
   a. Outer core contains lipid and a surface hepatitis B antigen (HbsAg),
   b. Inner core is released by nonionic detergent and is called core antigen (HbcAg),
   c. The e antigen (HbeAg) remains when the core is treated with the ionic detergent SDS,
   d. Presence of HbeAg = active viral replication.
2. Enters and replicates in hepatocytes but cannot be grown in tissue culture, survives in serum at 4°C for months but is killed by heating to 98°C.
3. Integrates into host DNA, may explain increased risk of hepatocellular carcinoma.

EPIDEMIOLOGY

Hepatitis B virus is primarily spread from person to person by blood and blood products. Blood transfusion remains one of the major modes of transmission in the United States; however, screening of donors has reduced the risk to 1 per 63,000 transfusions. Screening tests fail to exclude a small percentage of donors who have infectious viral particles in their blood despite a negative HbsAg. Hepatitis B virus is also found in other body fluids, including urine, bile, saliva, semen, breast milk, and vaginal secretions, but is not found in feces. Membrane contact with any of these body fluids can result in transmission. The virus can be spread to sexual partners and is prevalent in homosexual men as well as heterosexuals with multiple partners. It can be readily spread from mother to neonate at the time of vaginal delivery, a very common event in developing countries. Intravenous drug abusers have a high incidence of hepatitis B. Reuse of needles has also led to transmission of virus during placement of tattoos and ear piercing. Crowded environments, such as institutions

for the mentally handicapped, favor spread. Finally, the virus can been spread to a transplant organ recipient when the donated organ originates from a hepatitis B–infected donor. Hepatitis B virus infection is very common; 280,000 primary infections per year occur in the United States, and the virus is estimated to have infected approximately 5% of the world's population.

KEY POINTS

Epidemiology of Hepatitis B

1. Spread from person to person primarily by blood and blood products.
2. Intravenous drug abusers who share needles, reuse of needles for tattoos and ear piercing.
3. In other body fluids (urine, bile, saliva, semen, breast milk, and vaginal secretions).
4. Mucosal contact with infected body fluid can transmit infection to:
   a. Homosexual or heterosexual sexual partners of infected individuals,
   b. Neonate following vaginal delivery from an infected mother,
   c. Crowded environments such as institutions for the mentally handicapped.
5. 280,000 new cases per year in the U.S., estimated to have infected 5% worldwide.

CLINICAL MANIFESTATIONS AND DIAGNOSIS

The clinical picture of hepatitis B is similar to that of hepatitis A with two major differences: The average incubation period of 12 weeks is longer than that of hepatitis A, and hepatitis B is not always self-limited. Symptoms usually resolve over one to three months, and the transaminase values usually return to normal within one to four months. However, in a significant percentage of patients elevations in transaminase values persist for more than six months. This finding indicates progression to chronic active hepatitis. The percentage that progress to chronic disease is age dependent, being 90% in neonates, 20–50% in children ages one to five years, and 5–10% in adults.

A number of serum tests are available to assist in the diagnosis of hepatitis B, and these are based on our understanding of the virus's structure and life cycle (see Figures 8.4 and 8.5):

1. **The viral capsid surface antigen (HBsAg) and the antibody directed against the surface antigen (anti-HBs)**. The surface antigen was the first test available for detecting hepatitis B. HBsAg appears in serum within one to ten weeks after exposure and disappears within four to six months, indicating recovery (see Figure 8.5). The persistence of

HbsAg beyond six months indicates chronic disease. The disappearance of HBsAg may be preceded by the appearance of anti-HBs, and it is during this period that patients may develop a serum-sickness–like illness. In a large percentage of patients anti-HBs does not rise to detectable levels for several weeks to months after the disappearance of surface antigen. During this window both HBsAg and anti-HBs are negative (see Figure 8.5), and if these two tests alone are used for screening blood donors, a small percentage of infected donors may be missed. To prevent this occurrence, blood banks also test for IgM antibody directed against hepatitis B core antigen (see below). Anti-HBs rises slowly over six to

Figure 8.4

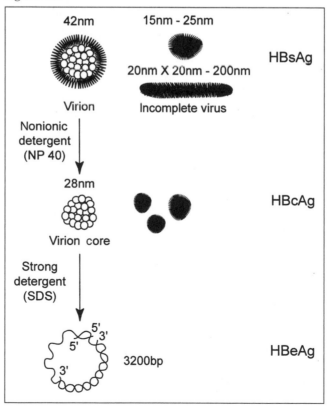

Schematic diagram of the different forms of hepatitis B virus antigen. (Adapted from *Hoeprich Infectious Diseases,* 1994.)

Figure 8.5

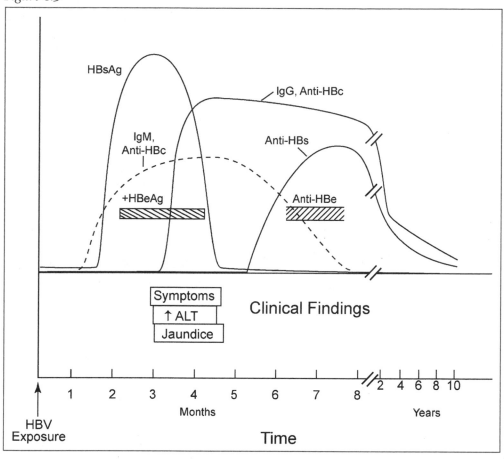

Clinical course of hepatitis B. (Adapted from *Hoeprich Infectious Diseases,* 1994.)

twelve months and usually persists for life, providing protection against reinfection.

2. **Antibody directed against the core antigen (anti-HBc).** The viral core antigen (HBcAg) is detected in infected hepatocytes but is not released into the serum; however, IgM antibody directed against the HBcAg (anti-HBc) is usually the earliest anti-hepatitis B antibody detected in the infected patient (see Figure 8.4). IgM anti-HBc is usually interpreted as a marker for early acute disease; however, in some patients anti-HBc IgM levels can for persist for up to two years after

acute infection, and in patients with chronic active hepatitis, IgM antibody levels can rise during periods of exacerbation. An anti-HBc IgM titer is particularly helpful for screening blood donors because this antibody is usually present during the window between HBsAg disappearance and anti-HBs appearance. IgG antibodies directed against the core antigen develop in the later phases of acute disease and usually persist for life.

3. **Hepatitis e antigen (HBeAg) and antibody (anti-HBe).** The e antigen is made up of the naked DNA strands and associated proteins

(see Figure 8.4). The presence of HBeAg in the serum indicates active viral replication. HBeAg persists in patients with chronic disease, and its presence correlates with infectivity. As the patient with acute hepatitis B recovers, HBeAg disappears, and antibody to e antigen appears. Seroconversion from HBeAg to anti-HBe usually corresponds with the disappearance of hepatitis B virus DNA from the serum.

4. **Hepatitis B DNA (HBV-DNA)**. Quantitation of viral DNA in serum is most commonly used in the assessment of patients with chronic active hepatitis. In the patient with acute hepatitis this test provides no significant advantages over the HBeAg test. Both indicate active viral replication. In patients with fulminant hepatitis, assays for HBV-DNA have been positive in the absence of other positive markers for hepatitis B.

KEY POINTS

Clinical Manifestations and Diagnosis of Hepatitis B

1. Incubation period: 12 weeks.
2. Acute disease similar clinically to hepatitis A; however, persistent infection can develop:
   a. 90% of infants,
   b. 20–50% children one to five years old,
   c. 5–10% adults.
3. Diagnosis is made by serological testing:
   a. HbsAg appears within 10 weeks of exposure, persists for four to six months, > 6 months = chronic disease,
   b. Anti-HBs often develops after HBsAg disappears; Anti-HBs usually persist for life. Anti-HBs and HbsAg may be negative during this "window" transition period,
   c. Anti-HBc IgM positive early is a marker for acute disease but can persist for two years and can increase during exacerbations of chronic active hepatitis. Used for blood screening,

   d. HBeAg indicates active viral replication. Disappearance HBeAg and appearance of HBeAb = clearance of virus,
   e. HBV-DNA: Quantitation of DNA used to assess responses to therapy of chronic disease.

TREATMENT AND PREVENTION

The approach to the treatment of acute hepatitis B is identical to that of hepatitis A, there being no therapeutic intervention to alter the course of acute disease. Prevention requires education of those who engage in high-risk behaviors, screening of the blood supply, and universal precautions by hospital personnel. High-titer hepatitis B immune globulin (HBIG) reduces the incidence of clinical hepatitis B. Immunoglobulin is prepared from the serum of patients with high titers of anti-HBs, and its administration is recommended after the following events:

♦ Accidental percutaneous inoculation or mucous membrane exposure to blood or body fluids from a patient who is HBsAg positive
♦ Intimate contact (living in the same household or having sexual contact) with a patient with acute hepatitis B or chronic active hepatitis B
♦ Birth of a neonate to a mother with acute hepatitis B

HBIG (0.05–0.07 ml/kg im) should be administered within 7 days of exposure. Ideally, the exposed person should receive HBIG immediately because maximum protection is afforded when the immunoglobulin is administered within 48 hours of exposure. A second dose is recommended in one month; however, the efficacy of a second dose has not been proven. In the majority of cases, hepatitis B vaccination should be initiated at the time of the first HBIG injection.

A safe and effective recombinant hepatitis B vaccine is available, and vaccination is now recommended for all neonates. In the United States vaccination is also recommended for all children who did not receive the vaccine as a neonate. Among adults vaccination is recommended for health care workers, laboratory workers who handle blood and blood products, patients who require repeated blood transfusions or clotting factors, hemodialysis patients, morticians, persons with multiple sexual partners, intravenous drug users, residents and staff of closed institutions such as prisons and institutions for the mentally handicapped, and household and sexual contacts of carriers. The vaccine should be given intramuscularly in three doses at months 0, 1–2, and 6–12. In neonates born to mothers with unknown or positive HBsAg, the first dose of vaccine should be given within 12 hours of delivery, and the booster doses should be given at one and six months.

KEY POINTS

Treatment and Prevention of Acute Hepatitis B

1. Treatment is the same as for hepatitis A: supportive measures.
2. Hepatitis B immune globulin (HBIG) should be given to:
   a. Needle-stick or mucosal exposure to blood or fluids from HbsAg-positive person,
   b. Intimate contact with someone who has acute or chronic hepatitis B,
   c. Neonates born to a hepatitis B–infected mother.
3. Recombinant vaccine is safe and efficacious and should be given to:
   a. Health care workers, laboratory workers who handle blood and blood products,
   b. Patients requiring repeated blood transfusions or clotting factors,
   c. Hemodialysis patients,
   d. Morticians,
   e. Persons with multiple sexual partners,
   f. Intravenous drug users,
   g. Residents and staff of closed institutions,
   h. Household and sexual contacts of carriers.

TREATMENT AND PROGNOSIS OF CHRONIC HEPATITIS B

Patients with a positive HBsAg for ≥20 weeks are defined as chronic HBsAg carriers. The carrier state develops in 5–10% of adults. The course of chronic disease depends on the balance between viral replication and the host's immune response. This chronic illness has several stages:

1. **Replicative phase, immune tolerance**. During this phase the virus actively replicates, and serum viral DNA levels are high and HBeAg is positive; however, liver functions are normal, and liver biopsies reveal minimal inflammation. The host immune system demonstrates tolerance to the virus, allowing active replication.
2. **Replicative phase, immune clearance**. In patients with neonatal disease the immune tolerance stage can last for 20–30 years. As this phase ends, the immune system recognizes the virus as a foreign antigen, and active inflammation ensues. Symptoms of hepatitis may develop, although most patients remain asymptomatic. During this period liver function tests become abnormal, indicating active hepatitis. Such exacerbations are often associated with a rise in anti-HBc IgM levels. During this phase HBeAg and viral DNA may clear from the serum. In others the viral replication may continue, and the patient is said to have had an episode of abortive immune clearance.
3. **Nonreplicative phase**. In this phase HBeAg is negative, and anti-HBe appears. HBsAg may persist in some of these patients and may be associated with progression of liver disease.

Patients with persistent HbsAg and ongoing hepatic inflammation can progress to cirrhosis and liver failure. Chronic carriage of hepatitis B is also associated with an increased risk of hepatocellular carcinoma, and HbsAg-positive individuals who develop cirrhosis have a 1.6% incidence of hepatocellular carcinoma per year. To prevent these complications, treatment is recommended in chronic carriers of hepatitis B virus with positive HBeAg. The goal of therapy is to achieve seroconversion from HBeAg positive to negative. Patients with normal transaminase values at the time of therapy have a poorer response rate, and many experts do not recommend treatment under these conditions. The treatment of chronic hepatitis B is rapidly evolving. At the present time three therapies are FDA approved:

1. **Lamivudine**. This antiretroviral drug causes premature termination during viral DNA replication. Lamivudine has been primarily used for the treatment of HIV (see Chapter 17). Treatment with lamivudine (100 mg po QD × 1 year) approximately doubles the seroconversion rate.

2. **Adefovir dipivoxil.** Placebo controlled trials have demonstrated improvements in liver function tests in a significant percentage of patients infected with both lamivudine-resistant and wild-type viral strains following treatment with adefovir dipivoxil (10 mg/day × 1 year). Exacerbations in hepatitis have been observed if the drug is discontinued and increased nephrotoxicity has been reported in patients with preexisting renal dysfunction.

3. **Interferon alpha**. This interferon has potent antiviral effects; however, it is expensive and is associated with a high incidence of unpleasant side effects (see Chapter 1). Treatment with interferon alpha (5–10 million units QD 3×/week for 12–24 weeks) is associated with a threefold higher seroconversion rate from HBeAg positive to negative compared to placebo controls. Seroconversion is often associated with normalization of liver function tests. This treatment is usually reserved for patients who have persistent HBeAg and elevated transaminase values.

Experience with antiretroviral treatment suggests that combination therapy will prove more efficacious, and preliminary trials combining lamivudine with famciclovir demonstrate improved response rates. On the other hand, lamivudine

combined with interferon alpha demonstrated responses comparable to those of single-agent therapy.

KEY POINTS
Chronic Hepatitis B

1. Defined as positive HbsAg ≥ 20 weeks.
2. Three stages:
   a. Replicative stage with immune tolerance, LFTs WNL, viral load high,
   b. Replicative stage with immune clearance, LFTs abnormal,
   c. Nonreplicative stage, HbeAg disappears, HbsAg may persist.
3. Chronic carriers can progress to cirrhosis and hepatic failure. Associated with an increased risk of hepatocellular carcinoma.
4. Treatment:
   a. Lamivudine doubles the seroconversion rate from HbeAg positive to negative,
   b. Adefovir dipivoxil improves LFTs in lumivudine-resistant virus,
   c. Interferon alpha triples seroconversion rate.

Hepatitis D

The hepatitis D virion is a small, single-stranded RNA virus that is surrounded by a single hepatitis D antigen and a lipoprotein envelope provided by hepatitis B. The hepatitis D virus, also called delta agent, can replicate only in the human host who is coinfected with hepatitis B, and when this virus is present, hepatitis B replication is suppressed. Hepatitis D virus replicates at very high levels in the nuclei of hepatocytes and during acute disease is thought to be directly responsible for cytotoxic damage in hepatocytes. Clinically, hepatitis D + B is indistinguishable from hepatitis B. A higher incidence of hepatic failure has been noted with combined infection in intravenous drug abusers. The rate of progression to chronic active hepatitis is the same. This virus is endemic in the Mediterranean basin, having been first discovered in Italy. There is also a high prevalence in eastern Asia (the Pacific Islands, Taiwan, Japan). The mode of person-to-person spread may be mucosal contact with infected body fluids or via injection of blood or blood products. Spread among household contacts is common and is associated with poor hygiene and a low socioeconomic status. The virus can be spread by sexual contact and is common among intravenous drug abusers. In the Western hemisphere the hepatitis D virus is uncommon, being found primarily in individuals requiring multiple blood transfusions or coagulation products and in those using intravenous drugs. Diagnosis is made by measuring anti-hepatitis D IgM and IgG serum titers. No test to detect hepatitis D antigen is commercially available, and there is no specific treatment for hepatitis D. Measures designed to prevent hepatitis B also eliminate the risk of this virus.

KEY POINTS
Hepatitis D (Delta Agent)

> 1. A single-stranded RNA virus that is surrounded by hepatitis B envelope.
> 2. Replicates only in the presence of hepatitis B virus.
> 3. Replicates rapidly in the host cell nucleus.
> 4. Clinically indistinguishable from other forms of acute hepatitis.
> 5. Person-to-person spread by body fluids and blood or blood products:
>   a. Sexual transmission,
>   b. Intravenous drug abusers,
>   c. In U.S., patients with multiple blood transfusions.
> 6. No commercially available test for hepatitis D.

Hepatitis C

VIROLOGY, PATHOGENESIS, AND EPIDEMIOLOGY

Hepatitis C (HCV) is a single-stranded RNA virus that is thought to be enveloped. As this RNA virus replicates, it demonstrates ineffective proofreading, generating multiple mutations and the production of virions in the blood, called quasispecies. These constant mutations allow the virus to evade the host's immune system and cause chronic disease. The virus cannot be propagated by routine methods, explaining the great difficulty in originally identifying the cause of non-A, non-B transfusion-associated hepatitis. Hepatitis C virus has a very narrow host range, infecting only humans and chimpanzees. Within the liver the virus infects only hepatocytes, leaving biliary epithelium and stromal cells uninfected. The virus may also infect hematopoietic cells. The mechanism of hepatocyte damage has not been clarified but probably involves both cytopathic and immune-mediated mechanisms. In addition to acute hepatitis the virus can cause chronic persistent hepatitis and chronic active hepatitis. The latter is characterized by periportal infiltration with lymphocytes and piecemeal necrosis and is often followed by fibrosis leading to cirrhosis.

This virus has a worldwide distribution, and in the United States seroprevalence ranges from 0.25% in low-risk blood donors to 2% among those who exhibit high-risk behaviors such as intravenous drug use. A similar range of seroprevalence is encountered internationally. Approximately 150,000 new cases develop annually in the United States, and 2–4 million people in this country are estimated to have chronic disease. The infection is primarily spread by the parenteral administration of blood or blood products and by needle sharing among intravenous drug abusers. Spread from an infected mother to her neonate is reported but is less common than is observed for hepatitis B. The risk is higher in mothers who are coinfected with HIV. Sexual transmission may occur but is less efficient than in hepatitis B virus or HIV. Coinfection with hepatitis C and HIV is common in the United States and has created new therapeutic challenges (see Chapter 17).

KEY POINTS
Pathogenesis and Epidemiology of Hepatitis C

1. Single-stranded RNA virus.
2. Viral replication is associated with inaccurate proofreading and multiple mutations, yielding multiple quasi-species. Mechanism for evading the immune system.
3. Infects only hepatocytes in the liver, infects only humans and chimpanzees.
4. 2–4 million chronically infected people in the U.S.
5. Spread by:
   a. Blood and blood products,
   b. Intravenous drug abuse,
   c. Mother to neonate less common than in hepatitis B,
   d. Sexual transmission is rare,
   e. Higher risk of infection in HIV-infected persons.

CLINICAL MANIFESTATIONS AND DIAGNOSIS

The incubation period for hepatitis C is six to ten weeks. A high percentage of acute attacks remain asymptomatic, only one quarter of infected patients experiencing the typical symptoms of acute hepatitis. Hepatitis C alone does not cause fulminant hepatitis. It has been estimated that 50–70% of acutely infected patients progress to chronic hepatitis C infection. Serum transaminase values fluctuate during chronic illness. During some periods they may be normal, and at other times they may increase to 7–10 times normal values.

Disease is detected by an ELISA assay designed to measure antibodies directed against specific hepatitis C antigens. The most recent generation of test has a greater than 95% sensitivity and a high positive predictive value. In low-risk populations the ELISA assay should be confirmed by recombinant immunoblot assay. This test has a higher specificity and, when positive, indicates true infection. PCR detection of serum viral RNA allows quantitation of the serum viral load, and some assays claim to detect levels as low as 100 copies/ml.

KEY POINTS
Clinical Manifestations and Diagnosis of Hepatitis C

1. Incubation period: 6–10 weeks.
2. Only 25% of patients develop symptoms of acute hepatitis.
3. 50–75% progress to chronic infection.
4. Diagnosis:
   a. ELISA that detects antibodies directed against specific hepatitis C antigens, 95% sensitivity,
   b. In low-risk populations confirm with recombinant immunoblot assay (RIBA),
   c. PCR methods are able to detect viral load.

TREATMENT AND PROGNOSIS

Unlike hepatitis B, which may spontaneously clear over time, spontaneous clearance is rare in hepatitis C. Approximately 20–25% of patients progress to cirrhosis over 20–30 years. Hepatitis C is one of the leading causes of hepatic failure, requiring liver transplant (20–50% of liver transplants in the United States). Like hepatitis B, chronic hepatitis C is associated with an increased incidence of primary hepatocellular carcinoma.

Treatment with interferon alpha (3 million units QD 3×/week for six months) results in normalization of serum transaminase values in 40–50% of patients compared to 0–6% of placebo controls. However, only 25% of patients demonstrate sustained reductions on discontinuation of interferon therapy. Pegylated interferon preparations have recently become available, allowing once per week therapy, and studies have demonstrated an improved response rate in comparison to standard three times per week therapy. Combining ribavirin (1–1.2 gm po QD) with interferon alpha improves response rates and now is recommended as initial therapy for hepatitis C. Ribavirin is a guanine analogue that inhibits both DNA and RNA viral replication (see Chapter 1). This agent is not recommended as monotherapy but is efficacious when combined with interferon alpha. The duration of combination therapy depends on the initial viral load. Patients with high viral loads, >2 million copies/ml, probably warrant treatment for 48 weeks, while in others 24 weeks of therapy is sufficient.

KEY POINTS

Treatment and Prognosis of Hepatitis C

1. 20–25% of patients with chronic hepatitis C progress to cirrhosis over 20–30 years.
2. One of the leading diseases requiring liver transplantation.
3. Increases the risk of hepatocellular carcinoma.
4. Treatment: Combined therapy has the highest cure rate:
   a. Pegylated interferon + ribovirin,
   b. Duration of therapy depends on initial viral load.

Additional Reading

Infectious Diarrhea

Glass, R.I., Noel, J., Ando, T., et al. The epidemiology of enteric caliciviruses from humans: a reassessment using new diagnostics. *J Infect Dis* 181 Suppl 2:S254-261, 2000.

Gonvers, J.J., Bochud, M., Burnand, B., Froehlich, F., Dubois, R.W., Vader, J.P. 10. Appropriateness of colonoscopy: diarrhea. *Endoscopy* 31:641-646, 1999.

Goodgame, R.W. Viral causes of diarrhea. *Gastroenterol Clin North Am* 30:779-795, 2001.

Gumbo, T., Hobbs, R.E., Carlyn, C., Hall, G., and Isada, C.M. Microsporidia infection in transplant patients. *Transplantation* 67:482-484, 1999.

Ilnyckyj, A. Clinical evaluation and management of acute infectious diarrhea in adults. *Gastroenterol Clin North Am* 30:599-609, 2001.

Okeke, I.N., and Nataro, J.P. Enteroaggregative *Escherichia coli*. *Lancet Infect Dis* 1:304-313, 2001.

Oldfield, E.C., 3rd., and Wallace, M.R. The role of antibiotics in the treatment of infectious diarrhea. *Gastroenterol Clin North Am* 30:817-836 2001.

Sirinavin, S., and Garner, P. Antibiotics for treating salmonella gut infections. *Cochrane Database Syst Rev* CD001167, 2000.

Antibiotic-Associated Diarrhea

Bartlett, J.G. Clinical practice. Antibiotic-associated diarrhea. *N Engl J Med* 346:334-339, 2002.

Yassin, S.F., Young-Fadok, T.M., Zein, N.N., and Pardi, D.S. Clostridium difficile-associated diarrhea and colitis. *Mayo Clin Proc* 76:725-730, 2001.

Primary Peritonitis

Navasa, M., and Rodes, J. Management of ascites in the patient with portal hypertension with emphasis on spontaneous bacterial peritonitis. *Semin Gastrointest Dis* 8:200-209, 1997.

Soares-Weiser, K., Paul, M., Brezis, M., and Leibovici, L. Evidence based case report. Antibiotic treatment for spontaneous bacterial peritonitis. *Br Med J* 324:100-102, 2002.

Secondary Peritonitis

Alapati, S.V., and Mihas, A.A. When to suspect ischemic colitis. Why is this condition so often missed or misdiagnosed? *Postgrad Med* 105:177-180, 183-184, 187, 1999.

Gupta, H., and Dupuy, D.E. Advances in imaging of the acute abdomen. *Surg Clin North Am* 77:1245-1263, 1997.

Liver Abscess

Ch Yu, S., Hg Lo, R., Kan, P.S., and Metreweli, C. Pyogenic liver abscess: treatment with needle aspiration. *Clin Radiol* 52:912-916, 1997.

Hepatitis A

Bornstein, J.D., Byrd, D.E., and Trotter, J.F. Relapsing hepatitis A: a case report and review of the literature. *J Clin Gastroenterol* 28:355-356, 1999.

Levy, M.J., Herrera, J.L., and DiPalma, J.A. Immune globulin and vaccine therapy to prevent hepatitis A infection. *Am J Med* 105:416-423, 1998.

Hepatitis B

Gitlin, N. Hepatitis B: diagnosis, prevention, and treatment. *Clin Chem* 43:1500-1506, 1997.

Lee, W.M. Hepatitis B virus infection. *N Engl J Med* 337:1733-1745, 1997.

Nakhoul, F., Gelman, R., Green, J., Khankin, E., and Baruch, Y. Lamivudine therapy for severe acute hepatitis B virus infection after renal transplantation: case report and literature review. *Transplant Proc* 33:2948-2949, 2001.

Hepatitis C

Moradpour, D., Wolk, B., Cerny, A., Heim, M.H., and Blum, H.E. Hepatitis C: a concise review. *Minerva Med* 92:329-339, 2001.

Shamoun, D.K., and Anania, F.A. Which patients with hepatitis C virus should be treated? *Semin Gastrointest Dis* 11:84-95, 2000.

Genitourinary Tract Infections and Sexually Transmitted Diseases (STDs)

Recommended Time to Complete: 2 days

Guiding Questions

1. What symptoms and signs help the clinician differentiate upper tract (pyelonephritis) from lower tract (cystitis) disease?

2. How useful is the urinary sediment in diagnosing UTI?

3. How valuable is urine Gram stain and what does a positive Gram stain mean?

4. When should a urine culture be ordered and what represents a true positive culture? What does 10^5 CFU/ml mean?

Urinary Tract Infection

Potential Severity: Often an outpatient infection; however, the development of pyelonephritis can lead to sepsis and death. These infections need to be treated promptly.

Urinary tract infections (UTIs) are the most common infection physicians see in their outpatient practice. The clinician must understand the different types of urinary tract infection and know how to diagnose and treat them.

Pathogenesis

In discussing urinary tract infection, it is important to take into account both bacterial virulence factors and host factors. The balance between the ability of a specific bacterium to invade the urinary tract and the ability of the host to fend off the pathogen determines whether the human host will develop a symptomatic urinary tract infection.

Bacterial Factors

Bacteria generally gain entry into the urinary system by ascending up the urethra into the bladder and in some cases then ascending up the ureters to the renal parenchyma. The most common organism to infect the urinary tract is *Escherichia coli,* and certain strains of *E. coli* are more likely to cause UTIs. These strains possess advantageous virulence characteristics, including increased ability to adhere to urethroepithelial cells, increased resistance to serum cidal activity, and hemolysin production. *E. coli* adhere by their fimbria. Pyelonephritis strains are most adherent, while cystitis strains tend to be intermediately adherent. The fimbria adhere to host epithelial cell receptors that contain mannose (mannose-sensitive receptors) and glycolipid (mannose-resist-

ant receptors). Trimethoprim-sulfamethoxazole, an agent used to prevent UTI, reduces the synthesis and expression of the fimbria adhesion molecules.

A number of other virulence factors contribute to the ability of urinary pathogens to survive and grow in the urinary tract. Because urine is an incomplete growth medium, for bacteria to grow in urine they must be capable of synthesizing several essential nutritional factors. Bacterial synthesis of guanine, arginine, and glutamine is required for optimal growth. Pathogenic *Proteus mirabilis* produces ureases that appear to play an important role in the development of pyelonephritis. Motile bacteria can ascend the ureter against the flow of urine. Endotoxins can decrease ureteral peristalsis, slowing the downward flow of urine and enhancing the ability of Gram-negative bacteria to ascend into the kidneys.

Host Factors

The urine contains high concentrations of urea and generally has a low pH. These conditions inhibit bacterial growth. The urine of pregnant women tends to be more suitable for bacterial growth. Diabetics often have glucose in their urine, making urine a better culture media. These factors help to explain why pregnant women and diabetics have an increased incidence of urinary tract infections.

Mechanical factors probably are the most important determinants for the development of urinary tract infections. Mechanical factors can be grouped into three risk categories:

1. **Obstruction**. The flushing mechanism of the bladder protects the host against infection of the urinary tract. When bacteria are introduced into the bladder, the organisms generally are cleared from the urine. Obstruction of urinary flow is one of the most important predisposing factors for the development of UTI. Prostatic hypertrophy and urethral strictures can lead to bladder outlet obstruction.

Defective bladder contraction associated with spinal cord injury also results in poor bladder emptying. These conditions result in a significant volume of urine remaining in the bladder after voiding (increased postvoid residual) and markedly increase the likelihood of infection. Intrarenal obstructions caused by renal calculi, polycystic kidney disease, and sickle-cell disease also increase the risk of renal infection. Proteus and other urea-splitting organisms can cause stone formation and can become entrapped within these stones. Another mechanical problem that increases the risk of upper tract disease is vesicoureteral reflux (defective bladder-ureteral valves).

2. **Urethral length**. Women have a short urethra, and this condition increases the risk of bacteria entering the bladder. The incidence of UTI in females (1–3% of women per year) is much higher than in males (0.1% or less until the later years). At least 10–20% of the female population develops symptomatic UTIs at some time during their life. Trauma to the urethra by sexual intercourse and use of a diaphragm increase the risk of UTI. Colonization of the vaginal area near the urethra is an important risk factor for UTI in women. This event is thought to precede the development of UTI. IgA and IgG antibodies against cell wall antigens have been described. The exact role of immunoglobulins in protecting against colonization and invasion of the urinary tract remains to be determined.

3. **Bypassing the urethra**. Bladder catheterization bypasses the urethra. Within 3–4 days of catheterization, cystitis generally develops unless a sterile closed drainage system is used. Unfortunately, even the most sterile handling of the bladder catheter only delays the onset of infection. All patients with a bladder catheter in place will eventually develop a UTI.

Once bacteria begin to actively grow in the bladder, they stimulate an acute inflammatory response. Polymorphonuclear leukocytes (PMNs) are attracted by chemoattractants released by epithelial cells and bacteria. Over time bacteria are capable of migrating up the ureters and reaching the kidney. The renal medulla is particularly susceptible to invasion by bacteria. The high concentrations of ammonia in the medulla inactivate complement, and the high osmolality in this region inhibits PMN migration. Once bacteria enter the renal parenchyma, they are able to enter the bloodstream and cause septic shock.

KEY POINTS

Pathogenesis of UTI

1. Bacterial characteristics that predispose to UTI:
   a. Adherence via fimbria that attach to mannose-sensitive and -insensitive host cell receptors,
   b. Hemolysin production,
   c. Resistance to serum cidal activity,
   d. Ability to synthesize essential amino acids arginine and glutamine,
   e. Urease production (*Proteus mirabilis*).
2. Host characteristics that predispose to UTI:
   a. Urine: Usually inhibits bacterial growth; exceptions: pregnant women and diabetics (glucose).
   b. Mechanical properties:
      (1) Obstruction, importance of flushing: prostatic hypertrophy, urethral strictures, defective bladder contraction, renal stones, vesicoureteral reflux,
      (2) Short urethral length and colonization of the vaginal area = higher risk in females (1–3% incidence/year versus < 0.1% in males),
      (3) Bladder catheterization: Bypasses the urethra.
   c. Renal medulla: High ammonia blocks complement; high osmolality inhibits PMNs.

Etiology

The majority of organisms that cause UTI come from the fecal and vaginal flora (see Table 9.1): *E. coli* is by far the most common pathogen in uncomplicated outpatient urinary tract infections. Klebsiella is the second most common pathogen, followed by Proteus. In young sexually active women *Staphylococcus saprophyticus* accounts for 5–15% of cases of cystitis. In patients who suffer with recurrent infections, who have been instrumented, who have anatomic defects, or who have renal stones, Enterobacter, Pseudomonas, and enterococci are more commonly cultured. Candida species are frequently encountered in hospitalized patients who are receiving broad-spectrum antibiotics and have a bladder catheter. Two other important nosocomial pathogens are *S. epidermidis* and Corynebacterium group D2. Ninety-five percent of UTIs are caused by a single organism. Patients with structural abnormalities are more likely to have polymicrobial infections.

Table 9.1

Common Urinary Pathogens

	Outpatient	Inpatient
E. coli	75%	Common
Klebsiella	15%	Common
Proteus	5%	Common
Enterococci	2%	Common
Staphylococcus epidermidis	<2%	Common
Group B Streptococcus	<2%	Common
Pseudomonas	Rare	Common

KEY POINTS
Etiology of UTI

1. *E. coli* is the most frequent pathogen, followed by Klebsiella and Proteus.

2. *Staphylococcus saprophyticus*: 5–15% of cystitis in young sexually active females.
3. Nosocomial infections: Enterobacter, Pseudomonas, enterococci, Candida, *S. epidermidis*, and Corynebacterium.

◆ CASE 9.1

A 23-year-old white female was admitted to the hospital with complaints of left flank pain × 4 days and fever × 2 days. One week prior to admission (four weeks after her honeymoon) she noted mild burning on urination. Four days prior to admission she noted left flank pain. Two days before admission she experienced fever associated with rigors and increasingly severe flank pain. She gave a past medical history of recurrent urinary tract infections over the past five years, generally requiring antibiotic treatment once per year. She denied vaginal discharge and was completing her menstrual cycle.

Physical examination: Temperature 100°F; except for mild left costovertebral angle tenderness within normal limits. No suprapubic tenderness. Pelvic exam within normal limits.

Laboratory data: WBC 10,200 (81% PMNs, 2 bands, 13 lymphs, 4 mono). Hct 36, BUN 3, Serum Creatinine 0.4. Urinalysis: SpG 1010, pH 5, 100 WBC per hpf (high power field, nl < 0-5), 0-2 rbc/hpf (nl). No protein or glucose detected. Urine culture: >10^5 *E. coli;* 2 of 2 blood cultures, *E. coli.*

Clinical Manifestations

Patients with cystitis usually experience the acute onset of dysuria (pain, tingling, or burning in the perineal area during or just after urination). Dysuria results from inflammation of the urethra. In addition, patients have to urinate frequently because inflammation of the bladder results in increasing suprapubic discomfort when the bladder is distended and may cause some bladder spasm interfering with bladder distention. Finally, some patients note blood in their urine caused by inflammatory damage to the bladder wall.

As illustrated in Case 9.1, the clinical manifestations of upper tract disease usually overlap with those of lower tract disease (see Table 9.2). However, in addition to symptoms of cystitis, patients with pyelonephritis are more likely to experience fever and chills, costovertebral angle pain, nausea and vomiting, and hypotension. Certain risk factors increase the likelihood of upper tract disease. Patients with diabetes mellitus often experience subacute pyelonephritis that clinically mimics cystitis. The elderly patient is more likely to develop upper tract disease and bacteremia. Finally, the patient with symptoms for more than 7 days is at increased risk for pyelonephritis. When antibiotic treatment for cystitis is delayed for this period, bacteria have time to migrate up the ureters and infect the kidneys.

Another clinical condition that is most commonly encountered in elderly females is called asymptomatic bacteriuria. This condition is defined as a positive urine culture without symptoms. Urinalysis shows no or an insignificant number of white blood cells. This form of bacteriuria does not need to be treated unless the patient is pregnant or a preschool child. Treatment is recommended in the pregnant female because this condition is associated with low-birth-weight neonates. Pregnant women with asymptomatic bacteriuria are also at increased risk of developing pyelonephritis. In preschool children asymptomatic bacteriuria can result in renal scarring and interfere with normal growth of the kidneys.

Urethritis, inflammation of the urethra, can be confused with cystitis. The primary symptom is burning on urination. Urine culture colony counts are less than 10^5 organisms/ml (see below), and the patient usually does not experience suprapubic pain or urinary frequency. Finally, woman with vaginitis can experience burning on urination. Therefore in the woman with symptoms suggestive of cystitis or urethritis accompanied by a vaginal discharge, a pelvic exam is warranted to exclude a pelvic infection.

The physical findings associated with urinary tract infection are usually minimal. Patients with cystitis may have suprapubic tenderness. Patients with pyelonephritis often are febrile and may be hypotensive and have an elevated heart rate. They often are acutely ill, appearing toxic. Costovertebral angle or flank tenderness may be noted as a result of inflammation and swelling of the infected kidney. In the elderly patient pyelonephritis and Gram-negative sepsis may lead to confusion and somnolence. Therefore urinalysis and urine culture should always be included in the workup of acute mental status changes in an elderly patient.

KEY POINTS

Clinical Manifestations of UTI

1. Overlap between the symptoms of cystitis and pyelonephritis.
2. Cystitis: Dysuria, urinary frequency, hematuria, suprapubic discomfort.
3. Pyelonephritis: Fever, chills, costovertebral angle pain and tenderness, nausea and vomiting. More likely in:
   a. Diabetics: Often have only symptoms of cystitis,
   b. Elderly: May present with confusion or somnolence,
   c. Cystitis symptoms for > 7 days.
4. Asymptomatic bacteriuria: + culture, no symptoms, without pyuria:

Table 9.2

Symptoms of Lower versus Upper Tract Disease

CYSTITIS	PYELONEPHRITIS
Burning	All cystitis symptoms +
Frequency, urgency	fever, chills
Suprapubic pain	CVA pain
Dysuria	Nausea and vomiting
	Hypotension

a. Treat pregnant females to prevent low-birth-weight neonates,

b. Treat adolescent children to prevent renal scarring.

5. Urethritis can be mistaken for cystitis, usually < 10^5 bacteria, no suprapubic tenderness.

6. Vaginitis can mimic cystitis; pelvic exam if symptoms associated with vaginal discharge.

Diagnosis

All patients should undergo a microscopic examination of their urinary sediment (see Figure 9.1). Following a careful cleaning of the perineal area, a midstream sample should be obtained and centrifuged for 5 minutes at 2000 rpm. On examination under a high-power lens (100 × oil immersion objective) each leukocyte represents 5–10 cells/ml of urine. Greater than 5–10 WBC/hpf is considered abnormal and represents pyuria. The dipstick leukocyte esterase test is rapid, sensitive, and specific for detecting pyuria. However, false-negative tests may occur, and in patients with a negative leukocyte esterase test and symptoms suggestive of urinary tract infection, a microscopic urinalysis is recommended. The finding of white blood cell casts is strong evidence for pyelonephritis (a rare finding) but does not exclude a noninfectious cause. Increased protein in the urine also commonly accompanies UTI. Unspun urinary Gram stain is very helpful and should be performed in all patients with suspected pyelonephritis. The presence of one or more bacteria per oil immersion field indicates $\geq 10^5$ organisms per milliliter. This bacterial concentration is unlikely to represent contamination and in combination with pyuria and appropriate symptoms indicates active infection.

Urine culture is not required as part of the initial evaluation in young sexually active females with suspected cystitis. However, in all other patients, urine culture should be obtained. Urine in the bladder is normally sterile. Since the urethra and periurethral areas are very difficult to sterilize, even carefully collected specimens are contaminated. By quantitating bacteria in midstream, clean-voided urine, it is possible to statistically differentiate contamination from true infection. In females infection is generally associated with $\geq 10^5$ organisms/ml, and in males, in whom the number of contaminating bacteria tends to be lower, true infection has been found to be associated with bacterial counts of $\geq 10^3$/ml. These statistical values are helpful guidelines; however, one third of young women with symptomatic lower tract infection have <10^5 organisms. The Infectious Disease Society of America recommends that in women with symptoms suggestive of a urinary tract infection, a colony count of 10^3 or greater should be considered significant. It is important that urine cultures be processed immediately or stored at 4°C for no longer than 24 hours before the sample is plated on growth media. Improper handling of urine samples renders colony counts unreliable, and under these conditions quantitative urine cultures cannot be used to differentiate true infection from contamination. Following the completion of antibiotic therapy, all patients should undergo a follow-up urine culture to document cure of their infection because symptoms may spontaneously resolve in the absence of cure. In patients with presumed cystitis a positive culture after short-course therapy strongly suggests either infection with an antibiotic-resistant organism or upper tract disease (see Figure 9.1).

Which patients should undergo imaging studies to exclude an anatomic defect of the urinary tract? Because anatomic defects are unlikely in young sexually active females with cystitis, imaging studies are not recommended in this population. However, women who relapse after therapy (indicative of upper tract disease) warrant investigation, as do all other patients with probable upper tract disease. Other patients who warrant investigation of the urinary tract anatomy include preschool girls after their second UTI and boys and men at any age.

Figure 9.1

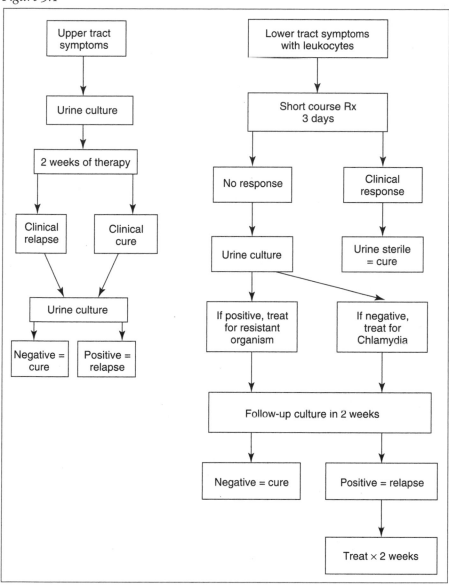

Schematic diagram of how to manage urinary tract infections.

Ultrasonography is recommended as the imaging study of choice. Urinary tract ultrasonography is sensitive, specific, inexpensive, and safe. Ultrasound can detect congenital anatomic abnormalities, renal stones, ureteral obstruction, hydronephrosis, kidney swelling, and bladder distention. An intravenous pyelogram may be required in some patients to further delineate the anatomic abnormalities demonstrated by ultrasonogram. Contrast-enhanced CT scan should be considered in patients who fail to respond to antibiotics after 48 hours of therapy to exclude the diagnosis of perinephric abscess. In the setting of renal failure or multiple myeloma, intravenous contrast often exacerbates renal dysfunction and should be avoided.

KEY POINTS

Diagnosis of UTI

1. Urinalysis should be performed in all patients with possible UTI:
   a. > 5–10 WBC/hpf = pyuria,
   b. Leukocyte esterase dip stick usually sensitive.
2. Unspun urine Gram stain helpful, 1 bacteria/hpf = $\geq 10^5$ organisms.
3. Urine culture requires quantitation to differentiate contamination from true infection:
   a. Not required in sexually active adult females with early symptoms of cystitis,
   b. Females: $\geq 10^5$/ml organisms = infection. Symptomatic females can have 10^3 organisms,
   c. Males: $\geq 10^3$/ml organisms = infection,
   d. Cultures must be processed immediately,
   e. After therapy all patients should have a follow-up culture.
4. Ultrasound is the imaging study of choice:
   a. Perform in patients with upper tract disease,
   b. Preschool females with second UTI, boys or men with UTI,
   c. IVP may be required to further delineate anatomic defects; avoid with multiple myeloma or renal failure,
   d. CT scan with contrast in patients who fail to respond to antibiotics within 48 hours.

Treatment

LOWER TRACT DISEASE

Short-course therapy is generally recommended. Although single-dose therapy may be effective, the preferred regimen is 3 days of antibiotics. Trimethoprim-sulfamethoxazole (1 DS BID), cephalexin, amoxicillin-clavulanic acid, norfloxacin, and ciprofloxacin are all generally effective treatment. Short-course therapy should not be used in men, patients with upper tract symptoms, elderly females (their infections are commonly upper tract and difficult to eradicate), women with more than 7 days of symptoms, or diabetics (who often have chronic pyelonephritis with lower tract symptoms).

UPPER TRACT DISEASE

These patients should receive a longer course of therapy. Two weeks of antibiotics are required. If the patient is not toxic and has not been vomiting, oral antibiotics can be used. Antibiotic treatment should be guided by a urine Gram stain. For Gram-positive cocci in chains (streptococci), amoxicillin is recommended. For Gram-positive cocci in clusters (most commonly *Staphylococcus aureus*), oral cephalosporins (cephalexin) are generally effective. For Gram-negative rods quinolones (ofloxacin or ciprofloxacin) are preferred; if sensitivity is confirmed, trimethoprim-sulfamethoxazole (1 DS BID), trimethoprim alone (100 mg BID), amoxicillin-clavulanic acid, or cephalexin can be used.

Patients with suspected bacteremia (high fever, shaking chills, hypotension) as well as patients with nausea and vomiting should be hospitalized for intravenous antibiotic therapy. Usually, the Gram stain reveals Gram-negative rods. Multiple antibiotic regimens are effective. Intravenous ciprofloxacin has been found to be superior to intravenous trimethoprim-sulfamethoxazole. Other effective regimens include gentamicin or tobramycin, a third- or fourth-generation cephalosporin (ceftazidime, cefepime, or ceftriaxone), aztreonam, and antipseudomonal penicillin (ticarcillin-clavulanate or piperacillin-tazobactam). In patients who demonstrate more severe, life-threatening septic shock, an aminoglycoside should be combined with a third- or fourth-generation cephalosporin, antipseudomonal penicillin, or a carbapenem (see Chapter 2, "The

Sepsis Syndrome"). If a patient relapses, a two-week course of therapy should be repeated. If relapse follows a second treatment, a four- to six-week course should then be given. All patients with relapse should be studied for anatomic defects or stones.

KEY POINTS
Treatment of UTI

1. Cystitis: Short course × 3 days, not for males, diabetics, women with 7 days of symptoms, or elderly.
   a. Trimethoprim-sulfamethoxazole,
   b. Cephalexin,
   c. Amoxicillin-clavulanic acid,
   d. Ciprofloxacin.
2. Pyelonephritis: Treat for 2 weeks; nontoxic, not vomiting can use oral antibiotics:
   a. Gram-positive cocci in chains (streptococci): Amoxicillin,
   b. Gram-positive cocci in clusters (*Staphylococcus aureus*): Oral cephalosporins,
   c. Gram-negative rods: Fluoroquinolones are preferred.
3. Suspected bacteremia with chills, toxic, hypotensive, vomiting: Hospitalize, iv antibiotics:
   a. Intravenous ciprofloxacin is superior to iv trimethoprim-sulfamethoxazole,
   b. Gentamicin or tobramycin is effective,
   c. Third- or fourth-generation cephalosporin (ceftazidime or cefepime, ceftriaxone),
   d. Aztreonam,
   e. Anti-pseudomonal penicillin.
4. Extremely ill patients: Usually treated with two antibiotics: aminoglycoside and a second antibiotic.

Prevention

Patients with frequent symptomatic recurrences should receive preventive therapy. In sexually active women voiding immediately after intercourse is often helpful. Administration of a single dose of trimethoprim-sulfamethoxazole immediately after intercourse is even more effective. In children and others with anatomic defects low-dose trimethoprim-sulfamethoxazole daily (1/2 tablet QD) or 50 mg of nitrofurantoin daily usually eliminates recurrent infection. Antibiotic prophylaxis for patients with indwelling bladder catheters is not effective and simply selects for antibiotic-resistant pathogens.

KEY POINTS
Prevention of UTI

1. Voiding and/or single-dose trimethoprim-sulfamethoxazole after intercourse reduces UTIs in females.
2. Anatomic defects that predispose to UTI: Daily low-dose trimethoprim-sulfamethoxazole or nitrofurantoin.
3. Antibiotic prophylaxis for bladder catheters is not recommended.

Prostatitis

Potential Severity: Acute prostatitis can lead to sepsis and requires acute empiric antibiotic therapy.

Guiding Questions

1. How is prostatitis contracted?
2. What organisms are most likely to cause prostatitis?
3. Should prostatic massage be performed in acute prostatitis?

4. How do the treatments of acute and chronic prostatitis differ?

Etiology and Pathogenesis

Gram-negative bacteria most commonly cause this infection. *E. coli* is most frequent, followed by Klebsiella, Proteus, Pseudomonas, and Enterobacter species and *Serratia marcescens*. Prostate infection is commonly associated with a urinary tract infection and may serve as a reservoir for recurrent UTIs. With the exception of enterococci, Gram-positive pathogens are uncommon. Cases of Staphylococcus species prostatitis have also been reported. The cause of culture-negative prostatitis has not been clarified. There is no significant evidence that Chlamydia, Mycoplasma, fungi, protozoa, or viruses are associated with this disease.

The mechanisms by which bacteria reach the prostate have not been clearly delineated. The most likely pathway is reflux of infected urine into the prostate. Other possibilities include ascending urethral infection, spread from infected lymphatics, invasion from the rectum, and hematogenous spread. The prostate contains a potent antibacterial substance called prostatic antibacterial factor. The production of this zinc-containing compound is markedly reduced during prostatitis, allowing active growth of bacteria. Infection results in influx of PMNs, edema, intraductal desquamation, and cell necrosis.

Symptoms and Clinical Manifestations

Patients with acute bacterial prostatitis experience fever, chills, dysuria, and urinary frequency. If the prostate becomes extremely swollen, bladder outlet obstruction may develop. On physical examination the patient often appears toxic and has a high fever. There is often moderate tenderness of the suprapubic region. On rectal exam the prostate is exquisitely tender and diffusely enlarged. In chronic prostatitis symptoms may be subtle. Back pain, low-grade fever, myalgias, and arthralgias are the most common complaints. These patients often present with recurrent urinary tract infections.

Diagnosis

In acute bacterial prostatitis, massage of the inflamed prostate is contraindicated because of the high risk of precipitating bacteremia. The etiologic agent can usually be identified by urine culture. Blood cultures may also prove to be positive. The diagnosis and treatment of chronic prostatitis are difficult and are best managed by an experienced urologist. Quantitative culturing of the first-void urine, midstream urine, and prostatic massage sample or postprostatic massage urine sample is required to differentiate cystitis and urethritis from chronic prostatitis.

Treatment

Initial empiric therapy for acute bacterial prostatitis should include coverage for Enterobacteriaceae, Pseudomonas, and enterococci. Ticarcillin-clavulanate or piperacillin-tazobactam provides reasonable coverage for these organisms. Another commonly used regimen is ampicillin and gentamicin (once-per-day dosing; see Chapter 1). Once the culture result is available, treatment can be modified. Therapy should be prolonged, approximately three weeks. It should be kept in mind that most antibiotics do not penetrate the lipophilic, acidic environment of the prostate; however, just as is observed in meningitis, marked inflammation allows antibiotic penetration in acute prostatitis, and patients usually respond quickly to therapy.

In chronic prostatitis antibiotic penetration is critical for effective treatment. Trimethoprim is lipid soluble and readily penetrates the prostate.

The fluoroquinolones have also proved effective for the treatment of chronic prostatitis. Treatment must be very prolonged. Trimethoprim-sulfamethoxazole (1 double-strength po BID) should be continued for four to 16 weeks, and fluoroquinolone therapy (ciprofloxacin or ofloxacin) for four to six weeks. Relapses are frequent, and prostatectomy may be required for cure.

Sexually Transmitted Diseases (STDs)

Potential Severity: Usually outpatient infections that can cause significant discomfort but are rarely life-threatening.

KEY POINTS

Prostatitis

1. Primarily caused by Gram-negative enteric organisms:
   a. *E. coli* most frequent,
   b. Klebsiella, Proteus, Pseudomonas, Enterobacter species and *Serratia marcescens* also cultured,
   c. Gram-positives rare except enterococcus.
2. Pathogenesis unclear:
   a. Reflux from urethra, often associated with UTI,
   b. Prostatic antibacterial factor (PAF) becomes depleted.
3. Clinical manifestations:
   a. Acute prostatitis: Fever, chills, dysuria, urinary frequency, bladder outlet obstruction. Prostate tender, do not massage, can precipitate bacteremia,
   b. Chronic prostatitis: Low-grade fever, myalgias and arthralgias, recurrent UTIs.
4. Diagnosis by urine or blood cultures.
5. Treatment:
   a. Acute disease: Ticarcillin-clavulanate or piperacillin-tazobactam or ampicillin + gentamicin,
   b. Chronic disease: Prolonged therapy with trimethoprim-sulfamethoxazole (4–16 weeks) or ciprofloxacin or ofloxacin (4–6 weeks). May require prostatectomy.

Guiding Questions

1. What are the most common causes of urethritis?
2. How is urethritis differentiated from cystitis?
3. Is Gram stain helpful in diagnosing urethritis?
4. Does delay in treating urethritis lead to any serious complications in women?
5. What physical findings accompany pelvic inflammatory disease?
6. Why should physicians have a low threshold for diagnosing and treating pelvic inflammatory disease?
7. What are the most common causes of genital ulcers?
8. Why can't *Treponema pallidum* be seen on routine microscopy and what techniques allow this organism to be visualized?
9. What are the three stages of syphilis and how are they treated?
10. How do the VDRL and RPR differ from the FTA-abs and how should these tests be utilized?
11. What is the leading cause of venereal warts and to what disease does this infection predispose?

Sexually transmitted diseases are a common outpatient problem and warrant continued public health measures, including education and tracking of secondary cases. The incidence of these infections rises in association with decreases in public health funding. The importance of aggressive case finding and early treatment cannot be overemphasized.

Urethritis

ETIOLOGY

Urethritis can be caused by *Chlamydia trachomatis* and *Neisseria gonorrhoeae*. These infections are associated with a purulent penile discharge in males and pyuria in females. *Ureaplasma urealyticum* as well as noninfectious causes (trauma, allergic, and chemical) also result in symptoms of urethritis but are not associated with pyuria.

◆ CASE 9.2

A 20-year-old college junior presents with dysuria and a urethral discharge which he first noted 6 days ago while vacationing in Fort Lauderdale. He admits to several sexual encounters during his vacation. On examination he has a urethral discharge which is yellow and thick. He has no palpable lymph nodes.

SYMPTOMS

As described in Case 9.2, patients with urethritis usually experience burning on urination but usually do not have other symptoms. The severity of dysuria varies greatly. Burning may be worse when passing concentrated urine or after drinking alcohol. This symptom is usually accompanied by a urethral discharge that often stains the undergarments. The urethral discharge may vary greatly in quantity and color and can be primarily purulent or can also contain significant mucus. Some patients note mucus strands in their urine.

CLINICAL MANIFESTATIONS

Examination reveals erythema of the urethral meatus, and milking of the urethra often yields a purulent material that can be cultured, used for DNA probe analysis, and applied to a slide for Gram stain. If a discharge cannot be expressed, a small calcium alginate urethral swab can be gently inserted at least 2 cm into the urethra. Because patients with urethritis often have multiple sexually transmitted diseases (STDs), the perineal area, inguinal nodes, and vagina or penis need to be carefully examined for skin and mucous membrane lesions (see below).

DIAGNOSIS

Gram stain of the urethral discharge is very helpful. A finding of more than four PMNs per oil immersion field is always abnormal and is seen in the majority of cases of acute symptomatic urethritis. In nearly all cases of gonoccocal urethritis, Gram-negative diplococci will be observed within PMNs. The absence of intracellular bacteria strongly suggests nongonococcal urethritis (NGU), caused primarily by *Chlamydia trachomatis*.

Urinalysis of the first 10 ml of urine followed by a midstream sample is useful for differentiating cystitis from urethritis. The finding of higher numbers of PMNs in the first-void sample than in the midstream sample strongly suggests the diagnosis of urethritis. In patients with cystitis, equal numbers of PMNs should be found in both samples. In many STD clinics DNA probes of urethral samples are used to diagnose *Neisseria gonorrhoeae* and *Chlamydia trachomatis*. However, culture may be used in some laboratories to diagnose *N. gonorrhoeae*. Neisseria requires 5% CO_2, and because this organism does not tolerate drying, samples must be immediately plated on selective Thayer-Martin plates. Culturing for *Ureaplasma urealyticum* is problematic and is not recommended. At the present time the diagnosis of this pathogen is usually presumptive and based on clinical findings. It must be kept in mind that many patients with gonococcal urethritis also have NGU.

Table 9.3

Treatment Regimens for STDS (CDC, 2002)

DRUG	DOSE	RELATIVE EFFICACY	COMMENTS
Gonococcal Urethritis			
Cefixime	400 mg po × 1	First-line	
Ceftriaxone	125 mg im × 1	First-line	Some discomfort with the im injection
Ciprofloxacin	500 mg po × 1	First-line	Increased resistance to fluoroquinolones in Honolulu, Hawaii
Ofloxacin	400 mg po × 1		
Levofloxacin	250 mg po × 1 (500 mg QD for disseminated disease)		
Combine with azithromycin (or) doxycycline	1 gm po × 1 100 mg po BID × 7 d		
Spectinomycin	2 gm im × 1	Alternative	
Ceftizoxime	500 mg im × 1	Alternative	
Cefoxitin	2 gm im with probenecid 1 gm po × 1	Alternative	
Disseminated Gonococcal Disease			
Ceftriaxone	1 gm iv or im QD	First-line	Continue for 24–48 hours after clinical improvement, switch to an oral regimen above to complete 7 days minimum
Cefotaxime (or)	1 gm iv Q8H	Alternative	Same duration and po regimen as for cef-triaxone
Ceftizoxime	1 gm iv Q8H		
Ciprofloxacin (or)	400 mg iv BID	Alternative	Same duration and po regimen as for cef-triaxone
Ofloxacin (or)	400 mg iv BID		
Levofloxacin	250 mg iv QD		
Spectinomycin	2 gm im QD	Alternative	Same duration and po regimen as for ceftri-axone
Nongonococcal Urethritis			
Azithromycin	1 gm po × 1	First-line	
Doxycycline	100 mg po BID × 7 d	First-line	
Erythromycin base	500 mg po QID × 7 d	Alternative	
Ofloxacin	300 mg po BID × 7 d	Alternative	
Levofloxacin	500 mg po QD × 7 d	Alternative	
Amoxicillin	500 mg po TID × 7 d	Alternative	In pregnancy only
Metronidazole	2 gm po × 1		Add if recurrent urethritis to treat *Trichomonas vaginalis*

(continued)

Table 9.3

Treatment Regimens for STDS (CDC, 2002) (continued)

DRUG	DOSE	RELATIVE EFFICACY	COMMENTS
Pelvic Inflammatory Disease			
"IV" Regimens			
A. Cefotetan (or)	2 gm iv Q12H	First-line	Continue for 24 hours
Ceftriaxone (+)	2 gm iv Q6H		after improvement
Doxycycline	100 mg po BID × 14 d		
B. Clindamycin (+)	500 mg iv Q8H	First-line	Continue iv for 24 hours
Gentamicin	1.5 mg/kg iv Q8H or		after improvement,
	7 mg/kg iv QD		then switch to clinda-
			mycin 450 mg po QID
			to complete 14 days
Ofloxacin (or)	400 mg iv Q12H	Alternative	Metronidazole adds
Levofloxacin (+/–)	500 mg iv QD		anaerobic coverage
Metronidazole	500 mg iv Q8H		
Ampicillin/sulbactam (+)	3 gm iv Q6H	Alternative	
Doxycycline	100 mg iv or po Q12H		
PID "Oral" Regimens			
A. Ofloxacin (or)	400 mg po BID	First-line	Metronidazole adds
Levofloxacin (+/–)	500 mg po QD		anaerobic coverage
Metronidazole	500 mg po BID × 14 d		
B. Ceftriaxone (or)	250 mg im × 1	First-line	Metronidazole adds
Cefoxitin (+)	2 gm im + probenecid 1 gm po × 1		anaerobic coverage
Doxycycline (+/–)	100 mg po BID × 14 d		
Metronidazole	500 mg po BID × 14 d		
Genital Ulcers			
Herpes Simplex, First Episode			
Acyclovir	400 mg po TID × 7–10 days	First-line	Less expensive
Acyclovir	200 mg po 5×/day × 7–10 days	First-line	Less expensive
Famciclovir	250 mg po TID × 7–10 days	First-line	
Valacyclovir	1 gm po BID × 7–10 days	First-line	
Episodic Therapy, HIV-negative			
Acyclovir	Same as first episode × 5 days	First-line	Less expensive
Acyclovir	800 mg po BID × 5 days	First-line	Less expensive
Famciclovir	125 mg po BID × 5 days	First-line	
Valacyclovir	500 mg po BID × 5 days	First-line	
Valacyclovir	1 gm po QD × 5 days	First-line	
EpisodicTherapy, HIV-positive			
Acyclovir	Same as first episode × 5–10 days	First-line	Less expensive
Famciclovir	500 mg po BID × 5–10 days	First-line	
Valacyclovir	1 gm po BID × 5–10 days	First-line	

(*continued*)

Table 9.3

Treatment Regimens for STDS (CDC, 2002) (continued)

DRUG	DOSE	RELATIVE EFFICACY	COMMENTS
Daily Suppressive Therapy, HIV-negative			
Acyclovir	400 mg po BID	First-line	Less expensive
Famciclovir	250 mg po BID	First-line	
Valacyclovir	500 mg po QD	First-line	
Valacyclovir	1 gm po QD	First-line	
Daily Suppressive Therapy, HIV-positive			
Acyclovir	400–800 mg BID or TID	First-line	Less expensive
Famciclovir	500 mg BID	First-line	
Valacyclovir	500 mg BID	First-line	
Chancroid			
Azithromycin	1 gm po × 1	First-line	Most convenient
Ceftriaxone	250 mg im × 1	First-line	im injection painful
Ciprofloxacin	500 mg po BID × 3 days	First-line	
Erythromycin base	500 mg po QID × 7 days	First-line	Least convenient
Lymphogranuloma venereum			
Doxycyline	100 mg po BID × 21 days	First-line	
Erythromycin base	500 mg po QID × 21 days	First-line	No data on azithromycin
Donovanosis			
Trimethoprim-sulfa	1 DS po BID × 21days	First-line	
Doxycycline	100 mg po BID × 21 days	First-line	
Ciprofloxacin	750 mg BID × 21 days	Alternative	
Erythromycin base	500 mg QID × 21 days	Alternative	
Azithromycin	1 gm po Q 1 week × 3	Alternative	
Syphilis			
Primary and Secondary			
Benzathine penicillin	2.4 million units im × 1	First-line	Retreatment Q1 week × 3
Doxycycline	100 mg po BID × 14 days	Alternative for PCN-allergic	
Tetracycline	500 mg po QID × 14 days	Alternative for PCN-allergic	
Erythromycin	500 mg po QID × 28 days	Alternative for PCN-allergic	Less effective; requires close follow-up
Latent Syphilis *Early, <1 year*			
Benzathine penicillin	2.4 million units im × 1	First-line	
Late or tertiary (except neurosyphilis)			
Benzathine penicillin	2.4 million units im Q 1 wk × 3	First-line	

(*continued*)

Table 9.3

Treatment Regimens for STDS (CDC, 2002) (continued)

DRUG	DOSE	RELATIVE EFFICACY	COMMENTS
Neurosyphilis			
Aqueous penicillin G	3-4 million units iv Q4H × 10-14 days	First-line	
Procaine penicillin + Probenecid	2.4 million units im QD + 500 mg po QID × 10-14 days	First-line	A painful regimen
Ceftriaxone	2 gm iv QD × 10-14 days	Alternative	

TREATMENT

When *Neisseria gonorrhoeae* is identified, treatment with a third-generation cephalosporin or a fluoroquinolone is recommended (see Table 9.3). Because of the high likelihood of concomitant NGU, this regimen should be accompanied by treatment with azithromycin or doxycycline in most cases (for doses, see Table 9.3). About 10% of *Ureaplasma urealyticum* strains are resistant to doxycycline; therefore if urethritis is refractory to doxycycline, a macrolide, a fluoroquinolone, or sparfloxacin is effective treatment (see Table 9.3).

KEY POINTS
Urethritis

1. Etiologies:
   a. *Chlamydia trachomatis* and *Neisseria gonorrhoeae* are associated with a purulent discharge,
   b. *Ureaplasma urealyticum* and noninfectious causes: nonpurulent.
2. Symptoms and signs:
   a. Burning on urination, worse with concentrated urine or after drinking alcohol,
   b. Staining of underwear, mucus in the urine,
   c. Meatus erythematous, milky discharge from penis.

3. Diagnosis:
   a. Primarily by DNA probes,
   b. Gram stain: In gonorrhea almost always find intracellular Gram-negative diplococci, negative Gram stain = NGU,
   c. Culture of *N. gonorrhoeae* using 5% CO_2, have to plate immediately.
4. Treatment:
   a. A third-generation cephalosporin or fluoroquinolone for gonorrhea,
   b. Macrolide, tetracycline, fluoroquinolone, or sparfloxacin for NGU.

Pelvic Inflammatory Disease

Etiology and Pathogenesis

Pelvic inflammatory disease (PID) is primarily a disease of young sexually active woman and is the most common gynecologic disease managed in emergency rooms. It has been estimated that 1 million cases are diagnosed annually in the United States. This disease is caused by spread of cervical microbes to the endometrium, fallopian tubes, ovaries, and surrounding pelvic structures. The vagina contains multiple organisms, lactobacillus being the predominant organism. The endocervical canal serves as a protective barrier, preventing the vaginal flora from entering the upper genital tract and maintaining a sterile environment. Menstruation allows the vaginal flora to bypass this barrier, and as a consequence most cases of PID begin within 7 days of menstruation. It is now thought that nearly all cases of community-acquired PID are sexually transmitted.

The organisms that most commonly cause PID are *Neisseria gonorrhoeae* and *Chlamydia trachomatis*. If treatment of urethritis is delayed, infection of the vaginal area can spread to the uterus and cause PID. Approximately 15% of both gonococcal and Chlamydia urethritis cases progress to PID. These two pathogens may be accompanied by the growth of other pathogenic organisms, most commonly *Streptococcus pyogenes* and *Haemophilus influenzae*. Other pathogens include Group B streptococci, *E. coli*, Klebsiella species, *Proteus mirabilis,* and anaerobes (primarily Bacteroides/Prevotella species, Peptococcus, and Peptostreptococcus species).

Factors that increase the risk of PID include younger age (sexually active teenagers have the highest incidence of the disease), multiple sexual partners, and a past history of PID. The use of condoms and the use of spermicidal agents protect against this infection. The placement of an IUD does not increase the risk for PID in women who are in a stable monogamous relationship.

KEY POINTS

Etiology and Pathogenesis of PID

1. Primarily caused by *Neisseria gonorrhoeae* and *Chlamydia trachomatis*. Other, less common pathogens:
   a. *Streptococcus pyogenes* and *Haemophilus influenzae* most frequently accompany gonorrhea and chlamydia,
   b. Group B streptococci, *E. coli*, Klebsiella species, *Proteus mirabilis*, and anaerobes are less common.

2. Cervical canal usually prevents vaginal flora from invading the endometrium:
   a. Menstruation allows bacteria to bypass the cervix, PID usually begins within 7 days after menstruation,
   b. Delayed treatment of urethritis leads to PID; 15% of cases of urethritis develop PID.
3. Risk factors for PID:
   a. Young age (sexually active teenagers at highest risk),
   b. Multiple sexual partners,
   c. Past history of PID.

◆ CASE 9.3

A 29-year-old woman presents with a 3-day history of lower abdominal pain, frequency, and severe dysuria. Except for two normal pregnancies, her past medical history was unremarkable. Her last menstrual period was normal and began 8 days ago. She was recently divorced. Her present boyfriend was treated for urethritis last week. Examination was normal except for an oral temperature of 100.7°F, lower abdominal tenderness, and moderate pain on lateral motion of the cervix. Severe abdominal tenderness precluded an adequate bimanual exam.

Symptoms and Clinical Manifestations

As described in Case 9.3, lower abdominal pain is the most common complaint of women with PID. Onset of pain often occurs during or immediately after menses. Pain may be worsened by jarring movements or sexual intercourse. Approximately one third of women experience uterine bleeding. Other complaints include fever and vaginal discharge. On physical examination only about half of patients are febrile. Abdominal exam usually reveals bilateral lower quadrant tenderness. Rebound and hypoactive bowel sounds may also be present. The finding of right upper quadrant tenderness suggests the development of perihepatitis (Fitz-Hugh-Curtis syndrome), noted in about 10 percent of cases. On pelvic exam cervical motion tenderness and a purulent endocervical discharge provide strong evidence for PID. Adnexal and uterine tenderness should also be present, or the diagnosis of PID should be questioned. Tenderness is usually symmetric in uncomplicated PID. The finding of increased tenderness in one adnexa and/or palpation of an adnexal mass suggests a tubo-ovarian abscess. Others diseases that may present with similar clinical findings should also be considered: appendicitis, ectopic pregnancy, diverticulitis, adnexal torsion, rupture or hemorrhage of an ovarian cyst, nephrolithiasis, pancreatitis, and perforated bowel.

KEY POINTS
Clinical Manifestations of PID

1. Lower abdominal pain during or immediately following menses:
   a. Made worse by jarring motions,
   b. In one third accompanied by vaginal bleeding,
   c. Vaginal discharge common.
2. On physical exam:
   a. Only half of patients have fever,
   b. Bilateral lower quadrant tenderness, cervical, uterine, and bilateral adnexal tenderness,
   c. Right upper quadrant tenderness = Fitz-Hugh-Curtis syndrome,
   d. Localized tenderness to one adnexa suggests tubo-ovarian abscess.

Diagnosis

A pregnancy test should be performed during the initial evaluation to exclude the possibility of tubo-ovarian pregnancy. A complete blood count should also be performed; however, an elevated peripheral WBC is observed in only half of the cases of PID. Erythrocyte sedimentation rate and C-reactive protein are more reliable in-

dicators of inflammation, and normal values make the diagnosis of PID unlikely. Urinalysis is recommended in all cases to exclude cystitis and pyelonephritis. Pyuria may also be present in patients with urethritis and PID; therefore if urethritis is suspected, a first-void urine sample should be compared to a midstream sample (see above). Microscopic examination of vaginal discharge usually reveals ≥3 WBC/hpf and has proved to be the most sensitive test (approximately 80%) for PID; however, a number of other disorders can also cause a purulent discharge, giving this test a low specificity (approximately 40%). Finally, tests for Chlamydia and gonococcus need to be performed in all patients with suspected PID. Ultrasound should be performed in patients with suspected tubo-ovarian abscess. Laparoscopy has high specificity for PID but low sensitivity, failing to reveal significant abnormalities in half of the cases. This test should be reserved for patients who are seriously ill and in whom a competing diagnosis such as appendicitis is suspected. This test should also be performed in the patient who remains acutely ill despite outpatient treatment or 72 hours of inpatient therapy.

There remains no gold standard for the diagnosis of PID. According to CDC guidelines, the definitive diagnosis of PID requires one of three findings:

1. Histologic evidence of endometritis in a biopsy
2. An imaging technique revealing thickened, fluid-filled oviducts with or without free pelvic fluid or tubo-ovarian swelling
3. Laparoscopic abnormalities consistent with PID

Because of the difficulty of definitively diagnosis and the potential harm to a woman's reproductive health, the CDC also recommends that "health care providers should maintain a low threshold for the diagnosis of PID." Young sexually active females with the appropriate risk factors and clinical findings should be presumptively managed as PID.

KEY POINTS

Diagnosis and Treatment of PID

1. There is no specific test for PID, usually a clinical diagnosis:
   a. ESR and C-reactive protein are elevated; normal values make this diagnosis unlikely,
   b. ≥3 WBC/hpf examination of the vaginal exudate, 80% sensitivity, 40% specificity.
2. Definitive diagnosis can be made by:
   a. Laparoscopy, low sensitivity, should be reserved for the seriously ill patient,
   b. Histologic evidence of endometritis on biopsy,
   c. An imaging technique revealing thickened, fluid-filled oviducts with or without free pelvic fluid or tubo-ovarian swelling.
3. Low threshold for treatment to prevent infertility and chronic pain:
   a. Outpatient treatment: Ofloxacin or levofloxacin + metronidazole × 14 days or ceftriaxone × 1 + doxycycline with or without metronidazole × 14 days,
   b. Inpatient treatment: Cefoxitin or cefotetan + doxycycline or clindamycin + gentamicin,
   c. Laparoscopy for tubo-ovarian abscess, laparotomy for ruptured abscess.

Treatment

To prevent the potential complications and minimize the sequelae of PID, prompt empiric antibiotic therapy is recommended. For outpatient therapy ofloxacin or levofloxacin plus metronidazole for 14 days is recommended. Alternatively, a single dose of ceftriaxone combined with a 14-day course of doxycycline with or without metronidazole is recommended by the CDC (see Table 9.3).

For inpatient therapy cefotetan or cefoxitin should be combined with doxycycline. This regimen should be continued for 24 hours after significant clinical improvement and should be followed by oral doxycycline to complete 14 days of therapy. An alternative inpatient regimen consists of clindamycin and gentamicin followed by oral clindamycin or doxycycline to complete 14 days of therapy (see Table 9.3). If tubo-ovarian abscess is suspected or the patient fails to respond within 72 hours, laparoscopy should be performed, and areas of loculated pus should be drained percutaneously or transvaginally. If a leaking or ruptured abscess is suspected, laparotomy should be performed immediately. The sequelae following PID can include infertility, chronic pelvic pain, and an increased risk of ectopic pregnancy.

Genital Ulcers

The most commonly diagnosed and treated venereal diseases of the skin and mucous membranes are genital ulcers.

Etiology

The most common cause of genital ulcers in the United States is herpes genitalis (usually due to herpes simplex type II), followed by syphilis (*Treponema pallidum*) and chancroid (*Haemophilus ducreyi*). Lymphogranuloma venereum (*Chlamydia trachomatis*) and Behçet's syndrome (unknown etiology) are rarer causes. In India, Papua New Guinea, the West Indies, and parts of Africa and South America, donovanosis or granuloma inguinale (*Calymmatobacterium granulomatosis*) is a major cause of genital ulcers. Trauma can also lead to ulceration. With the exception of Behçet's syndrome these diseases are sexually transmitted. Therefore a complete sexual history and a past history of sexually transmitted diseases must be obtained.

Clinical Manifestations

Certain clinical features tend to favor one etiologic agent over another. However, these rules should be applied with caution because the "classic" findings are seen in only one third of cases. Thus these physical findings, although specific, are insensitive (see Table 9.4).

NUMBER AND LOCATION

The number of ulcers has been purported to be helpful; however, because of the wide variability in ulcer number in each disease, recent studies indicate that this characteristic is not helpful. The one exception is herpes simplex virus (HSV), which frequently presents as a cluster of vesicles and ulcers. The location of the ulcers is helpful in differentiating Behçet's syndrome from other causes. This idiopathic inflammatory disease involves the mouth, conjunctiva, and joints in addition to the genitalia. In Behçet's syndrome ulcers usually form on the scrotum or vulva rather than the penis, anus, or vagina as observed with the venereal diseases.

ULCER SIZE

The size of the ulcers may also be helpful in differentiating the potential etiologies. The multiple ulcers of HSV tend to be the same size, while the ulcers associated with chancroid tend to vary in size and may coalesce to form a giant lesion.

ULCER TENDERNESS

Tenderness on palpation is most commonly noted in HSV and chancroid but is present in about one third of syphilitic ulcers.

Table 9.4

Clinical Characteristics of Genital Ulcers

DISEASES	NUMBER AND LOCATION	TENDERNESS	ULCER APPEARANCE	ADENOPATHY
HSV	Clusters of ulcers Labia and penis	Tender	Uniform size Clean base Erythematous border	Very tender inguinal nodes
Syphilis	One or two Vagina and penis	1/3 Tender	Clean base Indurated border	Rubbery, mildly tender
Chancroid	Labia and penis	Tender	Can be large Ragged and necrotic base Undermined edge	Very tender, fluctuant inguinal nodes
Lymphagransloma Venereum	Ulcer lasts 2–3 weeks Labia and penis	Painless	Ulcer spontaneously heals at time of fluctuant adenopathy	Fluctuant inguinal nodes, groove sign
Donovanosis	Kissing lesions Labia and penis	Painless	Clean, beefy red base Stark white heaped-up ulcer edges	Nodes usually firm, can mimic LGV
Behçet's syndrome	Mouth and scrotum or vulva	Painful	Yellow necrotic base	Adenopathy minimal

APPEARANCE OF ULCER BASE AND EDGES

The appearance of the base of the ulcer helps to differentiate chancroid and Behçet's syndrome from syphilis and herpes. The base is ragged and necrotic in chancroid and yellow and necrotic is Behçet's syndrome, while syphilitic and HSV ulcers have clean-appearing bases. Characteristics of the ulcer edge can also be helpful. In chancroid the edge tends to be undermined, and there is minimal induration. The edge is usually markedly indurated in cases of syphilis. An erythematous border is usually seen in HSV and chancroid. In donovanosis the edge has a unique stark white appearance.

INGUINAL ADENOPATHY

Inguinal lymphadenopathy is commonly encountered with genital ulcers. In chancroid and herpes genitalis inguinal nodes are often exquisitely tender, while in primary and secondary syphilis nodes tend to be rubbery and only minimally tender. In chancroid these nodes commonly become fluctuant and contain significant quantities of pus. Fluctuant nodes are also often encountered in lymphogranuloma venereum (LGV). In LGV the genital ulcer usually heals spontaneously, and three to six weeks later the patient develops markedly enlarged and tender inguinal nodes that become fluctuant (called secondary LGV). Infection also commonly spreads to the femoral nodes. The inguinal ligament that separates the inguinal from the femoral nodes forms a groove or indentation, resulting in the "groove sign," a classic sign associated with this disease.

Diagnosis

The CDC recommends that diagnosis be made clinically and that patients be treated empirically. At the present time the available diagnostic tests either have a low sensitivity or are impractical because of the time required to obtain results. In many instances follow-up is not possible; therefore diagnosis and treatment must occur during a single clinic visit. At a minimum patients with genital ulcers should have a VDRL or RPR drawn, and when possible, this test should be repeated in one month if negative. Because of the increased risk of HIV among patients with genital ulcers, all patients should receive HIV counseling and HIV antibody testing. In areas where chancroid is prevalent and ulcer appearance is suggestive, a Gram stain of the ulcer edge should be performed looking for Gram-negative rods arranged in parallel arrays having the appearance of a school of fish. It should be kept in mind this test is not very sensitive. Where available, culture should be performed using selective media. Also where available, a darkfield exam of an ulcer scraping should be performed looking for corkscrew appearing spirochetes (syphilis), a Tzank prep should be performed looking for multinucleated giant cells, and a viral culture (for HSV) should be performed. In areas where LGV is prevalent or classic findings are observed, an LGV serology should be ordered. A potentially highly sensitive and specific test that is currently available only for investigational purposes is called the multiplex polymerase chain reaction (M-PCR). M-PCR utilizes primers that are capable of identifying the three most common causes of genital ulcers: HSV, *Haemophilus ducreyi,* and *Treponema pallidum.*

Treatment

Empiric therapy depends on the clinical findings, the prevalence of STDs in the area, and the likelihood of follow-up. In most cases empiric therapy for HSV and syphilis is recommended. For the first episode of HSV, treatment should consist of 7–10 days of acyclovir, valacyclovir, or famciclovir (see Table 9.3). For primary syphilis penicillin is the drug of choice. The recommendations for treatment and follow-up are outlined below. In areas where chancroid is prevalent, coverage of *Haemophilus ducreyi* should also be included. Chancroid is effectively treated with a single dose of oral azithromycin or intramuscular ceftriaxone. Other effective regimens include erythromycin base and ciprofloxacin. If LGV is strongly suspected, doxycycline is the preferred treatment. Alternatively, this infection may be treated with erythromycin. Donovanosis is treated with trimethoprim-sulfamethoxazole or doxycycline.

KEY POINTS
Genital Ulcers

1. Six major etiologies: HSV, syphilis, chancroid, LGV, donovanosis, Behçet's syndrome.
2. Diagnosis usually made by clinical characteristics of the ulcer (not always reliable):
   a. Size and location,
   b. Pain and tenderness,
   c. Appearance of base and edges,
   d. Lymphadenopathy.
3. Laboratory studies: VDRL, HIV antibody, Gram stain if suspect chancroid, viral culture for HSV, LGV serum titers, dark field for syphilis.
4. Treatment:
   a. HSV: Acyclovir, valacyclovir, or famciclovir,
   b. Syphilis: Penicillin,
   c. Chancroid: Azithromycin or ceftriaxone,
   d. Donovanosis: Trimethoprim-sulfa or doxycycline,
   e. LGV: Doxycycline or erythromycin.

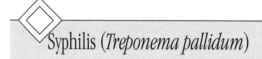

Syphilis (*Treponema pallidum*)

Potential Severity: Not life-threatening, but untreated primary infection can lead to debilitating complications 20–30 years later.

Epidemiology

Treponema pallidum is spread from person to person, primarily by sexual intercourse or by passage through the placenta, causing congenital disease. Less commonly, close contact with an active lesion, such as kissing, or transfusion of fresh blood from a patient with early disseminated disease can transmit the disease. The incidence of syphilis has waxed and waned over the past 50 years as a consequence of changing sexual practices and changing government commitments to public health. The history of syphilis is a rich one, and this spirochete is purported to have infected many famous political figures and artists, including Henry VIII, Frederick the Great, Pope Alexander VI, Oscar Wilde, Ludwig van Beethoven, and Franz Schubert. Syphilis abruptly appeared in Europe during the fifteenth century, and severe epidemics of secondary syphilis, then called "the great pox," were reported in the sixteenth century. It is estimated that by the late nineteenth century, 10% of the European population was infected with syphilis. In 1942, just before the use of penicillin became widespread, 575,000 new cases (approximately 4 per 1,000) of syphilis were reported in the United States. With testing and antibiotic treatment the number of new cases dropped to 6,500/year in the 1950s but then increased in the 1960s with the advent of the sexual revolution. With the rise of homosexual promiscuity in the late 1970s and early 1980s, 50% of new cases in the United States were reported in homosexual men. Many of these patients were also coinfected with HIV. Educational programs encouraging "safe sex" with condoms reduced the incidence in the homosexual community during the late 1980s and early 1990s. However, at the same time the incidence of syphilis increased dramatically in the heterosexual African American and Hispanic populations. By 1992, as a consequence of aggressive public health measures, the incidence of syphilis was reduced from 50,000/year to 28,000/year. Most recently, with the improved success of antiretroviral therapy, the fear of AIDS has decreased, and many individuals have falsely concluded that HIV is now easily treatable. With this reduced fear, "safe sex" practices have been ignored, and the incidence of syphilis has again begun to climb.

Pathogenesis and Clinical Manifestations

Syphilis is caused by *Treponema pallidum,* a fragile bacterium that is long (5–20 μm) and very thin (0.1–0.2 μm) and is a member of the spirochete family. Because it is so thin, it cannot be visualized by standard light microscopy but can be seen by darkfield or phase microscopy. These techniques utilize condensers that shine light at an oblique angle that accentuates the long, corkscrew morphology of the organism. The live spirochete moves gracefully by a characteristic flexing motion. This bacterium cannot be grown in vitro and requires cultivation in animals, rabbits being the most commonly used for live cultures. *T. pallidum* divides slowly by binary fission, with a doubling time of 30 hours (most conventional bacteria double every 60 minutes).

The natural history of syphilis can be broken down into three stages:

PRIMARY SYPHILIS

This slender organism is able to penetrate the skin following sexual intercourse and begins multiplying subcutaneously at the site of entry. The presence of the organism stimulates infiltration by PMNs, followed by T lymphocytes and the generation of specific antibodies. The development of this inflammatory response leads to skin ulceration and the formation of a painless chancre (see above) approximately three weeks after exposure. Spirochetes can be readily identified from skin scrapings of the ulcer by darkfield or phase microscopy.

SECONDARY SYPHILIS

Once the treponemes penetrate the skin, they quickly migrate to the lymphatics and gain entry to the bloodstream, widely disseminating throughout the body. Symptomatic secondary disease occurs in approximately 30% of patients. A skin rash is noted in 90% of patients and usually consists of pink to red macular, maculopapular, papular, or pustular lesions. The lesions usually begin on the trunk and spread to the extremities, often involving the palms and soles. In areas of increased moisture such as the groin area, the lesions may coalesce, producing painless, gray-white, erythematous, highly infectious plaques called condyloma lata. Patches of alopecia may result in a moth-eaten appearance of the eyebrows or beard. Rash is often accompanied by diffuse lymphadenitis. Enlargement of the epitrochlear nodes is particularly suggestive of secondary syphilis. The manifestations of secondary disease usually begin two to eight weeks after exposure. At this stage organisms can be found in the blood, skin, central nervous system, and aqueous humor of the eye. In addition to the skin and lymph nodes, virtually any organ in the body can be affected. Basilar meningitis may develop that can result in deficits of cranial nerves III, VI, VII, and VIII. These deficits are manifested as pupillary abnormalities, diplopia, facial weakness, hearing loss, and tinnitus. Anterior uveitis, immune-complex glomerulonephritis, syphilitic hepatitis, synovitis, and periostitis are other disease manifestations. Secondary syphilis has been called "the Great Imitator," and serologies for syphilis should always be ordered in a patient with unexplained skin rash, lymphadenopathy, lymphocytic meningitis, neurologic deficit, bone and joint abnormalities, glomerulonephritis, or hepatitis.

KEY POINTS

Secondary Syphilis

1. After skin penetration *Treponema pallidum* enters the lymphatics and bloodstream.
2. Disseminates throughout the body.
3. Pink to red, macular, maculopapular, or pustular rash, begins on trunk and spreads to extremities, palms, and soles. Less commonly skin lesions include:
    a. Condyloma lata in moist groin area,
    b. Areas of alopecia in eyebrows and beard.
4. Lymphadenopathy generalized, enlarged epitrochlear nodes suggest this diagnosis.
5. Basilar meningitis can cause ocular motor, pupillary, facial muscle, and hearing deficits.
6. Also causes anterior uveitis, glomerulonephritis, hepatitis, synovitis, and periostitis.
7. Called "the Great Imitator."

LATENT SYPHILIS

After dissemination is controlled by the immune system, the organisms can persist in the body without causing symptoms. During the latent period the spirochetes slow their metabolism and doubling time. Late syphilis is defined as the asymptomatic period of greater than one year after primary infection and often lasts 20–30 years. Prior to one year, patients are at risk of symptomatic relapse and are therefore considered infectious. During the latent period specific antibodies directed against *Treponema pallidum* can be detected by the fluorescent treponemal antibody absorption (FTA-abs) assay or by various hemagglutinin tests (see below).

TERTIARY OR LATE SYPHILIS

Patients who remain untreated for syphilis have a 40% risk of developing late syphilis. This disease causes four major syndromes.

LATE NEUROSYPHILIS   Arteritis can develop in the small vessels of the meninges, brain, and spinal cord, resulting in multiple small infarcts that can cause hemiparesis, generalized or focal seizures, and aphasia. This neurologic disease is called meningovascular syphilis and usually occurs 5–10 years after primary infection. Meningovascular syphilis should always be considered in the younger patient who suffers a cerebrovascular accident.

The spirochetes can also cause direct damage to the neural cells within the cerebral cortex and spinal cord. Cortical damage results in a constellation of clinical manifestations termed general paresis that usually develops 15–20 years after the primary infection:

1. Personality disorder, including emotional lability, paranoia, loss of judgment and insight, and carelessness in appearance
2. Psychiatric disturbances that may consist of delusions, hallucinations, and megalomania
3. Distinct neurologic abnormalities, including an abnormal pupillary response consisting of

small pupils that fail to react to light but accommodate to near vision by dilating, termed Argyll Robertson pupils; hyperreactive reflexes; tremors of the face, hands, and legs; seizures; speech disturbances, particularly slurred speech; and optic atrophy.

Demyelination of the posterior column, dorsal roots, and dorsal root ganglia gives rise to the constellation of symptoms and signs called tabes dorsalis:

1. Ataxic wide-based gait, with foot slap
2. Loss of position sense, vibratory, deep pain and temperature sensation
3. Lightninglike pains of sudden onset and rapid radiation
4. Argyll Robertson pupils
5. Loss of deep tendon reflexes
6. Impotence, loss of bladder function, and fecal incontinence
7. Neuropathy leading to Charcot's joints (caused by persistent trauma) and traumatic skin ulcers

KEY POINTS
Late Neurosyphilis

1. Meningovascular syphilis causes arteritis and cerebral infarction. A rare cause of stroke in younger patients. Occurs within 5–10 years of primary disease.
2. General paresis is due to direct damage of the cerebral cortex by spirochetes, 15–20 years after primary disease:
   a. Emotional lability, paranoia, delusions, hallucinations, megalomania,
   b. Tremors, hyperreflexia, seizures, slurred speech, Argyll Robertson pupils, optic atrophy.
3. Tabes dorsalis is caused by demyelination of the posterior column, 15–20 years after primary disease:

   a. Ataxic gait, loss of position sense, lightening pains, absent DTRs, loss of bladder function,
   b. Charcot's joints, skin ulcers.

CARDIOVASCULAR SYPHILIS Arteritis involves the feeding vessels of the aorta, the vasa vasorum, resulting in necrosis of the media of the vessels and progressive dilatation of the aorta that can lead to aortic regurgitation, congestive heart failure, and coronary artery stenosis causing angina. Less commonly, asymptomatic sacular aneurysms of the ascending aortic, transverse, and less commonly descending aorta may develop. Chest X-ray may demonstrate streaks of calcification in the aorta suggesting the diagnosis. Cardiovascular manifestations arise 15–30 years after primary infection in 10% of untreated patients.

LATE BENIGN GUMMAS A gumma is a nonspecific granulomatouslike lesion that can develop in the skin, bone, mucous membranes, or less commonly other organs. In the antibiotic era these lesions are rare with the exception of AIDS patients. In the skin the gumma can break down and form a chronic nonhealing ulcer. Bone gummas usually develop in the long bones and are associated with localized tenderness, bone destruction, and chronic draining sinuses. Visceral gummas can be found in any organ, most commonly presenting as mass lesions in the cerebral cortex, liver, and gastric antrum.

KEY POINTS
Cardiovascular Syphilis and Late Benign Gummas

1. Arteritis of the vasa vasorum causes damage to the aortic vessel wall 15–30 years after primary disease:
   a. Dilatation of the proximal aorta leading to aortic regurgitation and CHF,
   b. Sacular aneurysms primarily of the ascending and transverse aorta,

c. Chest X-ray may demonstrate linear calcifications of the aorta.

2. Gummas are granulomatouslike lesions, rare except for AIDS patients:
   a. Skin gummas can break down and form a chronic ulcer,
   b. Lytic bone lesions can cause tenderness and draining sinuses,
   c. Mass lesions of cerebral cortex, liver, and gastric antrum.

Diagnosis

The diagnosis of syphilis is complicated by the fact that *Treponema pallidum* cannot be cultured in vitro. Primary and secondary disease can be diagnosed by examining skin scrapings by darkfield microscopy. This test is not readily available in many laboratories and requires a skilled technician. More recently, fluorescently conjugated antitreponemal antibodies have proven to be more sensitive than darkfield, but their use is more technically demanding. This antibody can also be used to identify the spirochete in biopsy specimens. PCR identification of treponemal DNA is under development but is not commercially available. Serologic testing remains the primary method of making a diagnosis in most cases. The CDC has published extensive guidelines for the serodiagnosis and treatment of syphilis (see Additional Reading). There are two classes of serologic tests:

NONTREPONEMAL TESTS

These tests measure antibody levels to cardiolipin-cholesterol-lecithin antigen (previously called reagin). The most commonly used tests in this class are the VDRL and RPR; both measure the highest dilution of serum that causes the antigen to flocculate on a slide. In 2% of cases a prozone phenomenon is observed. That is, when the antibody titer is high, a flocculate is not observed in the undiluted sample, probably as a consequence of an imbalance between antigen and antibody. When the same sample is diluted, antibody-antigen ratios are more balanced, and a flocculate develops.

The VDRL or RPR titer is usually highest in secondary or early latent disease and following appropriate treatment usually decreases to <1:4; in one quarter of patients the VDRL or RPR becomes negative. In patients with primary or secondary syphilis there is usually a fourfold decline within six months of treatment and an eightfold decline by 12 months. In patients with late syphilis the decline is usually slower, fourfold over 12 months. A titer change of fourfold or greater is considered significant. The rate of titer decline is slower in patients with prolonged infection, a history of recurrent infection, and a high pretreatment titer. In a small number of patients the test remains persistently positive, and the patients are called chronic persisters. A persistent elevation represents a false positive, persistent active infection, or reinfection, particularly when the titer remains elevated above 1:4. False-positive tests are rarely encountered with the modern, more highly purified antigen, being most commonly observed in patients with connective tissue diseases or HIV infection. The nontreponemal test is recommended for screening and to monitor the response to antibiotic therapy.

SPECIFIC TREPONEMAL TESTS

These tests measure specific antibodies directed against the *Treponema pallidum* spirochete. The FTA-abs is the standard indirect immunofluorescent antibody test. Serum is absorbed with nonpathogenic treponemes to remove nonspecific cross-reactive antibodies. A 1:5 dilution of the serum is then mixed with pathogenic *T. pallidum* harvested from infected rabbits, and antibody binding is measured by subsequently incubating the spirochetes with a fluorescently conjugated anti-human IgG. This test is very specific but is difficult to quantify and does not predict active disease. A positive treponemal antibody test indicates only that the patient has been exposed to syphilis in the past. Other tests with similar specificity are the TPHA and MHATP test. The specific treponeme tests are used to verify a positive VDRL or RPR but cannot be used to follow the response to therapy. One of these tests should also be ordered in patients with suspected neurosyphilis who have a negative VDRL (see below).

CSF EXAMINATION

In patients with latent disease, cerebrospinal fluid should be examined if there are ophthalmic signs or symptoms, if there is evidence to suggest tertiary syphilis, if the patient's VDRL or RPR titer fails to decline following appropriate therapy, or if the patient develops HIV infection in association with late latent syphilis or syphilis of unknown duration. Neurosyphilis is accompanied by CSF white blood cell counts of 10–400/mm^3 with a predominance of lymphocytes and an elevated protein of 45–200 mg/dl. The CSF VDRL is positive in about half of active cases. The peripheral VDRL or RPR is negative in about one quarter of cases of neurosyphilis; however, the peripheral FTA-abs is usually reactive. Therefore when neurosyphilis is suspected, a specific antitreponemal test needs to be ordered to exclude this diagnosis.

KEY POINTS
Testing for Syphilis

1. Nontreponemal tests: VDRL and RPR test the ability of serum to flocculate a cardiolipin-cholesterol-lecithin antigen.
   a. Few false positives with modern tests, usually connective tissue disease,
   b. Prozone phenomenon observed in 2% of cases,
   c. Use as a marker for response to therapy.
2. Treponemal tests: Measure antibody directed against the treponeme.

   a. Specific and sensitive, antibody titers may persist for life,
   b. Not useful for assessing disease activity, used to verify a positive VDRL or RPR.
3. CSF examination:
   a. VDRL positive in the CSF in 1/2 of cases of neurosyphilis,
   b. Peripheral VDRL positive in 3/4 of cases,
   c. Specific treponemal test positive in all cases, order when considering neurosyphilis.

Treatment

Penicillin remains the treatment of choice for all forms of syphilis, and penicillin's efficacy is well documented. However, the optimal dose of penicillin and the duration of therapy have never been proven by well-designed studies. Because of the slow rate of *Treponema pallidum* growth, therapy for a minimum of two weeks and levels of 0.03 µg/ml or higher are thought to be important to ensure killing. Intramuscular benzathine penicillin maintains constant serum concentrations of antibiotic but might not maintain cidal serum levels. Therefore it is important that patients receiving conventional intramuscular benzathine penicillin receive appropriate follow-up testing to document cure.

The Jarisch-Herxheimer reaction is a well-described systemic reaction following initiation of antibiotic treatment in patients with syphilis. Patients experience the abrupt onset of fever, chills, muscle aches, and headache. These symptoms are often accompanied by hyperventilation, tachycardia, flushing, and mild hypotension. These symptoms usually begin 1–2 hours after the first dose of antibiotic is given and most commonly follow penicillin treatment. A Jarisch-Herxheimer reaction is reported in the majority of secondary syphilis cases (70–90%) but can occur with antibiotic treatment of any stage of syphilis (10–25%). Patients should be warned of the high likelihood of this reaction and should be informed that the symptoms are self-limited, lasting approximately 12–24 hours. The Jarisch-Herxheimer reaction can be aborted by simultaneously administering a single dose of prednisone (60 mg po) with the first dose of antibiotic. Prednisone pretreatment is recommended for pregnant women and patients with symptomatic cardiovascular disease or neurosyphilis. Aspirin every 4 hours for 24–48 hours will also ameliorate the symptoms.

The current recommendations for the treatment for the various stages of syphilis are listed below and summarized in Table 9.3:

1. **Primary and secondary syphilis**. A single intramuscular dose of benzathine penicillin G, 2.4 million units, remains the recommended treatment regimen. Patients should be reexamined at six months and one year. Treatment failure or reinfection is diagnosed if symptoms persist or recur or if the VDRL or RPR titer increases by fourfold. Under these circumstances the patient should be evaluated for HIV, a lumbar puncture should be performed, and the patient should be retreated with three doses of benzathine penicillin (2.4 million units im Q 1 week). In patients with penicillin allergy, doxycycline or tetracycline should be given for two weeks. In pregnant patients skin testing should be performed against penicillin. If positive, the patient should be desensitized and treated with penicillin.

2. **Latent syphilis.**
   a. Early latent (<1 year since documented exposure): A single dose of benzathine penicillin or in the penicillin-allergic patient doxycycline for four weeks.
   b. Late latent (>1 year or unknown duration): Three doses of benzathine penicillin; in the penicillin-allergic patient doxycycline for four weeks. If the symptoms of syphilis develop, the patient's VDRL or RPR titer increases by fourfold, or the initial titer is >1:32 and fails to decrease by fourfold over 12–24 months, a

lumbar puncture should be performed to exclude neurosyphilis, and the patient should be retreated.

3. **Neurosyphilis or ocular syphilis.** The preferred treatment is aqueous penicillin G 12–24 units QD in Q4H doses for 10–14 days. In the highly reliable patient outpatient treatment may be achieved with procaine penicillin (2.4 million units im QD) plus probenecid (500 mg po QID) for 10–14 days. In the penicillin-allergic patient desensitization is recommended.

4. **Late syphilis (other than neurosyphilis, i.e., gumma or cardiovascular syphilis).** Same as late latent syphilis.

Patients with HIV and syphilis at any stage should be treated as if they have neurosyphilis. Aggressive serologic follow-up is recommended, and if titers fail to drop, retreatment is usually recommended.

KEY POINTS
Treatment of Syphilis

1. Penicillin is the drug of choice:
   a. Therapy needs to be prolonged (2 weeks) because of the slow rate of growth of the treponeme,
   b. Jarisch-Herxheimer reaction is common: 10–25% in most stages, 70–90% in secondary disease.
2. Primary or secondary syphilis: im benzathine penicillin or PCN-allergic doxycycline × 2 weeks.
3. Early late syphilis (<1 year): im benzathine penicillin or PCN-allergic doxycycline × 4 weeks.
4. Late latent syphilis: im benzathine penicillin × 3 once per week or PCN-allergic doxycycline × 4 weeks.
5. Neurosyphilis: iv aqueous penicillin G × 2 weeks or im procaine penicillin + probenecid × 2 weeks.

6. Late syphilis (other than neurosyphilis): im benzathine penicillin × 3 once per week or doxycycline × 4 weeks.

Papular GU Lesions

In addition to ulcers, syphilis, LGV, chancroid, and herpes can cause papules. Condyloma acuminata or anogenital warts are a common form of venereal disease that form papules and are caused by human papillomavirus. Lesions are flesh- to gray-colored, raised, and often pedunculated. They can be less than a millimeter to several square meters in size. Lesions are seen on the penile shaft and in uncircumcised men on the prepuce. In homosexual men warts are commonly found in the perirectal region, while in women they are distributed over the lower perineum and can involve the labia and clitoris. Early lesions can be visualized by treating the skin with 3–5% acetic acid for 3–5 minutes and appear as flat, white plaques after this treatment. Infection with certain strains of papilloma virus predisposes to epithelial cancers, and infection of the cervix is a major risk factor for the subsequent development of cervical cancer. Oncogenic viral strains produce early proteins that impair the function of epithelial cell p53 protein, a negative regulator of cell growth. Multiple therapies are available. All regimens are palliative and include cryotherapy with liquid nitrogen, laser surgery, or topical therapy with 10% podophyllin, 0.5% podophyllotoxin (podofilox), or 5% 5-fluorouracil cream. Intralesional interferon has also been used with reasonable success. Given the complexity of therapy, the likelihood of relapse, and the risk of genital premalignant and malignant lesions, genital warts should be treated by a qualified specialist.

A rarer form of venereal wart is called molluscum contagiosum and is caused by a poxvirus. Lesions are usually discrete, firm, small, umbilicated papules. In normal hosts they often resolve spontaneously. However, in immunocompromised patients they may persist and spread. This infection can be particularly troublesome in patients with advanced AIDS. Several patients have been successfully treated with cidofovir, but to date there has been no controlled clinical trial confirming the efficacy of this treatment.

KEY POINTS
Venereal Warts

1. Condyloma acuminata, or anogenital warts, are caused by the human papillomavirus.
2. Vary in size and can be visualized by treatment with 3–5% acetic acid.
3. Predispose to epithelial cell cancers by altering the function of p53 protein.
4. Palliative treatment available:
   a. Cryotherapy with liquid nitrogen,
   b. Laser surgery,
   c. Topical therapy with 10% podophyllin, 0.5% podophyllotoxin (podofilox), or 5% 5-fluorouracil cream,
   d. Intralesional interferon.
5. Molluscum contagiosum is a rarer form of venereal warts due to a pox virus seen in AIDS patients.

Additional Reading

UTI

Bent, S., Nallamothu, B.K., Simel, D.L., Fihn, S.D., and Saint, S. Does this woman have an acute uncomplicated urinary tract infection? *JAMA* 287:2701-2710, 2002.

Gupta, K., Hooton, T.M., Roberts, P.L., and Stamm, W.E. Patient-initiated treatment of uncomplicated recurrent urinary tract infections in young women. *Ann Intern Med* 135:9-16, 2001.

Gupta, K., Scholes, D., and Stamm, W.E. Increasing prevalence of antimicrobial resistance among uropathogens causing acute uncomplicated cystitis in women. *JAMA* 281:736-738, 1999.

McIsaac, W.J., Low, D.E., Biringer, A., Pimlott, N., Evans, M., and Glazier, R. The impact of empirical management of acute cystitis on unnecessary antibiotic use. *Arch Intern Med* 162:600-605, 2002.

Scholes, D., Hooton, T.M., Roberts, P.L., Stapleton, A.E., Gupta, K., and Stamm, W.E. Risk factors for recurrent urinary tract infection in young women. *J Infect Dis* 182:1177-1182, 2000.

Prostatitis

Collins, M.M., Meigs, J.B., Barry, M.J., Walker Corkery, E., Giovannucci, E., and Kawachi, I. Prevalence and correlates of prostatitis in the health professionals follow-up study cohort. *J Urol* 167:1363-1366, 2002.

Collins, M.M., Stafford, R.S., O'Leary, M.P., and Barry, M.J. How common is prostatitis? A national survey of physician visits. *J Urol* 159:1224-1228, 1998.

Naber, K.G., Sorgel, F., Kinzig, M., and Weigel, D.M. Penetration of ciprofloxacin into prostatic fluid, ejaculate and seminal fluid in volunteers after an oral dose of 750 mg. *J Urol* 150:1718-1721, 1993.

PID

McNeeley, S.G., Hendrix, S.L., Mazzoni, M.M., Kmak, D.C., and Ransom, S.B. Medically sound, cost-effective treatment for pelvic inflammatory disease and tuboovarian abscess. *Am J Obstet Gynecol* 178:1272-1278, 1998.

Ness, R.B., Soper, D.E., Holley, R.L., et al. Effectiveness of inpatient and outpatient treatment strategies for women with pelvic inflammatory disease: results from the Pelvic Inflammatory Disease Evaluation and Clinical Health (PEACH) Randomized Trial. *Am J Obstet Gynecol* 186:929-937, 2002.

Scholes, D., Stergachis, A., Heidrich, F.E., Andrilla, H., Holmes, K.K., and Stamm, W.E. Prevention of pelvic inflammatory disease by screening for cervical chlamydial infection. *N Engl J Med* 1996; 334:1362-1366, 1996.

STDs

Centers for Disease Control. Sexually transmitted diseases Guidelines 2002. *MMWR* 51:1-77, 2002.

Daniel P. Lew and
Frederick S. Southwick

Chapter

10

Skin and Soft Tissue Infections

Recommended Time to Complete: 1 day

Guiding Questions

1. Which are the two most common bacteria causing skin infections?

2. Which skin and soft tissue infections require surgical intervention?

3. What clinical clues help to differentiate cellulitis from necrotizing fasciitis?

4. What conditions predispose to necrotizing fasciitis?

5. Which two organisms most commonly cause myonecrosis?

6. Should prophylactic antibiotics be given for human and animal bites?

7. When should tetanus toxoid vaccine and human tetanus immunoglobulin be given?

8. What is tinea and how is this infection treated?

Potential Severity: Can progress rapidly to shock and death. For deeper soft tissue infections, immediate antibiotic therapy is required, often accompanied by surgical debridement.

Classification of Skin and Soft Tissue Infections

Skin and soft tissue infections often produce an acute illness causing patients to seek medical attention in the emergency room. Cellulitis, which is

Figure 10.1

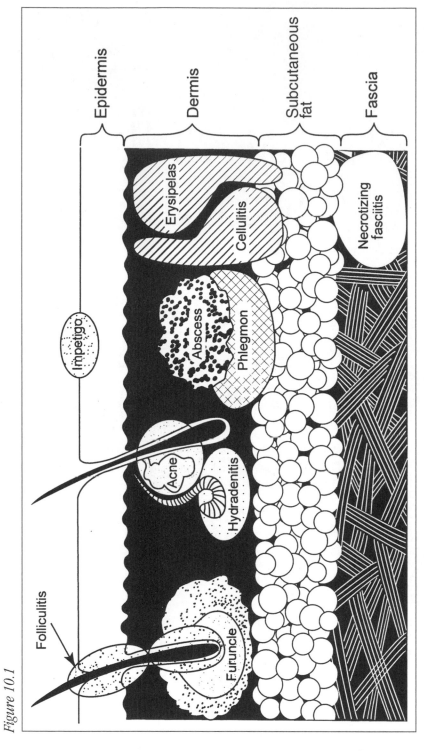

Schematic drawing of the anatomic sites of soft tissue infections. (Adapted from Saurat, J.-H., Grosshans, E., Laugier, P., and Lachapelle, J.-M.: *Dermatologic et Vénéréologic*, 2nd edition. Editions Masson, 1990, p. 109.)

a superficial, spreading infection involving subcutaneous tissue, is the most common skin infection leading to hospitalization. Two microorganisms are responsible for most cutaneous infections in immunocompetent patients: group A streptococcus (GAS) and *S. aureus*. Figure 10.1 depicts the different anatomic locations of skin and soft tissue infection. The symptoms and signs overlap; however, each infection has distinct clinical features.

More superficial infections include impetigo, erysipelas, and folliculitis. As they penetrate deeper, they may become furunculosis (associated with hair follicles), hidradenitis (associated with sweat glands), and skin abscess. Most superficial localized infections (impetigo, folliculitis, and furuncles) are caused by *S. aureus* or GAS, rarely require hospitalization, and may respond to local measures, and recurrence may be prevented by decreasing specific microbial carriage.

However, once these infections spread through subcutaneous tissues, as in the case of cellulitis, the infection may become fulminant and, if not treated energetically by parenteral antibiotics, may prove to be fatal. Delay in therapy as well as certain predisposing conditions can result in deeper extension of infection, vascular thrombosis, and tissue necrosis. In addition to antibiotic therapy these deeper infections require emergency surgical debridement. A very severe form of deep tissue infection called necrotizing fasciitis is usually due to GAS. Necrotizing fasciitis is associated with thrombosis of vessels in the fascia and requires fasciotomy. Severe streptococcal infection may also involve muscles and in this case it is defined as myonecrosis or necrotizing myositis. These severe infections, which can lead to sepsis and irreversible septic shock, have been largely published in the media as infections due to "flesh-eating bacteria."

KEY POINTS
Classification of Skin and Soft Tissue Infections

1. Superficial infections usually can be treated on an outpatient basis:

   a. Most superficial: impetigo, erysipelas, and folliculitis,

   b. Deeper localized infections: furunculosis, hidradenitis, and skin abscesses.

2. Deeper infections require hospitalization, parenteral antibiotics, and surgical debridement:

   a. Cellulitis is the most superficial and can be treated with systemic antibiotics alone,

   b. Necrotizing fasciitis involves the fascia and requires emergent surgery,

   c. Myonecrosis also requires rapid surgical debridement and is often fatal.

Severe Skin and Soft Tissue Infections

Cellulitis

Cellulitis is one of the more common infectious diseases and is managed by clinicians practicing in a wide variety of specialties. Cellulitis is an inflammatory process involving the skin and supporting tissues with some extension into the subcutaneous tissues. The most common location is the extremities. Not only is the infection common, but some patients develop frequent recurrences of cellulitis.

PREDISPOSING FACTORS

Several predisposing factors increase the likelihood of cellulitis:

1. Venous and/or lymphatic compromise secondary to surgery, previous thrombophlebitis, or previous trauma as well as right-sided congestive heart failure. This is the most common underlying condition leading to cellulitis.

2. Diabetes mellitus, which results in progressive peripheral neuropathy and small vessel occlusion. These conditions lead to inadvertent trauma, poor wound healing, and tissue necrosis.

3. Chronic alcoholism, which probably predisposes to cellulitis as a consequence of trauma to the skin and poor hygiene.

Not all patients with cellulitis have definable risk factors for the development of infection; about 50% of patients present without predisposing disease.

CLINICAL MANIFESTATIONS AND ETIOLOGY

◆ CASE 10.1

A 50-year-old Caucasian man arrived in the emergency room complaining of progressive warmth and erythema of his right leg. Three days earlier he accidentally hit his right shin on a tree stump. Approximately 24 hours later he noted increasing pain and erythema at the site of the small break in his skin. Erythema spread from his shin to his entire lower leg. He also noted fever and chills. On physical exam he appeared moderately ill. His right lower leg was diffusely red and edematous, sparing a small region of his posterior calf. The margins of erythema were indistinct. His right inguinal nodes were enlarged and tender. There was no crepitance; however, the leg was very tender. A small skin break was noted on the right anterior shin. Laboratory abnormalities included an elevated peripheral WBC of 15,500 (75% PMNs, 15% band forms). Blood cultures ×2 were positive for Group A, beta-hemolytic streptococci.

As observed in Case 10.1, there is swelling of the involved area and macular erythema that is largely confluent. On examination warmth and tenderness of the involved skin are most often found. Careful examination often reveals lymphangitis and tender regional lymphadenopathy. Presence of accompanying tinea pedis or other dermatologic abnormalities such as psoriasis or dyshidrosis in patients with lower extremity involvement should be sought because these are preventable ports of entry, and treatment of these dermatologic disorders may reduce the frequency of recurrent cellulitis. In patients presenting in the emergency room, systemic findings must be sought. Systemic toxicity including fever, chills, and myalgias is seen in patients presenting with severe cellulitis.

Cellulitis in the majority of patients is caused by beta-hemolytic streptococci, including groups A, B, C, and G. *Staphylococcus aureus* is also a common cause of cellulitis. *Haemophilus influenzae* in children can produce facial cellulitis or erysipelas.

SPECIAL FORMS OF CELLULITIS

ERYSIPELAS   Erysipelas represents a distinct form of superficial cellulitis that is associated with marked swelling of the integument with sharp demarcation between involved and normal tissues and often with prominent lymphatic involvement. It is almost always due to group A streptococci (uncommonly group C, G, or B). It is more common in young children and older adults. The majority of the lesions present in the lower extremities, but a significant proportion of cases present with lesions in the face. The erysipelas lesion is painful with a bright red, edematous, indurated appearance.

CLOSTRIDIAL CELLULITIS   This superficial infection is most often due to *Clostridium perfringens* and is usually preceded by local trauma or recent surgery. Gas is invariably found in the skin, but the fascia and deep muscle are spared. This entity differs from clostridial myonecrosis; nevertheless, thorough surgical exploration and debridement are required to distinguish between these entities. Magnetic resonance imaging (MRI) or CT scanning and measurement of the serum creatine kinase (CK) concentration can also help to determine whether muscle tissue is involved. However, imaging studies should not delay critical surgical therapy when there is crepitus on examination or clinical evidence of progressive soft tissue infection.

NONCLOSTRIDIAL ANAEROBIC CELLULITIS   This type of cellulitis is due to infection with mixed anaerobic and aerobic organisms that produce gas in tissues. Unlike clostridial cellulitis, this type of infection is usually associated with diabetes mellitus and often produces a foul odor. It must be distinguished from myonecrosis and necrotizing fasciitis by surgical exploration.

DIFFERENTIAL DIAGNOSIS OF CELLULITIS

The diagnosis of cellulitis is usually not difficult to make. Deep venous thrombosis can cause some of the same findings that characterize cellulitis, including fever, and is the primary illness to consider when confronted with a patient with lower extremity changes suggestive of cellulitis. Radiation therapy can cause erythema and swelling of the skin and associated structures and can be difficult to differentiate from cellulitis in some patients.

TREATMENT AND NATURAL HISTORY OF CELLULITIS

A mild early cellulitis may be treated with low doses of penicillin and, if staphylococcal infection is suspected, a penicillinase-resistant penicillin (nafcillin 1–1.5 gm intravenously every 4 hours or, for milder cases, dicloxacillin orally 0.25 or 0.5 gm every 6 hours) (see Table 10.1). A first-generation cephalosporin (cefazolin 1–1.5 gm iv Q8H) also effectively covers GAS and methicillin-sensitive *Staphylococcus aureus*. Vancomycin (1 gm Q12H) intravenously is an alternative for highly penicillin-allergic patients. Initial local care of cellulitis includes immobilization and elevation of the involved limb to reduce swelling and a cool, sterile saline dressing to remove purulent exudate and decrease local pain. Resolution of local findings with treatment is typically slow and can require one to two weeks of therapy. Local desquamation of the in-

volved area can be seen during the early convalescence.

KEY POINTS
Cellulitis

1. An infection of the skin with some extension to the subcutaneous tissues.
2. Predisposing factors: Venous or lymphatic insufficiency, diabetes mellitus, and alcoholism.
3. Erythema, edema, diffuse tenderness, indistinct border, lymphadenopathy.
4. Caused by streptococci and *Staphylococcus aureus*. *Haemophilus influenzae* in children.
5. Subclasses of cellulitis include:
   a. Erysipelas: More superficial, very sharp raised border,
   b. Clostridia cellulitis: Associated with crepitance, no muscle involvement,
   c. Anaerobic cellulitis: Foul smelling, more common in diabetics.
6. Treatment: Penicillinase-resistant penicillin (oxacillin, nafcillin) or first-generation cephalosporin (cefazolin). Vancomycin for the penicillin-allergic patient.

Necrotizing Fasciitis

Necrotizing fasciitis is a rare and often fatal soft tissue infection involving the superficial fascial layers of the extremities, abdomen, or perineum. It is a deep-seated infection of the subcutaneous tissue that results in progressive destruction of fascia and fat but may spare the skin.

PREDISPOSING FACTORS AND ETIOLOGY

Necrotizing fasciitis typically begins with trauma; however, the inciting event may be as seemingly innocuous as a simple contusion, minor burn, or insect bite. It also may be associated with a bacterial superinfection of varicella. An association between the use of nonsteroidal anti-inflamma-

Table 10.1

Antibiotic Treatment of Skin and Soft Tissue Infections

DRUG	DOSE	RELATIVE EFFICACY	COMMENTS
Cellulitis	See text for duration		
Nafcillin or oxacillin	1–1.5 gm iv Q4H	First-line	
Cefazolin	1–1.5 gm iv Q8H	First-line	Inexpensive, less frequent dosing
Vancomycin	1 gm iv Q12H	Alternative	For PCN-allergic patient
Necrotizing fasciitis	See text for duration		
Penicillin G (+)	4 million units iv Q4H	First-line	PCN dose for adults > 60 kg
clindamycin	600–900 mg iv Q8H		and normal renal function
Piperacillin-tazobactam (or)	3/0.375 gm iv Q6H	Alternative	Useful forms of monotherapy
Ticarcillin-clavulanate (or)	3.1 gm iv Q4–6H	Alternative	
Imipenam	500 mg iv Q6H	Alternative	
Myonecrosis	See text for duration		
Penicillin G (+)	4 million units iv Q4H	First-line	PCN dose for adults > 60 kg
clindamycin	600–900 mg iv Q8H		and normal renal fucntion
Impetigo	Treat × 10 days		Treatment prevents post-strep-tococcal complications
Erythromycin	250 mg po QID	First-line	May cause GI toxicity
Dicloxacillin	250 mg po QID	First-line	
Cephalexin	250 mg po QID or 500 mg po BID	Alternative	
Mupirocin	Polyethylene glycol ointment, apply BID	Alternative	
Skin abscesses			
Clindamycin	150 mg po QID	First-line	
Dicloxacillin	250 mg po QID	First-line	

tory drugs and the progression or development of GAS necrotizing infection has also been suggested.

Classic necrotizing fasciitis is caused by GAS (*Streptococcus pyogenes*). Necrotizing fasciitis caused by GAS was previously called "streptococcal gangrene" or streptococcal toxic shock syndrome. In recent years there has been a dramatic increase in the number of invasive infections such as necrotizing fasciitis caused by GAS. Most cases are community-acquired, but a significant proportion may be nosocomial or acquired in a nursing home. Although GAS is the most common bacterial isolate, a polymicrobial infection with a variety of Gram-positive and Gram-negative aerobic and anaerobic bacteria is also quite common. The polymicrobial form usually contains four or five bacterial isolates. Infecting organisms include aerobic (*Staphylococcus aureus,* GAS, and *Escherichia coli*) and anaerobic (Peptostreptococcus, Clostridia, Prevotella, Porphyromonas, and Bacteroides species) Gram-positive and Gram-negative bacteria.

The bacteria associated with necrotizing fasciitis depend on the underlying conditions leading to infection. Three important clinical conditions are associated with this form of skin infection:

1. **Diabetes mellitus**. Necrotizing fasciitis with a mixed flora occurs most often in diabetic patients. These infections usually occur on the feet, with rapid extension along the fascia into the leg. Necrotizing fasciitis should be considered in diabetic patients with cellulitis who also have systemic signs of infection such as tachycardia, leukocytosis, marked hyperglycemia, or acidosis. Diabetic patients can also develop necrotizing fasciitis in other areas, including the head and neck region and the perineum.

2. **Fasciitis of the head and neck**. Cervical necrotizing fasciitis can result from a breach of the integrity of mucous membranes after surgery or instrumentation or from an odontogenic infection. In the head and neck region, bacterial penetration into the fascial compartments can result in a syndrome known as Ludwig's angina, a rapidly expanding inflammation in the submandibular and sublingual spaces, or in necrotizing fasciitis.

3. **Fournier's gangrene**. In the perineal area penetration of the gastrointestinal or urethral mucosa can cause Fournier's gangrene, an aggressive infection. These infections begin abruptly with severe pain and may spread rapidly onto the anterior abdominal wall, into the gluteal muscles, and in males onto the scrotum and penis.

CLINICAL MANIFESTATIONS AND EARLY DIAGNOSIS

◆ CASE 10.2

A 63-year-old African American male presented to the emergency room with a one-day history of mild swelling of his right foot and ankle that was extremely tender to palpation. He had a long history of alcohol abuse and had a history of cirrhosis. He was afebrile at that time and was sent home with po Keflex. Two days later he returned complaining of fever and increased swelling. He was admitted to the hospital, and iv clindamycin and gentamicin were begun. Despite this therapy his leg swelling and erythema failed to improve. Physical exam on the third hospital day: He ap-

peared severely ill and toxic. Temperature 103.2°F, pulse 120, blood pressure 90/70. Marked erythema, edema of the right ankle that extended up the front and lateral regions of the leg, halfway to the knee. A new 1 × 1 cm patch of dark, reddish-purple skin was noted that was exquisitely tender to the touch. No lymphadenopathy was observed. Laboratory studies revealed a WBC of 25,000 (90% PMNs). An emergency surgical exploration revealed an area of necrotic fascia consistent with necrotizing fasciitis. Intraoperative cultures grew *Streptococcus pyogenes*.

Early diagnosis of necrotizing fasciitis is critical because, as is observed in Case 10.2, there may be a remarkably rapid progression from an inapparent process to one associated with extensive destruction of tissue. Differentiating necrotizing infections from common soft tissue infections such as cellulitis and impetigo is both challenging and critically important. A high degree of suspicion may be the most important aid in early diagnosis. Prompt diagnosis is imperative because necrotizing infections typically spread rapidly and can result in multiple organ failure, adult respiratory distress syndrome, and death.

As is noted in Case 10.2, unexplained pain that increases rapidly over time may be the first manifestation of necrotizing fasciitis. In some patients, however, signs and symptoms of infection are not initially apparent. Erythema may be present diffusely or locally, but in some patients excruciating pain in the absence of any cutaneous findings is the only clue for infection. Within 24–48 hours, erythema may develop or darken to a reddish-purple color, as observed in Case 10.2, frequently with associated blisters and bullae; bullae can also develop in normal-appearing skin. The bullous stage is associated with extensive deep soft tissue destruction that may result in necrotizing fasciitis or myonecrosis; such patients usually exhibit fever and systemic toxicity. In addition to pain and skin findings, fever, malaise, myalgias, diarrhea, and anorexia may develop during the first 24 hours. Hypotension may be present initially or develop over time.

Necrotizing fasciitis must be distinguished from gas gangrene, pyomyositis, and myositis. Early frozen biopsy of the skin and subcutaneous tissue has proven useful for the diagnosis of early necrotizing fasciitis. However, any of the abnormalities described above should be of sufficient concern to prompt consideration of surgical exploration. It is critical to proceed with surgery rather than to delay to obtain an imaging study; indeed, necrotizing fasciitis and myositis are diseases that are diagnosed by surgeons in the operating room and often lead to extensive debridement. Imaging studies, such as soft tissue X-rays, CT scan, and MRI are most helpful if there is gas in the tissue.

TREATMENT

Intensive-care physicians and orthopedic surgeons are often the first physicians to evaluate patients with such infections and therefore need to be familiar with this potentially devastating disease and its management. Prompt diagnosis, immediate administration of appropriate antibiotic, and emergent aggressive surgical debridement of all compromised tissues are critical to reduce the morbidity and mortality of these rapidly progressive infections.

SURGERY The best indication for surgical intervention is severe pain, toxicity, fever, and elevated CK with or without radiographic findings. If necrotizing fasciitis is a possibility, the only definitive method of diagnosis is surgical exploration. After initial debridement, the infection can continue to progress if there is residual necrotic tissue. Therefore surgical reexploration is often required and should be performed as often as necessary.

ANTIBIOTICS Some recent studies suggest that clindamycin is superior to penicillin in the treatment of experimental necrotizing fasciitis/myo-

necrosis due to GAS. Clindamycin may be more effective because this antibiotic is not affected by inoculum size or the stage of growth, suppresses toxin production, facilitates phagocytosis of *Streptococcus pyogenes,* and has a long postantibiotic effect. Currently, most experts recommend the administration of combined therapy with penicillin G (4 million units iv Q4H in adults >60 kg in weight and with normal renal function) and clindamycin (600–900 mg iv Q8H) (see Table 10.1).

In a diabetic patient or a patient with Fournier's gangrene, antibiotic treatment should be based on Gram stain, culture, and sensitivity. However, early empiric treatment is necessary: ampicillin (combined with clindamycin or metronidazole) or ampicillin-sulbactam is appropriate. Broader Gram-negative coverage might be necessary if the patient has had prior hospitalization or if antibiotics have been used recently. This can be accomplished with ticarcillin-clavulanate, piperacillin-tazobactam, or imipenem as monotherapy.

ADDITIONAL MEASURES Because of intractable hypotension and diffuse capillary leak in patients with shock, massive amounts of intravenous fluids (10–20 l/day) are often necessary to maintain tissue perfusion combined with vasopressors such as dopamine or epinephrine. Several recent case reports and a case series suggest the beneficial effect of high-dose immunoglobulins, and it is the author's opinion that in the case of a severe infection this form of therapy is warranted. Unfortunately, even with optimal therapy necrotizing fasciitis is associated with considerable mortality.

KEY POINTS
Necrotizing Fasciitis

> 1. Deep subcutaneous infection that causes necrosis of the fascia and subcutaneous fat.

2. Caused by GAS or due to a mixed infection with Gram-positive and Gram-negative aerobes and anaerobes.
3. Severe pain is often the earliest symptom; toxic appearance and tachycardia are also suggestive.
4. Surgical exploration or punch biopsy is required for diagnosis.
5. Treatment must include:
   a. Aggressive and often repeated surgical debridement,
   b. Systemic antibiotics: GAS: penicillin and clindamycin; mixed infection: ticarcillin, clavulanate, piperacillin-tazobactam, or imipenem,
   c. Volume replacement and vasopressors.

Myonecrosis

Myonecrosis (also called necrotizing myositis) is an uncommon infection of muscle that develops rapidly and is life threatening. Early recognition and aggressive treatment are essential. The vast majority of infections resulting in necrosis of muscle are due to Clostridium species (gas gangrene). Spontaneous gangrenous myositis is another invasive infection caused by GAS, which often has overlapping features with necrotizing fasciitis. These infections typically evolve from either contiguous spread from an area of trauma or surgery or spontaneous spread from hematogenous seeding of muscle.

PREDISPOSING FACTORS AND ETIOLOGY

Clostridial gas gangrene due to *C. perfringens* occurs after deep, penetrating injury (e.g., knife or gunshot wound or crush injury that classically occurs in war wounds). Other conditions associated with traumatic gas gangrene may be bowel surgery and postabortion with retained placenta. Clostridial gas gangrene may be spontaneous and nontraumatic and is often associated with *C. septicum* (See Case 10.3 below). Many of the

spontaneous cases occur in patients with gastrointestinal portals of entry such as adenocarcinoma.

Several other clinical entities may be associated with muscular injury and should be considered in patients presenting with myositis:

◆ Tropical pyomyositis due to *Staphylococcus aureus* and is less often caused by other organisms. These organisms produce a primary muscle abscess (pyomyositis) in the absence of an apparent port of entry. Pyomyositis is more common in tropical areas.
◆ Necrotizing infections due to *Vibrio vulnificus* can involve the skin, fascia, and muscle and are most common among patients with cirrhosis, consumers of raw seafood, or inhabitants of coastal regions.
◆ A number of viral infections, such as acute influenza type A, can also produce skeletal muscle injury that produces rhabdomyolysis.

PATHOPHYSIOLOGY OF CLOSTRIDIAL INFECTIONS

The initiating trauma introduces organisms (either vegetative or spore forms) directly into deep tissue but, at the same time, through tissue damage, produces an anaerobic environment with low oxidation-reduction potential and acid pH, which is optimal for growth of clostridial organisms. Necrosis progresses within 24–36 hours of the traumatic injury. Shock associated with gas gangrene may be partly attributable to direct and indirect effects of toxins. Clostridial theta toxin destroys host tissues and inflammatory cells when elaborated in high concentrations at the site of infection. As the toxin diffuses into surrounding tissues or enters the systemic circulation, adhesive interactions of PMNs and endothelial cells are disrupted, and leukocytes are primed for increased respiratory burst activity. These actions lead to vascular leukostasis, endothelial cell injury, and regional tissue hypoxia. Alpha toxin, a phospholipase C, directly suppresses myocardial contractility and may contribute to profound hypotension via a sudden reduction in cardiac output. This toxin also lyses cell membranes, causing hemolysis and the destruction of leukocytes, fibroblasts, and intact muscle cells.

CLINICAL MANIFESTATIONS AND DIAGNOSIS

◆ **CASE 10.3**

A 54-year-old truck driver presented to the emergency room with the sudden onset of severe left shoulder pain. On exam severe tenderness of the left shoulder was elicited, and he was given a pain medication for presumed bursitis. Four hours later he returned to the emergency room. He appeared toxic and confused. Pulse was 125/min, and blood pressure was 80/50. A large blister was noted over the left deltoid, and the skin had a bronze appearance. Aspiration revealed brownish fluid, and Gram stain demonstrated Gram-positive rods and no PMNs (see Figure 10.2). Intravenous penicillin was initiated; however, despite antibiotic therapy, edema and erythema marched down his arm and within one hour had spread to the elbow. Crepitance was readily palpated, and subcutaneous air in the arm and left chest wall was noted on X-ray. His hematocrit dropped from 45 to 23 over the same time period. In the operating room the arm was amputated, and the left chest wall was debrided. In many areas muscle was necrotic and had a cooked meat appearance, failing to contract with electrical stimulation. Despite aggressive debridement, multiple blood transfusions, and respiratory support, the patient developed irreversible shock and died 18 hours after admission. Blood cultures and tissue cultures were positive for *Clostridia septicum*. Autopsy revealed an early carcinoma of the cecum.

As illustrated in Case 10.3, the first symptom in traumatic or bacteremic gas gangrene is usually the sudden onset of severe pain at the site of infection; the mean incubation period may be less than 24 hours but ranges from 6 hours to several days, probably depending on the size of the bacterial inoculum and the extent of vascu-

lar compromise. The skin over the infected area may initially appear pale but quickly changes to bronze and then to purplish-red and becomes tense and exquisitely tender with overlying bullae (see Figure 10.2). An important local sign is the presence of crepitus. As was observed in Case 10.3, signs of systemic toxicity quickly develop and include tachycardia and low-grade fever followed by shock and multiorgan failure. When clostridial bacteremia occurs, it may be associated with extensive hemolysis. Gas within the soft tissue can be detected by physical examination, radiography, computerized tomographic (CT) scan, or magnetic resonance imaging (MRI). Definitive diagnosis is associated with the presence of large, Gram-positive or Gram-variable rods at the site of injury.

TREATMENT

Penicillin, clindamycin, metronidazole, and a number of cephalosporins have excellent activity in vitro against *Clostridium perfringens* and other Clostridia. As was described above for streptococcal gangrene, the combination of penicillin and clindamycin has been recommended in this condition: penicillin (3–4 million units iv Q4H), clindamycin (600–900 mg iv Q8H) (see Table 10.1).

Aggressive surgical debridement is urgent if one wants to improve the chance of survival and preserve tissue. It is critical that all necrotic tissue be resected and that margins of resection contain bleeding healthy tissue. Clearly, an extremity is easier to debride than is the trunk. In Case 10.3 the infection extended to the chest wall, making full debridement impossible. If anaerobic gas gangrene is diagnosed and hyperbaric oxygen facilities are available this therapeutic modality should be considered. The fulminant nature of this infection and extensive toxin production make Clostridia myonecrosis a particularly lethal infection. If early aggressive debridement is not accomplished, a fatal outcome is to be expected.

Figure 10.2

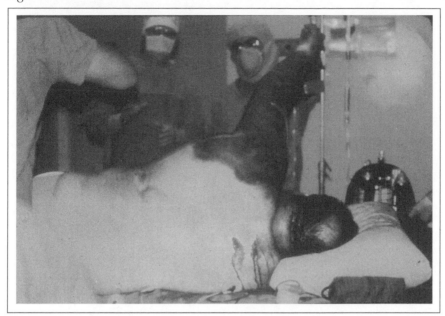

A

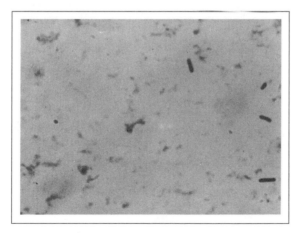

B

Clostridia myonecrosis. (A) Patient from Case 10.3 undergoing surgical debridement. Note the brownish-red discoloration of the skin on his left arm and shoulder. See also Color Plate 2. (B) Gram stain of brown fluid obtained from the large blister on his arm. Note the large Gram-positive rods and an absence of inflammatory cells.

Myonecrosis

1. Primarily caused by *Clostridia perfringens* and *C. septicum* (the latter associated with bowel carcinoma).
2. Clostrida toxins depress myocardial contractility, lyse WBCs and RBCs, and cause tissue necrosis.
3. Skin becomes bronze colored, followed by bullae; on palpation crepitant and extremely tender. Systemic toxicity, tachycardia, and hypotension are common.
4. X-rays reveal subcutaneous gas.
5. Treatment must be rapid, and outcome is often fatal:
   a. Removal of all necrotic tissue and amputation of the infected limb,
   b. Intravenous penicillin and clindamycin,
   c. Hyperbaric oxygen where available.

Burn Infections

PATHOLOGY OF BURNS

All burn wounds become colonized with microorganisms. Burn eschar is composed of dead and denatured dermis in which a wide variety of microbes can flourish. The quantity of organisms, their intrinsic virulence, and the degree to which they invade host tissues determine their significance. Whereas microbial colonization should be expected, invasion of surrounding tissue is a dangerous sign. The organisms associated with invasive infection vary from institution to institution and also vary over time. Common pathogens include *Enterobacter cloacae, Staphylococcus aureus, S. epidermidis, Enterococcus faecalis, E. coli, Pseudomonas aeruginosa, Klebsiella pneumoniae,* and *Acinetobacter baumanii.* Aggressive wound care and extreme vigilance are required to control the concentration of organisms in the burn wound in an effort to protect patients from invasive burn wound sepsis.

Burn wound infections are generally classified as invasive or noninvasive. If a burn wound is allowed to remain *in situ* and is treated with adequate debridement and topical antibiotics, after two to three weeks the naturally occurring microorganisms that colonize the wound will promote separation of the eschar by producing bacterial collagenases. A layer of granulation tissue forms where the eschar separates, and the improved blood supply and wound hypermetabolism help to limit the proliferation of microbes.

When burn wound infections become invasive, the concentration of microorganisms rises to greater than one million per gram of tissue. Developing granulation tissue becomes edematous and pale, with subsequent occlusion and thrombosis of new blood vessels. Lack of bleeding is evident on surgical exploration of the wound. As the infection advances, the surface becomes frankly necrotic, and the infection spreads rapidly.

Containment of invasive burn wound sepsis requires a very low threshold of suspicion, aggressive attempts at early detection, and extremely vigorous therapy. Fortunately, the advent of aggressive surgical removal of the burn wound has made burn wound sepsis a rare event.

CLINICAL MANIFESTATIONS

The presence of microorganisms in the wound and ongoing tissue necrosis in the burn eschar result in the continuous elaboration of endogenous pyrogens. As a consequence persistent fever almost always accompanies burns. Therefore fever is usually not a helpful sign for determining whether or not a burn patient has an invasive infection. Systemic antibiotics play little role in the prophylaxis of infections confined to the burn wound, since the avascular wound prevents adequate delivery of antibiotics to the bacteria. Fortunately, early burn excision has greatly diminished, although not eliminated, this problem. Topical antibacterial preparations have also reduced the extent of colonization. Systemic infection is the most common cause of death in the burn patient, when infections at all sites are combined (lung, wound, and other). The high fatality rate associated with infection is explained by a combination of immune suppression, lung parenchymal damage from smoke inhalation, and the fact that, while massive burns can be excised, it is not possible to immediately cover the wound to provide an effective barrier to infection. The burn patient manifests signs of sepsis as do other critically ill patients, except that the burn patient's "normal" hyperdynamic state mimics some of the typical signs of sepsis. Changes in status, rather than the presence or absence of specific abnormalities, are most helpful in deciding whether or not the burn patient has developed an invasive infection.

TREATMENT

Successful treatment of burn wound infections is extremely difficult. Appropriate systemic antibiotics may ameliorate some systemic manifestations but do little to treat the primary infection in the burn wound. Emergent excision of infected burn eschar is the primary treatment modality. Excision removes the source of infection but may lead to severe bacteremia during the operation; therefore specific antibiotic coverage is necessary. Operations performed in patients with deteriorating cardiovascular status and pulmonary function are extremely hazardous.

KEY POINTS
Burn Infections

> 1. Burned skin provides a fertile environment for bacterial growth.
> 2. Organisms associated with invasive infection include:
>   a. Gram-positive aerobic bacteria: *Staphylococcus aureus*, *S. epidermidis*, enterococcus,

>   b. Gram-negative aerobic bacteria: Enterobacter, *E. coli*, Klebsiella, Pseudomonas, and Acinetobacter.
> 3. Burn patients are often febrile and have sinus tachycardia; a sudden worsening often indicates sepsis.
> 4. Debridement and topical antimicrobial therapy are the mainstays of therapy.
> 5. Broad-spectrum antibiotics are given when sepsis is suspected.

Less Severe, More Common and Localized Skin Infections

Impetigo

Impetigo is a very superficial vesiculopustular skin infection that occurs primarily on exposed areas of the face and extremities. The infection usually occurs in warm, humid conditions and is common in children. Poverty, crowding, and poor personal hygiene promote impetigo, which is easily spread within families. Carriage of GAS and *Staphylococcus aureus* predisposes to subsequent impetigo.

Impetigo due to GAS, *Staphylococcus aureus,* or both cannot be distinguished clinically. In the typical case, vesiculopustules form that subsequently rupture and become crusted. Affected patients usually develop multiple red and tender lesions in exposed areas at sites of minor skin trauma such as insect bites or abrasions. Impetigo results in little or no systemic toxicity but may be accompanied by local lymphadenopathy. Poststreptococcal glomerulonephritis is a rare complication that can be prevented by early antibiotic treatment.

Impetigo may be treated topically; however, when there are multiple lesions, systemic oral therapy is appropriate. Although penicillin was the treatment of choice for impetigo in past years, this antibiotic is no longer recommended because *S. aureus* strains almost universally produce beta-lactamase, which inactivates penicillin. Therefore amoxicillin-clavulanate, erythromycin, cephalexin, dicloxacillin, and topical mupirocin ointment are effective and should be used, provided that local strains of staphylococci do not harbor resistance to the selected agent. The general treatment of choice is erythromycin (250 mg or, in children, 2.5–12.5 mg/kg po QID for 10 days) or mupirocin ointment in a polyethylene glycol base applied locally. An alternative is cephalexin (250 mg po QID or 500 mg po BID for 10 days) (see Table 10.1).

Folliculitis

Folliculitis is a pyoderma that is localized to hair follicles. Several factors predispose to the development of folliculitis: Individuals with nasal carriage of *Staphylococcus aureus* have a higher incidence of folliculitis. Exposure to whirlpools, swimming pools, and hot tubs with inadequate chlorination can become contaminated with *Pseudomonas aeruginosa* and cause "whirlpool" folliculitis. Antibiotic administration and corticosteroid therapy predispose to Candida folliculitis. The lesions of folliculitis are often small and multiple. They are erythematous and may have a central pustule at the peak of the raised lesion. Folliculitis does not cause systemic toxicity. Lesions may spontaneously drain or resolve without scarring. The most common pathogen responsible for folliculitis is *S. aureus* but may include *P. aeruginosa* and Candida species.

Systemic antibiotics do not appear to be helpful in treating folliculitis. Topical therapies such as warm saline compresses and topical antibacterial or antifungal agents are usually sufficient. The monthly use of mupirocin ointment applied to the anterior nares bilaterally twice a day for 5 days each month reduces the incidence of both nasal colonization with *Staphylococcus aureus* and recurrence of either folliculitis or furunculo-

sis in immunocompetent patients who carry *S. aureus* and present with frequent recurrences of folliculitis. Progressive infection due to *Pseudomonas aeruginosa* can occur in immunocompromised hosts and folliculitis is occasionally complicated by furunculosis.

KEY POINTS
Impetigo and Folliculitis

1. Impetigo causes superficial vesicular lesions that crust over:
   a. Caused by GAS and *Staphylococcus aureus,*
   b. Treat with amoxicillin-clavulanate, dicloxacillin, cephalexin, or erythromycin. Localized disease may use topical mupirocin.
2. Folliculitis: infection localized to the hair follicles:
   a. *S. aureus* most common, often associated with nasal carriage,
   b. *Pseudomonas aeruginosa* associated with "whirlpool" folliculitis,
   c. Candida usually follows the use of broad-spectrum antibiotics,
   d. Treated with topical antibiotics or antifungals, systemic antibiotics not recommended.

Furunculosis and Carbuncles

Furunculosis is an inflammatory nodule involving the hair follicle that usually follows an episode of folliculitis. A carbuncle is a series of abscesses in the subcutaneous tissue that drain via hair follicles. *Staphylococcus aureus* is the most common cause of both lesions.

Furuncles and carbuncles arise when areas of skin containing hair follicles are exposed to friction and perspiration. The back of the neck, face, axillae, and buttocks are commonly involved. Factors that predispose to the development of these lesions include obesity and corticosteroid therapy.

Although defects in neutrophil function have been proposed as an explanation for this condition, abnormalities in function are rarely found. Furunculosis is a nodular lesion that is painful and usually drains pus spontaneously. Systemic symptoms are uncommon. Systemic symptoms such as fever are more common in patients with carbuncles, which represent a deeper infection.

Most patients with furuncles can be treated with warm compresses to promote spontaneous drainage. For carbuncles or furuncles in a patient with fever, antimicrobial therapy should be directed against *Staphylococcus aureus*. Dicloxacillin (500 mg po QID) is a reasonable first choice. Cephalexin (250 mg po QID) or clindamycin (150 mg po QID) can be used in penicillin-allergic patients. Surgical drainage may be required in cases in which spontaneous drainage does not occur and antibiotic treatment does not achieve resolution of the lesion(s). In the presence of recurrent or continuous furunculosis, chlorhexidine solution for bathing; attention to personal hygiene; appropriate laundering of garments, bedding, and towels; and careful wound-dressing procedures are recommended. Elimination of nasal carriage of *S. aureus* should be attempted in patients with recurrent episodes of furuncles or carbuncles who have documented nasal carriage of the organism. Mupirocin nasal ointment or oral antibiotic regimens of rifampin (600 mg/day) plus dicloxacillin (500 mg QID) or ciprofloxacin (500 mg BID) for 10 days can be added to mupirocin nasal therapy if an initial course of mupirocin is not effective. Low-dose clindamycin therapy is an alternative suppressive regimen.

Carbuncles are the most important complication of furunculosis, and surgical intervention may be necessary for debridement of affected tissues. Furuncles involving the nose and perioral area can be complicated by cavernous sinus infection due to venous drainage patterns. Bacteremia with development of secondary distant sites of infection can occur (particularly if the furuncle is manipulated) and result in considerable morbidity or mortality.

KEY POINTS

Furuncles and Carbuncles

1. Furuncles are nodular lesions that are result of progression from folliculitis.
2. Carbuncles are larger subcutaneous abscesses that represent a progression from furuncles.
3. Both infections are caused by *S. aureus*.
4. Treatment may include:
   a. Hot compresses to promote spontaneous drainage,
   b. Oral antibiotics if fever develops: dicloxacillin, cephalexin, clindamycin,
   c. Surgical drainage if spontaneous drainage fails to occur.
5. Prevention: Chlorhexidine solutions, mupirocin in the nose to prevent carriage, prophylactic antibiotics.
6. Can be dangerous:
   a. On the face, can lead to cavernous sinus infection,
   b. Bacteremia can occur if the lesions are manipulated.

Skin Abscess

Skin abscess is a common infection that is usually managed in the ambulatory setting. The infection is characterized by a localized accumulation of polymorphonuclear leukocytes with tissue necrosis involving the dermis and subcutaneous tissue. Large numbers of microorganisms are typically present in the purulent material. Skin abscesses and carbuncles are similar histologically, but carbuncles, like furuncles, arise from infection of the hair follicles. Skin abscesses can arise from infection tracking in from the skin surface but are usually deeper than carbuncles (see Figure 10.1). This infection, in contrast to carbuncles, also can be seen as a complication of bacteremia. Relatively minor local trauma such as injection of a drug can also be a risk factor for skin and soft tissue infections. Skin abscess is the most common skin infection in drug abusers who administer their drugs by injection. Nasal or skin carriage of *Staphylococcus aureus* further predisposes to the formation of skin abscess. Skin abscess can be due to a variety of microorganisms and may be polymicrobial. However, the most common single organism is *S. aureus.*

The most common findings with a skin abscess are local pain, swelling, erythema, and regional adenopathy. Spontaneous drainage of purulent material also frequently occurs. Fever, chills, and systemic toxicity with skin abscess are unusual except in patients with concomitant cellulitis. Patients may have single or multiple skin abscesses, and cellulitis around the skin abscess can occasionally occur. Skin abscess commonly involves the upper extremity in drug abusers but can be located at any anatomic site. Patients with recurrent episodes of skin abscess often suffer anxiety due to the discomfort and cosmetic effects of the infections.

Initial antibiotic therapy should always include coverage for *Staphylococcus aureus* regardless of the anatomic area of involvement. Results of microbiologic studies, including Gram stain and routine culture, should direct subsequent treatment. Clindamycin (150 mg po QID) is a reasonable empiric choice because it provides good coverage for both *S. aureus* and anaerobes. Parenteral nafcillin (or another semisynthetic penicillin with activity against *S. aureus*), cefazolin, or clindamycin should be used in patients with associated cellulitis and signs of systemic toxicity. Once the culture results are obtained, dicloxacillin (500 mg po QID) or cephalexin (250 mg po QID) can be given for the treatment of skin abscess caused by *S. aureus.* Clindamycin or macrolides (erythromycin, azithromycin, and clarithromycin) are alternative forms of therapy in patients with a history of life-threatening reaction to penicillin or other beta-lactam antibiotics. Broad-spectrum therapy should be selected as initial empiric therapy for skin abscess in the oral, rectal, and vulvovaginal areas. Amoxicillin-clavulanate (875 mg po TID) is a suitable option for oral therapy of patients with skin abscess in these sites. Surgical incision

and drainage can be performed if the abscess feels fluctuant or has "pointed"; spontaneous drainage can obviate the need for surgery.

Preventive efforts are directed at patients with recurrent episodes of skin abscess. Although the results of testing will usually be negative, metabolic and immunologic screening should be performed in patients with recurrent abscess formation in the absence of another predisposing factor. These tests should include determinations of the fasting blood glucose and, if high-normal or elevated, followed by hemoglobin A1C. Neutrophil number and eventually function as well as immunoglobulin levels also should be evaluated. Elevated IgE levels in association with eczema defines the Job or hyperimmunoglobulinemia E syndrome, a disease that is characterized by recurrent furunculosis, carbuncles, and skin abscesses.

Most patients with skin abscess respond to therapy and do not develop serious complications. Bacteremia can occur, however, and metastatic sites of infection including endocarditis and osteomyelitis can develop. Individuals who are at high or moderate risk for endocarditis should be given antimicrobial prophylaxis prior to incision and drainage of potentially infected tissue. Parenteral administration of an anti-staphylococcal antibiotic (either oxacillin 2 gm or cefazolin 1–2 gm Q6–8H) is recommended as prophylactic therapy in this setting. Vancomycin, 1 gm Q12H, should be given if the patient has had prior colonization or infection with methicillin-resistant *Staphylococcus aureus.*

KEY POINTS
Skin Abscesses

1. Localized infection of the dermis and subcutaneous tissue, usually deeper than carbuncles.
2. Can arise from local trauma, iv drug abuse, and bacteremic seeding.
3. *Staphylococcus aureus* most common.
4. Therapy should include:

    a. Oral clindamycin (adds anaerobic coverage) or dicloxacillin,
    b. If cellulitis, iv clindamycin, nafcillin, oxacillin, or cefazolin,
    c. Perirectal, oral, or vaginal area: amoxicillin-clavulanate.
  5. Preventive measures:
    a. If recurrent furunculosis, carbuncles, or abscesses exclude diabetes mellitus, neutrophil dysfunction, and hyperimmunoglobulinemia E syndrome,
    b. Prophylactic antibiotics prior to incision and drainage if high risk for endocarditis.

Tetanus

Tetanus is an uncommon problem in the United States as a result of immunization policies. Approximately 70 cases per year are reported, most occurring in individuals over 60 years who have waning immunity. The incidence is much higher in developing countries, mortality rates associated with tetanus being as high as 28 per 100,000. In developed countries most cases develop following punctures or lacerations. *Clostridium tetani* spores can contaminate these wounds and germinate in the anaerobic conditions created by a closed wound. The growing bacterium produces an exotoxin called tetanospasmin. This metalloprotease degrades a protein required for docking of neurotransmitter vesicles that normally inhibit the firing of motor neurons. As a consequence muscle spasms develop, and patients experience masseter muscle trismus, or "lockjaw," as well as generalized muscle spasm leading to arching of the back (opisthotonus), flexion of the arms, and extension of the legs. Spasms may be triggered by any sensory stimulus and are very painful. Spasm of the diaphragm and throat can lead to respiratory arrest and sudden death. Autonomic dysfunction can lead to hypertension or hypotension and to bradycardia or tachycardia and is the leading cause of death. Neonatal tetanus develops following infection of the umbilical stump and is most commonly reported in developing countries. Neonates present with generalized weakness followed by increased rigidity, and mortality exceeds 90%.

Patients should receive human tetanus immunoglobulin (HTIG) 500 IU im. Diphtheria-pertussis-tetanus vaccine (DPT, 0.5 ml) should also be administered intramuscularly. Metronidazole (500 mg iv Q6H) should be given for 7–10 days to eradicate *Clostridium tetani* from the wound. Intravenous diazepam is recommended for the control of muscle spasms, and tracheostomy should be performed after endotracheal intubation in anticipation of prolonged respiratory compromise. Sympathetic hyperactivity should be controlled with short-acting beta-blockers, and hypotension should be treated with saline infusion combined with dopamine or norepinephrine. Two additional doses of DPT vaccine are recommended: one dose at the time of discharge and a third dose four weeks later. The mortality rate ranges from 6% in milder cases to 60% in severe disease.

The devastating consequences of this disease emphasize the importance of prevention. Tetanus toxoid vaccination provides complete immunity for at least five years. Routine boosters are recommended every ten years. Tetanus spores can be inoculated into any wound; however, certain wounds are at higher risk: wounds contaminated with dirt, saliva, or feces; puncture wounds; unsterile injections; frostbite; bullet or shrapnel wounds; crush injuries; and compound fractures. If a patient with one of these types of wounds has not received immunization in the past five years or is immunocompromised, he or she should receive passive immunization with HTIG as well as active immunization with a tetanus toxoid booster.

KEY POINTS

Tetanus

  1. Rare in the U.S. but common in developing countries.

2. *Clostridium tetani* produces tetanospasmin, blocks normal inhibition of motor neurons.
3. Associated with severe muscle spasm, jaw trismus, opisthotonus, and respiratory failure.
4. Treatment:
   a. Tetanus immunoglobulin (HTIG),
   b. Tetanus toxoid vaccine,
   c. Metronidazole iv,
   d. Diazepam, short-acting beta-blockers, vasopressors, fluids,
   e. Intubation and tracheostomy.
5. Prevention;
   a. Tetanus toxoid vaccine Q10 years,
   b. Potential contaminated wound, give booster vaccine after 5 years,
   c. High-risk wound or immunocompromised patient also give HTIG.

Animal and Human Bites

Animal bites caused by pet dogs and cats are a common problem, representing approximately 1% of visits to emergency rooms. The incidence tends to be highest among children. Dog bites most frequently occur in young boys, while cat bites more commonly occur in young girls and women. Dog and cat bites can result in soft tissue and bone infections, particularly on the hands. The teeth of cats are very sharp and commonly penetrate the skin and puncture the underlying bone, increasing the risk of osteomyelitis. The most common organism associated with pet animal bites is Pasteurella species (found in 50% of dog bites and 70% of cat bites); *Pasteurella canis* is most common in dog bites, while *P. multocida* is most commonly associated with cat bites. *Staphylococcus aureus,* streptococcal species, *Capnocytophaga canimoris,* and anaerobic bacteria are also frequently cultured from these wounds. These infections are usually polymicrobial.

Because of the high likelihood of infection, cat and dog bite wounds should not be closed pri-marily. Antibiotic prophylaxis is usually recommended, consisting of a single parenteral dose of ampicillin-sulbactam (3 gm iv × 1) followed by amoxicillin-clavulanate (875 mg po BID × 3 days). Alternative regimens in patients with penicillin allergy include clindamycin (900 mg iv followed by 300 mg po Q6H) plus ciprofloxacin (400 mg iv, followed by 500 mg po BID). In children clindamycin combined with trimethoprim-sulfamethoxazole is recommended. The same regimens are also recommended for treatment. The duration of intravenous and oral antibiotic treatment depends on the rate of response of the infection, the degree of tissue damage, and the likelihood of bone or joint involvement. Patients who have defects in lymphatic or venous drainage, who are receiving corticosteroids, or who are otherwise immunocompromised are at higher risk of developing sepsis and need to be followed closely. First-generation cephalosporins, dicloxacillin, and erythromycin should be avoided because a number of bacteria that cause animal bite infections, including *Pasteurella multocida,* are resistant to these antibiotics. If the animal bite was unprovoked, rabies vaccination or quarantined observation of the animal is the standard of care (see Chapter 6). Finally, prophylaxis for tetanus must be provided (see above).

KEY POINTS
Animal Bites

1. A leading cause of visits to the emergency room.
2. More common in children, dog bites more common in males, cat bites more common in females.
3. *Pasteurella* species important pathogens in dog and cat bites.
4. Prophylaxis recommended:
   a. iv ampicillin-sulbactam followed by amoxicillin-clavulanate × 3–5 days,
   b. iv followed by oral clindamycin + ciprofloxacin in penicillin-allergic patients.

5. Treatment:
   a. Same antibiotic regimens as prophylaxis but more prolonged, 10–28 days,
   b. Rabies prophylaxis,
   c. Tetanus prophylaxis.

Human bites most commonly arise as a consequence of closed fist injuries during a fight. Human mouth flora can also be inoculated into the skin as result of nail biting or thumb sucking. Love nips and actual bites in association with an altercation are also encountered. Alcohol, other drugs, or a medical condition leading to confusion is often associated with human bite injuries. Multiple aerobes and anaerobes can be cultured from the human mouth, and infections associated with human bites are usually polymicrobial. Aerobic organisms include *Streptococcus viridans* and *Staphylococcus aureus*. Important anaerobes include *Eikenella corrodens*, Bacteroides species, Fusobacterium species, and peptostreptococci. *E. corrodens* is a particular concern because this organism is resistant to oxacillin, nafcillin, clindamycin, and metronidazole and is variably resistant to cephalosporins. Prophylaxis with amoxicillin-clavulanate is recommended. Treatment with intravenous ampicillin-sulbactam, ticarcillin-clavulanate, or cefoxitin is usually effective. As noted in the discussion of animal bites, the duration of therapy depends on the rate of improvement, the degree of soft tissue damage, and the likelihood of bone involvement. In clenched fist injuries, bone and tendon involvement is common and usually warrants more prolonged antibiotic therapy for presumed osteomyelitis.

KEY POINTS
Human Bites

1. Often associated with alcohol or other drugs, clenched fist injuries most common.

2. Polymicrobial infections, often includes *Eikenella corrodens*.
3. Prophylaxis and treatment:
   a. Ampicillin-sulbactam, ticarcillin-clavulanate, cefoxitin,
   b. Avoid oxacillin, nafcillin, clindamycin, metronidazole, many cephalosporins,
   c. Duration depends on response, tissue damage, and bone involvement.

Dermatophytosis

The dermatophytes are molds that can invade the stratum corneum of the skin or other keratinized tissues derived from epidermis, such as hair and nails. They may cause infections at most skin sites, although the feet, groin, scalp, and nails are most commonly affected. There are three genera of pathogenic dermatophyte fungi: Trichophyton, Microsporum, and Epidermophyton.

The classic lesion of dermatophytosis is an annular scaling patch with a raised margin showing a variable degree of inflammation, the center usually being less inflamed than the edge. This clinical form is sometimes described as tinea circinata. The word "tinea" is used to refer to dermatophyte infections, and it is usually followed by the Latin description of the appropriate site. The clinical appearances of the infection vary with the site, the fungal species involved, and the host's immune response.

TINEA PEDIS

Tinea pedis is usually caused by infection with either *Trichophyton rubrum* or *T. mentagrophytes* (*interdigitale*), less commonly by *Epidermophyton floccosum*. Tinea pedis is usually seen in young adults or teenage children. It is particularly common in institutions or places where common bathing facilities are used. The clinical manifestations of infection are altered in patients with T lymphocyte abnormalities, including those with AIDS, in whom there is often extensive spread of the lesions onto the dorsal surface of the foot. Scaling between the toes is often referred to as athlete's foot.

TINEA CRURIS

The most common dermatophytes associated with groin infections are *Trichophyton rubrum* and *Epidermophyton floccosum*. This infection is also called jock itch. The infection starts with scaling and irritation in the groin. The rash usually involves the anterior aspect of the thighs and, less commonly, the scrotum. The leading edge extending onto the thighs is prominent and may contain follicular papules and pustules.

TREATMENT

The usual approach to the management of dermatophyte infections is to treat with topical therapy if possible, but most nail and all hair infections and widespread dermatophytosis are best treated with oral drugs (see Chapter 1). The main topical agents used for dermatophytosis are the keratolytics and compounds with specific antifungal activity. The keratolytic agent that is used most frequently is Whitfield's ointment (salicylic and benzoic acid compound). This is particularly effective in infections that are confined to heavily keratinized areas such as the soles or palms. It is inexpensive but messy to use, although a cream formulation of benzoic acid compound is available in some countries.

More attention has been focused on one particular group of antifungal drugs, the azoles, which include miconazole, clotrimazole, econazole, and ketoconazole. These are active against all the common skin fungi, and many can be given once daily. Generally, topical therapy for tinea pedis has to be continued for at least two weeks and possibly four weeks. The topical form of the allylamine terbinafine can be used to clear lesions of tinea pedis in 1–7 days.

The main oral antifungals used for dermatophytosis are terbinafine, itraconazole, and fluconazole. Griseofulvin is an alternative treatment but is still the treatment of choice for most cases of tinea capitis. Terbinafine is given for two weeks for tinea cruris or tinea corporis, six weeks for fingernail infections, and twelve weeks for toenail infections. It produces rapid and long-lasting remissions for dry-type dermatophytosis and other skin infections.

Onychomycosis caused by dermatophytes can be treated with oral therapy. Terbinafine and itraconazole have replaced griseofulvin for this indication. For instance, terbinafine produces 70–80% cure rates in six weeks for fingernails and twelve weeks for toenails. Daily itraconazole (200 mg QD) for three months is also effective in toenail infections. But it is more commonly administered as a pulsed treatment given for one week of each month (400 mg QD), the week's course being repeated once more for fingernail infections (two pulses) and twice or three times for toenail disease (three or four pulses). Reported remission rates are above 60%. Intermittent regimens using fluconazole in the treatment of onychomycosis have been also used.

KEY POINTS
Dermatophytosis

1. Molds: Trichophyton, Microsporum, and Epidermophyton, invade the stratum corneum.
2. Tinea pedis = mold infection of the feet.
3. Tinea cruris = mold infection of the groin area.
4. Topical therapy except for nail infections:
   a. Topical azoles,
   b. Allylamine terbinafine effective after shorter periods.
5. Nail infections: oral therapy recommended:
   a. Griseofulvin rarely used,
   b. Terbinafine daily for 6–12 weeks,
   c. Pulsed itraconazole or fluconazole.

Cutaneous Candida Syndromes

Candida species can generate a variety of cutaneous infections, including the following:

1. **Generalized cutaneous candida infection**. This condition is an unusual form of cutaneous candidiasis and is characterized by widespread eruptions over the trunk, thorax, and extremities with increased severity in the genitocrural folds, anal region, axillae, hands, and feet. The process begins as individual lesions that spread into large confluent areas. It occurs in both adults and children.
2. **Erosio interdigitalis blastomycetica**. This term applies to Candida infection occurring between the fingers or toes. It has a red base, may extend onto the sides of the digits, is painful, and is predisposed to by maceration.
3. **Candida folliculitis**. Infection at the hair follicles with Candida can occur. Rarely, the condition may become extensive. It must be distinguished from folliculitis caused by the dermatophytes and tinea versicolor.
4. **Intertrigo**. This common skin condition affects any site in which skin surfaces are in close proximity and provide a warm, moist environment. It begins as vesicopustules, which enlarge and rupture, causing maceration and fissuring. The area of involvement has a scalloped border with a white rim consisting of necrotic epidermis, which surrounds an erythematous, macerated base. Frequently, satellite lesions are found that may coalesce and extend the affected area. A variant form of cutaneous candidiasis in the intertriginous region has a miliary appearance resembling miliaria rubra with erythematous macules or vesicopustules.
5. **Paronychia and onychomycosis**. Candida is one of the most common causes of paronychia. Many skin bacteria, as well as Candida, can usually be recovered by culture of the infected area. The appearance of the reaction is that of a relatively well-localized area of inflammation that becomes warm, glistening,

and tense and may extend under the nail. Unless the disease process is stopped, secondary thickening, ridging, and discoloration occur, and nail loss may result.

These infections are usually effectively treated with topical or oral azoles. Duration of therapy depends on the site and associated underlying diseases.

KEY POINTS
Cutaneous Candidiasis

> 1. Generalized cutaneous candidiasis can spread over the entire body.
> 2. Erosio interdigitalis blastomycetica refers to infection between the toes and fingers.
> 3. Candida folliculitis results from infection of the hair follicles.
> 4. Intertrigo refers to infections on skin regions that are moist and in close approximation.
> 5. Paronychia and onychomycosis. Candida is one of the most common causes of paronychia.
> 6. Treated with oral or topical azoles.

Ectoparasites

SCABIES

The causative agent of human scabies, *Sarcoptes scabiei,* is a 0.4-mm-long, round-bodied, eight-legged mite. Most of the clinical symptoms associated with scabies result from infestation by the adult female. Following mating with the smaller adult male, the female burrows into the epidermis and lays two to three eggs daily until she dies approximately one month later; the male dies shortly after mating. The eggs hatch in three to four days, releasing larvae that emerge on the skin surface. The larvae then pass through a nymphal stage, mature into adult mites in two to three weeks, and mate. Human scabies infestation predominantly results from person-to-person contact, with fomite transmission playing a much less important role. Intimate interpersonal contact with a scabies-infested individual, especially sexual contact, poses a greater risk of transmission than does casual contact. Other risk factors associated with acquiring scabies include poor hygiene and overcrowding.

Scabies commonly manifests itself as a highly pruritic skin eruption that presumably results from the host's immune response to the mite excreta. In general, pruritus is particularly troublesome at night and after the patient's showers. Studies have demonstrated that symptomatic disease typically begins an average of four weeks after initial infestation but almost immediately if reinfestation occurs. Among immunocompetent adults infestation generally occurs below the neck, and the average number of mites per patient is fewer than 15. Accordingly, mites are difficult to find. Nevertheless, they can often be found by a diligent search for burrows in high-yield areas, namely, the fingerweb spaces, wrists, elbows, periumbilical region, feet, and genitalia. The burrows typically appear as slightly elevated, linear or wavy dark lines that measure 5–20 mm in diameter. Frequently, a vesicle or black dot at one end of the burrow can be seen; this corresponds to the location of the mite. Other helpful findings on physical examination include the presence of vesicles, small erythematous papules, and nodules. The scabetic nodules, which appear as reddish-brown nodules 3–10 mm in diameter, are most often located on male genitalia, the groin, or axillae. All types of scabies lesions can become secondarily infected, especially following overly vigorous scratching.

A definitive diagnosis of scabies requires finding a mite, egg, or scybala (barrel-shaped brown fecal pellets) on a skin scraping of a burrow. To more readily identify a burrow, one can spread ink from a black fountain pen over a suspect area, wipe the skin with an alcohol pad, and then look for ink outlining the burrow. The burrow should be scraped with a scalpel blade (or a similar device) followed by transfer of the material to a glass slide. Mineral oil or 10–20% potassium hydroxide is then added. With Norwegian scabies, scraping any hyperkeratotic area will yield multiple mites.

First-line therapy for scabies usually consists of using 5% permethrin cream. The patient should thoroughly massage it into the skin from the neck down and then wash it off 8–12 hours later. To avoid reinfection, bed linens and recently worn clothes should be washed using the hot cycle of the machine (or dry cleaned). If objects cannot be laundered or dry-cleaned, they should be placed in a tightly closed plastic bag for at least 7 days. In addition, close contacts should receive simultaneous treatment even if they have no symptoms.

KEY POINTS
Scabies

1. Caused by an 8-legged female mite that burrows under the skin and lays eggs.
2. Person-to-person spread by intimate contact or poor hygiene.
3. Eggs cause intense itching, can become superinfected.
4. Look for burrows or small nodules in the fingerweb spaces, wrists, elbows, periumbilical region, feet, and genitalia.
5. Treat with permethrin cream; launder or dry-clean all cloths and linens; treat close contacts.

Lice Infestation (Pediculosis and Diseases Caused by Lice)

Lice are blood-requiring, six-legged, wingless insects that cause human disease either by directly infesting the skin or by injecting antigenic secretions into the skin. In addition, they can serve as a vector for transmitting infectious microorganisms. Lice have a worldwide distribution and traditionally flourish in conditions associated with overcrowding, poor hygiene, and poverty. Transmission predominantly occurs by person-to-person contact, although in some instances fomites may play a role. In general, lice live about two months, but if away from the host for more than 10 days, they will die of starvation. Three different subspecies of lice commonly infect humans, and each type has a predilection for distinct body locations: *Pediculus humanus* var. *capitus,* or the head louse, prefers the scalp; *P. humanus* var. *corporis,* or the body louse, prefers the trunk, axillae, and groin; and *Phthirus pubis,* also known as the pubic louse, prefers short hairs found at the pubis, trunk, axillae, beard, eyebrows, eyelashes, and occiput.

HEAD LICE

Although *Pediculus humanus* var. *capitus,* the head louse, most often affects children, individuals of any age can become infested. The infestation can result from either direct person-to-person contact or by indirect means, such as by sharing contaminated grooming devices. Infested patients typically develop an intense pruritus of the scalp, although rare patients remain asymptomatic. As a result of the pruritus and subsequent scratching, patients can develop impetigo or furunculosis. When searching for head lice on a patient, one should carefully look at the base of hair shafts near the ears or neck. When found, the adult head lice appear elongated and small (1–3 mm in diameter). The adult female louse can lay up to three eggs (nits) per day, cementing each egg to the base of a hair shaft. In general nits are found more readily than the adult lice. As the hair grows, the nit remains firmly attached, allowing one to estimate the duration of infestation (the average hair grows 1 cm per month).

Control of head lice requires killing of both the adult and egg forms. Permethrin 1% liquid is the generally accepted treatment of choice, mainly because it is safe and kills both the eggs and the lice. Before applying this medication, patients should wash, rinse, and towel-dry their hair. Next they should apply the permethrin, leave it on for 10 minutes, and then rinse it off. The other most commonly used and effective treatment consists of vigorously massaging lindane 1% shampoo into the scalp for 4–5 minutes, followed by thorough rinsing. Nits should be removed with a fine-tooth comb.

PUBIC LICE (CRABS)

Transmission of *Phthirus pubis,* also known as pubic lice or crabs, predominantly occurs though sexual intercourse, although fomite transmission can occur. The diagnosis of pubic lice should lead one to investigate concomitant sexually transmitted diseases. Likewise, the presence of pubic lice in the eyelashes of a child should serve as a marker for possible sexual abuse. Pubic lice are broader than body or head lice and clasp onto hairs with their large hind-leg claws. Typically, they attach to the base of short body hairs located on the trunk, thighs, axillae, beard, eyebrows, eyelashes, or occiput. The nits cement themselves to the base of the hair shaft and grow out with the hair. Clinically, patients tend not to manifest symptoms during the incubation period (30 days) but subsequently will develop pruritus and 2- to 3-mm blue macules (*maculae cerulea*).

The treatment of pubic lice requires applying lindane 1% shampoo to the affected area, leaving it on for 4 minutes, and then thoroughly washing it off. Alternatively, permethrin 1% cream rinse can be used in a similar manner, except that it is left on for 10 minutes. The presence of lice or nits on the eyelashes requires application of a thick coat of an occlusive eye ointment twice daily for 10 days.

KEY POINTS

Lice

1. A small wingless insect; three types infect humans: the head louse, body louse, and pubic louse.

2. Person-to-person spread, poor hygiene, may also be spread by fomites.
3. Head lice cause intense itching, more common in children, spread by contaminated hair-grooming instruments. Eggs or nits deposited at base of hair shaft.
4. Pubic lice spread by sexual contact, causes pruritus and small blue macules.
5. Treatment: Topical lindane or permethrin, remove nits with a fine-tooth comb.

Additional Reading

Duvanel, T., Auckenthaler, R., Rohner, P., Harms, M., and Saurat, J.H. Related articles. Quantitative cultures of biopsy specimens from cutaneous cellulitis. *Arch Intern Med,* 149(2):293–296, 1989.

Hay, R.J. Dermatophytosis and other superficial mycoses. In Mandell, G.L., Bennett, J.E., and Dolin, R. (Eds.). *Principles and Practice of Infectious Diseases,* 4th edition, Churchill Livingstone, New York, 1995.

Schwartz, M.N. Cellulitis and subcutaneous tissue infections. In Mandell, G.L., Bennett, J.E., and Dolin, R. (Eds.), *Principles and Practice of Infectious Diseases,* 4th edition. Churchill Livingstone, New York, 1995.

Stamenkovic, I., and Lew, P.D. Early recognition of potentially fatal necrotizing fasciitis: The use of frozen-section biopsy. *N Engl J Med,* 310(26):1689–1693, 1984.

Daniel P. Lew

Bone and Joint Infections

Recommended Time to Complete: 1 day

Guiding Questions

1. How does one distinguish between acute and chronic bone infection?
2. What are the most frequent pathogens in osteomyelitis?
3. Is a bone biopsy necessary to guide treatment in osteomyelitis?
4. How long should osteomyelitis be treated?
5. Are oral antibiotics ever the appropriate treatment for osteomyelitis or septic arthritis?
6. What are the indications for surgical debridement?
7. How long should septic arthritis be treated?

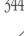

Osteomyelitis

Potential Severity: A subacute to chronic infection that can cause severe disability if improperly managed.

Osteomyelitis is a progressive infectious process that can involve one or multiple components of bone, including the periosteum, medullary cavity, and cortical bone. The disease is characterized by progressive, inflammatory destruction of bone, necrosis, and new bone formation.

Classification

It is helpful to classify osteomyelitis because the different types of osteomyelitis have differing prognoses and are treated in different ways.

ACUTE VERSUS CHRONIC OSTEOMYELITIS

Acute osteomyelitis evolves over several days to weeks; chronic osteomyelitis is a disease characterized by clinical symptoms that persist for several weeks. Chronic osteomyelitis can also evolve over months or even years and is characterized by the persistence of microorganisms, low-grade inflammation, the presence of necrotic bone (sequestra) and foreign material, and fistulous tracts. The terms "acute" and "chronic" do not have a sharp demarcation and are often used somewhat loosely. Nevertheless, they are useful clinical concepts in infectious disease, as they describe two different patterns of the same disease caused by the same microorganisms but with different rates of progression.

OSTEOMYELITIS OF HEMATOGENOUS ORIGIN OR DUE TO A CONTIGUOUS FOCUS OF INFECTION

Hematogenous osteomyelitis is the result of bacteremic spread with seeding of bacteria in bone. It is seen mostly in prepubertal children and elderly patients. Osteomyelitis secondary to a contiguous focus of infection follows trauma, perforation, or an orthopedic procedure. As the name implies, infection first begins in an area adjacent to bone, eventually spreading to the bone. A second category of osteomyelitis due to contiguous spread is found in the diabetic. Diabetic foot infection commonly spreads to bone and is often associated with vascular insufficiency.

KEY POINTS

Classification of Osteomyelitis

1. Acute osteomyelitis develops over days to weeks.
2. Chronic osteomyelitis develops over weeks to months and can persist for years.
3. Hematogenous osteomyelitis occurs in the children and the elderly.
4. Infections at continguous sites can spread to bone. Traumatic injury, penetrating injuries, postoperative orthopedic surgery infections, and diabetic as well as other forms of ischemic ulcer can spread infection to bone.

Hematogenous Osteomyelitis of Long Bones and Vertebral Bodies

PATHOGENESIS

Hematogenous osteomyelitis most commonly occurs in children and usually results in a single focus of infection involving the metaphysis of long bones (particularly the tibia and femur). In adults hematogenous osteomyelitis most frequently involves the vertebral bodies These locations are favored because of their vascular supply. In the case of the long bones bacteria tend to lodge in small end vessels that form sharp loops near the epiphyses. In the case of vertebral bodies small arteriolar vessels are thought to trap bacteria. The vertebral arteries usually bifurcate and supply two adjacent vertebral bodies, a situation that may explain why hematogenous vertebral osteomyelitis usually involves two adjacent bone segments and the intervening disc. Infection may also spread from one vertebra to the intervening disc and then to the adjacent vertebral body. In addition to being supplied by small arteries, the vertebrae are surrounded by a plexus of veins lacking valves, called Batson's plexus. This venous system drains the bladder and pelvic region and on occasion can also transmit infection to the vertebral bodies. The lumbar segments are most commonly infected, followed by the thoracic regions; the cervical region is only rarely involved.

MICROBIOLOGY

Bacteria responsible for hematogenous osteomyelitis reflect essentially their bacteremic incidence as a function of age, so the organisms that are most frequently encountered in neonates include *Staphylococcus aureus* and group B streptococci; in infants the majority of infections are due to *S. aureus*, coagulase-negative staphylococci, and various streptococci. Later in life, *S. aureus* predominates; in elderly persons, who are frequently subject to Gram-negative bacteremias, an increased incidence of vertebral osteomyelitis due to Gram-negative rods is found. Fungal osteomyelitis is a complication of intravenous device infections, neutropenia, of profound immune deficiency; *Pseudomonas aeruginosa* hematogenous osteomyelitis is often seen in drug addicts and has a predilection for the cervical vertebrae (see Table 11.1).

◆ CASE 11.1

An 86-year-old white female underwent cardiac catheterization three months before admission. Several days after her catheterization she noted a fever that lasted for 2–3 days. Approximately three weeks after her catheterization she began experiencing dull pain in the lumbosacral region that progressively worsened over the next two months. Pain was not relieved by over-the-counter pain medications and became so severe that she sought medical attention in the emergency room. She reported a 25-lb weight loss over the three months.

Physical examination: Temperature 36.4°C, pulse 84. General appearance: Elderly woman complaining of back pain. A II/VI systolic ejection murmur was heard along the left sternal border (previously described). Moderate tenderness to palpation over the L–S spine area. Motor and sensory exams of the lower extremities within normal limits.

Laboratory findings: ESR 119, WBC 8.1 (52% PMNs, 12.8% lymphocytes, 10.8% monocytes), Plts 537K. CT scan L4–L5 marked decalcification of the vertebral bodies, moth-eaten appearance of the vetebral end plate in L5. CT scan guided aspirate: No growth, and a repeat aspirate was performed that demonstrated an acute inflammatory reaction and the culture positive for *Staphylococcus aureus*. Blood cultures × 2: No growth.

CLINICAL MANIFESTATIONS

The clinical features of hematogenous osteomyelitis in long bones include chills, fever, and malaise reflecting the bacteremic spread of microorganisms. Pain and local swelling subsequently develop at the site of local infection. Patients with vertebral osteomyelitis complain of localized back pain and tenderness that may mimic an early herniated disk; however, the presence of fever should always raise the possibility of infection. It should be pointed out that fever may not be present at the time of presentation (as noted in Case 11.1), particularly in more chronic cases of osteomyelitis. The erythrocyte

Table 11.1

The Microbiology of Osteomyelitis

TYPE OF OSTEOMYELITIS	COMMON PATHOGENS
Hematogenous (usually one organism)	
Infant (<1 year)	*Staphylococcus aureus*
	Group B streptococci
	Escherichia coli
Children (1–16 years)	*S. aureus*
	S. pyogenes
	Haemophilus influenzae
Adults (>16 years)	*S. aureus*
	Coagulase-negative staphylococci
	Gram-negatives: *E. coli,* Pseudomonas, Serratia
Contiguous spread (polymicrobial)	
Microbiology depends on the primary site of infection.	*S. aureus*
	S. pyogenes
	Enterococcus
	Coagulase-negative staphylococci
	Gram-negatives
	Anaerobes
Diabetic foot (polymicrobial)	*S. aureus*
	Streptococcus species including enterococcus
	Gram-negatives: *Proteus mirabilis,* Pseudomonas
	Anaerobes

sedimentation rate (ESR) is commonly elevated, and in a patient with back pain and a high ESR, vertebral osteomyelitis should be considered.

KEY POINTS

Pathogenesis, Microbiology, and Clinical Manifestations of Hematogenous Osteomyelitis

1. Bacteria are trapped in small end vessels:
   a. At the metaphysis of long bone in children,
   b. In vertebral bodies in the elderly. Also can spread via Batson's venous plexus.
2. Microbiology reflects the causes of bacteremia in the two age groups:
   a. Children: *Staphylococcus aureus*, group B streptococcus, other streptococci, and coagulase-negative staphylococci,
   b. Elderly: Gram-negatives and *S. aureus*,
   c. Immunocompromised: Fungi,
   d. IV drug abusers: *Pseudomonas aeruginosa*.
3. Clinical manifestations :
   a. Long bones: Fever, chills, and malaise + soft tissue swelling and pain, usually children,
   b. Vertebral osteomyelitis: Back pain and localized tenderness + high ESR.

DIAGNOSIS

In most cases the peripheral white blood cell count is normal. If the infection has continued for a prolonged period, the patient may have a normochromic normocytic anemia (anemia of chronic disease). The diagnosis of osetomyelitis is usually made radiologically. Standard bone films generally show demineralization within two to three weeks of the onset of infection. X-rays generally require a loss of 50% of the bone calcium before demineralization can be detected, a fact that explains the low sensitivity early in the course of infection. In long bone infections, in addition to areas of reduced calcium (lytic lesions), periosteal elevation may develop and soft tissue swelling is apparent (see Figure 11.1). In chronic osteomyelitis areas of increased calcification or bone sclerosis are also seen. In vertebral osteomyelitis early plain X-rays might reveal no

abnormalities, and obvious changes might not develop for six to eight weeks. At this time the bony plate of the vertebra becomes eroded and appears irregular or "moth-eaten." Collapse of the disc space usually is seen as the infection progresses and is most readily seen on CT scan (see Figure 11.2). Metastatic neoplastic bone lesions can also cause erosions on the vertebral margin. One critical finding helps to distinguish between these two diseases. In osteomyelitis, infection almost always involves two adjacent vertebral bodies and the disc space, while most neoplastic processes involve a single vertebral body and do not extend across the disc space.

CT scan is helpful in defining the extent of bone damage in both vertebral osteomyelitis and long bone osteomyelitis and is more sensitive than plain films are. This procedure is commonly used to guide the needle biopsy in vertebral osteomyelitis. If surgical debridement is being considered, CT scan is often used to help to decide the extent of debridement. MRI is also increasingly used to detect areas of dead bone, also termed sequestrum. When long bones become

Figure 11.1

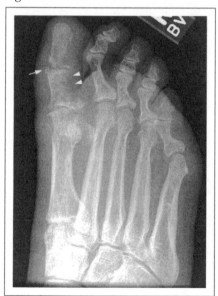

Plane X-ray showing changes of osteomyelitis of the great toe. Arrow points to fragmentation of the distal interphalangeal joint. Arrowheads outline the expected location of the medial margin of the proximal phalangeal bone. Multifocal areas of cortical destruction and ill defined lytic areas are found throughout the distal first metatarsal and both first toe phalanges. (Courtesy of Maria T. Calimano, MD and Andres R. Acosta, MD, University of Florida.)

Figure 11.2

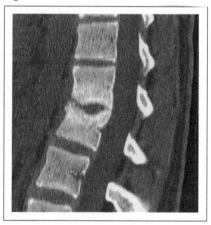

Sagittal CT scan showing typical changes of vertebral osteomyelitis. Obliteration of the disc space is seen with marked irregularity and sclerosis of the cortical endplates. (Courtesy of Maria T. Calimano, MD and Andres R. Acosta, MD, University of Florida.)

necrotic, the bone marrow dies, producing a unique MRI signal. This diagnostic tool very effectively guides the orthopedic surgeon and allows a more complete surgical debridement of sequestrum. MRI has also proved to be more sensitive than CT scan for detecting early osteomyelitis. Decreased signal intensity of the disc and infected vertebral bodies is observed on T2-weighted images, and loss of end plate definition is noted on T1 images. Contrast enhancement of the infected regions is also observed (see Figure 11.3). MRI also is helpful in detecting the spread of vertebral infection to the epidural space (a rare event in the modern antibiotic era; see Chapter 6).

Bone scan may be useful in detecting early infection; however, in many circumstances MRI has proved to be the study of choice in early osteomyelitis. Three-phase technetium bone scan is sensitive but produces false-positive results in patients with fractures or overlying soft tissue infection. False-negative results are occasionally observed in early infection or when bone infarction accompanies osteomyelitis. Gallium imaging is more specific and sensitive in cases of vertebral

ostoemyelitis and demonstrates intense uptake in the disc space and adjacent vertebral bodies.

To define the microbiology, two or three blood cultures should be drawn. However, blood cultures are positive in only a small percentage of cases; therefore in most patients a deep tissue sample should be obtained for aerobic and anaerobic culture as well as for Gram stain and histopathology examination. Often children are treated empirically because any operative intervention near the epiphyseal plate can result in impaired bone growth. In the rare adult with long bone infection, debridement and/or incision and drainage of soft-tissue abscesses are usually required, and also allow acquisition of deep-tissue samples for culture. In vertebral osteomyelitis the number of potential pathogens is large, and effective antimicrobial therapy needs to be guided by culture results. Needle biopsy using CT guidance is currently the procedure of choice for obtaining culture samples. Needle aspirates should be submitted in parallel for bacteriologic and pathologic evaluation. Pathology is particularly useful in patients with previous antibiotic

Figure 11.3

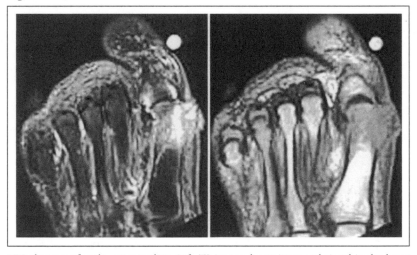

MRI changes of early osteomyelitis. *Left:* T2 image shows increased signal in the bone marrow of the metatarsal and the surrounding soft tissue. *Right:* T1 post contrast image showing loss of the bone marrow fat signal and cortical margins in the metatarsal. (Courtesy of Maria T. Calimano, MD and Andres R. Acosta, MD, University of Florida.)

therapy, in which cultures may be negative, and in patients with suspected mycobacterial disease. If the first biopsy is culture negative, a second biopsy guided by CT scan should be obtained. For patients in whom the second sample fails to establish a diagnosis, the physician is faced with the options of beginning empiric therapy or requesting an open surgical biopsy for diagnosis.

KEY POINTS
Diagnosis of Hematogenous Osteomyelitis

1. Plain films require two to three weeks to become positive (require a 50% loss of bone calcium), in vertebral osteomyelitis can take six to eight weeks. They may show:
   a. Periosteal elevation,
   b. Areas of demineralization and loss of a sharp bony margin, "moth eaten" appearance,
   c. Soft tissue swelling,
   d. Late stages areas of increased calcification or sclerosis.
2. CT scan: More sensitive.
3. MRI: Able to detect early changes.
4. Bone scan: Can detect early disease, false positives common. Gallium preferred for vetebral osteomyelitis.
5. Tissue sample for culture and histopathology should be obtained except when blood culture is culture-positive:
   a. Long bone infection in children may be treated empirically,
   b. Long bone infection in adults usually requires operative culture,
   c. Vertebral osteomyelitis: CT-guided needle biopsy.

TREATMENT

In long bone infections parenteral administration of an antimicrobial regimen may be begun as empiric therapy aimed at the clinically suspected pathogens(s) (see Table 11.2). Once one or more organisms are isolated, in vitro susceptibility testing can be performed as a guide to treatment.

The current standard of care is parenteral antimicrobial treatment for four to six weeks. The start of therapy must be dated from the day on which effective antimicrobial therapy, as judged by in vitro susceptibility, was begun. Surgical debridement is rarely required in long bone hematogenous osteomyelitis if antibiotic therapy is started early in the course of the illness. However, if a large area of necrotic bone is identified, surgical removal may be required for cure.

Empiric coverage of vertebral osteomyelitis is generally not recommended. The choice of an antimicrobial drug should be guided by the results of cultures of blood, as well as bone and soft tissue specimens obtained by biopsy or debridement before treatment. For patients who traveled to endemic areas, Brucella serology may be useful. Depending on the pharmacologic characteristics of a specific drug, the drug may be administered by the oral or the parenteral route. The antimicrobial agent should be given for four to six weeks. The duration of treatment is usually dated either from the initial use of an effective antimicrobial agent or from the last major debridement. The indications for surgery in vertebral osteomyelitis are failure of medical management, formation of soft tissue abscesses, impending instability, or neurologic signs indicating spinal cord compression. In the latter case surgery becomes an emergency procedure (see Chapter 6, "Central Nervous System Infections"). The neurologic status of the patient must therefore be monitored at frequent intervals. Eventual fusion of adjacent infected vertebral bodies is a major goal of therapy.

KEY POINTS
Treatment of Hematogenous Osteomyelitis

1. Empiric antibiotic therapy is usually avoided. Treat for four to six weeks.
   a. *S. aureus*: Methicillin-sensitive nafcillin or oxacillin, MRSA, vancomycin,

Table 11.2

Antibiotic Treatment of Hematogenous Osteomyelitis in Adults

Microorganisms Isolated	Treatment of Choice (IV unless specified)	Alternatives
Staphylococcus aureus		
Penicillin-sensitive	Penicillin G (4 million units every 6 hours)	A second-generation cephalosporin, clindamycin (600 mg every 6 hours) or vancomycin
Penicillin-resistant	Nafcillin[a] (2 gm every 6 hours)	A second-generation cephalosporin, clindamycin (600 mg every 6 hours) or vancomycin
Methicillin-resistant	Vancomycin (1 gm every 12 hours)	Teicoplanin[b] (400 mg every 24 hours, first day every 12 hours)
Various streptococci (group A or B beta-hemolytic; *Streptococcus pneumoniae*)	Penicillin G (3 million units every 4–6 hours)	Clindamycin (600 mg every 6 hours), erythromycin (500 mg every 6 hours), or vancomycin
Enteric Gram-negative rods	Quinolone (ciprofloxacin, 500–750 mg every 12 hours, IV or oral)	A third-generation cephalosporin
Serratia sp., P. aeruginosa	Piperacillin[c] (2–4 gm every 4 hours) and gentamicin (1.5 mg/kg/every 8 hours)	A third-generation cephalosporin[c] or a quinolone (with aminoglycosides)
Anaerobes	Clindamycin (600 mg every 6 hours)	Ampicillin-sulbactam (2.2 gm every 8 hours) or metronidazole for Gram-negative anaerobes (500 mg every 8 hours)
Mixed infection (aerobic and anaerobic microorganisms)	Ampicillin-sulbactam (2.2 gm every 8 hours)	Imipenem[d] (500 mg every 6 hours)

[a]Flucloxacillin in Europe; [b]Teicoplanin is currently only available in Europe; [c]Depends on sensitivities; piperacillin/tazobactam and imipenem are useful alternatives; [d]In cases of aerobic Gram-negative microorganisms resistant to ampicillin-sulbactam.

    b. Streptococci: Penicillin G,
    c. Enteric Gram-negatives: Ciprofloxacin,
    d. *Serratia* or *Pseudomonas aeruginosa*: Piperacillin-tazobactam + gentamicin,
    e. Anaerobes: Clindamycin or metronidazole.
2. Surgical debridement not necessary if early treatment:
    a. Required to remove necrotic long bone,
    b. Rarely required in vertebral osteomyelitis; if instability, cord compression, drainage of soft tissue abscess.

Osteomyelitis Secondary to a Contiguous Infection

CLINICAL MANIFESTATIONS AND ASSOCIATED PRIMARY INFECTIONS

The clinical picture is more complex in cases of osteomyelitis associated with a comminuted fracture. Bacteria are often introduced at the time of trauma. Following initial corrective surgery, pain improves, and the patient progressively mobilizes the injured limb. As the patient begins to bear weight, pain reappears. A mild fever is noted, and the wound becomes more erythematous, accompanied by a slight discharge. No other clinical signs point toward the diagnosis of osteomyelitis, and no radiographic examination or other imaging procedure is fully diagnostic.

Other forms of osteomyelitis due to contiguous spread include the following:

1. Acute purulent frontal sinusitis spreading to the frontal bone and causing edema of the forehead (Pott's puffy tumor)
2. Dental root infection leading to local bone destruction
3. Deep-seated pressure sores spreading to underlying bone, usually the sacrum

In all these conditions the inflammatory reaction may be mild, and the extent of bone destruction may be difficult to assess

ETIOLOGY

This infection is usually polymicrobial. *Staphylococcus aureus* remains the most frequently reported microorganism in osteomyelitis secondary to contiguous spread (see Table 11.1). However, various types of streptococci, Enterobacteriaceae, and *Pseudomonas aeruginosa* (the latter mostly in the setting of chronic osteomyelitis, comminuted fractures, and puncture wounds to the heel) are encountered. Finally, osteomyelitis of the mandible and osteomyelitis secondary to pressure sores frequently contain an abundance of anaerobic flora. Anaerobes also are common pathogens in osteomyelitis caused by human and animal bites (see Chapter 10).

KEY POINTS

Osteomyelitis Due to Contiguous Spread

1. Clinical manifestations subtle:
   a. Increasing pain,
   b. Mild fever and minimal drainage.

2. Imaging procedures are often difficult to interpret.
3. Microbiology may reveal multiple organisms:
   a. *Staphylococcus aureus* most common,
   b. Streptococci,
   c. Enterobacteriaceae, *Pseudomonas aeruginosa*,
   d. Anaerobes.

Diabetic Foot Infection: Osteomyelitis Secondary to Vascular Insufficiency

Clinical Manifestations

Osteomyelitis secondary to vascular insufficiency is a special entity observed in patients with diabetes and/or vascular impairment and is located almost exclusively on the lower extremities. The disease starts insidiously in a patient who has complained of intermittent claudication in an area of previously traumatized skin. Cellulitis may be minimal, and infection progressively burrows its way to the underlying bone (e.g., toe, metatarsal head, tarsal bone). Physical examination elicits either no pain (with advanced neuropathy) or excruciating pain if bone destruction has been acute. An area of cellulitis may or may not be present; crepitus can be felt occasionally, which points toward the presence of either anaerobes or Enterobacteriaceae. Physical examination includes a careful examination of the vascular supply to the affected limb and the evaluation of a concomitant neuropathy.

ETIOLOGY, DIAGNOSIS, AND TREATMENT

Here again, the whole gamut of human pathogenic bacteria can be isolated, often in multiple combinations. *Staphylococcus aureus* still predominates, but any other Gram-positive or Gram-negative, aerobic or anaerobic bacteria may be involved, particularly in more severe infections (see Table 11.1).

The ability to reach bone by gently advancing a sterile surgical probe combined with a plain radiography is the best initial approach to the diagnosis of osteomyelitis. If bone is detected on probing, treatment for osteomyelitis is recommended. If bone cannot be detected by probing and the plain radiography does not suggest osteomyelitis, the recommended treatment is a course of antibiotics directed at soft tissue infection. Because occult osteomyelitis may be present, radiography should be repeated in two weeks. Further studies such as MRI are recommended in doubtful cases.

The prognosis for cure of osteomyelitis associated with vascular insufficiency is poor because of the impaired ability of the host to assist in the eradication of the infectious agent and the inability of systemic antibiotics to gain entry into the site of infection. The vascular insufficiency may be the result of trauma, atherosclerotic peripheral vascular disease, secondary manifestations of diabetes mellitus, or some combination of these processes. It is important to determine the amount of vascular compromise. This assessment can be made by measurement of transcutaneous oximetry (once inflammation has been controlled) and of pulse pressures with Doppler ultrasonography. If serious ischemia is suspected, arteriography of the lower extremity including the foot vessels should be performed.

Treatment includes antimicrobial therapy, debridement surgery, or ablative surgery. The type of treatment that is offered depends on the oxygen tensions of tissue at the infected site, the extent of osteomyelitis and duration of damage, the potential for revascularization, and the patient's preference. Revascularization often proves to be useful before amputation is considered. There is no convincing evidence that hyperbaric oxygen is useful for the treatment of diabetic osteomyelitis. Debridement and a four- to six-week course of antimicrobial therapy may benefit the patient with localized osteomyelitis and good oxygen tension at the infected site. In such patients in the presence of a well-defined pathogen (usually *Staphylococcus aureus*), six weeks of parenteral therapy sometimes followed by oral antibiotics can lead to a high cure rate. If these conditions do not exist, the wound often fails to heal, and an amputation of infected bone is ultimately required. Digital and ray resections, transmetatarsal amputations, and midfoot disarticulations allow the patient to walk without prosthesis. The patient should be treated with antimicrobial agents for four weeks when infected bone is transected surgically. Two weeks of anti-infective therapy should be given when the infected bone is completely removed because there may be some residual soft tissue infection. When the site of amputation is proximal to infected bone and soft tissue, the patient is given standard antimicrobial prophylaxis. In contrast, prolonged therapy is recommended for tarsal or calcaneal osteomyelitis, since the infected bone is debrided and not totally removed.

KEY POINTS
Diabetic and Ischemic Osteomyelitis

1. Most common clinical presentation: Painless ulcer that extends to bone.
2. Mild cellulitis, crepitance with anaerobes or Enterobacteriaceae.
3. Probe the ulcer; if probe reaches bone, the diagnosis is osteomyelitis.
4. Microbiology: Mixed Gram-positives, Gram-negatives, and anaerobes.
5. Treatment:
   a. Revascularization when possible, hyperbaric oxygen is of no benefit,
   b. Amputation or debridement is required,
   c. Antibiotics for four to six weeks; duration depends on the extent of amputation.

General Principles for the Management of Osteomyelitis

The many pathogenic factors, modes of contamination, clinical presentations, and types of orthopedic procedures for osteomyelitis have precluded a very scientific approach to therapy, with well-controlled, statistically valid studies. There are three critical principles for the management of osteomyelitis:

1. **Obtain adequate tissue for culture and histopathology**. If there is one area in which adequate sampling for bacteriology is important, it is in the case of osteomyelitis, because treatment will be given for many weeks, most often by a parenteral route following the results of the initial culture. Adequate sampling of deep infected tissue is therefore extremely useful (in contrast to specimens obtained superficially from ulcers or from fistula, which are often misleading). After clinical evaluation a bone biopsy should be performed, and the sample that is obtained should be submitted for aerobic and anaerobic cultures and histopathologic evaluation. Results of Gram stain and culture, ideally obtained before therapy, should be carefully analyzed.

2. **Design a specific antimicrobial regimen**. When possible, the patient should receive antimicrobial agents only after the results of cultures and susceptibility tests become available. However, if immediate debridement is required and there is significant risk of precipitating bacteremia or spread of infection, the patient may receive empiric antimicrobial therapy before the bacteriologic data are reported (see Table 11.2). This antimicrobial regimen can be modified if necessary on the basis of culture and susceptibility results.

Experimental models have clarified some basic principles of antibiotic therapy. Except for the fluoroquinolones, which penetrate unusually well into bone, bone antibiotic levels 3–4 hours after administration are usually quite low in comparison to serum levels; therefore maximal doses of parental antibiotics should be used. Since revascularization of bone after debridement takes three to four weeks, prolonged antimicrobial therapy is required to treat viable infected bone and to protect bone that is undergoing revascularization. Parenteral therapy is generally recommended for four to six weeks. In cases of severe bone necrosis, parenteral therapy may be prolonged to 12 weeks. The start of this therapy is usually dated from the last major debridement. Early antibiotic treatment, given before extensive bone destruction has occurred, produces the best results.

Single-agent chemotherapy is usually adequate for the treatment of osteomyelitis due to hematogenous spread. A conventional choice of antimicrobial agents for the most commonly encountered microorganisms is given in Table 11.2. In recent years, new approaches to antimicrobial therapy have been developed experimentally and validated clinically. Thus in hematogenous osteomyelitis of childhood, parenteral administration of antibiotics may be followed with an equal success rate by oral therapy for several weeks, provided that the organism is known, clinical signs abate rapidly, patient compliance is good, and serum antibiotic levels can be monitored. Another approach that is gaining acceptance because of its reduced cost is outpatient parenteral administration of antibiotics. Outpatient parenteral therapy requires a team of dedicated nurses and physicians.

Long-term oral therapy extending over months and more rarely years is aimed at palliation of acute flare-ups of chronic, refractory osteomyelitis. Local administration of antibiotics, either by instillation or by gentamicin-laden beads, has its advocates both in the United States and in Europe, but it has not been submitted to critical, controlled studies. Antibiotic diffusion is limited in time and space but may be of some additional benefit in osteomyelitis secondary to a contiguous focus of infection. Among new classes of drugs, fluoroquinolones have been one of the most important advances for the treatment of osteomyelitis. They have been shown to be effective in experimental infections and in several randomized and nonrandomized studies in adults. Whereas their efficacy in the treatment of osteomyelitis due to most Enterobacteriaceae (which are very sensitive to fluoroquinolones) seems undisputed, their advantage over conventional therapy in osteomyelitis due to Pseudomonas or Serratia species as well as Gram-positive organisms (in particular *Staphylococcus aureus*) remains to be demonstrated.

3. **Proper surgical management**. A combined antimicrobial and surgical approach should at least be discussed in all cases. Whereas at one end of the spectrum (e.g., hematogenous osteomyelitis) surgery usually is unnecessary, at the other end (a consolidated infected fracture) cure may be achieved with minimal antibiotic treatment provided that the foreign material is removed. Proper surgical management includes drainage, thorough debridement, and obliteration of dead space. Ideally, specific antimicrobial therapy is initiated before debridement is undertaken. Debridement includes removal of all orthopedic appliances except those deemed absolutely necessary for stability. Often, debridement must be repeated at least once for the removal of all nonviable tissue.

   Wound protection is also an important surgical management principle. Open wounds must be covered to prevent bacteria from reinfecting the bone. Posttraumatic infected fractures are especially difficult to treat. A variety of techniques have evolved for management of the exposed bone and/or the dead space(s) created by the trauma and debridement, that is, use of local tissue flaps and of vascularized tissue transferred from a distant site. Other experimental modalities that are occasionally employed include cancellous bone grafting and implantation of acrylic beads impregnated with one or more antibacterial agents. Finally, in patients with osteomyelitis the Ilizarov fixation device allows

major segmental resections, in combination with new bone growth, to fill in the defect.

ASSESSMENT OF CLINICAL RESPONSE

Assessing the response to therapy can be difficult because bed rest or modification of physical activity by itself can temporarily improve symptoms. Second, despite appropriate antibiotic therapy the radiologic and MRI changes of osteomyelitis can worsen for several weeks. Therefore during antibiotic therapy serial radiologic or MRI studies are not recommended. The ESR is probably the most helpful objective criterion and, combined with the monitoring of symptoms, should be used to monitor the response to therapy.

Because of the protracted clinical course of osteomyelitis, cure is defined as the resolution of all signs and symptoms of active disease at the end of therapy and after a minimal posttreatment observation period of one year. By contrast, failure is defined as a lack of apparent response to therapy as evidenced by one or more of the following: (1) persistence of drainage; (2) recurrence of a sinus tract or failure of a sinus tract to close; (3) persistence of systemic signs of infection (chills, fever, weight loss, bone pain); and (4) progression of bone infection shown by imaging methods (e.g., radiography, CT, MRI).

KEY POINTS
Management of Osteomyelitis

1. Adequate tissue must be obtained for culture and histopathology.
2. Empiric antibiotic therapy should usually be avoided:
   a. Prolonged therapy for four to six weeks,
   b. Outpatient parenteral therapy often utilized,
   c. In children, hematogenous osteomyelitis may be treated orally.

3. Surgery is often required for drainage, debridement, obliteration of dead space, and wound coverage.
4. Assessment of response and cure is difficult:
   a. ESR and symptomatic improvement are the best parameters, imaging study improvement can be very delayed,
   b. Cure = resolution of signs and symptoms for >1 year.

Infections in Prosthetic Joints

Pathogenesis and Microbiology

Infections following total replacement of the hip joint are divided into three categories on the basis of time course and pathogenesis:

1. Acute contiguous infections are recognized within the first six months after surgery and are often evident within the first few days or weeks. These infections result directly from infected skin, subcutaneous tissue, or muscle and/or from operative hematoma.
2. Chronic contiguous infections are diagnosed 6–24 months after surgery, usually because of persistent pain. In the majority of cases infection is believed to result from contamination at the time of surgery with microorganisms of lower pathogenicity. The infection progresses slowly to a chronic form before it is recognized.
3. Hematogenous infections, as discussed above, are diagnosed more than two years after surgery and arise from late transient bacteremia with selective persistence of the microorganisms in the joint.

Coagulase-positive and coagulase-negative staphylococci are the microorganisms that are most often isolated from infected prosthetic hip joints and account for three fourths of the bacteria that are cultured.

KEY POINTS
Pathogenesis, Microbiology, Clinical Manifestations, and Diagnosis of Prosthetic Joint Infections

1. Three forms:
   a. Acute contiguous infection (≤6 months after surgery),
   b. Chronic contiguous infection (6–24 months after surgery),
   c. Hematogenous spread (>2 years after surgery).
2. Microbiology: Three quarters due to Staphylococcus:
   a. Coagulase-negative Staphylococcus most common,
   b. *S. aureus*.
3. Clinical manifestations are difficult to differentiate from mechanical loosening:
   a. Joint pain,
   b. Fever often not present.
4. Diagnosis by joint aspiration with quantitative culture and Gram stain.

◆ CASE 11.2

A 75-year-old Caucasian male with a history of diabetes mellitus × 38 years presented with fever and severe right knee pain × 10 days. He had suffered with osteoarthritis for many years, and five years before admission had bilateral placement of hip prostheses followed two years later by replacement of both knees. Four months prior to admission he began to experience right knee pain that steadily worsened until 10 days prior to admission, when he began experiencing very severe pain accompanied by fever to 102°F and increased warmth and erythema of the right knee.

Physical findings included a temperature of 39°C and a pale, chronically ill-appearing general appearance. Right knee exam revealed marked edema, erythema, and warmth with decreased range of motion secondary to pain. No instability of the knee joint was noted.

Laboratory findings: WBC 13,000 (87% PMNs, 5% band forms), Hct 29, ESR >100 mm. Knee aspirate: Gram stain: many PMNs and Gram-positive cocci in chains; culture: Group B streptococci.

Clinical Manifestations and Diagnosis

Most patients have no elevation in temperature and present with a painful joint that is found to be unstable by physical examination and/or radiography. Because of the difficulty of distinguishing loosening of the joint based on mechanical failure from that based on infection, a positive culture of fluid aspirated from the artificial joint space and/or of bone from the bone-cement interface is required (as was performed in Case 11.2) and remains the diagnostic method of choice. Since the microorganisms responsible for these infections colonize the skin, Gram stain and quantitative cultures obtained from deep tissues are very useful to distinguish contamination from infection.

Treatment

Two approaches to treatment exist. With one-stage exchange arthroplasty the infected components are excised, surgical debridement is performed, and a new prosthesis is immediately put into place. Several proponents of this technique use cement containing an antimicrobial drug, a factor that may contribute to the high success rate reported for the procedure. A second approach, described by investigators at the Mayo Clinic, requires surgical removal of all foreign bodies, debridement of the bone and soft tissues, and a minimum of four weeks of parenteral antimicrobial therapy. Reconstruction is performed three months or more after the com-

pletion of therapy for "less virulent infections" but is delayed for at least one year for "a more virulent infection." In the early stage of infection, when the prosthesis is still firmly in place, it is possible to attempt to achieve cure only with antibiotics without removal of the prosthesis.

This infection is difficult to cure. The relapse rate is approximately 10% at three years and 26% after ten years.

KEY POINTS

Diagnosis and Treatment of Prosthetic Joint Infections

1. Removal of the prosthesis is usually required. There are two approaches:
   a. One-step procedure that includes antibiotic impregnated cement,
   b. Removal, debridements, and a minimum of 4 weeks of antibiotic therapy.
      (1) With less virulent pathogens: Replacement > 3 months,
      (2) More virulent pathogens : Replacement > 1 year.
2. A stable joint with early infection may occasionally be cured with antibiotics alone.

Septic Arthritis
(Excluding Reactive Arthritis)

Potential Severity: Delays in appropriate therapy can lead to irreversible joint damage.

Infectious arthritis is a serious condition because of its potential to lead to significant joint morbidity and disability if not detected and treated early.

Pathogenesis, Predisposing Factors, and Microbiology

Septic arthritis primarily arises because of hematogenous spread of bacteria to the synovial membrane lining the joint. An acute inflammatory reaction results in infiltration of polymorphonuclear leukocytes (PMNs). Bacteria and inflammatory cells quickly spread to the synovial fluid, leading to joint swelling and erythema. Cytokines and proteases are released into the synovial fluid and if not quickly treated causes cartilage damage and eventually joint space narrowing. Causes of bacteremia leading to septic arthritis include urinary tract infection, intravenous drug abuse, intravenous catheters, and soft tissue infections. Patients with bacterial endocarditis, particularly when caused by *Staphylococcus aureus* or enterococcus, can present with septic arthritis. Patients with underlying joint disease are at higher risk for developing infection of the previously damaged joint. Patients with rheumatoid arthritis and osteoarthritis most commonly develop this complication. Patients with HIV infection have a higher risk of septic arthritis and are more likely to be infected with a fungus or mycobacteria. Sometimes the predisposing factor is minor trauma or an upper respiratory infection. Unfortunately, a common medically induced cause is the intra-articular injection of corticosteroids leading to bacterial superinfection.

Staphylococcus aureus remains the most common cause of infectious arthritis. Other common causes include, in young adults, *Neisseria gonorrhoeae* (presenting sometimes as disseminated gonococcal infection; see below) and Gram-negative bacilli in the elderly (often secondary to urinary tract infection). Certain viruses such as parvovirus B19, hepatitis B, rubella, mumps, and HIV can be causes of acute arthritis. Mycobacterial and fungal infections commonly cause chronic monoarticular arthritis. Lyme arthritis caused by *Borrelia burgdorferi* is a diagnosis to be considered in the appropriate epidemiologic setting; it may occur as an acute transient arthritis and more rarely as a late chronic arthritis (see Chapter 13).

◆ CASE 11.3

A 19-year-old African American female presented to her physician with a 3-day history of progressive swelling of her left knee. The knee was hot to touch, and painful to move. She denied any sexual contacts in the past year. She also denied fever or chills. On physical exam she was afebrile. No skin rashes. The only positive finding was a swollen left knee that was erythematous and warm to touch. Fluid was readily palpable. Any movement of the knee caused moderate pain. Laboratory findings: Peripheral WBC 7,100 (71% PMNs), needle aspiration of the joint: 102,000 WBC (95% PMNs), Gram stain: many PMNs, Gram-positive cocci, culture + for *Staphylococcus aureus*. Blood cultures: negative.

Clinical Manifestations, Diagnosis, and Treatment

As illustrated by Case 11.3, the primary manifestations of septic arthritis are swelling and pain in a single joint accompanied by fever. Elderly patients may be afebrile at the time of presentation. Connective tissue diseases usually present with bilateral joint involvement; therefore any patient with monoarticular arthritis should be considered to have septic arthritis until proven otherwise. In addition to being swollen, the infected joint is usually warm to touch, and any movement of the joint is accompanied by exquisite pain. The most commonly involved joints in adults are the knee (40–50%) and hip (15–20%), followed by shoulder, wrist, ankle, and elbow. In children the hip joint is most commonly affected (60%), followed by the knee joint (35%). Nearly half of patients who develop septic arthritis have underlying chronic joint disease, such as rheumatoid arthritis and osteoarthritis. It is likely that damage to the synovial membrane increases the likelihood of bacterial invasion.

The critical diagnostic test is the analysis of the synovial fluid. The synovial fluid leukocyte count is normally <180 cells/mm^3, and a count that exceeds 200 is generally considered inflammatory. In acute infections the count is often (but not always) over 50,000 with a predominance of PMNs. Gram stain smears are positive in 75–80% of patients with Gram-positive microorganisms but lower in the presence of Gram-negative or *Neisseria gonorrhoeae* infection. Blood cultures are positive in a significant proportion of cases. Selected gonococcal media may be useful to plate from pharyngeal, rectal, cervical, or urethral specimens when *N. gonorrhoeae* infection is suspected. PCR has been used with success to detect *Borrelia burgdorferi* DNA and gonococcal arthritis. Crystals should be sought because crystal arthropathy may be inflammatory in the absence of infection or may even coexist with infection.

The therapy of infectious arthritis has two important components. The first is complete drainage and washing of the purulent exudate when possible by arthroscopy (for example, in the knee joint) or, when not possible, by surgery (for example, in the hip joint) in particular for *Staphylococcus aureus* or Gram-negative infection. If the activated PMNs are allowed to remain in the joint space, these cells will continue to mediate a powerful inflammatory response that can lead to irreversible cartilaginous damage. The second component of therapy is the administration of the most appropriate antibiotic based on Gram stain, bacterial culture results, or clinical presentation. The antibiotic regimens are identical to those used for osteomyelitis (see Table 11.2); however, the duration of treatment after appropriate drainage is usually shorter, three to four weeks. Despite the development of more effective antibiotics, the outcome of septic arthritis has not improved. One third of patients suffer significant residual joint damage. An adverse outcome is more likely in the elderly and in patients with preexisting joint disease or infection in a joint containing synthetic material.

KEY POINTS
Septic Arthritis

> 1. Usually results from hematogenous spread.
> 2. *Staphylococcus aureus*, Gram-negative rods, and *Neisseria gonorrhoeae*.
> 3. Acute monoarticular arthritis is septic arthritis until proven otherwise.
> 4. Joint fluid usually has >50,000 WBC (mainly PMNs); Gram stain and culture are usually positive.
> 5. Therapy should include:
>   a. Joint drainage,
>   b. Systemic antibiotics × 3–4 weeks; nafcillin or oxacillin for *S. aureus*, third-generation cephalosporin or fluoroquinolone for Gram-negative.

Disseminated Gonococcal Infection

One to 3 percent of patients infected with *Neisseria gonorrhoeae* develop disseminated disease. The most common manifestation of this complication is monoarticular or polyarticular arthritis.

Pathogenesis and Predisposing Factors

Progression of localized gonococcal disease to disseminated disease requires that the bacterium gain entry into the bloodstream. The most important factor predisposing to bacteremia is the delay in antibiotic treatment. Most patients who develop disseminated disease have a mucosal infection that is asymptomatic. Women are more likely to have asymptomatic disease than men, and women are three times more likely to develop disseminated disease than men. Dissemination often follows menstruation, and it is likely that bacteria can more readily invade the bloodstream during endometrial bleeding. Similarly, asymptomatically infected women who are postpartum are more likely to develop disseminated disease. The terminal complement cascade plays an important role in killing Neisseria species, and patients who have congenital or acquired deficiencies (including patients with systemic lupus erythematosus) of the terminal complement components (C5–C8) have a higher risk of developing disseminated gonococcal as well as meningococcal infection. Bacterial virulence factors are also likely to play a role in dissemination. *Neisseria gonorrhoeae* strains that fail to express the outer membrane protein II and form transparent colonies on culture plates are more likely to disseminate. Compared to strains that cause urethritis, most strains associated with disseminated disease are penicillin-sensitive.

Clinical Manifestations, Diagnosis, and Treatment

This is primarily a disease of sexually active young adults or teenagers. Patients usually present with one of two syndromes:

1. **Tenosynovitis, dermatitis, and polyarthritis syndrome**. The first manifestations of discase are fever, malaise, and arthralgias. Subsequently, inflammation of the tendons in the wrist, the fingers, and less commonly the ankles and toes is noted. On examination tenderness is noted over the tendon sheaths, and pain is exacerbated by movement. The development of tenosynovitis in a young person is virtually pathopneumonic for disseminated gonococcemia. Pustular, vesiculopustular, and, less commonly, hemorrhagic or papular skin lesions accompany the onset of tenosynovitis. Lesions are often periarticular, relatively few in number (usually 4–10, rarely more than 40 lesions), and transient, spontaneously resolving over 3–4 days. If untreated, patients with this syndrome may progress to purulent arthritis.

2. **Purulent arthritis without skin lesions**. This form of arthritis is similar to other forms of septic arthritis with high numbers of PMNs being found in the synovial fluid.

Blood cultures should be drawn in all patients with suspected disseminated gonococcal disease and are positive in about half of cases. Blood cultures are more frequently positive in patients with the tenosynovitis-dermatitis-polyarthritis syndrome. Cultures and Gram stains of joint aspirates should also be performed but are frequently unrevealing. Cultures and Gram stains of cervical and urethral exudate as well as skin lesions should also be obtained.

Because of the increasing incidence of penicillin-resistant strains, disseminated gonococcal infection is usually treated with parenteral ceftriaxone (1 gm iv or im/day), which should be continued for 24–48 hours after clinical improvement. Patients can then be switched to an oral regimen such as cefixime, ciprofloxacin, ofloxacin, or levofloxacin to complete 7–10 days of therapy. Alternative regimens including parenteral administration of other third-generation cephalosporins, a fluoroquinolone, or spectinomycin are also available (see Table 9.3). Management of purulent joint effusions is identical to that of other forms of septic arthritis. Compared to *S. aureus* and Gram-negative bacilli, residual joint damage is unusual following *Neisseria gonorrhoeae* infection.

KEY POINTS
Disseminated Gonococcal Disease

1. Most commonly occurs in patients with asymptomatic mucosal infections:
   a. More common in females,
   b. Higher incidence following menstruation or postpartum,

c. Higher incidence in patients with terminal complement deficiencies.
2. Two clinical syndromes are associated with dissemination:
    a. Tenosynovitis, dermatitis, polyarthritis: Tenosynovitis is pathpneumonic. Pustular skin lesions range from 4 to 40 lesions, periarticular,
    b. Purulent arthritis.
3. Treatment with IV ceftriaxone followed by oral cefixime or a fluoroquinolone.

Additional Reading

Caputo, G.M., Cavanagh, P.R., Ulbrecht, J.S., Gibbons, G.W., and Karchmer, A.W. Assessment and management of foot disease in patients with diabetes. *N Engl J Med* 331(13):854–860, 1994.

Gentry, L.O. Approach to the patient with chronic osteomyelitis. In *Current Clinical Topics in Infectious Diseases*, Vol. 8. McGraw-Hill, New York, 62–83, 1987.

Lew, D.P., and Waldvogel, F.A. Osteomyelitis. *N Engl J Med* 336:999–1007, 1997.

Lew, D.P., and Waldvogel, F.A. Use of quinolones in osteomyelitis and infected septic arthritis. *Drugs* 158(Suppl. 2):85–91, 1999.

Mader, J.T., Norden, C., Nelson, J.D., and Calandra, G.B. Evaluation of new anti-infective drugs for the treatment of osteomyelitis in adults. Infectious Diseases Society of America and the Food and Drug Administration. *Clin Infect Dis* 15(Suppl. 1):S155–S161, 1992.

O'Brien, J.P., Goldenberg, D.L., and Rice, P.A. Disseminated gonococcal infection: A prospective of 49 patients, and a review of the pathophysiology and immune mechanisms. *Medicine* 62:395, 1983.

Parasitic Infections

Recommended Time to Complete: 2 Days

What does the infectious disease specialist mean by parasitic infection? In reality most infectious agents fulfill the definition of a parasite: an organism that grows, feeds, and is sheltered on or in a different organism and contributes nothing to the host. However, medical science has created the classification "parasite" to include a complex group of nonfungal eukaryotic human pathogens. Unlike fungi, parasites have no cell wall and are often motile. In addition many parasites require two or more host species to complete their life cycle and reproduce both sexually and asexually. The host in which sexual reproduction takes place is called the definitive host, and the host in which reproduction occurs asexually is termed the intermediate host.

Previously, parasitic infections were a health problem almost exclusively in developing countries with poor sanitation. However, with the marked rise in international travel these infections are now increasingly being diagnosed in the United States, Europe, and other developed countries. The incidence of symptomatic parasitic infections has also increased because of the ever-increasing population of immunocompromised hosts. Organ transplant, cancer chemotherapy, and infection with human immunodefi-

ciency virus all lead to depressed cell-mediated and humoral immunity, allowing dormant parasites to reactivate and cause disease. Now, more than ever before, thorough travel and exposure histories are critical steps in accurately diagnosing parasitic infections. An awareness of geography and environmental conditions and a familiarity with the life cycles of parasites are all required for proper diagnosis and treatment.

Blood Protozoa

Malaria

Guiding Questions

1. Which form of malaria is most dangerous and why?

2. What disease does malaria most commonly mimic?

361

3. How is malaria diagnosed? Is there a particular time in the course of illness when diagnostic studies should be performed?

4. Why are many people of black African descent more resistant than other ethnic groups to some forms of malaria?

5. What are the current recommendations for malaria treatment and what factors dictate the regimen of choice?

6. When should chemoprophylaxis be begun and how long after completion of a trip to an endemic area should preventive therapy be continued?

Potential Severity: Hours can make the difference between life and death. Rapid diagnosis and treatment are critical.

PREVALENCE

The deteriorating political and economic conditions of countries in sub-Saharan Africa as well as the development of chloroquine drug resistance in many parts of the world have resulted in a resurgence of malaria. The worldwide annual incidence of malaria is between 300 and 500 million cases, causing 2–3 million deaths. Countries with significant numbers of malaria cases include Africa, the Middle East, India, Southeast Asia, South America, Central America, and parts of the Caribbean. Chloroquine resistance is now the rule in most countries. *Plasmodium falciparum* in Southeast Asia is frequently resistant not only to chloroquine, but also to pyrimethamine-sulfadoxine, mefloquine, and halofantrine. Areas where *P. falciparum* remains sensitive to chloroquine include Central America and the Caribbean, in particular Haiti. Because the sensitivity patterns of malaria continue to change annually, the Centers for Disease Control should be consulted for the most up-to-

date statistics (Internet address: www.cdc.gov/ travel).

EPIDEMIOLOGY AND LIFE CYCLE

Humans contract malaria after being bitten by the female Anopheles mosquito. Only the female mosquito takes a blood meal, because blood is required for the development of the mosquito egg. Certain strains appear to be more efficient transmitters of disease. In particular *Anopheles gambiae* and *A. funestus* are thought to account for the high transmission rates in sub-Saharan Africa. These strains are not present in South America and Southeast Asia, where transmission rates are lower. Clearly, the larger the number of mosquito bites a person acquires, the greater the risk of contracting malaria. Therefore in addition to chemoprophylaxis (see below), mosquito netting, long-sleeved shirts, long pants, insect repellant, and staying in a protected environment during the times of the day when the mosquito population is highest are recommended as preventive measures.

The female anopheline mosquito introduces sporozoites into the human bloodstream that quickly travel to the liver and invade hepatocytes (see Figure 12.1). Sporozoites contain a specific protein that is thought to be critical for binding and entry into hepatocytes (circumsporozoite protein), and this protein binds to specific host cell membrane receptors (heparin sulfate proteoglycans and low-density lipoprotein receptor–related protein). Within hepatocytes sporozoites mature to tissue schizonts. Some sporozoites become dormant, form hypnozoites, and take six to eleven months to activate into tissue schizonts. Each schizont-infected hepatocyte then produces 10,000–30,000 merozoites, which are released into the blood stream following cell lysis. Each merozoite in turn can invade a single red blood cell and asexually replicate five times over 48–72 hours to produce 32 merozoites. The production of merozoites is followed by red blood cell lysis, and release of these newly formed merozoites then can infect

Figure 12.1

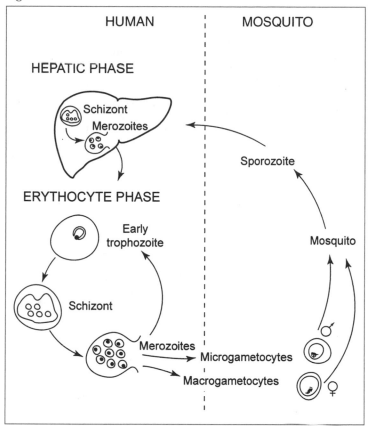

HUMAN   MOSQUITO

HEPATIC PHASE

Schizont
Merozoites

Sporozoite

ERYTHOCYTE PHASE

Early
trophozoite

Mosquito

Schizont

Merozoites
Microgametocytes
Macrogametocytes

Life cycle of plasmodium.

additional red blood cells. Under ideal conditions a single sporozoite theoretically could account for the infection of nearly 1 million red blood cells. (Many of the free merozoites are intercepted by host macrophages, thus reducing the efficiency of red cell infection.) As is observed with sporozoite entry into hepatocytes, a specific protein on the merozoite surface (erythrocyte-binding antigen 175 in *Plasmodium falciparum* and Pv135 in *P. vivax*) binds to a specific red blood cell membrane receptor (glycophorin A in *P. falciparum* and Duffy factor in *P. vivax*), allowing attachment and entry. Once the merozoite enters the red blood cell, it matures to a trophozoite. This form looks like a signet ring

and can be readily seen in parasitized red blood cells following Giemsa or Wright staining (see Figure 12.2). As the trophozoite matures, it loses its discrete signet ring morphology, becoming larger and subsequently developing into a red blood cell schizont, which then splits into multiple merozoites.

On entry into the red blood cell, some merozoites mature into sexual forms called gametocytes rather than asexual forms. The male form is smaller and is called a microgametocyte; the larger female form is called a macrogametocyte. Sexual mating does not occur in the human host but only in the mosquito; therefore the mosquito is considered the

Figure 12.2

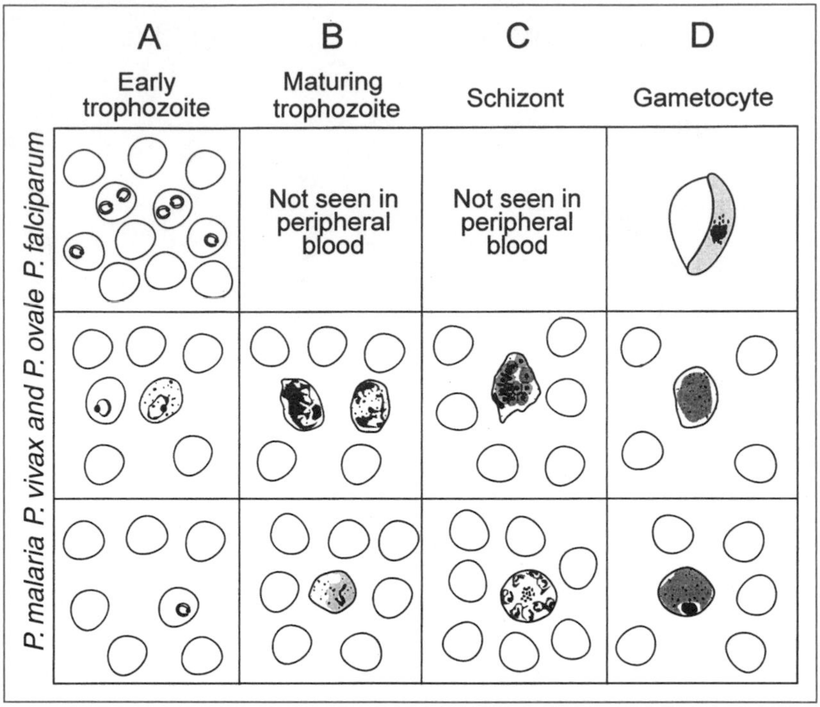

Typical blood smear findings of the different strains of malaria. (Adapted from Schaechter, M., Engleberg, N.C., Eisenstein B.I., and Medoff, G. (Eds.), *Mechanisms of Microbial Disease.* Lippincott Williams & Wilkins, Baltimore, 1999.)

definitive host and the human the intermediate host. Once fertilization occurs, a zygote is formed that subsequently develops into an oocyst. The oocyst then forms thousands of infectious sporozoites that gain entry into the mosquito salivary gland, where they are transmitted to the human host.

DIFFERENCES IN THE LIFE CYCLE AMONG THE DIFFERENT PLASMODIUM SPECIES

Plasmodium falciparum is the most common form of malaria and is the most dangerous. Unlike other strains, all sporozoites that enter the liver remain active and develop into tissue schizonts that go on to form thousands of merozoites. Also unlike other strains, the *P. falciparum* merozoite can

infect red blood cells of all ages, explaining the high level of parasitized red blood cells observed in this infection. In comparison to the other forms of malaria, in which only a single merozoite gains entry into cells, multiple *P. falciparum* merozoites can infect and mature within a single red blood cell. Once within the red blood cell, merozoites rapidly mature, asexually divide, and within 48 hours lyse the host red blood cell. This rapid asexual reproduction results in a rapid rise in the percentage of infected host red blood cells, and as the percentage of parasitized red blood cells increases, the risk of death or serious complications also increases. *P. falciparum* is especially harmful to the host because invasion by this strain is uniquely associated with the formation of red blood cell membrane knobs that tightly adhere to the vascular endothelium. These adherent red blood cells block blood flow in small blood vessels, causing severe hypoxic damage, particularly to the brain and kidneys. Because red blood cell adherence develops as the merozoite matures beyond the early trophozoite stage, other maturation stages of the parasite (with the exception of the banana-shaped gametocytes) are rarely seen in the peripheral blood (see Table 12.1 and Figure 12.2).

Table 12.1

Differences in Malaria Strains

MALARIA STRAIN	TRAITS
Plasmodium falciparum	No dormant phase in the liver
	Multiple signet ring trophozoites per cell
	High percentage (>5%) of parasitized RBCs
	Development stages other than the early ring trophozoite and mature gametocyte not seen
P. vivax and *P. ovale*	Dormant liver phase
	Single signet ring trophozoites per cell
	Schuffner's dots in the cytoplasm
	Low percentage (<5%) of parasitized RBCs
	All developmental stages seen
	RBCs often appear enlarged in the later stages
P. malariae	No dormant phase
	Single signet ring trophozoites per cell
	Very low level of parasitemia
	All developmental stages seen
	RBCs normal size

Life Cycle of *Plasmodium falciparum*

Plasmodium falciparum is the most dangerous form of malaria because it:

1. Infects red blood cells of all ages and causes high levels of parasitemia.
2. Induces the formation of knobs on the RBC surface that adhere to vessel walls causing obstruction and local hypoxia.
3. Can cause severe hemolysis, renal failure, central nervous system damage, and pulmonary edema.

Plasmodium vivax is the next most common form of malaria. *P. malariae* is less common, and *P. ovale* is a rare human infection. *P. vivax* and *P. ovale* can form hypnozoites that can remain dormant within the liver for months before becoming active tissue schizonts. This explains the ability of these strains to relapse six to eleven months after initial treatment. *P. malariae* has no dormant liver phase but can persist as a low level infection for up to 30 years. *P. vivax* and *P. ovale* merozoites bind only young red blood cells, having the highest affinity for reticuloytces, while *P. malariae* tends to infect older red blood cells. The inability of these strains to infect a broad age range of red blood cells explains their low level of parasitemia. Furthermore, these three strains do not form knobs and do not obstruct the microcirculation, features that explain their milder clinical manifestations.

GENETIC DETERMINANTS OF SUSCEPTIBILITY TO MALARIA

Two genetic traits have been associated with reduced susceptibility to malaria. First, the absence of the Duffy blood group antigen blocks invasion of *Plasmodium vivax*. This strain of malaria must bind to this blood group antigen to gain entry into red blood cells. A significant number of black Africans are Duffy-negative and are resistant to *P. vivax*. Second, individuals with sickle-cell hemoglobin are resistant to *P. falciparum,* and it is likely that this deadly strain of malaria has served as a powerful selective force, giving individuals with sickle-cell trait a survival advantage in endemic areas. When parasitized red blood cells containing sickle-cell hemoglobin form membrane knobs and become trapped in small vessels, oxygen tension decreases, and sickle-cell hemoglobin polymerizes, resulting in sickling of these red blood cells. The polymerization of hemoglobin S kills the *P. falciparum* parasite, preventing this infection from progressing. As a consequence individuals with sickle-cell trait and sickle-cell disease are resistant to *P. falciparum*. Because the other strains of malaria do not form knobs and do not become trapped in blood vessels, sickle-cell hemoglobin does not protect against *P. vivax, P. ovale,* or *P. malariae*.

KEY POINTS

Genetic Traits That Protect Against Malaria

1. Sickle-cell disease and trait are resistant to *Plasmodium falciparum.*
2. Negative Duffy blood group antigen blocks invasion by *P. vivax.*

◆ CASE 12.1

Mr. and Mrs. R. were sailing in the Caribbean near Jamaica with their three children. They lived primarily on their boat but took several day trips to a small island off the coast of Jamaica. They noted some mosquito bites and ate some fruits on the island. Both Mr. and Mrs. R. suddenly came down with fevers, chills, muscle aches, and loss of appetite. About 3 days into the illness Mr. R. became jaundiced and began passing dark urine. They sought treatment from a local Jamaican physician,

who diagnosed hepatitis secondary to ingestion of a toxic food. Two days later Mr. R. became comatose and died. Mrs. R. was referred to the University Hospital for a possible liver transplant. On further questioning it was learned that none of her children were sick despite having eaten the same diet. The family had taken malaria prophylaxis. However, Mr. and Mrs. R. had developed side effects from the chloroquine and had discontinued their prophylaxis 2 weeks before the onset of their illness. A thin smear of her blood revealed many signet ring trophozoites, and the parasitemia level was estimated to be 10%. She was treated with intravenous quinine and rapidly improved. In retrospect her husband had died of untreated blackwater fever.

Clinical Presentation

As described in Case 12.1, the clinical manifestations of malaria are nonspecific, and if the proper exposure history is not elicited, this infection can be mistaken for other febrile illnesses. The incubation period is generally 9–40 days but cases of non–*Plasmodium falciparum* malaria may be prolonged (6–12 months in *P. vivax,* years for *P. malariae* and *P. ovale*). The hallmark of all forms of malaria is fever. Fever can occur at regular 2- to 3-day intervals in *P. vivax* and *P. malariae* or a more irregular pattern in *P. falciparum*. Fever generally occurs soon after the lysis of the red blood cells and release of merozoites. Three classic stages of the febrile paroxysms have been described. First comes the "cold stage," which occurs 15–60 minutes prior to the onset of fever. During this period the patient feels cold and has shaking chills. These symptoms are followed by the "hot stage," during which the body temperature rises to 39–41°C. Fever is associated with lassitude, loss of appetite, and vague pains in the bones and joints. In nonendemic areas these symptoms are most commonly mistaken for influenza. The clinician must always consider malaria in individuals who develop flulike symptoms after returning from a developing country. Other symptoms associated with malarial fever include tachycardia, hypotension, cough, headache, back pain, nausea, abdominal pain, vomiting, diarrhea, and altered consciousness. Usually within 2–6 hours symptoms progress to the third, "sweating," stage, at which time the patient develops marked diaphoresis followed by resolution of fever, profound fatigue, and a desire to sleep.

Other symptoms depend on the strain of malaria. In cases of *Plasmodium vivax, P. ovale,* and *P. malariae* there are few additional symptoms. However, depending on the prior immune status of the host, individuals with *P. falciparum* can develop a severe fatal illness similar to that described in Case 12.1. Because *P. falciparum* can infect red blood cells of all ages and induces the formation of knobs on the red blood cell surface that adhere to endothelial cells and obstruct small vessels, this parasite can cause severe damage, particularly to the kidneys, brain, and lungs. Tourists who have no prior immunity to *P. falciparum,* as well as individuals who have undergone splenectomy can develop very high levels of parasitemia that result in profound hemolysis. The marked release of hemoglobin can exceed the metabolic capacity of the liver, resulting in a rise in unconjugated bilirubin in the bloodstream and jaundice. Hemoglobin also may be excreted into the urine, causing the urine to become dark. The combination of jaundice and hemoglobinuria has been called blackwater fever. Severe malaria is commonly complicated by renal failure. Heavy infections with *P. falciparum* also result in vascular obstruction of small arteries in the central nervous system (CNS), leading to hypoxia. Hypoglycemia may also contribute to CNS dysfunction. Confusion and obtundation can rapidly progress to coma. Grand mal seizures may also develop. Pulmonary edema is a less common complication of *P. falciparum* infection and is the result of fluid leakage from pulmonary capillaries into the alveoli.

KEY POINTS

Clinical Presentation of Malaria

> Always consider malaria in the traveler from a developing country who:
> 1. Presents with an influenzalike syndrome.
> 2. Presents with jaundice.
> 3. Presents with confusion or obtundation.

DIAGNOSIS

Microscopic examination of Giemsa-stained blood smear remains the primary way of identifying malaria. In *Plasmodium falciparum* blood smears are best taken just after the fever peak when early ring forms are most abundant in peripheral red blood cells. At other times *P. falciparum* becomes trapped in the capillaries and might not be found in the peripheral blood. In *P. vivax, P. malariae,* and *P. ovale* various stages of the parasite are present at all times; therefore smears can be performed at any time. Because parasites can be absent between attacks, the blood should be examined on 3 or 4 successive days before malaria can be ruled out. The presence of pigment in peripheral monocytes and/or neutrophils should encourage a continued search for parasites. Thin smears need to be examined for at least 15 minutes using a high-power oil objective (1000× magnification). Thick smears are the most reliable method for detecting malaria. A 5-minute search will generally yield the diagnosis. The clinician's primary goal is to differentiate potentially fatal *P. falciparum* from other, more benign forms of malaria (see Table 12.1). For this purpose three new assays have been developed: an enzyme-linked immunoabsorbance assay (ELISA) for histidine-rich *P. falciparum* antigen, an immunoassay for species-specific parasite lactic dehydrogenase isoenzymes, and polymerase chain reaction (PCR) amplification of parasite DNA or mRNA.

Laboratory Diagnosis of Malaria

> 1. The clinician must focus on differentiating *Plasmodium falciparum* from other forms of malaria.
> 2. Blood smear remains the preferred method; however, ELISA and PCR are now available.
> 3. In *P. falciparum* ring forms are most abundant on peripheral smear immediately after a fever spike.

Anemia, elevated lactic dehydrogenase levels, and increased reticulocytes are associated with red blood cell hemolysis. An elevated unconjugated bilirubin level without a significant increase in hepatic enzymes is also observed when hemolysis is severe. Thrombocytopenia is common. Elevated serum creatinine, proteinuria, and hemoglobinuria levels are found in severe cases of *Plasmodium falciparum*. Hypoglycemia may also complicate severe cases of *P. falciparum*, requiring close monitoring of blood sugars during the acute illness.

PROPHYLAXIS AND TREATMENT

Drug treatment exploits unique targets in the parasite that are not found in host cells. The aminoquinolines, chloroquine, quinine, mefloquine, and halofantrine inhibit proteolysis of hemoglobin in the food vacuole and inhibit the plasmodium heme polymerase required for production of malaria pigment. Inhibition of these functions kills the organism. In recent years many areas of Africa, northern South America, India, and Southeast Asia have become populated with chloroquine-resistant *Plasmodium falciparum*. These strains contain an energy-dependent chloroquine efflux mechanism that prevents the drug from concentrating in the parasite. Resistance to mefloquine and halofantrine has also developed, being seen primarily in Southeast Asia.

Chemoprophylaxis should be given two weeks before departure to an endemic area and be continued for four weeks after return. Because of the continual changes in resistance patterns, up-to-date prophylactic and treatment regimens should be reviewed on the Centers for Disease Control (CDC) web page (*www.cdc.gov/travel*). For areas with chloroquine-susceptible *Plasmodium falciparum* chloroquine is the drug of choice. The adult dosage is 300 mg base (500 mg of chloroquine phosphate) orally per week. In areas of chloroquine-resistance treatment consists of oral mefloquine 250 mg (228 mg of base) per week, oral doxycycline 100 mg per day, primaquine 0.5 mg base/kg/day, oral atovaquone 250 mg combined with 100 mg proguanil (a combination tablet called Malarone) per day, or the above dose of chloroquine with proguanil 200 mg/day. A vaccine is not available, and the immune response required to protect the host against malaria is poorly understood, making the development of an effective vaccine a formidable task.

Malaria Prophylaxis

> 1. Determine whether the traveler will be in areas with chloroquine resistance (check *www.cdc.org/travel*).
> 2. Begin prophylaxis 2 weeks before travel to ensure that there are no intolerable side effects.
> 3. Continue prophylaxis for 4 weeks after return.

All individuals with *Plasmodium falciparum* without previous immunity should be hospitalized because their clinical course can be unpredictable. Patients with *P. vivax, P. ovale,* or *P. malariae* can usually be treated as outpatients if there is reliable follow-up. The treatment for these three strains as well for chloroquine-susceptible *P. falciparum* is the same: chloroquine 600 mg base (1000 mg of the phosphate) po initially, followed 6 hours later by 300 mg of base (500 mg of phosphate) and again on days 2 and 3. To prevent relapse of *P. vivax* or *P. ovale,* these infections also require treatment with primaquine phosphate 15.3 mg base (26.5 mg phosphate salt) po for 14 days or 45 mg base (79 mg salt) per week for eight weeks. This agent kills dormant hepatic hypnozoites, preventing their subsequent development into infective schizonts. Prior to administration of this drug all patients should be tested for glucose-6-phosphate dehydrogenase (G6PD) deficiency because patients with G6PD deficiency are at risk of severe hemolysis during primaquine treatment.

KEY POINTS

Choosing Chemotherapy

1. Determine whether the traveler came from a chloroquine-resistant area (requires quinine or an equivalent regimen).
2. Determine whether the patient is too ill to take oral medicines (requires intravenous quinidine).
3. Determine whether the patient has *Plasmodium vivax* or *P. ovale* (requires primaquine if not G6PD deficient).

Individuals who contract malaria in regions with chloroquine-resistant *Plasmodium falciparum* should be treated with quinine 650 mg every 8 hours for 3–7 days plus doxycycline 100 mg BID × 7 days. A number of alternative regimens have been recommended, including quinine plus piramethamine sulfadoxine (three tablets on the last day of quinine therapy), quinine plus clindamycin (900 mg TID × 5 days), a single dose of mefloquine (1250 mg), halofantrine (500 mg every 6 hrs × 3 doses repeated in one week), atovaquone (1000 mg daily) plus proquanil (400 mg daily) (four Malarone tablets)

× 3 days, and artesunate (4 mg/kg/day × 3) plus mefloquine (750 mg followed in 12 hours by 500 mg). Halofantrine should not be used in patients who have developed malaria while on mefloquine because cross-resistance is common. Also the toxicities of these two drugs can be additive. Use of a higher than recommended dose of halofantrine, recent treatment with mefloquine, and thiamin deficiency are associated with an increased risk of a halofantrine-induced prolonged QT interval or ventricular arrythmias. A single high dose of mefloquine (1250 mg) alone frequently causes intolerable side effects including vertigo (10–20%), gastrointestinal disturbances, seizures, and, less commonly, psychosis.

If a patient is too ill to take oral medicines, intravenous quinidine is the treatment of choice. This drug is three to four times more active than intravenous quinine, and serum levels can be measured. Furthermore, parenteral quinine is no longer available in the United States. Quinidine gluconate 10 mg salt/kg loading dose (maximum 600 mg) in normal saline should be infused slowly over 1–2 hours followed by a continuous infusion of 0.02 mg/kg/min until the patient is able to take oral medications.

The risk of end organ damage and death increases with the level of parasitemia. Patients with levels above 5% constitute a medical emergency and require intensive treatment. Patients with no immunity and levels of *Plasmodium falciparum* parasitemia above 10–15% should be considered for exchange transfusion. This measure can be life-saving; however, patients with levels of parasitemia greater than 50% have survived without blood exchange. Volume status, renal function, and serum glucose must be carefully monitored, and respirator support may be required in cases of severe pulmonary edema. Intravenous steroids have been shown to be harmful in cases of cerebral malaria and therefore should not be used. Because of the risk of arrhythmias associated with quinine, quinidine, mefloquine, and halofantine, patients who are treated with these agents should be cardiac monitored.

Managing Patients with *Plasmodium falciparum*

1. Levels of parasitemia >5% constitute a medical emergency and require immediate institution of antimalaria treatment.
2. Hematocrit, blood sugar, volume status, cardiac rhythm, renal function, CNS function, and arterial oxygenation must all be closely monitored.
3. In the nonimmune host the course of *P. falciparum* infection is not predictable.
4. The severity of organ damage and risk of death correlate with the level of parasitemia.

Babesiosis

Guiding Questions

1. How is babesiosis contracted?
2. Why has the incidence of this infection increased in the United States?
3. How does Babesia's life cycle differ from that of Plasmodium and how might the differences relate to the clinical manifestations of babesiosis and malaria?
4. What other infection do patients with babesiosis often contract at the same time and why?
5. Is this blood protozoon treated in the same way as malaria?

Potential Severity: Usually causes mild disease but can be fatal in splenectomized patients.

PREVALENCE, EPIDEMIOLOGY, AND LIFE CYCLE

Babesiosis, an infection caused by protozoa of the genus Babesia, was once thought to be only a disease of cattle and wild animals. However, in the last 30 years this organism has been found to occasionally infect humans. Over 100 cases of human babesiosis have been described, many of the early cases occurring in Massachusetts on the islands of Nantucket and Martha's Vineyard. Subsequently, cases have been described throughout New England and in New York, Maryland, Virginia, Georgia, Wisconsin, Minnesota, Washington State, and California.

Like the agents that cause malaria, Babesia is a blood protozoon. It has a life cycle similar to that of Plasmodium; however, the organism is transmitted by the deer tick, *Ixodes scapularis* (see Figure 12.3). Curiously, deer do not become infected by Babesia. However, its intermediate host, the white-footed mouse, is readily infected by *Babesia microti,* the primary strain that causes human disease in the United States. In endemic areas the percentage of these rodents infected by Babesia can reach 60%. During its larval and nymph phases the deer tick lives on the white-footed mouse, from which it obtains blood meals. The nymph can leave the mouse and attach to humans. After attachment this tiny tick (2 mm in diameter) eats a blood meal and introduces the Babesia sporozoite, which enters human red blood cells. The mature signet ring–shaped trophozoite multiplies asexually by binary fission, forming characteristic tetrads, and subsequently lyses its host red blood cell. Because multiplication is asynchronous, massive hemolysis is not seen. Also, unlike Plasmodium, Babesia does not have a hepatic phase.

The Babesia Life Cycle

1. Babesia uses the small nymph form (2 mm in diameter) of the deer tick, *Ixodes scapularis*, to carry it from white-footed mice to humans.
2. In human red blood cells the mature signet ring trophozoite multiplies by binary fission, forming characteristic tetrads.
3. Multiplication is asynchronous, and therefore RBC lysis is never massive.
4. Babesiosis has no hepatic phase.

The rise in incidence of babesiosis in the United States has been attributed to the decreased popularity of deer hunting and the associated increase in the deer and deer tick populations. Also Americans' move to the suburbs has brought humans in close proximity to the mouse reservoirs that harbor the infectious *Ixodes scapularis* nymph. This infection is contracted by humans during the months of May through September when the nymphs are feeding.

KEY POINTS
Babesia Epidemiology

1. Endemic in areas where the deer population is abundant.
2. Requires the presence of the white-footed deer mouse, which harbors the infectious deer tick (*Ixodes scapularis*) nymphs.
3. Human infections occur during the period of nymph feeding (May–September).

CLINICAL PRESENTATION

♦ **CASE 12.2**

Mrs. S. was a 65-year-old white female who presented with intermittent fevers for the past two months associated with intermittent myalgias and fatigue. She had just returned from a two-month summer vacation on Martha's Vineyard, Massachusetts. She denied any history of tick bites. One month earlier she was diagnosed with Lyme disease. However, despite appropriate treatment, her fevers did not resolve. Aside from a mild anemia, her routine blood tests were normal; however, Giemsa stain of her peripheral blood revealed occasional red blood cells containing ring forms, some in tetrads. Treatment with clindamycin and quinine caused a rapid resolution of her fever.

The symptoms of babesiosis are nonspecific, making the disease difficult to diagnose clinically. Generally, patients present one to three weeks after exposure with a flulike illness.

Fever, chills, myalgias, arthralgias, fatigue, and anorexia are most common. The illness presents during the summer months as a "summer flu." In endemic areas the clinician should inquire about recent hiking in tick-infested areas, particularly areas with tall grasses and brush. Patients often do not give a history of tick bites, failing to detect the attached nymph because of its small size (the diameter of a small freckle). In the normal host the disease may cause minimal symptoms and spontaneously resolve. However, in patients who have undergone splenectomy or are elderly, infection can be more severe and persistent. Cases of adult respiratory distress syndrome and hypotension have been reported, and on rare occasion patients have died. In Europe cases have strictly involved splenectomized patients, and the clinical presentation has been more fulminant, being associated with severe hemolysis and death.

Patients with babesiosis may also have symptoms suggestive of Lyme disease, particularly the skin rash of erythema migrans. *Ixodes scapularis* is also the vector for *Borrelia burgdorferi,* and in one series of cases 54% of patients with babesiosis possessed antibodies against the Lyme spirochete, a finding suggesting that these patients had dual infections (see Chapter 13).

KEY POINTS
Clinical Presentation of Babesiosis

1. Presents as the "summer flu" one to three weeks after exposure.
2. History of hiking in tick-infested areas.
3. Often no history of tick bite, because the *Ixodes scapularus* nymph is mistaken for a small freckle.
4. More serious disease occurs in splenectomized patients and the elderly.
5. Patients with babesiosis may also have Lyme disease because *I. scapularis* transmits both infections.

DIAGNOSIS AND TREATMENT

Giemsa stain of thick and thin smears from the peripheral blood need to examined under an oil immersion objective. Small ring forms often in the form of tetrads (see Figure 12.3) are the only form seen. Babesiosis is frequently mistaken for *Plasmodium falciparum* infection. The classic tetrad is not observed in Plasmodium infection, and the banana-formed gametocytes that are observed in *P. falciparum* infection are never observed in babesiosis. An indirect immunofluorescent antibody titer that measures antibody against the primary form causing babesiosis in the United States, *Babesia microti,* is available through the CDC. Significant increases in antibody titer develop three to four weeks after the infection is contracted. Treatment should be initiated in splenectomized patients as well as other patients with serious disease. Clindamycin, 300–600 mg every 6 hours intravenously or intramuscularly, combined with oral quinine, 650 mg every 6–8 hours for 7–10 days, is effective. Chloroquine, often initiated when babesiosis is mistaken for *P. falciparum* infection, is not effective. Also doxycycline, pentamidine, primaquine, and pyrimethamine-sulfadoxine are not efficacious. A potentially effective regimen, atovaquone and azithromycin, may be considered in the quinine-allergic patient.

KEY POINTS

Diagnosis and Treatment of Babesiosis

1. Giemsa stains of the peripheral blood remain the best way to make the diagnosis.
2. Only ring forms are seen.
3. Frequently mistaken for *Plasmodium falciparum*.
4. Tetrad ring forms strongly support the diagnosis of babesiosis.

Figure 12.3

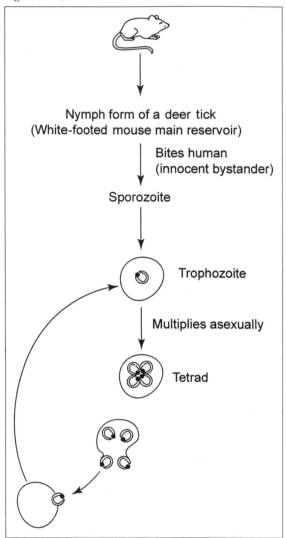

Life cycle of Babesia.

5. Many malaria regimens, including chloroquine and primaquine, are not effective in babesiosis.
6. Clindamycin and oral quinine × 7–10 days are recommended.

Tissue Protozoa

Leishmaniasis

Guiding Questions

1. How is leishmaniasis contracted and where is this disease most commonly found?

2. What form of immunity is most important for protecting against Leishmania and are HIV-positive patients and organ transplant patients at increased risk for developing leishmaniasis?

3. How do patients with visceral leishmaniasis usually present clinically and what diseases can this infection mimic?

4. Where are lesions of cutaneous leishmaniasis usually located and why?

5. What is the FDA-approved therapy for visceral leishmaniasis?

Potential Severity: Visceral disease is a chronic disease that can cause severe morbidity and death in debilitated and immunocompromised hosts.

PREVALENCE, EPIDEMIOLOGY, AND LIFE CYCLE

Leishmania has caused major epidemics in eastern India, Bangladesh, and East Africa. Urban outbreaks have been reported in the cities of northeastern Brazil. A small number of American military personnel contracted leishmaniasis during the Persian Gulf War in 1991. Rarely, indigenous cases have been reported in the United States, but most U.S. cases result from travel to a tropical country. Leishmaniasis has emerged as an opportunistic infection in patients with human immunodeficiency virus

and in persons who have had organ transplants.

This parasite is transmitted by the female phlebotomine sandfly. Sandflies breed in cracks in the walls of dwellings, rubbish, and rodent burrows. Because they are weak fliers, they remain close to the ground near their breeding sites, resulting in localized pockets of infectious insects. Humans and other animals infected with Leishmania serve as reservoirs. The sandfly bites the infected host and ingests blood containing the nonflagellated form, called an amastigote. In the digestive tract of the insect the amastigote develops into a flagellated spindle-shaped promastigote. When the infected fly takes its blood meal from an uninfected human, the promastigote enters the host's bloodstream. The promastigote then binds to complement receptors on macrophages and is ingested. Within the phagolysome the promastigote differentiates into an amastigote. The amastigote is resistant to lysozyme damage and depends on the low pH of the phagolysosome for uptake of nutrients. The parasite multiplies by simple division and eventually is released to infect other cells.

Cell-mediated immunity plays an important role in controlling leishmaniasis. Interferon gamma activates macrophages to kill the amastigote by inducing the production of nitric oxide. Resolution of leishmanial infection is associated with the expression of CD4+ T cells of the Th-1 type, which secrete interferon-γ and interleukin-2 (IL-2). Progression of infection is associated with Leishmania-induced expansion of CD4+ cells of the Th-2 type that produce interleukin-4 (IL-4), a cytokine that inhibits the production of Th-1 cells and the activation of interferon-γ production.

KEY POINTS

Epidemiology and Life Cycle of Leishmania

1. Contracted in tropical areas where the phlebotomine sandfly is common, rare in the

U.S. Found in South America, India, Bangladesh, the Middle East, and East Africa.
2. Flagellated promastigote introduced by the sandfly is ingested by macrophages.
3. In the macrophage, develops into a nonflagellated amastigote that lives happily within the macrophage phagolysosome.
4. This intracellular parasite is controlled by activation of the Th-1 cell-mediated immune response, which increases interferon-γ.
5. Leishmaniasis can be an opportunistic infection in HIV and transplant patients.

CLINICAL PRESENTATION

There are three forms of leishmaniasis: visceral, cutaneous, and mucosal. A single species can produce more than one syndrome, and each syndrome is produced by multiple different species.

VISCERAL LEISHMANIASIS (KALA AZAR)   In different areas of the world certain species tend to be most commonly associated with this disorder: *Leishmania donovani* in India, *L. infantum* in the Middle East, *L. chagasi* in Latin America, and *L. amazonensis* in Brazil. After inoculation of promastigotes into the skin, a small papule may be noticed. Leishmania amastigotes subsequently silently invade macrophages throughout the reticuloendothelial system. Usually, three to eight months pass before the burden of organisms increases to a level that causes symptoms. The onset of symptoms can be gradual or sudden. In subacute cases the patient will experience slow but progressive enlargement of the abdomen as a result of hepatosplenomegaly. Increased abdominal girth is accompanied by intermittent fever, weakness, loss of appetite, and weight loss. This presentation can be mistaken for lymphoma, infectious mononucleosis,

brucellosis, chronic malaria, and hepatosplenic schistosomiasis. In acute cases there is an abrupt onset of high fever and chills mimicking malaria or an acute bacterial infection. On exam the spleen may be massively enlarged, hard, and nontender. Hepatomegaly is also present. The skin tends to be dry and thin and in light-skinned individuals takes on a grayish tint. This characteristic accounts for the Indian name "kala-azar," which means black fever. On laboratory examination anemia, leukopenia, and hypergammaglobulinemia are common. Diagnosis is made by biopsying lymphatic tissue or bone marrow and demonstrating amastigotes on Wright or Geimsa stain. ELISA assays usually demonstrate high antileishmanial antibody titers. However, this test frequently cross-reacts with antibodies to other pathogens. Patients with HIV infection frequently fail to develop antibody titers. Splenomegaly might not be present in these patients, and infection may disseminate to the lungs, pleura, gastrointestinal tract, or bone marrow (causing aplastic anemia). In HIV patients amastigotes may be identified in macrophages from bronchoalveolar lavage, pleural effusion, bone marrow aspiration, or even buffy coat samples of the peripheral blood.

KEY POINTS
Visceral Leishmaniasis

1. Incubation period is three to eight months.
2. Subacute onset: Increased abdominal swelling due to massive splenomegaly and hepatomegaly, intermittent fever, weight loss; can be mistaken for lymphoma or infectious mononucleosis.
3. Acute onset: Persistent high fever mimicking bacteremia or malaria.
4. Anemia, leukopenia, and hypergammaglobulinemia are common.

5. Diagnosis is made by biopsy and Giemsa stain showing amastigotes.
6. HIV patients may have disseminated disease without splenomegaly.

CUTANEOUS LEISHMANIASIS   This form of disease is widespread and is most commonly a problem for farmers, settlers, troops, and tourists in the Middle East and Central and South America. The species that are most commonly associated with cutaneous disease are *Leishmania major* and *L. tropica* in the Middle East, India, Pakistan, and Asia and *L. mexicana, L. braziliensis, L. amazonensis,* and *L. panamensis* in Central and South America. *L. mexicana* has been reported in Texas. After a sandfly bite, significant skin lesions generally take two weeks to several months to develop. Lesions usually develop on exposed areas, primarily the arms, legs, and face. Amastigotes multiply in mononuclear cells within the skin and cause a granulomatous inflammatory reaction. Single or multiple lesions may be found, and their morphology varies. Lesions may be crusted and dry or moist with an exudate. Ulcers may develop that are shallow and circular with sharp, raised borders that progressively increase in size and develop a pizzalike appearance as a result of the beefy red appearance of the ulcer base associated with yellow exudate. Lesions may become secondarily infected with staphylococci or streptococci. Diagnosis is made from biopsy of the raised border of the skin lesion, where Leishmania-infected macrophages are most abundant. Amastigotes are seen on Giemsa stain.

MUCOSAL LEISHMANIASIS   This is a less common manifestation and is primarily caused by *Leishmania braziliensis*. Only 2–3% of patients with skin lesions develop this complication. Organisms invade mononuclear cells of the mucosa. The nose is most commonly involved, resulting in nasal stuffiness, discharge, pain, or epistaxis. Later the nasal septum is destroyed, and the nose collapses. Involvement of the genital mu-

cosa and trachea have also been reported. Diagnosis is made by biopsy.

KEY POINTS

Cutaneous and Mucosal Leishmaniasis

1. A problem for farmers, settlers, troops, and tourists.
2. Found throughout the world, cases reported in Texas.
3. Lesions occur primarily on exposed areas, incubation period: 2 weeks to 2 months.
4. Dry or moist in appearance, ulcers have sharp, raised borders, pizzalike lesions are common.
5. Mucosal disease is rarer, usually involves the nose.
6. Diagnosis by biopsy, always biopsy the border of skin lesions.

TREATMENT

The only drug that has been approved for treatment of leishmaniasis in the United States is liposomal amphotericin B, 3 mg/kg body weight/day on days 1–5, 14, and 21 for visceral leishmaniasis in immunocompetent patients. The course can be repeated if the parasite persists. For an immunocompromised host the recommended regimen is 4 mg/kg/day given on days 1–5, 10, 17, 24, 31, and 38. Relapses are common in HIV-positive patients. Outside the United States, pentavalent antimony continues to be used; however, this treatment is associated with many side effects, including abdominal pain, anorexia, nausea and vomiting, and myalgias. Amylase and lipase often increase. Treatment of cutaneous leishmaniasis depends on the location. Because the lesions can heal spontaneously, they can be followed without therapy or treated topically with 15% paromomycin and 12% methylbenzethomium chloride if there is no mucosal involvement and they are located in areas of no cosmetic concern. Patients with mucosal involvement, progressive lesions, or lesions in cosmetically sensitive areas require treatment with pentavalent antimony (20 mg/kg/day for 20 days) or ketoconazole (400–600 mg/day for 4 weeks).

KEY POINTS

Treatment of Leishmaniasis

1. Visceral disease: Liposomal amphotericin B is the only approved therapy.
2. Cutaneous: May spontaneously heal. If mucosal involvement or in cosmetically sensitive site or if fails to heal, ketoconazole or pentavalent antimony is recommended.

Trypanosomiasis

CHAGAS' DISEASE

Guiding Questions

1. What insect is responsible for transmitting Chagas' disease and is this disease commonly transmitted to tourists? Why or why not?
2. How does this insect's defecation habits affect transmission to the human host?
3. What organs are most commonly affected by chronic Chagas' disease?

Potential Severity: A chronic disorder that can lead to fatal cardiomyopathy.

PREVALENCE, EPIDEMIOLOGY, AND LIFE CYCLE   Chagas' disease, which is caused by *Trypanosoma cruzi,* is found throughout Central and South America. Sixteen to 18 million people worldwide are infected with *T. cruzi,* and nearly one half million· die from Chagas' disease annually. With improvement of substandard housing the incidence among young people is decreasing. The parasite is transmitted by reduviid bugs that suck blood from their host. This insect contains trypomastigotes in its gut. At the time it bites the host it also defecates, depositing trypomastigotes on the skin. The human host then scratches the bite, introducing the parasite into the wound and subsequently the bloodstream. Mucous membranes, the conjunctiva, and breaks in the skin are common sites of entry. Once in the bloodstream, the trypomastigotes enter host cells and differentiate into amastigotes that multiply, filling the cell cytoplasm. They then differentiate again into trypomastigotes, and the cell ruptures, spreading the parasite to adjacent cells and into the bloodstream. Asymptomatic parasitemia occurs in humans, and in endemic areas the parasite can be transmitted by blood transfusions. Because the reduviid bug takes up residence in the cracks of primitive homes, this infection occurs almost exclusively among poor rural people. Transmission of the disease most commonly occurs in young children. This disease has not been reported in tourists because they are unlikely to be exposed to primitive living quarters.

KEY POINTS

The Life Cycle of *Trypanosoma cruzi*

1. Transmitted by the reduviid bug, which carries the trypomastigote in its feces.
2. The host allows the parasite to enter the bloodstream by scratching and rubbing the infected feces into the skin.
3. The reduviid bug lives in the cracks of substandard housing.
4. A disease of poor rural people, not tourists.

CLINICAL PRESENTATION   Acute Chagas' disease often causes minimal symptoms. About a week after the parasite enters the skin, an area of localized swelling called a chagoma develops, often being associated with local lymph node swelling. Entry of the parasite via the conjunctiva causes periorbital edema (Romaña's sign). Onset of local edema is quickly followed by fever, malaise, anorexia, and edema of the face and legs. Occasionally, myocarditis or encephalitis may develop. Years to decades after the primary infection 10–30% of patients go on to develop chronic Chagas' disease. The heart is the primary organ that is damaged. Severe cardiomyopathy results in thromboembolism, congestive heart failure, and life-threatening arrhythmias. Esophageal involvement can lead to megaesophagus associated with dysphagia, regurgitation, and aspiration pneumonia. Chagasic megacolon is another manifestation of chronic disease causing constipation and bowel obstruction that can lead to perforation and bacterial sepsis. In immunocompromised hosts such as organ transplant patients and AIDS patients, *Trypanosoma cruzi* can reactivate, presenting with manifestations of chronic Chagas' disease. Unlike normal hosts, the immunocompromised patient is also at risk for developing *T. cruzi* brain abscesses.

KEY POINTS

Clinical Presentation of Chagas' Disease

1. Acute disease is associated with localized areas of swelling called chagomas.
2. Chronic disease develops decades after initial infection in 10-30% of cases.
3. Chronic disease affects:
   a. The heart causing a cardiomyopathy associated with CHF, emboli, and arrhythmias,
   b. The GI tract causing megaesophagus and megacolon.

DIAGNOSIS   Acute disease can be diagnosed by examining Giemsa-stained blood or buffy coat smears. Trypomastigotes, whose length is approximately twice the diameter of a red blood cell, can be readily seen by microscopy. In chronic disease diagnosis is made by detecting IgG antibodies. A number of serologic tests are available that are sensitive; however, they frequently yield false-positive results. In the United States the U.S. Food and Drug Administration has approved two ELISA assays for detecting clinical disease, but they are not approved for screening the blood supply. PCR testing has demonstrated promise but is not commercially available.

TREATMENT   This parasite is not sensitive to most antiparasitic drugs. Nifurtimox 8–10 mg/kg body weight per day divided into four oral doses for 90–120 days cures about 70% of acute cases. This drug causes gastrointestinal and neurologic side effects in many patients. Benznidazole 5 mg/kg/day for 60 days has a similar cure rate. Peripheral neuropathy, granulocytopenia, and rash are the most common side effects of this agent. Treatment with these same agents is now recommended for chronic Chagas' disease. Recent studies have shown that treatment slows the progression of heart disease.

KEY POINTS

Diagnosis and Treatment of Chagas' Disease

1. Acute disease is diagnosed by Giemsa stain of a peripheral blood smear.
2. Chronic disease can be diagnosed by an ELISA assay that detects IgG antibody to *Trypanosoma cruzi*.
3. Both acute and chronic disease should be treated with nifurtimox or benznidazole.
4. Treatment reduces mortality and progression of chronic disease.

TRYPANOSOMA BRUCEI COMPLEX

Potential Severity: Over weeks to months can progress to coma followed by death.

Trypanosoma brucei complex refers to several Trypanosoma subspecies that are spread by the bloodsucking tsetse fly. Unlike *Trypanosoma cruzi,* which takes up residence within cells, *T. brucei* trypomastigotes multiply within the bloodstream, evading the humoral immune system indefinitely by changing their surface antigens every 5 days. This disease is confined to Africa. Fewer than one case per year is imported into the United States. After the initial bite, the infection progresses slowly, systemic symptoms of fever and lymph node swelling being noted weeks to months later. In the West African form, neurologic manifestations do not develop until months to years after the initial symptoms. In East African trypanosomiasis, onset of systemic complaints may develop days after the insect bite, and CNS complaints may develop within weeks. Symptoms include somnolence (explaining the name "sleeping sickness"), choreiform movements, tremors, and ataxia mimicking Parkinson's disease. Coma and death frequently ensue. Diagnosis is made by Giemsa-stained peripheral blood thick and thin smears. Trypomastigotes can also be found in the cerebro spinal fluid. The treatment for disease caused by *T. brucei* is complex and depends on the species of infecting parasite, whether or not there is CNS involvement, and the patient's ability to tolerate the side effects of the treatment regimen. Potential medications include eflornithine, suramin alone or combined with the arsenical tryparsamide, pentamidine, and the arsenical melarsoprol.

Intestinal Helminths

Guiding Questions

1. In what two ways do intestinal helminths gain entry into the human host?
2. How does the life cycle of Ascaris differ from that of Trichuris and how does this difference manifest itself clinically?

3. How is Strongyloides able to persist in the human host for three to four decades?
4. What conditions precipitate the Strongyloides hyperinfection syndrome and why?
5. Which helminth most commonly causes iron deficiency anemia and why?

Potential Severity: Infections are often asymptomatic. In the immunocompromised host Strongyloides can progress to a fatal hyperinfection syndrome.

Helminths include roundworms (nematodes), flukes (trematodes), and tapeworms (cestodes). These parasites are large, ranging from 1 cm to 10 m in length, and often live in the human gastrointestinal tract without causing symptoms. Only when the infection is very heavy or the worm migrates to extraintestinal sites do patients seek medical attention. Transmission to humans in most cases results from contact with human waste. Diagnosis is generally made by examining the stool for eggs, larvae, or adult worms (see Figure 12.4).

Intestinal Nematodes (Roundworms)

Nematodes can be classified in two groups: those that gain entry to the host by egg ingestion (Trichuris, Ascaris, and Enterobius) and those capable of producing larvae that penetrate the skin of their host (Strongyloides and hookworm). The life cycles of the roundworm can also be classified into two groups. One group, Trichuris and Enterobius, attach and grow in the intestine soon after being ingested. The second group, Ascaris, Strongyloides, and hookworm, first penetrate the venous system, enter the lungs, migrate up the trachea, are swallowed, and then take up residence in the gastrointestinal tract (see Figure 12.5). These differences in life cycle account for some of the unique clinical characteristics of different species of nematodes.

Figure 12.4

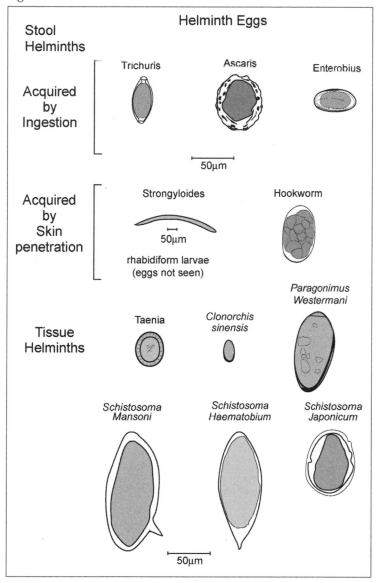

Helminth eggs. All eggs are drawn to scale. In Strongyloides only the rhabidiform larvae are usually seen.

Nematodes Acquired by Ingestion

TRICHURIS TRICHIURA (WHIPWORM)

This is one of the most prevalent helminths. Over 2 million people are estimated to be infected in the United States. This parasite is most commonly found in the rural Southeast and particularly Puerto Rico, where the appropriate moisture and temperature favor egg maturation. Worldwide, this worm commonly causes infection in poor rural communities with poor sanita-

Figure 12.5

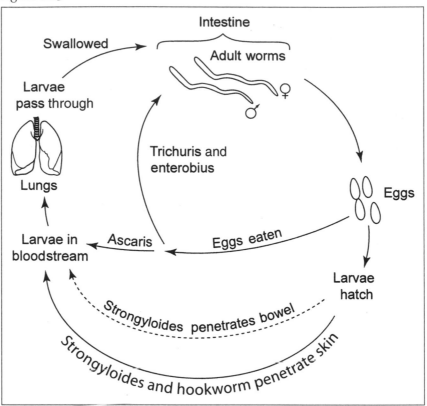

Comparative life cycles of intestinal nematodes. (Adapted from Schaechter, M., Engleberg, N.C., Eisenstein B.I., and Medoff, G. (Eds.), *Mechanisms of Microbial Disease*. Lippincott Williams & Wilkins, Baltimore, 1999.)

tion. Humans are the principal host, and infection results from ingestion of embryonated eggs. After eggs are excreted in the stool, under optimal conditions of shade and moisture embryonic development takes place within two to four weeks, and when the eggs are ingested by humans, larvae break out of the eggshell and penetrate the intestinal villi of the small intestine. Over 3–10 days they migrate down to the cecum, and over one to three months they develop into egg-producing adults. Most *Trichuris trichiura* infections are asymptomatic. Heavy infections can result in iron deficiency as well as abdominal pain and tenderness. Bloody diarrhea, growth retardation, and rectal prolapse are

potential complications of heavy infection. Diagnosis is made by fecal smear. The ovum has a classic lemon shape with pluglike ends (see Figure 12.4). Mebendazole 100 mg twice a day for 3 days is highly effective treatment and is rarely associated with side effects.

ASCARIS

This is the most common helminthic infection of humans and is estimated to infect over 1 billion humans worldwide. In the United States infections are found predominantly in the Southeast, where weather conditions favor egg embryonation. Like Trichuris, Ascaris is a parasite of humans, the infection being contracted by ingesting material contaminated with human feces. Within 5–10 days under proper temperature and moisture conditions eggs develop into infective embryos. When ingested, the parasites hatch in the small intestine. Embryos then penetrate the intestinal wall and enter the venous bloodstream. On reaching the capillaries of the lung, they break into the alveoli, crawl up through the bronchi and trachea, and then are swallowed and reenter the gastrointestinal tract, where they mature over two months. Each mature gravid female can produce 200,000 eggs per day. As with other roundworm infections most patients are asymptomatic. However, patients with high worm burdens can suffer from obstruction of the small intestine accompanied by vomiting and abdominal pain. Patients may vomit worms during such attacks or pass them in their stool. Heavy infections may also be associated with malabsorption, steatorrhea, and weight loss. A single ascaris worm can migrate up the biliary tree and obstruct the common bile duct, precipitating symptoms of cholecystitis, including epigastric abdominal pain, nausea, and vomiting. As the worms migrate into the lungs, some patients experience respiratory symptoms and develop pneumonia on chest X-ray accompanied by peripheral eosinophilia (sometimes called Löffler's syndrome). Worms on occasion can migrate to other sites in the body, causing local symptoms. Because of the large number of eggs that are excreted daily, this infection is easily diagnosed by stool smear (see Figure 12.4). Ascaris infection is effectively cured with mebendazole 100 mg twice a day for 3 days.

ENTEROBIUS (PINWORM)

This is the most common worm infection in countries within the temperate zone. This infection is very common in children of all socioeconomic groups in the United States. The eggs of this parasite resist drying and can contaminate bedclothes and dust. As a result, infection in one young child can lead to infestation of the entire family. After ingestion the eggs hatch in the duodenum and jejunum, and larvae mature in the cecum and large intestine. At night gravid females migrate to perianal area, where they lay eggs and cause localized itching. When this area is scratched, eggs are trapped under fingernails and are subsequently ingested by the host, resulting in repeated autoinfection. The major clinical manifestation of pinworm is nocturnal itching of the perianal area that often interferes with sleep. This parasite rarely causes other symptoms. Because Enterobius rarely migrates through tissue, this infection is not associated with peripheral eosinophilia. Diagnosis is made by pressing adhesive cellophane tape onto the perianal area in the early morning. Small, white, threadlike worms and eggs become attached to the tape and can be easily identified by using a low-power (100×) microscope. A single 100-mg dose of mebendazole repeated in two weeks is curative. All symptomatic family members should be treated simultaneously.

KEY POINTS

Nematodes Acquired by Ingestion

1. Tend to cause minimal symptoms and are not life-threatening.
2. Contracted by contact with fecal material.
3. *Trichuris trichiura* can cause iron deficiency anemia, excretes lemon-shaped ova.
4. Ascaris passes through the lung and can initially cause respiratory symptoms, also can cause biliary obstruction, excretes round, thick-walled ova.
5. Enterobius is common in children and readily spreads by dust and contaminated linen. Diagnosed by the adhesive tape test demonstrating worms in the anal area.
6. Mebendazole is effective treatment.

Nematodes Acquired by Skin Penetration

STRONGYLOIDES

PREVALENCE, EPIDEMIOLOGY, AND LIFE CYCLE   Strongyloides infection is less common than the other roundworm infections; however, strongyloidiasis is widely distributed throughout the tropics and infects people in the southern United States. Because Strongyloides can cause a fatal hyperinfection syndrome in the immunocompromised host, clinicians need to be familiar with this parasite. The filariform larvae excreted in the feces are capable of penetrating the skin. Humans become infected as a result of skin exposure to feces or soil contaminated by feces. Walking barefoot on contaminated soil is the most common way of contracting this infection. After skin penetration the larvae enter the bloodstream and lymphatics. Subsequently, they become trapped in the lungs, where they enter the alveoli and are coughed up and swallowed, and then enter the gastrointestinal tract. The larvae mature in the upper gastrointestinal tract, where females are able to penetrate the bowel mucosa and deposit their eggs. Eggs hatch in the mucosa, releasing filariform larvae that either penetrate the bowel wall, resulting in autoinfection, or are passed in the feces. Because Strongyloides can reinfect the human host, this infection can persist for 35–40 years. The intensity of infection depends not only on the initial inoculum of organisms, but also on the degree of autoinfection. In the immunocompromised host autoinfection can be intense and cause severe illness.

KEY POINTS

Epidemiology and Life Cycle of Strongyloides

1. Endemic in warm areas, including the southeast United States.
2. Larvae in fecally contaminated soil penetrate the skin of bare feet.

3. Larvae enter the bloodstream, invade the lung, crawl up the trachea, are swallowed, and mature in the small intestine.
4. Adult worms deposit eggs in the bowel wall, where they hatch.
5. Larvae in the bowel can enter the bloodstream, causing autoinfection.
6. Infection can persist for 35-40 years.

CLINICAL PRESENTATION

◆ CASE 12.3

A 43-year-old white female who had lived her entire life in Florida presented to the hospital with a two-year history of loss of energy, weight loss, and anorexia. She was found to have pericarditis. Multiple serologic tests for connective tissue diseases confirmed the diagnosis of lupus erythematosus. Subsequently, her illness was complicated by the development of left hemiparesis due to central nervous system vasculitis diagnosed by arteriography. Her neurologic symptoms improved after treatment with 100 mg/day of prednisone. During the third week of high-dose prednisone she began experiencing severe shortness of breath. Over 3 days she became increasingly hypoxic (arterial pO_2 = 50), requiring intubation and positive end-expiratory pressure. Her chest X-ray showed diffuse pulmonary infiltrates. Her hematocrit dropped from 40 to 20, and her peripheral white blood cell count dropped from 7,000 to 1,800. No peripheral eosinophils were noted. Lung biopsy revealed histologic findings of a hemorrhagic pneumonia, and in one field a small nematode was seen in the alveolar space (see Figure 12.6). Many small nematodes were also seen in a sputum sample. The patient died soon after the diagnosis of Strongyloides hyperinfection was made. At autopsy multiple worms were found throughout the small intestine.

As is observed with other roundworms, the majority of patients with Strongyloides infection have no symptoms because they harbor only a small number of worms. Heavier infestations can cause symptoms that relate to the parasite's life cycle. When the filariform larvae first penetrate

Figure 12.6

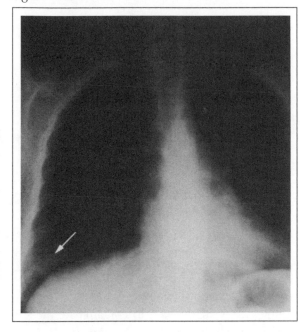

A

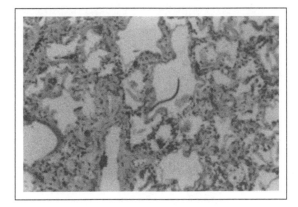

B

Strongyloidiasis hyperinfection syndrome. (A) Chest X-ray: Demonstrates only a small area of atelectasis (arrow). (B) Lung biopsy: Hematoxylin and eosin stain showing inflammatory cells within the alveoli and a rhabidiform larva (middle of the field).

the skin, they can cause itching as well as a papular erythematous rash. Migration into the lungs can cause respiratory symptoms, pneumonia, and peripheral eosinophilia (Löffler's syndrome). Once Strongyloides takes up residence in the gastrointestinal tract, the parasite can cause burning abdominal pain that mimics peptic ulcer disease or colicky abdominal pain that mimics gallbladder disease. Abdominal pain may be associated with diarrhea and the passage of mucus. Malabsorption, nausea, vomiting, and weight loss may also be present. Because the female worm penetrates the bowel mucosa and filariform larvae can migrate through the bowel wall, the host responds by producing eosinophils, and peripheral eosinophilia is a prominent finding in strongyloidiasis. When larvae penetrate the perianal area, a localized snakelike urticarial rash may be seen. A generalized urticarial rash may also be seen.

As described in Case 12.3, when asymptomatic individuals who harbor small numbers of organisms receive immunosuppressives such as high-dose corticosteroids or develop depressed cell-mediated immunity because of severe malnutrition or AIDS, the level of autoinfection can increase markedly, resulting in a hyperinfection syndrome. Symptoms may include diffuse pulmonary infiltrates, severe abdominal pain, meningitis, and Gram-negative sepsis as a result of filariform larvae compromising the integrity of the bowel wall. As in Case 12.3, eosinophilia is usually absent in this syndrome. When an immunocompromised patient presents with this clinical constellation and grew up in the rural South or previously lived in a tropical region, hyperinfection with Strongyloides needs to be considered.

KEY POINTS

Clinical Presentation of Strongyloidiasis

1. Many patients are asymptomatic.
2. Skin penetration can cause an itchy erythematous rash.

3. Lung invasion can produce Löffler's syndrome (cough, wheezing, pneumonia, and eosinophilia).
4. Heavy infection can cause abdominal pain and eosinophilia.
5. Treatment with high-dose steroids can cause a fatal hyperinfection syndrome (accelerated autoinfection).
6. Hyperinfection causes diffuse pneumonia, meningitis, abdominal pain, and Gram-negative sepsis. Eosinophilia is absent.

KEY POINTS

Diagnosis and Treatment of Strongyloidiasis

1. Diagnosis is difficult (stools do not contain ova).
2. Larvae found in the stool; duodenal aspiration may be required.
3. Peripheral eosinophilia may be the only finding.
4. Treat asymptomatic infections.
5. Thiabendazole is the drug of choice.

DIAGNOSIS AND TREATMENT Because the eggs usually hatch in the gastrointestinal tract, the Strongyloides egg is rarely seen on stool smear. Diagnosis depends on identifying filariform larvae in the feces or duodenal fluid. Diagnosis requires expertise because hookworm larvae can easily be misdiagnosed as Strongyloides. At least three stools need to be examined under a low-power (100×) microscope, and if they are negative, the Entero-Test should be used to sample the duodenal contents for larvae. Serodiagnosis and molecular probes are currently under development to improve the diagnostic yield. Another important clue is the presence of peripheral eosinophilia, which may increase to 10–20% of the peripheral white blood cells. However, lack of eosinophilia, particularly in the hyperinfection syndrome, does not exclude the diagnosis of strongyloidiasis.

Thiabendazole is the drug of choice. The recommended dose is 25 mg/kg twice a day for 2 days (maximum dose 3 gm/day). All patients infected with Strongyloides, even the asymptomatic patient, should be treated because of the potential danger of severe autoinfection. Patients who develop the hyperinfection syndrome should be treated for two to three weeks. However, mortality associated with this syndrome remains high despite treatment. Therefore patients with a past history of Strongyloides should be thoroughly examined and treated before receiving immunosuppressive therapy.

HOOKWORM (*ANCYLOSTOMA DUODENALE AND NECATOR AMERICANUS*)

PREVALENCE, EPIDEMIOLOGY, AND LIFE CYCLE Hookworm has been estimated to infect nearly one quarter of the world's population, being found throughout the tropical and subtropical zones. Infection is prevalent in areas where untreated human feces are allowed to contaminate the soil and people walk barefoot. *Necator americanus,* or New World hookworm, is found primarily in the Western hemisphere but also in southern Asia, Indonesia, Australia, and the Pacific Islands. *Ancylostoma duodenale,* or Old World hookworm, is found predominantly in the Mediterranean region, northern Asia, and the west coast of South America. As a result of sanitary waste disposal policies this infection has a low prevalence in the United States, being found primarily in the Southeast. The life cycle of hookworm is very similar to that of Strongyloides. As with Strongyloides, filariform larvae penetrate the skin, enter the bloodstream and lymphatics, pass into the lung, migrate to the trachea, are swallowed, and finally take up residence in the upper small intestine (see Figure 12.5). They attach by a buccal capsule that is used to suck blood from the host. A single *N. americanus* worm can remove 0.03 ml of blood per day, and a single *A. duodenale* worm can remove 0.2 ml. Worldwide, hookworm is a major cause of iron deficiency anemia and is responsible for an estimated blood loss of 7 million liters per day, or the total blood volume of over 1 million people!

Hookworm's life cycle differs from that of Strongyloides in several important ways, which account for hookworm's milder clinical manifestations. The Strongyloides egg matures quickly, hatching in the bowel wall of the host; while the hookworm egg matures more slowly, requiring several days of incubation in warm, moist, shady soil. This explains why human hookworm infestation is confined to areas with a warm climate. Also as a consequence of hookworm eggs' longer maturation time, autoinfection does not occur, and infection by fresh feces is not possible.

CLINICAL PRESENTATION   When hookworm larvae penetrate the skin, they can cause intense pruritus, sometimes called "ground itch." Itching is associated with local erythema and a papular rash at the site of penetration. Subsequently, as is observed with both Ascaris and Strongyloides, as the worm penetrates the lung, respiratory symptoms and patchy pneumonia associated with peripheral eosinophilia (Löffler's syndrome) can develop. The most common abnormalities associated with hookworm are iron deficiency and protein malnutrition. These abnormalities depend on the worm burden as well as the nutritional status of the patient. Other complaints may include abdominal pain, diarrhea, and weight loss.

DIAGNOSIS AND TREATMENT   Adult female worms release 10,000–20,000 eggs per day and make diagnosis by stool smear simple. The eggs are readily seen by using a low-power (100×) microscope (see Figure 12.4). Quantitation of the egg count allows the clinician to estimate the worm burden. Mebendazole 100 mg twice a day for 3 days is usually curative.

KEY POINTS

Hookworm (*Necator americanus* and *Ancylostoma duodenale*)

1. Larvae from the soil penetrate the skin, causing a pruritic rash.

2. Larvae pass through the lung and can cause Löffler's syndrome.
3. Eggs hatch outside of the host in soil, no autoinfection.
4. Adult worms attach to bowel wall and suck blood.
5. Iron-deficiency anemia is the most common manifestation.
6. Diagnosis is made readily by seeing ova in the stool.
7. Mebendazole is the treatment of choice.

Tissue and Blood Helminths

Guiding Questions

1. Which tissues do Trichinella, Echinococcus, and *Taenia solium* prefer to infect?
2. Why is Trichinella uncommon in the United States?
3. What is a hydatid cyst and how is it treated?
4. Why does treatment with praziquantel often exacerbate the manifestations of neurocysticercosis?

TRICHINELLA

Potential Severity: Usually asymptomatic, but heavy infections can lead to severe myocarditis, pneumonia, and encephalitis that can be fatal.

PREVALENCE, EPIDEMIOLOGY, AND LIFE CYCLE   Trichinosis is found worldwide wherever contaminated meat is undercooked. Trichinella is a roundworm whose larvae are released from cyst walls in contaminated meat by acid-pepsin digestion in the stomach. On entering the small intestine, larvae invade the intestinal microvilli and develop into adult worms. Females then release larvae, which enter the bloodstream and seed skeletal and cardiac muscle. The larvae grow in individual muscle fibers and eventually become surrounded by a cyst wall. Once encysted, larvae can remain viable for many years. If the cyst-containing muscle tissue is ingested, Trichinella is able to take up residence in the new host. The primary domestic animal that becomes infected with Trichinella is the pig. In many countries, including the United States, pigs are fed with grain, explaining the low incidence of trichinosis. In the United States laws were enacted to prevent the feeding of uncooked garbage to pigs, and as a result fewer than 100 cases are reported annually in the United States. The majority of cases of trichinosis result from improperly processed pork; however, undercooked bear, walrus, and cougar meat as well as wild boar and horse meat have also been sources of Trichinella infection.

CLINICAL PRESENTATION   Symptoms correlate with the load of worms in tissues. Because the number of cysts ingested is often low, the majority of infections are asymptomatic. Heavier infestations can result in diarrhea, abdominal pain, and vomiting during the intestinal phase, followed in one to two weeks by fever, periorbital edema, subconjunctival hemorrhages, and chemosis. Muscle pain, swelling, and weakness are common. The extraocular muscles are frequently involved first, followed by the neck and back, arms, and legs. Occasionally, a macular or petechial diffuse body rash may be seen. These symptoms usually peak within two to three weeks but may be followed by a prolonged period of muscle weakness. Death is uncommon but can result from severe myocarditis leading to congestive heart failure. Fatal encephalitis and pneumonia have also been reported.

DIAGNOSIS AND TREATMENT   An elevated peripheral eosinophil count associated with periorbital edema, myositis, and fever strongly suggests the diagnosis. Eosinophil counts are often very high. Serum creatine phosphokinase reflecting muscle damage is also elevated. A specific diagnosis requires muscle biopsy of a symptomatic muscle

to demonstrate Trichinella larvae. Because an exposure history and the clinical manifestations are usually distinct, a biopsy is rarely required. Antibody to Trichinella increases within three weeks and can be detected by ELISA. There is no effective treatment for trichinosis. If exposure to tainted meat is verified within one week of ingestion, thiabendazole, 25 mg/kg/day, can be given for one week. This drug is active against intestinal worms but is ineffective for treating muscle larvae. In critically ill patients corticosteroids may be helpful, but there have been no controlled trials proving efficacy. Cooking meat above 55°C until all pink flesh is browned kills encysted larvae and prevents trichinosis.

KEY POINTS
Trichinosis

1. Caused by ingesting larvae cysts, primarily from pork.
2. Uncommon in countries that don't feed pigs uncooked garbage.
3. Larvae infect skeletal and cardiac muscle.
4. Light infections are often asymptomatic.
5. Heavy infection causes diarrhea, abdominal pain, and diarrhea followed by fever, periorbital edema, muscle pain (ocular muscles first), and myocarditis associated with marked eosinophilia and increased serum creatine phosphokinase.
6. Diagnosis is made by muscle biopsy, ELISA, or clinically.
7. Thiabendazole for intestinal phase.
8. Corticosteroids may be helpful in severe myocarditis.

Echinococcus (Echinococcosis)

Potential Severity: Rarely fatal. Clinical symptoms are often delayed for many years and result from the mass effect of the hydatid cyst.

PREVALENCE, EPIDEMIOLOGY, AND LIFE CYCLE

Echinococcus is a member of the cestode or tape-worm family. Infections with *E. granulosus* are found worldwide including Africa, the Middle East, southern Europe, Latin America, and the southwestern United States. A second species, *E. multilocularis,* is found in northern Europe, Asia, the northern United States, and the Arctic regions. Humans represent an inadvertent inter-mediate host, infection being contracted by in-gestion of food contaminated with viable para-site eggs. Echinococcus is carried in the feces of sheep, goats, camels, horses, and domestic dogs that live around livestock. In the south-western United States most cases are contracted from sheepdogs. Because eggs are partially re-sistant to drying and can remain viable for many weeks, food can become contaminated without coming into direct contact with infected animals. Ingested eggs hatch in the intestine, forming oncospheres that penetrate the bowel wall, enter the bloodstream, and are deposited in various organs, most commonly the liver and lungs and less frequently the brain, heart, and bones. Oncospheres then encyst, forming hy-datid cysts that consist of a germinal membrane that produces multiple tapeworm heads and also undergoes budding to form multiple sep-tated daughter cysts within the primary cyst (see Figure 12.7). Cysts can survive in the host for decades.

♦ CASE 12.4

A 33-year-old woman who was an immigrant from Jordan presented with a chief complaint of bloody cough and shortness of breath × 2 weeks. At age 22 she had undergone a CT scan of the abdomen as part of her workup for polycystic ovaries. She

Figure 12.7

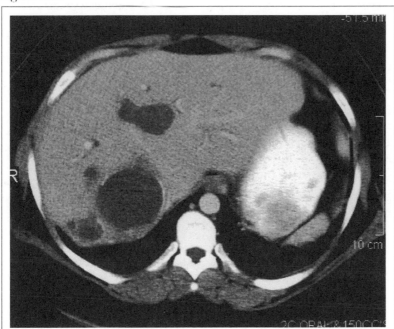

CT scan showing multiple echinococcal hepatic abscesses. CT was performed after both oral and IV contrast. (Courtesy of Dr. Pat Abbitt, University of Florida College of Medicine.)

was noted at that time to have a large liver cyst consistent with Echinococcus. Although she was asymptomatic, resection of the left lobe of the liver was performed that year. Despite surgical resection she suffered with recurrent cysts and on three occasions underwent percutaneous aspiration followed by injection of hypertonic saline. One month prior to admission, 6 years after her last aspiration and injection procedure, she began coughing up blood and began noting shortness of breath. She received several courses of oral antibiotics but failed to improve. She began coughing up gelatinous, foul-smelling serosanguineous fluid. Pulmonary exam revealed decreased breath sounds and dullness to percussion at the right base. Bronchial breath sounds and e to a changes were noted in the right posterior midlung field. The liver was not palpable. CT scan of the chest and abdomen revealed a fluid collection over the dome of the liver as well as an 8 × 5 cm abscess in the right lower lobe of the liver that contained an air-fluid level.

CLINICAL PRESENTATION

Most patients with echinococcosis are asymptomatic, infection being detected incidentally on an imaging study. Symptoms generally develop when the hydatid cyst reaches a size of 8–10 cm in diameter and begins compressing vital structures or erodes into the biliary tract or a pulmonary bronchus as occurred in Case 12.4. The cysts can also become superinfected, resulting in a bacterial abscess. Cyst leakage or rupture can result in an anaphylactic reaction causing fever and hypotension.

DIAGNOSIS AND TREATMENT

Ultrasonography, CT scan, or MRI reveals a characteristic hydatid cyst with a distinct septated structure representing daughter cysts (see Figure 12.7). Often, tapeworm heads can also be visualized. The diagnosis can be confirmed by ELISA, which is highly sensitive for liver cysts but less sensitive for cysts in other organs.

Surgical resection of the hydatid cyst is the treatment of choice. The cyst should be removed intact, taking great care that it not rupture and spread the infection by daughter cysts. To reduce the risk of spread, aspiration of the cyst is recommended with removal of a fraction of the contents and instillation of hypertonic saline (30% NaCl solution), iodophor, or 95% ethanol to kill the germinal layer and daughter cysts. Thirty minutes after instillation, surgical resection should be performed. In cases with biliary communication such cidal agents are not recommended because of the risk of inducing sclerosing cholangitis. Treatment in the perioperative period with three or four cycles of albendazole 400 mg twice a day for four weeks followed by a two-week rest period is generally recommended to limit the risk of intraoperative dissemination. The same medical therapy is recommended for patients with inoperable hydatid cysts. Computed tomography has been used to guide needle aspiration and instillation of cidal agents to sterilize inoperable lesions. However, experience with this procedure is limited.

KEY POINTS

Echinococcus

1. Spread primarily by sheepdogs that excrete eggs in their feces. Eggs survive in dust and contaminate food.
2. Eggs hatch in the intestine, and onchospheres enter the bloodstream spreading to the liver, lung, and, less commonly, the brain, forming hydatid cysts.
3. Hydatid cysts survive and grow over decades, causing symptoms when they reach 8–10 cm in diameter.
4. Diagnosis by CT scan, MRI, or ultrasound.
5. Treatment: Albendazole and when possible surgical resection preceded by instillation of an agent cidal to the germinal layer.

Taenia solium (Cysticercosis)

Potential Severity: Causes neurologic complications in a significant number of infected patients many years after the initial infection.

PREVALENCE, EPIDEMIOLOGY, AND LIFE CYCLE

Taenia solium is also a cestode, or tapeworm. Infections are common in Central and South America, Mexico, the Philippines, Southeast Asia, India, Africa, and southern Europe. Like Echinococcus, this parasite can be contracted by ingesting viable eggs, or infection may be contracted by eating raw or undercooked pork containing encysted larvae. Once ingested, the eggs hatch or encysted larvae are released in the stomach and develop in the intestine into adult worms that can reach 8 m in length. Autoinfection can occur as a result of regurgitation of eggs into the stomach or accidental ingestion of eggs from the host's own feces.

CLINICAL PRESENTATION

◆ CASE 12.5

A 33-year-old Indian male was admitted to the hospital following a grand mal seizure. Two years prior to admission he had noted some vertigo and a CT scan demonstrated a calcified lesion in the left temporal-parietal region. The lesion enhanced with contrast. As a child he had lived in an area of India that was endemic for cysticercosis and frequently ate pork. His brother had had a seizure several years earlier. On the day of admission he was talking on the phone when he suddenly had difficulty speaking and experienced a sudden loss of consciousness. Fellow employees noted generalized tonic clonic seizures that lasted 10 minutes. Repeat CT scan demonstrated new localized cerebral edema around the previously identified ring enhancing lesion as well as a second contiguous ring

Figure 12.8

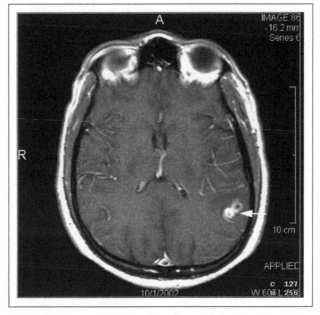

CT scan with contrast of the cerebral cortex showing typical ring enhancing lesions of neurocysticercosis.

enhancing legion (See Figure 12.8). He was treated with intravenous followed by oral phenytoin (Dilantin) and a 5-day course of corticosteroids. Initially he was noted to have mild right arm weakness that resolved over 4 hours. He was continued on phenytoin and has had no additional seizures. ELISA titer was positive for antibodies directed against *Taenia solium*. It was elected not to treat him with praziquantel or albendazole

Adult intestinal worms rarely cause symptoms. However, larvae can penetrate the intestine, enter the bloodstream, and eventually encyst in the brain, causing neurocysticercosis. Cysts may lodge in the cerebral ventricles causing hydrocephalus, in the spinal cord resulting in cord compression and paraplegia, in the subarachnoid space causing chronic meningitis, or in the cerebral cortex causing seizures. As in Case 12.5, cysts may remain asymptomatic for many years, becoming clinically apparent only when the larvae die, an event that is associated with cyst swelling and increased inflammation. Larvae also encyst in other tissues but rarely cause symptoms.

DIAGNOSIS AND TREATMENT

Computed tomography and nuclear magnetic resonance scan are the preferred diagnostic studies and demonstrate discrete cysts that may be enhanced following the administration of contrast media, depending on the degree of surrounding inflammation (see Figure 12.8). In the central nervous system multiple lesions are generally detected. However single lesions may be seen, particularly in cases from India. Older lesions are often calcified. In the absence of cerebral edema, lumbar puncture can be performed, and cerebrospinal fluid analysis usually reveals lymphocytes or eosinophils accompanied by a low glucose level and an elevated protein level. Serologic tests that detect antibody directed against *Taenia solium* may be positive, particularly in patients with multiple cysts.

Treatment for neurocysticercosis is complex and controversial. Praziquantel and albendazole may kill living cysts, but death of larvae results in increased inflammation and edema and may exacerbate symptoms. When possible, surgical resection of the symptomatic cyst is the preferred treatment. In Case 12.5 it was elected not to treat with antiparasitic medications, and because of the location in a vital region of the brain surgical resection was not possible. Corticosteroids may be helpful for reducing edema and inflammation, and antiepileptic medications should be utilized to control seizures.

KEY POINTS
Cysticercosis (*Taenia solium*)

1. Contracted by eating eggs from fecally contaminated food or encysted larvae from undercooked pork.
2. Larvae enter the bloodstream, encysting primarily in the brain.
3. Symptoms develop after many years when larvae die, causing increased inflammation.
4. Can cause seizures, hydrocephalus, paraplegia, and meningitis.
5. Diagnosis by CT scan or MRI, serology.
6. Treatment: Surgical resection, corticosteroids; praziquantel or albendazole controversial.

Schistosomiasis

Guiding Questions

1. Why doesn't primary schistosomiasis occur in the United States?
2. How is schistosomiasis contracted?
3. What strain of Schistosoma causes swimmer's itch?

4. What is Katayama fever?
5. In late disease, how does egg deposition cause clinical symptoms?

Potential Severity: Usually a chronic disorder resulting in debilitating complications. Occasionally fatal during the early stage of infection as a result of a severe serum sickness syndrome.

PREVALENCE, EPIDEMIOLOGY, AND LIFE CYCLE

Schistosoma mansoni, S. haematobium, and *S. japonicum* are members of the fluke or trematode family. Schistosomes are estimated to infect between 200–300 million people worldwide. Primary infection does not occur in the United States because the critical intermediate host, a specific type of freshwater snail, is absent. However, there are approximately 400,000 imported cases in immigrants from Puerto Rico, South America (particularly Brazil), the Middle East, and the Philippines. The parasite is contracted by exposure to fresh water containing infectious cercariae. The fork-tailed cercariae are able to swim to and penetrate human skin of persons wading in infested stagnant freshwater pools or rice paddies. Once within the host, cercariae lose their tails, maturing to schistosomulae that enter the bloodstream and then penetrate the lung and liver, where over six weeks they mature to adult worms. The adult worms then migrate through the venous plexus to different sites depending on the strain of Schistosoma: *S. mansoni* worms take up residence in the inferior mesenteric veins responsible for venous drainage of the large intestine, *S. japonicum* in the superior mesenteric veins that drain the small intestine, and *S. haematobium* in the vesicular plexus that drains the urinary bladder. Here worms can live for decades, releasing eggs into the bowel or bladder. Improper handling of contaminated stool and urine leads to egg contamination of water. Eggs hatch in fresh water, forming miracidia that contain cilia enabling them to swim and infect freshwater snails. Each species of Schistosoma requires a specific freshwater snail intermediate, a fact that explains the geographic distribution of the strains. Within the snail, miracidia multiply, and within four to six weeks they release large numbers of cercariae that are capable of infecting humans. *S. mansoni* is found primarily in South America, the Caribbean, Africa, and Arab countries, *S. haematobium* in Africa and the Middle East, and *S. japonicum* in China and the Philippines. Two other strains have more recently been found to cause disease: *S. intercalatum* in western and central Africa and *S. mekongi* in Indochina.

KEY POINTS

The Life Cycle of Schistosomiasis

1. Cercariae swimming in fresh water can penetrate human skin.
2. Cercariae mature to schistosomulae, which enter the bloodstream, liver, and lung, where they mature.
3. Mature worms migrate to the venous system of the small intestine (*Schistosome japonicum*), large intestine (*S. mansoni*), or bladder venous plexus (*S. haematobium*).
4. Worms release eggs for many years into stool or urine, resulting in contamination of fresh water.
5. Freshwater snails are infected by miracidia and are necessary for the production of cercariae and human infection.

◆ CASE 12.6

A 32-year-old man was evaluated for a lesion of the urinary bladder. He had been well until 16 months earlier. At that time, soon after returning from a one-week vacation in Malawi, he had an episode of perineal pain associated with painful ejaculation and a brown-colored ejaculate. His condition improved after treatment with ciprofloxacin. Four months before the evaluation he began experiencing urinary frequency with intermittent passage of small blood clots in the urine. His symptoms failed to improve on treatment with ciprofloxacin.

Epidemiology: Frequent travel outside the United States. He most recently traveled to Malawi with his wife. While there, he had repeatedly swum in a lake that he was assured was "safe."

Laboratory findings: Peripheral white blood cell count and differential were normal. Urinalysis: hematuria. Cytologic examination: no malignant cells. A urogram and ultrasound demonstrated a round structure, 8 × 10 mm in diameter, adherent to the bladder wall. Cystoscopic examination disclosed multiple slightly raised, polypoid lesions that were less than 5 mm in diameter. They were erythematous, with focal yellow areas. Bladder biopsies revealed on low-power microscopic examination a polypoid inflammatory lesion of the bladder mucosa with a dense inflammatory infiltrate surrounding clusters of eggs in the submucosa.

Figure 12.9

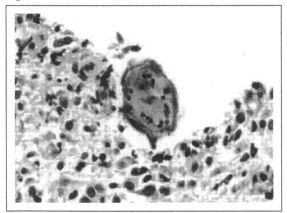

Bladder mucosal biopsy showing a *Schistosoma haematobium* egg. (From Case Records of the Massachusetts General Hospital. Weekly clinicopathological exercises. Case 31-2000. A 32-year-old man with a lesion of the urinary bladder. *N Engl J Med* 342:1105–1111, 2001.) See also Color Plate 2.

At higher magnification the granulomas were found to contain clusters of helminthic eggs surrounded by epithelioid histiocytes, chronic inflammatory cells, and eosinophils. The eggs were oval and had a terminal spine, characteristic of *Schistosoma haematobium* (see Figure 12.9). His wife was subsequently examined, and schistosoma eggs were found in her urine. Both were treated with praziquantel, and eggs have disappeared from their urine. (Adapted from Case Records of the Massachusetts General Hospital: Weekly clinicopathological exercises. Case 31-2000. A 32-year-old man with a lesion of the urinary bladder. *N Engl J Med* 342: 1105–1111, 2001.)

CLINICAL PRESENTATION

There are three stages of disease, which correspond to the life cycle of the parasite in the human host. The first stage occurs at the time of penetration and is commonly termed "swimmers' itch." A very itchy macular papular rash develops within 24 hours of cercariae penetrating the skin. Swimmers' itch is a common complaint in the Great Lakes region of the north central United States as well as among swimmers in freshwater lakes in Europe. It is caused by an avian strain of Schistosoma that is not capable of entering the bloodstream. These skin manifestations spontaneously resolve.

The second stage of clinical disease occurs four to eight weeks later when the worms mature and begin releasing eggs. Patients develop a serum sickness–like syndrome with elevated IgE levels and peripheral eosinophilia as they react to egg antigens. Fever, headache, cough, chills, and sweating are accompanied by lymphadenopathy and hepatosplenomegaly. This clinical constellation has been called Katayama fever and is most commonly associated with *Schistosoma japonicum*. Symptoms usually resolve spontaneously; however, in heavy infections this acute reaction can be fatal.

The third, chronic stage results from granulomatous reactions to egg deposition in the intestine, liver, bladder, and, less commonly, lungs and central nervous system. Granulomatous reactions in the bowel can lead to chronic diarrhea, abdominal pain, and blood loss. Eggs may enter the portal venous system and gain entry to the liver, where chronic inflammation is followed by fibrosis leading to portal hypertension, splenomegaly and bleeding esophageal varices. Because the hepatic parenchyma is rarely compromised, liver function tests are usually normal. Peripheral eosinophilia is commonly encountered. Hepatosplenomegaly with normal liver function tests, peripheral eosinophilia, and a history of residence in an endemic area should raise the possibility of chronic hepatic schistosomiasis. The development of collateral venous channels in association with portal hypertension can result in egg deposition in the pulmonary arteries causing pulmonary hypertension and right-sided congestive heart failure. Deposition of eggs in the central nervous system is less common and can cause seizures or, if eggs are deposited in the spinal cord region, transverse myelitis. In *S. haematobium* eggs are deposited in the bladder wall leading to hematuria, bladder obstruction, hydronephrosis, and recurrent urinary tract infections. Bladder cancer may also complicate chronic *S. haematobium* infection.

KEY POINTS

Clincal Presentation of Schistosomiasis

> 1. Skin penetration causes "swimmers' itch."
> 2. A serum sickness syndrome with eosinophilia and high IgE may follow and is called Katayama fever.
> 3. Granulomatous reaction to egg deposition leads to chronic diarrhea, portal hypertension and hepatosplenomegaly, and pulmonary hypertension in *Schistosoma mansoni* and *S. japonicum.*
> 4. Eggs deposited in the bladder can lead to hematuria, bladder obstruction, hydronephro-

> sis, recurrent UTIs, and bladder cancer in cases of *S. haematobium.*

DIAGNOSIS AND TREATMENT

Demonstration of eggs in the stool or urine allows a specific diagnosis to be made. Quantitative egg counts are helpful in assessing the intensity of infection. Urine is best collected between 12:00 and 2:00 P.M. and passed through a 10-micron filter to concentrate the eggs. As observed in Case 12.6, eggs may also be identified on tissue biopsies. Rectal biopsy is particularly helpful in diagnosing *Schistosoma mansoni*. The eggs of *S. mansoni, S. japonicum,* and *S. haematobium* have distinct morphologies, allowing them to be readily identified by using a low-power (100×) microscope (see Figure 12.4). In chronic disease the egg burden may be low, making the diagnosis difficult. Antischistosome antibody tests are now available for detecting chronically infected patients; however, their specificity and sensitivity limit their value. Furthermore, these tests cannot be used in lifelong residents of endemic areas because serologies are frequently positive in the absence of active infection.

Praziquantel is effective treatment for all forms of schistosomiasis. For *Schistosoma mansoni* and *S. haematobium* 20 mg/kg given twice over one day and for *S. hematobium* 20 mg/kg given three times in one day are recommended. Side effects of treatment are mild and include fever, abdominal discomfort, and headache.

KEY POINTS

Diagnosis and Treatment of Schistosomiasis

> 1. Characteristic eggs in the stool or urine (check between 12:00 and 2:00 P.M.) or on tissue biopsy are diagnostic; consider rectal biopsy in *Schistosoma mansoni.*
> 2. Eggs may not be seen in chronic disease; antischistosome antibody test may be helpful.
> 3. Praziquantel is the treatment of choice.

Other, Less Common Tissue Flukes

These flukes have a similar life cycle to that of Schistosoma, requiring snails as the intermediate host. Cercariae, rather than gaining entry by penetrating the human skin, take up residence in other food sources and become encysted. Infection is contracted when the human host eats cercaria-contaminated food.

Clonorchis sinensis (or Chinese liver fluke) infections results from the ingestion of raw or undercooked freshwater fish. Infections occur in China, Hong Kong, and Vietnam. Worms gain entry into the biliary tract via the ampulla of Vater. Infection can be complicated by cholangitis and later cholangiocarcinoma. Infections are effectively treated with praziquantel.

Fasciola hepatica, another liver fluke, is found in sheep-raising areas of the world, including South America, Australia, China, Africa, and Europe. Ingestion of vegetables contaminated with encysted cercariae is the most common route of infection. This fluke is treated with bithionol.

Paragonimus westermani (lung fluke) is contracted by eating raw or pickled crawfish or freshwater crabs. This parasite is found in Central and South America, West Africa, India, and the Far East. The parasite first enters the gastrointestinal tract and subsequently penetrates the diaphragm, entering the pleural cavity and lungs and causing respiratory symptoms. Praziquantel is the treatment of choice.

FILARIASIS (*WUCHERERIA BANCROFTI* AND *BRUGIA MALAYI*)

Guiding Questions

1. How is this infection transmitted?
2. What key characteristic helps to differentiate inflammatory filariasis from bacterial cellulitis?
3. Is elephantiasis an early or late manifestation of filariasis?
4. At what time of day are blood smears most likely to be positive?

Potential Severity: A chronic debilitating infection that can cause severe disfiguring complications by blocking lymphatic drainage.

PREVALENCE, EPIDEMIOLOGY, AND LIFE CYCLE Microfilaria is less common than many parasites, being estimated to infect approximately 120 million individuals. Several strains of worm can cause this disease. *Wuchereria bancrofti* is found throughout the tropics, while *Brugia malayi* is restricted to the southern regions of Asia. A third strain, *B. timori,* is found only in Indonesia. Infectious larvae are transmitted by the bite of a mosquito. Larvae pass from the skin into the lymphatic system, where over several months they mature in the lymph nodes. Adult worms (40–100 mm in length) are then released into the bloodstream. In *W. bancrofti* the highest concentration of worms in the blood is generally found in the middle of the night, a fact explaining why midnight blood smears are recommended for diagnosis. If a mosquito bites an infected human, worms are ingested and develop into infective larvae that can be transmitted to a new human host. The percentage of mosquitoes containing infective larvae has been estimated to be only 1% in endemic areas. Therefore repeated mosquito bites are generally required to contract this infection. This may explain why adults, particularly men, more commonly contract this infection.

KEY POINTS

The Life Cycle of *Wuchereria bancrofti* and *Brugia malayi*

1. Transmitted by the bite of an infected mosquito.
2. Repeated mosquito bites are required.

> 3. Microfilaria live in the lymphatic system, and worms enter the bloodstream at midnight (except in the South Pacific).
> 4. Mosquitoes are infected by biting humans.

CLINICAL PRESENTATION

Asymptomatic Filariasis Many individuals have asymptomatic infection. Peripheral eosinophilia and palpable lymphadenopathy may be the only clinical manifestations. Children usually experience no symptoms, despite high numbers of microfilariae in their blood.

Inflammatory Filariasis Adults more commonly react to the invasion of worms by strong allergic reactions that begin approximately a year after exposure. Fever, chills, vomiting, headache, and malaise may be associated with lymphangitis of an extremity, orchitis, epididymitis, or scrotal swelling. The affected extremity becomes hot, swollen, erythematous, and painful, mimicking cellulitis. These symptoms are associated with a peripheral leukocytosis and an increased percentage of eosinophils (6–25%). Attacks may occur monthly and do not respond to antibiotics. The granulomatous response in the lymphatic tissue is thought to be the host's inflammatory reaction to dying worms.

Obstructive Filariasis Over time, chronic inflammation leads to fibrosis and permanent obstruction of lymphatic flow. This syndrome occurs over years as a result of continuous microfilaria infection. Persistent lymphatic obstruction and edema lead to marked skin thickening and deposition of collagenous material, eventually causing elephantiasis. Patients suffer with debilitating enlargement of their legs or massive enlargement of their scrotal tissue, making walking difficult. Recurrent cellulitis due to Streptococcus or *Staphylococcus aureus* may periodically occur, requiring antibiotic treatment. Rupture of the lymphatics into the kidney or bladder can result in chyluria, and rupture into the peritoneum can cause chylous ascites.

KEY POINTS

Clinical Presentation of Filariasis

> 1. Many people, particularly children, are asymptomatic.
> 2. Inflammatory filariasis is associated with periodic erythema, warmth, pain, and swelling mimicking cellulitis (associated with peripheral eosinophilia).
> 3. Obstructive disease results in chronic limb swelling due to lymphatic fibrosis causing elephantiasis.
> 4. Obstructive disease can lead to recurrent bacterial cellulitis.
> 5. Rupture of lymphatics can cause chyluria or chylous ascites.

DIAGNOSIS AND TREATMENT Giemsa- or Wright-stained peripheral smears should be obtained at midnight in all cases except those from the South Pacific. Identification of adult worms in the blood is definitive. However, in early and late disease worms often are not seen. Antibody titers are available but do not differentiate between past and current infection. A PCR test for *Wuchereria bancrofti* is under development. Biopsies of infected lymph nodes are generally not recommended but, when performed in addition to granuloma, may reveal adult worms. Ultrasound of dilated lymphatics in the spermatic cord have revealed motile worms. In early infection and during the inflammatory stage, peripheral eosinophilia is commonly seen. During the chronic stages of disease eosinophilia generally is not present. If worms cannot be identified, the diagnosis has to be made on clinical grounds. Diethylcarbamazine 6 mg/kg daily by mouth for two weeks kills some adult worms but not all. A reduction in the level of microfilariae in the blood is usually observed. Treatment may increase inflammation and might not halt progression to fibrosis and lymphatic obstruction. Ivermectin 200–400 μg/kg combined with albendazole 400 mg as a single dose is a more recent treatment regimen that may more effectively kill the adult worms. Anti-inflammatory agents may be used to reduce the extent of inflammation, and elastic support stockings can be helpful in reducing moderate lymphedema.

KEY POINTS

Diagnosis and Treatment of Filariasis

1. Midnight blood smear demonstrating worms allows definitive diagnosis.
2. In early and late disease worms might not be seen.
3. Ultrasound of dilated lymphatics may demonstrate worms.
4. Peripheral eosinophilia is common.
5. Antibody titers may be helpful but do not prove active disease.
6. Diethylcarbamazine or ivermectin plus albendazole are used for treatment. Treatment can exacerbate symptoms.

DIROFILARIASIS (DOG HEARTWORM)

Humans are an accidental host of this worm. Dirofilaria is most commonly found in the southeastern United States and is transmitted by mosquitoes. After developing in the subcutaneous tissue, the young adult filariae migrate to the right side of the heart and right pulmonary vessels, where they survive in the dog. However, in humans the young forms migrate to the lung but fail to develop and die, producing local granulomatous inflammation. Most human cases present as an asymptomatic pulmonary coin lesion mimicking an early neoplasm. Lung biopsy reveals a dead worm. Treatment of human cases is not necessary.

ONCHOCERCIASIS (ONCHOCERCA VOLVULUS)

This parasite is found primarily in Africa, where it infects approximately 20 million people. Rare cases are seen in Central and South America. This infection is transmitted by a black fly that swarms around the face, often biting around the eyes and depositing onchocerca larvae onto the skin. These larvae penetrate and crawl through the skin and connective tissue. The worms initially cause an itchy erythematous rash. Later fibrous skin nodules develop.

Worms often migrate into the anterior chamber of the eye, causing inflammation and blindness. Because the offending black fly is commonly found near streams, this disease has been called "river blindness." Diagnosis is made by skin snips or visualizing worms by slit lamp examination of the eyes. The treatment of choice is ivermectin 150 μg/kg orally as a single dose repeated at three-month intervals until symptoms resolve. Fever, itching, and an urticarial rash may develop as a result of dying microfilariae.

LOIASIS (LOA LOA)

This microfilaria is also transmitted by a fly and is found in western and central Africa. The microfilariae migrate through the skin, causing localized edema called Calabar swellings. Several hours before swelling occurs, local itching and pain are noted. Occasionally, the microfilariae can be seen migrating through the subconjunctiva, causing intense conjunctivitis. Active microfilaria migration is associated with marked peripheral eosinophilia. Diagnosis is made by daytime blood smear. Diethylcarbamazine or ivermectin is recommended as treatment. Diethylcarbamazine can precipitate encephalitis in heavily infected patients.

Additional Reading

General Reading

O'Brien, D., Tobin, S., Brown, G.V., and Torresi, J. Fever in returned travelers: Review of hospital admissions for a 3-year period. *Clin Infect Dis* 33:603–609, 2001.

Malaria

Angus, B.J. Malaria on the World Wide Web. *Clin Infect Dis* 33:651–661, 2001.

Bruneel, F., Gachot, B.,Wolff, M., Regnier, B., Danis, M., and Vachon, F. Resurgence of blackwater fever in long-term European expatriates in Africa: Report of 21 cases and review. *Clin Infect Dis* 32:1133–1140, 2001.

Kockaerts, Y., Vanhees, S., Knockaert, D., Verhaegen, J., Lontie, M., and Peetermans, W. Imported malaria in the 1990s: A review of 101 patients. *Eur J Emerg Med* 8:287–290, 2001.

Wellems, T.E., and Plowe, C.V. Chloroquine-resistant malaria. *J Infect Dis* 184:770–776, 2001.

Babesia

Hatcher, J.C., Greenberg, P.D., Antique, J., and Jimenez-Lucho, V.E. Severe babesiosis in Long Island: Review of 34 cases and their complications. *Clin Infect Dis* 32:1117–1125, 2001.

Homer, M.J., Aguilar-Delfin, I., Telford, S.R., 3rd, Krause, P.J., and Persing, D.H. Babesiosis. *Clin Microbiol Rev* 13:451–469, 2000.

White, D.J., Talarico, J., Chang, H.G., Birkhead, G.S., Heimberger, T., and Morse, D.L. Human babesiosis in New York State: Review of 139 hospitalized cases and analysis of prognostic factors. *Arch Intern Med* 158:2149–2154, 1998.

Leishmania

Berenguer, J., Gomez-Campdera, F., Padilla, B., Rodriguez-Ferrero, M., Anaya, F., Moreno, S., and Valderrabano, F. Visceral leishmaniasis (kala-azar) in transplant recipients: Case report and review. *Transplantation* 65:1401–1404, 1998.

Herwaldt, B.L. Leishmaniasis. *Lancet* 354:1191–1199, 1999.

Murray, H.W. Treatment of visceral leishmaniasis (kala-azar): A decade of progress and future approaches. *Int J Infect Dis* 4:158–177, 2000.

Rosenthal, E., Marty, P., del Giudice, P., Pradier, C., Ceppi, C., Gastaut, J.A., Le Fichoux, Y., and Cassuto, J.P. HIV and Leishmania coinfection: A review of 91 cases with focus on atypical locations of Leishmania. *Clin Infect Dis* 31:1093–1095, 2000.

Trypanosomiasis

de Oliveira, R.B., Troncon, L.E., Dantas, R.O., and Menghelli, U.G. Gastrointestinal manifestations of Chagas' disease. *Am J Gastroenterol* 93:884–889, 1998.

Rassi, A., Jr., Rassi, A., and Little, W.C. Chagas' heart disease. *Clin Cardiol* 23:883–889, 2000.

Sinha, A., Grace, C., Alston, W.K., Westenfeld, F., and Maguire, J.H. African trypanosomiasis in two travelers from the United States. *Clin Infect Dis* 29:840–844, 1999.

Intestinal Helminths

Grencis, R.K., and Cooper, E.S. Enterobius, trichuris, capillaria, and hookworm including *Ancylostoma caninum*. *Gastroenterol Clin North Am* 25:579–597, 1996.

Juckett, G. Common intestinal helminths. *Am Fam Physician* 52:2039–2048, 2051–2052, 1995.

Liu, L.X., and Weller, P.F. Strongyloidiasis and other intestinal nematode infections. *Infect Dis Clin North Am* 7:655–682, 1993.

Tanowitz, H.B., Weiss, L.M., and Wittner, M. Diagnosis and treatment of common intestinal helminths. II: Common intestinal nematodes. *Gastroenterologist* 2:39–49, 1994.

Strongyloides

Mahmoud, A.A. Strongyloidiasis. *Clin Infect Dis* 23:949–952; quiz 953, 1996.

Sarangarajan, R., Ranganathan, A., Belmonte, A.H., and Tchertkoff, V. *Strongyloides stercoralis* infection in AIDS. *AIDS Patient Care and STDS* 11:407–414, 1997.

Siddiqui, A.A., and Berk, S.L. Diagnosis of *Strongyloides stercoralis* infection. *Clin Infect Dis* 33:1040–1047, 2001.

Zaha, O., Hirata, T., Kinjo, F., and Saito, A. Strongyloidiasis: Progress in diagnosis and treatment. *Arch Intern Med* 39:695–700, 2000.

Trichinella

Bruschi, F., and Murrell, K.D. New aspects of human trichinellosis: The impact of new Trichinella species. *Postgrad Med J* 78:15–22, 2002.

Capo, V., and Despommier, D.D. Clinical aspects of infection with Trichinella spp. *Clin Microbiol Rev* 9:47–54, 1996.

Clausen, M.R., Meyer, C.N., Krantz, T., Moser, C., Gomme, G., Kayser, L., Albrectsen, J., Kapel, C.M., and Bygbjerg, I.C. Trichinella infection and clinical disease. *Q J Med* 89:631–636, 1996.

Echinococcus

Balik, A.A., Basoglu, M., Celebi, F., Oren, D., Polat, K.Y., Atamanalp, S.S., and Akcay, M.N. Surgical treatment of hydatid disease of the liver: Review of 304 cases. *Arch Surg* 134:166–169, 1999.

Bosanac, Z.B., and Lisanin, L. Percutaneous drainage of hydatid cyst in the liver as a primary treatment: Review of 52 consecutive cases with long-term follow-up. *Clin Radiol* 55:839–848, 2000.

Burgos, R., Varela, A., Castedo, E., Roda, J., Montero, C.G., Serrano, S., Tellez, G., and Ugarte, J. Pulmonary hydatidosis: Surgical treatment and follow-up of 240 cases. *Eur J Cardiothorac Surg* 16: 628–634; discussion 634–635, 1999.

Eckert, J., Conraths, F.J., and Tackmann, K. Echinococcosis: An emerging or re-emerging zoonosis? *Int J Parasitol* 30:1283–1294, 2000.

Taenia solium

Garcia, H.H., and Del Brutto, O.H. Taenia solium cysticercosis. *Infect Dis Clin North Am* 14:97–119, ix, 2000.

Garg, R.K. Neurocysticercosis. *Postgrad Med J* 74: 321–326, 1998.

White, A.C., Jr. Neurocysticercosis: Updates on epidemiology, pathogenesis, diagnosis, and management. *Annu Rev Med* 51:187–206, 2000.

Schistosomiasis

Bichler, K.H., Feil, G., Zumbragel, A., Eipper, E., and Dyballa, S. Schistosomiasis: A critical review. *Curr Opin Urol* 11:97–101, 2001.

Ross, A.G., Sleigh, A.C., Li, Y., Davis, G.M., Williams, G.M., Jiang, Z., Feng, Z., and McManus, D.P. Schistosomiasis in the People's Republic of China: Prospects and challenges for the 21st century. *Clin Microbiol Rev* 14:270–295, 2001.

Siddiqui, A.A., and Berk, S.L. Diagnosis of *Strongyloides stercoralis* infection. *Clin Infect Dis* 33:1040–1047, 2001.

Talaat, M., El-Ayyat, A., Sayed, H.A., and Miller, F.D. Emergence of *Schistosoma mansoni* infection in upper Egypt: The Giza governorate. *Am J Trop Med Hyg* 60:822–826, 1999.

Whitty, C.J., Mabey, D.C., Armstrong, M., Wright, S.G., and Chiodini, P.L.. Presentation and outcome of 1107 cases of schistosomiasis from Africa diagnosed in a non-endemic country. *Trans R Soc Trop Med Hyg* 94:531–534, 2000.

Filariasis

Cunningham, N.M. Lymphatic filariasis in immigrants from developing countries. *Am Fam Physician* 55:1199–1204, 1997.

Dunn, I.J. Filarial diseases. *Sem Roentgenol* 33:47–56, 1998.

Shah, M.K. Human pulmonary dirofilariasis: Review of the literature. *South Med J* 92:276–279, 1999.

Onchocerciasis

Burnham, G. Onchocerciasis. *Lancet* 351:1341–1346, 1998.

Hall, L.R., and Pearlman, E. Pathogenesis of onchocercal keratitis (river blindness). *Clin Microbiol Rev* 12:445–453, 1999.

Malatt, A.E., and Taylor, H.R. Onchocerciasis. *Infect Dis Clin North Am* 6:963–977, 1992.

Chapter 13

Zoonotic Infections

Recommended Time to Complete: 2 days

Guiding Questions

1. Why have zoonotic infections become more common over the past two decades?

2. What type tick is responsible for spreading Lyme disease and how long must the tick be attached to transmit the disease?

3. What early skin lesion is pathognomonic for Lyme disease, and what manifestations may develop later in the course of infection?

4. Is antibiotic prophylaxis ever recommended for Lyme disease?

5. How is leptospirosis spread and what activities increase the risk of contracting this illness?

6. What are the typical manifestations of Weil's syndrome?

7. What clinical findings suggest the diagnosis of Rocky Mountain spotted fever and why is it important to recognize this illness quickly?

8. Which rickettsial disease is frequently mistaken for chickenpox?

9. What hematologic findings usually accompany Ehrlichiosis?

10. What organism causes cat scratch disease and how is this infection usually contracted?

11. How is brucella spread to humans and which individuals are at highest risk for developing brucellosis?

As a consequence of increased outdoor activities, increasing populations of deer in close proximity to urban areas, and the spread of housing to more rural settings, humans increasingly come into contact with animals and with disease-spreading insect vectors. As a consequence, the natural spread of infection from lower mammals to humans, termed zoonotic infections, has greatly increased over the past three decades. Zoonotic infections represent one of the most important classes of emerging infectious diseases. A number of newly discovered zoonotic diseases have been identified by combining our new understanding of the genomic structures of pathogens with highly sensitive and specific polymerase chain reaction (PCR) detection methods (for example, Bartonella and Ehrlichia).

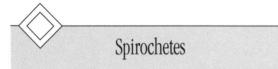

Spirochetes

Lyme Disease (Borrelia burgdorferi)

Potential Severity: Can present acutely or result in a chronic disease that is rarely life-threatening.

EPIDEMIOLOGY

Lyme disease is the most common insect-borne infection in the United States. More than 10,000 cases are reported annually in the United States between the months of May and September. Cases are concentrated in three areas of the country: the Northeast, Massachusetts to Maryland; the Midwest, primarily Wisconsin; and the far West, primarily California and Oregon. Lyme disease is also found in the temperate regions of Europe, Scandinavia, parts of the former Soviet Union, China, Korea, and Japan. Children and middle-aged adults are at greatest risk of acquiring this infection.

ETIOLOGY AND PATHOGENESIS

Lyme disease is caused by the spirochete *Borrelia burgdorferi,* the longest and narrowest member of the Borrelia species, being 20–30 μm in length and 0.2–0.3 μm in width. Like other spirochetes it is microaerophilic and fastidious, but it can be grown in vitro by using Barbour-Stoener-Kelly (BSK-2) media. *B. burgdorferi* expresses a number of lipoproteins on its outer surface (called Osp, or outer surface proteins) that are thought to help the organism survive within the tick as well as within mammals and birds. A fibronectin-binding protein, flagellar antigen, and two heat shock proteins have also been described. These heat shock proteins cross-react with human proteins and may play a role in the development of the rheumatologic complaints that are commonly associated with late Lyme disease.

Like Babesia, *Borrelia burgdorferi* is transmitted by the deer tick *Ixodes scapularis.* Other Ixodes species are responsible for transmission in the far western United States, Europe, and Asia. The increased incidence of Lyme disease over the past two decades is thought to be the result of the rise in the deer population in suburban areas. The deer and other large mammals are the primary host for the adult tick but do not play a direct role in transmission of the spirochete. The adult Ixodes tick does not transmit Lyme disease to humans. As is observed with Babesia (see Chapter 12), infection is spread to humans by the young Ixodes nymph. These small ticks survive primarily on the white-footed mouse but can also be found on other rodents. They attach to humans as they walk through brush or tall grass. Because the nymph is the size of a small freckle, it often is not detected and is allowed to remain attached for 36–48 hours, the period that is required to efficiently transmit infection. As the tick feeds, spirochetes escape from the salivary gland of the insect into the skin of human host. As is observed with primarily syphilis, *B. burgdorferi* multiplies locally in the skin and after an incubation period of 3–32 days begins to form a distinct, slowly expanding circular erythematous lesion call erythema migrans. The organism then disseminates throughout the body, and during the dissemination stage the organism can be cultured from blood and cerebrospinal fluid (CSF). Initially, the immune response is suppressed; however, over days to weeks cell-mediated immunity is activated, and macrophages are stimulated to produce the proinflammatory cytokines tumor necrosis factor and interleukin-1. During this period IgM and IgG antibodies are slowly generated. IgM levels usually peak between three and six weeks after the initial infection, while IgG levels gradually rise over months. Sites of infection are infiltrated by lymphocytes and plasma cells, and evidence of small vessel vasculitis is often apparent. However, despite these immune responses, *B. burgdorferi* can survive for years in the synovial fluid, nervous system, and skin of the untreated patient.

KEY POINTS

Epidemiology, Etiology, and Pathogenesis of Lyme Disease

1. The most common insect-borne disease in the United States. Found in:
   a. Northeast U.S., Wisconsin, California, and Oregon,
   b. Temperate regions of Europe, Scandinavia, former Soviet Union, China, Korea, and Japan.
2. Caused by *Borrelia burgdorferi,* microaerophilic spirochete, grows on BSK-2 media:
   a. Expresses lipoproteins on its surface (Osps), which help the organism survive in hosts,
   b. Produces fibronectin-binding protein, flagellar antigen, and two heat shock proteins that cross-react with human proteins.

3. Transmitted by Ixodes nymph tick. From deer to white-footed mouse to humans:
   a. Size of a freckle, commonly missed,
   b. Must attach for 36–48 hours to transmit the spirochete.
4. Begins in the skin, then disseminates.
5. Induces cell-mediated and humoral immunity, can survive for years in the joint fluid, CNS, and skin of untreated humans.

CLINICAL MANIFESTATIONS

♦ CASE 13.1

A young man sought medical attention because of neck stiffness, shoulder pain, and a rash on his leg. On examination he was noted to have a macular erythematous circular lesion on one leg. Further examination revealed a wood tick attached to his other leg, indicating recent tick exposure. The tick was subsequently identified as *Ixodes pacificum*. Western Blot assay demonstrated specific IgG and IgM antibodies to *Borrelia burgdorferi*. He was treated with doxycycline, and his symptoms resolved. (Adapted from an Internet case report by E.K. Murakami, N. Shojania, and S. Christie.)

Just as is observed in syphilis (see Chapter 9), Lyme disease can be divided into three stages:

1. **Early localized infection (primary Lyme disease)**. The patient in Case 13.1 presented with erythema migrans, the hallmark of Lyme disease, noted in 90% of patients (see Figure 13.1). The lesion begins within a month of exposure as a red macule or papule at the site of the tick bite and then expands over days, forming a bright red flat border at the advancing edge. As the lesion expands, there may be central clearing, and in some cases the site takes on the appearance of a target. However, in many patients the lesion remains diffusely erythematous. Erythema migrans are usually large, reaching an average size of 15 cm in diameter (range: 3–70 cm). They are commonly located in moist, warm areas of

Figure 13.1

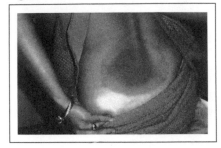

Erythema migrans of Lyme disease. See also Color Plate 2.

the body where ticks prefer to feed (axilla, behind the knees, and at the belt line). Despite their size, warmth, and bright color, the lesions are usually painless but can cause burning or itching.

2. **Early disseminated disease (secondary Lyme disease)**. Several days after the onset of erythema migrans, small annular satellite lesions may be observed, reflecting early dissemination. Also at this time patients often experience a viral-like syndrome consisting of malaise, fatigue, myalgias, arthralgias, and headache. They may also develop generalized lymphadenopathy. Migratory joint, tendon, muscle, and bone pain are common complaints. In a significant percentage of patients symptoms involving the nervous system and heart commonly develop at this stage. *Nervous system involvement*: The spirochete often disseminates to the nervous system, initially causing a severe generalized headache that waxes and wanes. If the disease is not treated, about 10% of cases develop more serious neurologic manifestations. Frank meningitis can result in neck stiffness, CSF lymphocytic pleocytosis (usually about 100 cells/mm^3), and elevated CSF protein with a normal CSF glucose. Cranial nerve deficits can accompany meningitis, bilateral Bell's palsies being the most common cranial nerve dysfunction. Lymphocytic infiltration of small vessels supplying axons can lead to axonal degeneration and peripheral neuritis. The

triad of meningitis, cranial nerve deficits, and radiculoneuritis has been termed Bannwarth's syndrome. This syndrome is more commonly reported in Europe than in the United States. *Cardiovascular involvement*: Five to eight percent of untreated patients develop cardiac manifestations within several weeks of the onset of illness. Spirochetes can directly infiltrate the myocardium, causing lymphocytic inflammation. Conduction defects are most common, and an EKG should be ordered in all patients with symptomatic Lyme disease. First-degree heart block is most common; second degree and complete heart block may also develop. However, complete heart block rarely persists for longer than 7 days and does not usually require placement of a pacemaker. More severe myocarditis accompanied by congestive heart failure is rare.

KEY POINTS

Primary and Secondary Lyme Disease

1. Hallmark of primary disease is erythema migrans:
   a. Macular expanding erythematous lesion, central clearing,
   b. Begins one month after the tick bite,
   c. Mean diameter: 15 cm,
   d. Painless, can cause itching.
2. Dissemination associated with small annular lesions and a flulike illness:
   a. CNS involvement can cause waxing and waning headache. CSF lymphocytosis (100 cells/mm^3), cranial nerve deficits (Bell's palsy), and peripheral neuritis = Bannwarth's syndrome,
   b. Cardiovascular: Spirochetes infiltrate the myocardium, causing conduction defects.

3. **Late Disease (tertiary Lyme disease)**. Late disease develops months to years after primary infection. Some patients never experienced symptoms in the earlier stages. Muscu-

loskeletal complaints are most common at this stage; however, neurologic complaints, skin disease, and generalized symptoms may also occur. *Musculoskeletal manifestations:* Approximately 60–80% of untreated patients experience musculoskeletal symptoms. Migrating arthralgias or frank arthritis causing joint swelling most commonly involves the knees and other large joints. Less commonly, small joints may be affected. Joint aspiration may reveal white cell counts of 500–110,000 cells/mm³ with a predominance of polymorphonuclear leukocytes (PMNs). The presence of spirochetes in the joint fluid can be detected in the joint fluid by PCR in most patients, and arthritis usually resolves after antibiotic therapy. *Neurologic manifestations:* Just as is observed in syphilis, *Borrelia burgdorferi* may invade the cerebral cortex and cause a chronic encephalopathy associated with mood, cognitive, and sleep disorders. Subtle language disturbances have also been observed. The CSF may reveal elevated protein levels and increased CSF antibody titers to *B. burgdorferi*. Patients may also develop peripheral neuropathies leading to paresthesias and radicular pain. The evaluation of neurologic complaints can be complicated, and the neurocognitive complaints associated with fibromyalgia are often misdiagnosed as central nervous system Lyme disease. The response to antibiotic therapy is variable. *Other manifestations:* Acrodermatitis chronica atrophicans can develop years after erythema migrans. It begins as a bright red skin lesion that later becomes atrophic, mimicking localized scleroderma. *B. burgdorferi* can be cultured from these lesions up to 10 years after their onset. A very difficult management problem arises from the small percentage of patients who suffer with persistent diffuse aches and pains. Some patients with Lyme disease develop a fibromyalgia-like syndrome, and others may experience a chronic fatigue–like syndrome. The contribution of *B. burgdorferi* infection to these complaints remains controversial, and many patients with these complaints fail to improve after antibiotic therapy.

KEY POINTS

Late or Tertiary Lyme Disease

1. Symptomatic disease develops months to years after primary disease.
2. Musculoskeletal complaints are most common:
   a. Migrating arthritis and arthralgias,
   b. Joint fluid 500–110,000 cells/mm³, primarily PMNs,
   c. Usually improves with antibiotics.
3. CNS: Encephalopathy causing mood, cognitive, and sleep disorders:
   a. Elevated CSF protein and antibody against *Borrelia burgdorferi*,
   b. Response to antibiotics variable.
4. Acrodermatitis chronica atrophicans: A chronic skin infection containing spirochetes.
5. Fibromyalgia-like or chronic fatigue–like syndrome, controversial, antibiotics not helpful.

DIAGNOSIS

Although the organism can be grown in vitro, cultures are rarely positive because the number of organisms in skin lesions, blood, and CSF is very low. The diagnosis is based on clinical manifestations and a history of possible tick exposure in an endemic area combined with serologic testing. In considering the diagnosis, it is important to keep in mind that many patients with confirmed Lyme disease deny having been bitten by a tick. The enzyme-linked immunosorbent assay (ELISA) test uses a sonicate of *Borrelia burgdorferi* as the antigen and detects IgG and IgM antibodies directed against the spirochete. Acute and convalescent titers spaced two to four weeks apart should be collected. In early disease a significant rise in antibody titer is detected in only 60–70% of patients. Therefore negative titers at this stage do not exclude Lyme disease. Also antibiotic therapy can abort a full antibody response, further complicating serologic diagnosis. For these reasons ELISA testing is not recommended for patients with classic erythema migrans because this lesion is pathognomonic for Lyme disease. IgM titers begin to rise within two weeks, but a significant rise might not be detected for six to eight weeks. IgM levels usually peak at six to eight weeks and decline over two to three months. IgG titers rise later, being first detected at six to eight weeks and peaking at four to six months. A significant IgG titer usually persists for life. False-positive tests occur 3–5% of the time and are more common in patients with syphilis, leptospirosis, malaria, bacterial endocarditis, viral infections, and connective tissue diseases. Western blot analysis is recommended to verify all positive ELISA tests. This test detects serum antibodies directed against specific polypeptide components of *B. burgdorferi*. Infected patient serum most commonly contains antibodies directed against the 23-kDa OspC protein and the 41-kDa flagellar antigen but may also cross-react with other Osp proteins and the heat shock proteins. Strict criteria for interpretation of Western blots have been established by the Centers for Disease Control and Prevention (CDC). A number of other diagnostic tests have been described; however, their usefulness has not been substantiated. Serologic tests are best utilized for the patient with suspected early disease who does not have erythema migrans or in the patient with symptoms of late disease. A negative serology in early disease may require follow-up testing because of the delay in the rise of antibody titers in some patients. In the patient with suspected late disease a negative IgG titer virtually excludes the diagnosis.

KEY POINTS
Diagnosis of Lyme Disease

1. Cultures are rarely positive and are not recommended.

2. Diagnosis made by combining epidemiology, clinical manifestations, and serology.
3. Many patients with Lyme disease deny a tick bite.
4. ELISA assay detects IgG and IgM antibodies:
   a. Not recommended if classic erythema migrans; this finding is pathognomonic,
   b. Titer rise is aborted by early antibiotic treatment,
   c. IgM begins to rise at two weeks, declines by two to three months,
   d. IgG rises at six to eight weeks, persists for life, negative IgG titer excludes late disease,
   e. 3–6% false positive rate.
5. Western blot recommended to confirm all (+) ELISA tests:
   a. 23-kDa OspC protein and the 41-kDa flagellar antigen most commonly cross-react,
   b. Strict criterion for (+) Western blot have been established by the CDC.

TREATMENT

For the treatment of early disease amoxicillin (500 mg po TID) and doxycycline (100 mg BID) for 21–28 days are equally effective (see Table 13.1). The ideal duration of therapy has not been determined, and many physicians opt for the longer course of therapy. Cefuroxime axetil (500 mg po BID) is an effective alternative. Erythromycin (250 mg po QID) and azithromycin (500 mg po QD) have proved to be less effective. For early disseminated disease with isolated seventh nerve palsies, multiple erythema migrans lesions, or carditis with first-degree heart block, doxycycline (100 mg po BID × 21 days) and ceftriaxone (2 gm im QD × 14 days) are effective. A Jarisch-Herxheimer–like reaction may be observed in up to 15% of patients during the first 24 hours of therapy for disseminated disease. In patients with meningitis or other neurologic abnormalities and in patients who are experiencing carditis with high-degree heart

Table 13.1

Antibiotic Treatment of Zoonotic Infections

DRUG	DOSE	RELATIVE EFFICACY	COMMENTS
Lyme disease			
- Early	Duration 21–28 days		
Amoxicillin (or)	500 mg po TID	First-line	
Doxycycline	100 mg po BID		
Cefuroxime	500 mg po BID	Alternative	
- Early disseminated			
Doxycycline (or)	100 mg BID × 21 days		Jarisch-Herxheimer
Ceftriaxone	2 gm im QD × 10 days		reaction common
- Heart block or meningitis	Duration 14–30 days		
Ceftriaxone (or)	2 gm iv QD		
Penicillin G	4 million units iv Q4H		
- Chronic arthritis	Duration 30–60 days		
Doxycycline (or)	100 mg po BID		
Amoxicillin (or)	500 mg po TID		
Rx of heart block and meningitis			
Leptospirosis	See text for duration		
- Severe			
Penicillin G (or)	1.5 million units iv Q6H		Jarisch-Herxheimer
Ampicillin	0.5–1 gm iv Q6H		reaction common
- Mild			
Doxycycline (or)	100 mg po BID		
Amoxicillin	875 mg po TID		
Rocky Mountain spotted fever	See text for duration		
Tetracycline (or)	500 mg po Q6H	First-line	
Doxycycline	100 mg po or iv Q12H		
Chloramphenicol	500 mg po or iv Q6H	Alternative	
Typhus	See text for duration		
Tetracycline (or)	500 mg po Q6H	First-line	
Doxycycline	100 mg po or iv Q12H		
Chloramphenicol	500 mg po or iv Q6H	Alternative	
Add rifampin in areas with	600–900 mg po QD		
resistant strains			
Erlichia	See text for duration		
Doxycyline	100 mg po or iv Q12H		Also preferred for
			children
Q fever	See text for duration		
Doxycycline (+)	100 mg po or iv BID		Add hydroxychloro-
Hydroxychloroquine	200 mg po TID		quine for endocarditis
Bartonella	See text for duration		
- Lymphatic disease			
Azythromycin (or)	500 mg po × 1, then		All equally effective
	250 mg		
Clarithromycin (or)	500 mg po BID		
Doxycycline (or)	100 mg po BID		
Ciprofloxacin	500 mg po BID		

(continued)

Table 13.1

Antibiotic Treatment of Zoonotic Infections (continued)

DRUG	DOSE	RELATIVE EFFICACY	COMMENTS
- Severe disease	See text for duration		
Azythromycin (+)	500 mg po QD		Efficacy not proven
Rifampin	600 mg po or iv QD		
Brucellosis	See text for duration		
Doxycycline (+)	100 mg po BID	First-line	Single-drug therapy not
Rifampin	600–900 mg po BID		recommended
Doxycycline (+)	100 mg po BID	Alternative	
Gentamicin	5 mg/kg iv QD		

block, intravenous ceftriaxone (2 gm QD × 14–30 days) or high-dose penicillin (20 million units iv divided in six doses per day × 14–30 days) is recommended. Patients with intermittent or chronic arthritis may be treated with a very prolonged course of doxycycline (100 mg po BID × 30–60 days) or amoxicillin (500 mg po QID × 30–60 days), or treated with intravenous ceftriaxone or penicillin (same doses as above).

A rare but difficult management problem arises in the patient who complains of persistent symptoms despite appropriate therapy. Patients must be warned that symptoms can linger for up to six months after treatment. In the patient whose symptoms persist for more prolonged periods, objective evidence for relapse is rarely found. Repeat antibiotic therapy rarely relieves symptoms. The wisest course of action is reevaluation rather than retreatment because the most likely explanation for a lack of response to therapy is misdiagnosis.

PREVENTION

Because of the extensive publicity surrounding Lyme disease, people often panic when they sustain a tick bite. In endemic areas frantic calls to the physician's office are a frequent occurrence during the summer months. A logical approach to the management of tick bites will reduce unnecessary administration of antibiotics.

Assessment of the risk of contracting Lyme disease requires a careful history of the nature of the tick bite. The questioner needs to inquire about the following:

1. **The size of the tick**. Lyme disease is primarily spread by the *Ixodes scapularis* nymph. This tick is very small, about the size of a small freckle. Larger ticks are unlikely to transmit Lyme disease.
2. **Attachment**. If the tick fails to attach to the skin, it cannot transmit disease. The likelihood of being bitten by a tick can be reduced by wearing long pants and shirts when walking in areas with brush and high grasses. In endemic areas public health officials recommend that on returning from the outdoors, the individual perform a complete body check for ticks. Removing ticks before they attach is an excellent preventive measure. If an attached tick is discovered, the duration of attachment needs to be estimated. If attachment is less than 24 hours, the risk of disease transmission is low.
3. **Engorgement**. If the tick is engorged with blood, this finding suggests prolonged attachment and an increased risk of disease transmission.

Prophylactic antibiotics consisting of a single dose of doxycycline (200 mg po) within 72 hours of the tick bites can prevent the development of Lyme disease. The incidence of Lyme disease is approximately 1/100 in areas where a high percentage of ticks harbor *Borrelia burgdorferi,* and prophylaxis should be strongly considered in these locations. A more targeted approach of administering prophylactic antibiotics to the individual who reports attachment of a small tick for >24 hours or finds an engorged tick may prove more efficacious. In patients who do not fulfill these criteria, a careful explanation of the risk and natural progression of Lyme disease will usually calm the concerned caller.

KEY POINTS
Treatment and Prevention of Lyme Disease

1. Early disease: Amoxicillin or doxycycline × 21–28 days.
2. Disseminated disease with mild carditis (first-degree heart block) or seventh nerve palsy: Doxycycline × 21 days) or im ceftriaxone × 14 days.
3. Meningitis or carditis with high-degree block: iv ceftriaxone or penicillin × 14–30 days.
4. Chronic arthritis: Doxycycline or amoxicillin × 30–60 days or meningitis regimen.
5. Failure to improve on antibiotics suggests another diagnosis.
6. Prophylactic antibiotics recommended if a small tick attached > 24 hours or an engorged tick is found.

Leptospirosis

Potential Severity: Can cause a life-threatening systemic illness. Early diagnosis and treatment reduce the severity of the disease.

EPIDEMIOLOGY

This disease is rarely diagnosed in the United States with the exception of Hawaii, where annual rates of 128 per 100,000 have been reported.

Leptospirosis is found throughout the world in temperate and tropical climates. Infection often follows flooding and hurricanes in Central and South America as well as the Caribbean islands. In endemic areas the incidence of leptospirosis is 5–20% per year. The acute illness often causes nonspecific symptoms that never require medical attention, explaining the low incidence detected by passive surveillance studies. Dogs, livestock, and rodents as well as amphibians and reptiles can become infected. They often harbor leptospira in their renal tubules, excrete the pathogen in the urine, and contaminate both soil and water, where the organism can persist for weeks to months. Humans who are at risk of becoming infected include trappers and hunters, dairy farmers, livestock workers, veterinarians, military personnel, and sewer workers. Infection has also been associated with outdoor activities in fresh water, including wading, swimming, white-water rafting, kayaking, and canoeing. In cities humans may become inadvertently exposed to rat and dog urine.

KEY POINTS
Epidemiology of Leptospirosis

1. Found in temperate and tropical climates:
   a. Rare in U.S., except for Hawaii,
   b. Follows flooding, particularly in Central and South America, Caribbean Islands.
2. Dogs, livestock, rodents, amphibians excrete in urine, contaminating soil and water.
3. Trappers, hunters, dairy farmers, livestock workers, veterinarians, military, and sewer workers at risk.
4. Outdoor, freshwater activities predispose to disease.

PATHOGENESIS

Leptospirosis is caused by *Leptospira interrogans,* a tightly spiraled spirochete with 18 or more coils per cell. Like other spirochetes it is narrow (0.1 μm in width) and long (6–12 μm in length) and is best visualized by darkfield microscopy. Leptospira are obligate aerobes and grow slowly. There are over 200 serovars of *L. interrogans,* and different serovars have a predilection for different animals.

These thin organisms gain entry to the human host through cuts, abrasions, and skin softened by prolonged water exposure. Mucous membranes and conjunctivae are other portals of entry. Inhalation of aerosolized droplets can lead to pulmonary invasion. Once in the host, the spirochetes spread to the lymphatic system and then enter the bloodstream, disseminating throughout the body. The organisms' outer wall is coated with lipopolysaccharide (LPS), which serves as a major antigenic stimulus. The spirochete releases a glycolipoprotein toxin that displaces long-chain fatty acids from host vascular endothelial cells, causing breakdown of the vessel walls and fluid leakage and allowing the organisms to escape from the bloodstream to the tissues. The host generates IgM and IgG antibodies directed against the leptospira LPS. These antibodies are opsonins that enhance phagocytosis by macrophages in the reticuloendothelial system and enhance clearing of the organisms from the bloodstream.

KEY POINTS

Pathogenesis of Leptospirosis

1. Caused by *Leptospira interrogans,* a tightly coiled spirochete, slow-growing obligate aerobe.
2. Penetrates breaks in skin or softened skin after prolonged water exposure, conjunctiva, or mucous membranes, less commonly aerosolized entering via the lungs.
3. Disseminates after traveling to the lymphatics and bloodstream.
4. Outer surface coated with LPS. Glycoprotein toxin damages endothelial cells.
5. Induces IgM and IgG antibodies directed against LPS, killed by macrophages.

CLINICAL MANIFESTATIONS

◆ CASE 13.2

A 25-year-old male presented to the hospital with complaints of fever and headache of 3 days duration. His symptoms began three days after completing a 12-day survival race with three teammates held in Sabah State on Borneo Island, Malaysia. The day before admission, one of his teammates was admitted to the hospital with similar complaints. Physical examination revealed a body temperature of 37.9°C and a pulse rate of 90/minute (regular). Conjunctiva were hyperemic but nonicteric. Lymph nodes were not palpable, and a skin eruption was not seen. Neurologic exam was normal. WBC: 13,100/μl (neutrophils, 91%); Hb: 14.8 g/dl; platelet: 190,000/μl; total bilirubin: 0.5 mg/dl; GOT: 63 IU/l; GPT: 66 IU/l; LDH: 420 IU/l; BUN: 12.5 mg/dl; creatine: 0.9 mg/dl.

Minocycline was administered intravenously on the third hospital day, and fever subsided over 48 hours. Intravenous minocycline was continued for a week, followed by 2 weeks of oral doxycycline. Acute sera was negative for Leptospira antibody, while convalescent serum two weeks later revealed a 1:160 titer of antibody directed against *L. interrogans* serovar *hebdomadis.*

Further investigation revealed that 51 of 78 participants in the race had developed symptoms consistent with leptospirosis. Activities had included jungle trekking, canoeing, kayaking, rafting, scuba diving, mountain biking, and cave exploring. Local rivers were flooded at the time of the race. (Adapted from Sakamoto, M., Sagara, H., Koizumi, N., and Watanabe, H. A leptospirosis case returning from the Eco-Challenge on Borneo Island, Malaysia, September 2000. *Infectious Agent Surveillance Report,* 22:5–6, 2001.)

The incubation period for leptospirosis is usually 5–14 days but can take up to 30 days. The severity of illness varies greatly and probably depends on the degree of exposure and the infecting serovar. Certain serovars from cows cause mild disease, while others contracted from rats are more likely to cause severe disease. Classically, there are two phases of symptomatic disease: the bacteremic phase and the immunologic phase; however, fewer than half of patients actually experience a biphasic illness. Over 90% of cases are self-limited; however, a small percentage experience a severe, sometimes fatal illness called Weil's syndrome.

As is illustrated in Case 13.2, the onset of illness is usually sudden. Symptoms may include fever, rigors, sweating, headache, photophobia, and severe myalgias accompanied by marked tenderness of the calves, thighs, and mid-back. Other manifestations can include epistaxis, cough, and sore throat. Severe abdominal pain can mimic an acute surgical abdomen. Nausea, vomiting, and diarrhea may also develop. On examination the vessels in the conjunctiva are often very prominent owing to vascular dilatation. Transient skin rashes may be noted. Capillary fragility can result in macular, maculopapular, purpuric, or urticarial lesions as well as diffuse skin redness. During the acute phase leptospirosis can be cultured from the blood and CSF.

Resolution of fever may herald the onset of the second, immune phase of the illness, which can last 4–30 days. Blood cultures turn negative at this time. Prominent conjunctivitis with or without hemorrhage is seen, accompanied by photophobia, retrobulbar pain, neck stiffness, diffuse lymphadenopathy, and hepatosplenomegaly. Aseptic meningitis with or without symptoms is characteristic of this stage and is immune mediated. CSF reveals lymphocytes (<500 mm^3), moderate protein elevation (50–100 mg/ml), and a normal glucose.

Weil's syndrome can develop after the acute phase and consists of hemorrhage, jaundice, and renal failure. Severe hemorrhagic pneumonitis may also develop. Jaundice is caused by vascular injury to the hepatic capillaries without significant hepatocellular necrosis. Transaminase levels rarely exceed 200 U/L, and an elevated prothrombin time is uncommon. Creatine phosphokinase (CPK, MM fraction) reflecting myositis is often disproportionately high in comparison to the serum transaminase values. Marked elevations in conjugated bilirubin are the hallmark of liver involvement and can reach levels of 80 mg/dl, associated with mild to moderate elevations of alkaline phosphatase. The constellation of a high direct bilirubin, mild elevation in alkaline phosphatase, mild elevation in transaminase values, and high CPK should always raise the possibility of Weil's syndrome. Liver biopsy reveals hypertrophy and hyperplasia of Kupffer cells accompanied by cholestasis. The hepatic architecture usually remains intact, and there is little evidence of hepatic necrosis. Acute renal failure is associated with oliguria and usually develops during the second week of illness at the same time that jaundice is noted. Thrombocytopenia may accompany renal failure in the absence of disseminated intravascular coagulopathy. Renal biopsy demonstrates acute interstitial nephritis, and immune-complex glomerulonephritis may also be seen. Pulmonary disease can develop in the absence of hepatic or renal involvement. This hemorrhagic pneumonia is generally associated with a bloody cough, and chest X-ray reveals nodular densities in the lower lobes. Histopathology reveals damage to the capillary endothelium and intra-alveolar hemorrhage. Cardiovascular collapse can develop suddenly. The mortality rate for severe leptospirosis ranges from 5% to 40%.

KEY POINTS
Clinical Manifestations of Leptospirosis

1. Incubation period 5–14 days, severity depends on inoculum and serovar, rat serovars more severe.
2. Two phases in fewer than half of patients:
   a. Bacteremic phase: Sudden onset, fever, rigors, headache, photophobia, and severe myalgias; dilated conjunctival vessels; marked tenderness in calves, thighs, and mid-back; macular rash,
   b. Immunologic phase (4–30 days): Conjunctivitis, photophobia, retrobulbar pain, neck stiffness, diffuse lymphadenopathy,

> hepatosplenomegaly, and aseptic menin-
> gitis with CSF lymphocytosis.
> 3. Weil's syndrome rare, severe, mortality rate
>   5–40%:
>   a. High direct bilirubin, mild elevation in al-
>   kaline phosphatase, mild elevation in
>   transaminase values combined with a
>   high CPK,
>   b. Renal failure accompanied by thrombo-
>   cytopenia,
>   c. Hemorrhagic pneumonia.

DIAGNOSIS AND TREATMENT

Even in endemic areas the early clinical diagnosis of leptospirosis is difficult to make because
the clinical manifestations are often nonspecific.
Leptospira can be cultured in vitro on special
media (Fletcher's, Ellinghausen's, or polysorbate
80 media). Significant growth may be detected
after one to two weeks but can take up to three
months. Blood, CSF, and urine are positive during the first 7–10 days of illness, and urine remains positive during the second and third
weeks of the illness.

The sensitivity of culture is low; therefore the
diagnosis usually must be made by measuring
acute and convalescent antibody titers. The microscopic agglutination test is the most specific
test and allows identification of serum antibodies
to specific serovars. Live leptospires are placed
on a slide, and the highest serum dilution at
which >50% of the spirochetes agglutinate on
darkfield microscopy is defined as the positive titer. Antibody titers can be detected as early
as 3 days into the illness but usually take two
weeks and continue to rise for three to four
weeks. A fourfold or greater rise in titer is defined as serologic confirmation of leptospirosis. A
single titer of ≥1:800 in combination with appropriate symptoms is considered indicative of active
disease, while a single titer of 1:200 or a persistent titer of 1:100 is suggestive evidence. This test
is technically demanding and potentially hazardous and is performed only by CDC reference

laboratories. An ELISA test for IgM antibodies is
commercially available and has a sensitivity that
varies from 100% to 77% and a specificity of
93–98%. PCR methods are under development
but are currently only experimental.

Penicillin G (1.5 million units iv Q6H) or ampicillin (0.5–1 gm iv Q6H) are recommended for
severe disease. In severe disease penicillin treatment has been shown to reduce the duration of
illness. As observed in the treatment of other
spirochetes, therapy may be associated with a
Jarisch-Herxheimer reaction. For mild leptospirosis oral doxycycline (100 mg BID) or amoxicillin
(875 mg Q8H) may be administered. When exposure in endemic areas is anticipated, prophylaxis
with doxycycline (200 mg po QD) has been
shown to be efficacious (see Table 13.1).

KEY POINTS
Diagnosis and Treatment of Leptospirosis

> 1. Can be cultured from blood, CSF, and urine.
>   Low yield.
> 2. Serologies most helpful:
>   a. Microscopic agglutination test (only in
>   CDC reference labs), (+) two weeks,
>   rises three to four weeks: ≥fourfold rise
>   diagnostic, titer of ≥1:800 + symptoms =
>   active disease, 1:200 suggestive,
>   b. ELISA for IgM antibodies commercially
>   available, good sensitivity and specificity.
> 3. Intravenous penicillin or ampicillin for se-
>   vere disease, oral doxycycline or amoxicillin
>   for milder disease.
> 4. Prophylaxis in endemic areas, doxycycline.

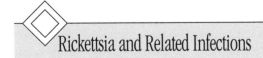

Rickettsia and Related Infections

There are two genera in the Rickettsiaceae family: *Rickettsia* and *Ehrlichia*. These organisms
are small Gram-negative coccobacilli (0.3-μm-

diameter coccal forms, 0.3 × 1- to 2-μm-diameter bacillary forms) that possess a cell wall that consists of a peptidoglycan layer sandwiched between two lipid membranes. They are all obligatory intracellular pathogens. Rickettsia gain entry by inducing host cells to phagocytose them. Some strains (e.g., *Rickettsia rickettsii*) produce a phospholipase that dissolves the confining phagolysosome membrane, allowing them to escape into the cytoplasm. Other strains multiply and survive within the phagolysosome by blocking release of toxic enzymes into the phagolysosome (e.g., Ehrlichia species). All rickettsial diseases are spread to humans by arthropods: ticks, mites, lice, and fleas.

Clinically, the Rickettsial family of diseases have been classified into the spotted fever group, which includes *R. rickettsii* (causes Rocky Mountain spotted fever), *R. conorii* (boutonneuse fever), *R. australis* (Queensland tick typhus), *R. sibrica* (North Asian tick typhus), and *R. akari* (rickettsialpox); the typhus group, which includes *R. prowazekii* (louse-borne or epidemic typhus and Brill-Zinsser disease), *R. typhi* (murine typhus), and *Orienta tsutsugamushi* (scrub typhus); and the Ehrlichia group, which consists of *E. chaffeensis* (human monocytic ehrlichiosis) and *E. phagocytophila* (human granulocytic ehrlichiosis). The final disease, Q fever, does not fall into any of the above categories and is caused by *Coxiella burnetii*.

Rocky Mountain Spotted Fever and Other Spotted Fevers

Potential Severity: Untreated Rocky Mountain spotted fever can be fulminant and fatal.

EPIDEMIOLOGY

Rocky Mountain spotted fever (RMSF) is the most severe disease in the spotted fever group of rickettsial diseases. RMSF is found throughout the United States, Mexico, and Central and South America. Although it was first recognized in the Rocky Mountains, the disease is most commonly reported in the southeastern and south central United States. There are small endemic areas in Long Island and Cape Cod. Cases have also been reported in urban parks. The disease occurs in the late spring and summer, the seasons when ticks feed. In the South, the dog tick (*Dermacentor variabilis*) is the primary vector, and in states west of the Mississippi the wood tick is primarily responsible for transmitting disease.

PATHOGENESIS

After the tick has been attached to the host for several hours to a day, it injects the rickettsiae into the dermis. Once exposed to the warmer temperature and mammalian blood, *Rickettsia rickettsii* activates and proliferates in the skin. The organism resides in the cell cytoplasm, where it divides by binary fission and spreads from cell to cell by a mechanism similar to that used by *Listeria monocytogenes*. Both organisms induce host cell actin filament assembly to propel them to the periphery of the cell, where they are ingested by adjacent cells and form plaques of necrotic cells. *R. rickettsii* contains outer membrane proteins (called Omps) as well as lipoproteins that stimulate cell-mediated immunity, resulting in the infiltration of lymphocytes and macrophages. After multiplying in the skin, the organism disseminates via the bloodstream, where it prefers to invade vascular endothelial cells. Damage to endothelial and vascular smooth muscle cells results in a vasculitis that can involve the lungs, heart, and central nervous system. Discrete areas of hemorrhage can be found in these organs as well as in the skin, intestine, pancreas, liver, skeletal muscle, and kidneys. Hemorrhage often leads to platelet consumption and thrombocytopenia; however, disseminated intravascular coagulopathy is rare. Increased vascular permeability and fluid leakage result in edema, low serum protein levels, hypovolemia, and shock. Decreased intravascular volume can induce antidiuretic hormone secretion and hyponatremia. Shock can also precipitate acute tubular necrosis and renal failure in severe cases.

KEY POINTS

Epidemiology and Pathogenesis of Rocky Mountain Spotted Fever

1. Found throughout the United States, Mexico, Central and South America:
   a. Most common in the southeastern and south central U.S.,
   b. Areas of Cape Cod, Long Island, and some urban parks.
2. Injected into the skin by dog and wood ticks in the late spring and summer.
3. Proliferates in the skin, disseminates via the bloodstream:
   a. Survives in the host cell cytoplasm, spreads cell to cell, producing plaques of necrotic cells,
   b. Causes hemorrhage in skin, intestine, pancreas, liver, skeletal muscle, and kidneys.

CLINICAL MANIFESTATIONS

◆ CASE 13.3

A 56-year-old white man arrived in the hospital for elective surgery. Overnight he developed a fever associated with headache, generalized malaise, chills, nausea, and vomiting, forcing cancellation of surgery. Fever continued. The following day, a diffuse macular rash was noted on the trunk and extremities. A petechial eruption was also noted around both ankles. Laboratory studies revealed a normal WBC count (9.3×10^9/l) and urinalysis; chest X-ray film was unremarkable. Results of liver function tests and serum electrolyte values were normal. Platelet count was 219×10^9/l. The patient had no history of tick bites; however, during the week before admission he had been in a wooded area where ticks are common. Skin biopsy revealed perivascular lymphocyte infiltrates around dermal blood vessels. Direct immunofluorescence staining of the biopsy specimen showed organisms consistent with spotted fever group rickettsiae. Therapy with oral tetracycline (500 mg QID) was started. Two days later, the fever had disappeared and the patient was discharged home. (Adapted from an Internet case report by M.A. Eloubeidi, C.S. Burton, and D.J. Sexton, Duke University Medical Center.)

As Case 13.3 illustrates, the incubation period averages 7 days but can vary from 2 to 14 days. The early symptoms and signs of RMSF are nonspecific. Patients complain of fever, headache, malaise, myalgias, and nausea. Some patients experience severe abdominal pain, particularly children, suggesting the diagnosis of cholecystitis, appendicitis, or bowel obstruction. A rash usually develops within 5 days of the onset of illness; it was a rash that alerted the physicians in Case 13.3 to the possibility of RMSF. However, in up to 10% of patients a rash may never appear, and in dark-skinned individuals lesions may be difficult to recognize. "Spotless" fever occurs more commonly in the elderly and in African Americans. Patients often seek medical attention prior to the development of rash, and therefore the physician may fail to consider the diagnosis. Lesions are nonpruritic. They are usually first noted on the ankles and wrists, subsequently spreading centrally and to the palms and soles. Initially, they are macular or maculopapular, subsequently becoming petechial. The presence of urticarial lesions or a pruritic skin rash makes RMSF unlikely.

As the disease progresses, headache may become an increasingly prominent complaint. Severe headache can be accompanied by neck stiffness and photophobia, suggesting meningitis, and the CSF may contain lymphocytes or PMNs and the CSF protein may be elevated; however, a low CSF glucose is unusual. Conjunctivitis may be noted, and funduscopic examination may reveal the manifestations of the small vessel vasculitis, flame hemorrhages, and arterial occlusion as well as venous engorgement and papilledema. Respiratory complaints may become prominent, and chest X-ray may reveal alveolar infiltrates or pulmonary edema, indicating the development of adult respiratory distress syndrome. Gangrene of the digits can also develop in severe cases as a sequence of occlusion of small arterioles.

Laboratory findings tend to be nonspecific. The peripheral white cell count can be normal, elevated, or depressed. Thrombocytopenia is common in more severe cases. Elevations in BUN and serum creatinine may be noted, and hyponatremia develops in patients with hypotension. Transaminase values and bilirubin levels may be elevated as well. If appropriate therapy is not given within the first 5 days, RMSF can progress and cause death within 8–15 days.

KEY POINTS

Clinical Manifestations of Rocky Mountain Spotted Fever

1. Incubation period 2–14 days.
2. Acute onset of nonspecific symptoms: fever, headache, malaise, myalgias, and nausea. Abdominal pain may mimic cholecystitis or appendicitis.
3. 5 days after symptoms begin, macular, petechial rash begins on ankles and wrists and spreads to trunk:
   a. Spotless infection in 10%; occurs in elderly and African Americans,
   b. Urticaria or pruritic rash makes RMSF unlikely.
4. Aseptic meningitis, conjunctivitis, fundoscopic hemorrhages, acute respiratory distress syndrome in severe disease.

DIAGNOSIS

Because of the rapid course of this disease and the inability of most laboratories to culture the organism, the diagnosis of Rocky Mountain spotted fever is usually made on the basis of epidemiology and clinical manifestations. A significant percentage of patients deny a tick bite, making the diagnosis particularly difficult. In the first few days RMSF is most commonly mistaken for a viral syndrome. If penicillin or a cephalosporin is mistakenly prescribed during this period, the subsequent rash of RMSF may be mistaken for a drug allergy. Severe headache and abnormalities in the CSF may suggest viral meningoencephalitis. The development of petechial skin lesions may raise the possibility of meningococcemia or leptospirosis. During the spring and summer months the clinician must always treat patients in endemic areas for RMSF pending culture results. Skin biopsy is helpful in confirming the diagnosis. As is illustrated in Case 13.3, immunofluorescence staining using specific antibodies directed against *R. rickettsii* can be helpful and has a 70% sensitivity and 100% specificity. If antibiotics for RMSF have been initiated, skin biopsy is not recommended because organisms are difficult to identify after treatment has been initiated. Acute and convalescent serum antibody titers can be measured by indirect immunofluorescence (IFA), latex agglutination, or complement fixation, and a significant rise in titer allows a retrospective diagnosis. However, these tests are of no help in managing the acutely ill patient. The Weil-Felix test, which detects cross-reactive antibodies to *Proteus vulgaris,* is nonspecific as well as insensitive and is no longer recommended.

TREATMENT

Because of the unpredictable course of Rocky Mountain spotted fever, physicians in endemic areas should have a low threshold for initiating doxycycline or tetracycline therapy in patients who have a nonspecific febrile illness of greater than two days during the spring and summer. RMSF responds rapidly to antibiotic therapy and patients usually defervesce within 48–72 hours. Therapy with tetracycline (500 mg po Q6H) or doxycycline (100 mg po or iv Q12H) is the treatment of choice (see Table 13.1). Chloramphenicol (500 mg po or iv Q6H) is also effective and is recommended in pregnancy as well as for children (50 mg/kg po or iv Q6H) with developing teeth. Antibiotic therapy should be continued for at least 3 days after the patient has defervesced. The mortality rate in untreated patients varies depending on the strain and inoculum but in one retrospective series was 22% in untreated patients and 6% in patients who received treatment within 5 days of the onset of their illness.

OTHER SPOTTED FEVERS

There are six other Rickettsial species that cause skin rashes and fever in humans. *R. conorii* shares 90% DNA homology with *R. rickettsii*, shares many of the same proteins, and causes boutonneuse fever. This tick-borne illness is found in southern Europe, Africa, and the Middle East and is very similar clinically to Rocky Mountain spotted fever. A black eschar called a *tache noire* may be noted at the site of the tick bite and

is caused by vascular endothelial damage that leads to dermal and epidermal necrosis. A diffuse macular papular rash develops within 3–5 days of the onset of the febrile illness; however, as is observed with RMSF, some patients fail to develop a black eschar or rash. Rickettsialpox, caused by *R. akari,* is transmitted by a blood-sucking mite that normally lives on mice; however, on rare occasions it does bite humans. When mouse populations are reduced by extermination campaigns, these mites are more likely to infest humans and cause disease. Rickettsialpox has been reported in urban areas of the United States, including Boston, Pittsburgh, and Cleveland, as well as in Arizona and Utah. This disease is not considered by many U.S. physicians and is often mistaken for chickenpox. The disease has also been reported in Mexico, where it may be initially mistaken for dengue fever. Rickettsialpox is also found in South Africa, the Ukraine, Croatia, and Korea. The incubation period is 10–14 days and the illness is characterized by the development of an eschar at the site of the mite bite, abrupt onset of fever, chills, myalgias, and headache, followed by a papulovesicular rash. The rash initially is maculopapular, later becoming papulovesicular. Lesions then scab over and heal without scars. The number of skin lesions varies, and they can involve the face, mucous membranes, palms, and soles. The disease spontaneously resolves within two to three weeks and is never fatal. Treatment with doxycycline or tetracycline is associated with resolution of symptoms within 24–48 hours. The diagnosis can be made by direct immunofluorescence staining of biopsy material from the eschar or by acute and convalescent antibody titers.

    b. Found in Europe, Africa, and the Middle East.

2. Rickettsialpox, caused by *R. akari*, transmitted by a blood-sucking mouse mite:

    a. Causes papulovesicular rash, often mistaken for chickenpox,

    b. In U.S. found in Boston, Pittsburgh, and Cleveland as well as in Arizona and Utah,

    c. Also found in Mexico, South Africa, the Ukraine, Croatia, and Korea,

    d. Self-limited disease, quickly responds to tetracycline or doxycycline.

Typhus

Potential Severity: Patients can become extremely toxic, develop shock and organ failure, and die.

This group of diseases received the name typhus because the illness caused by these species of Rickettsia clinically mimics typhoid fever (see Chapter 8).

EPIDEMIOLOGY, PATHOGENESIS, AND CLINICAL MANIFESTATIONS

Rickettsia prowazekii causes the most serious form of typhus. This disease has been called louse-borne typhus as well as epidemic typhus and is spread from person to person by body lice. High concentrations of Rickettsia are harbored in the louse's alimentary canal. When the infected louse bites the human and ingests a blood meal, it also defecates, releasing the organisms onto the skin. The unwitting host scratches the site and inoculates the infected feces into the wound or onto mucous membranes. This disease has most commonly been encountered during periods of war and famine. During World War II louse-borne typhus was common in Eastern European and North African concentration camps. Over the past 20 years infections have most commonly been reported in Africa and less commonly in South and Central America. Rare cases have been reported in the eastern and central United States and are thought to have been transmitted by lice or fleas from flying squirrels.

The incubation period is approximately one week, followed by the abrupt onset of high fever, severe headache, and myalgias. The headache is retro-orbital and bifrontal, comes on suddenly, and is unremitting. As is observed with severe Rocky Mountain spotted fever, tissue necrosis develops as a result of small vessel vasculitis, and this process involves multiple organs, including the lungs, liver, gastrointestinal tract, central nervous system, and skin. Skin rash is observed in 60% of patients and begins on the trunk, spreading outwardly over 24–48 hours. Lesions are initially macular but quickly progress to maculopapular lesions and then to petechiae. Peripheral gangrene can develop as a consequence of small vessel occlusion. Central nervous system involvement can lead to drowsiness and confusion and in severe cases can result in grand mal seizures and focal neurologic deficits. Louse-borne typhus has been associated with 30–70% mortality.

After primary infection *R. prowazekii* can remain latent for decades and then reactivate after physical or psychological stress, particularly in the elderly. This reactivated form of typhus is called Brill-Zinsser disease and is similar in clinical presentation to primary disease; however, the disease is milder. *R. typhi* responsible for flea-borne typhus (other names are murine or endemic typhus) also causes a milder form of typhus and is found throughout the world. The prognosis for Brill-Zinsser disease and flea-borne typhus is much better than that for primary louse-borne typhus, mortality rates being less than 5% for both diseases.

A third form of typhus, called scrub typhus, is caused by *R. tsutsugamushi* and is transmitted by mite larvae (commonly called chiggers). These insects crawl on vegetation and then attach themselves to small mammals and humans as they pass through the brush. Agricultural workers and military personnel in endemic areas most often contract this disease. Scrub typhus is found in Japan, eastern Asia, Australia, and the western and southwestern Pacific islands. The incubation period is similar to that for other rickettsial diseases (6–21 days); however, the onset is usually gradual rather than sudden. Headache, high fever, chills, and anorexia are the most common symptoms. Diffuse lymphadenopathy, splenomegaly, conjunctivitis, and pharyngitis are common physical findings. Within a week of the onset of symptoms a high percentage of patients develop a maculopapular skin rash. A black eschar may be noted at the site of the chigger bite in approximately half of patients.

KEY POINTS

Epidemiology, Pathogenesis, and Clinical Manifestations of Typhus

1. Louse-borne typhus, caused by *Rickettsia prowazekii,* most serious form:
   a. Person-to-person spread by lice, common during World War II,
   b. Now found in Africa and, less commonly, in South and Central America,
   c. Rare in eastern and central United States, transmitted by lice or fleas from flying squirrels,
   d. Causes small vessel vasculitis, petechial skin rash on trunk, multiple organ failure, peripheral gangrene, encephalitis, 30–70% mortality.
2. Brill-Zinsser disease: Reactivation of *R. prowazekii,* milder but similar to primary disease.
3. Flea-borne typhus caused by *R. typhi,* milder form of typhus, worldwide distribution.
4. Scrub typhus caused by *R. tsutsugamushi* and transmitted by mite larvae (chiggers):

   a. Found in Japan, eastern Asia, Australia, and Pacific Islands,
   b. More gradual onset, black eschar at chigger bite site in half of patients, rash common.

DIAGNOSIS AND TREATMENT

The diagnosis of these febrile illnesses is presumptive and based on clinical and epidemiologic findings. Acute and convalescent antibody titers to the specific forms of Rickettsia can be performed, and the specific diagnosis may be made retrospectively. Immunofluorescence staining of the primary eschar where available can yield a more rapid diagnosis. The once popular Weil-Felix Proteus agglutination test is no longer recommended because of its poor sensitivity and lack of specificity. The treatment for all forms of typhus is identical to that for the spotted fever group: tetracycline (500 mg po QID), doxycycline (100 mg po or iv BID), or chloramphenicol (500 mg po or iv QID) (see Table 13.1). Therapy should usually be continued for 3–5 days after defervescence. In some regions where antibiotic resistance has developed, rifampin (600–900 mg po QD) may more efficacious. Early treatment aborts the antibody response, and as a consequence relapse may occur after treatment is completed. Patients respond well to retreatment.

KEY POINTS

Diagnosis and Treatment of Typhus

1. Presumptive diagnosis must be made by clinical and epidemiologic findings.
2. Antibody titers available, immunofluorescence staining of primary lesion helpful.
3. Weil-Felix Proteus agglutination is no longer recommended.
4. Treatment with tetracycline, doxycycline, or chloramphenicol; may relapse, requiring retreatment.

Ehrlichia

Potential Severity: Can cause severe multisystemic disease that is usually not fatal.

There are two forms of ehrlichiosis: human monocytotropic ehrlichiosis (HME), caused by *Ehrlichia chaffeensis,* and human granulocytotropic ehrlichiosis (HGE), caused by *E. phagocytophila.*

EPIDEMIOLOGY

Both species of Ehrlichia are transmitted to humans by ticks, and the seasonal nature of these diseases is identical to that of other tick-borne illnesses. The majority of cases of human monocytotropic ehrlichiosis are associated with bites from the Lone Star tick (*Amblyomma americanum*). This tick also infests the white-tailed deer, the natural reservoir for *E. chaffeensis.* This disease is very common in the Southeast, and attack rates have been estimated to be 5 per 100,000; however, in certain endemic areas incidences as high as 660 per 100,000 have been reported. In addition to hikers and outdoor workers, golfers are at risk for contracting this disease. Human granulocytotropic ehrlichiosis was first reported in 1994; therefore an understanding of its epidemiology is still evolving. To date, cases have been associated with tick bites from *Ixodes scapularis,* the same tick that transmits Lyme disease and babesiosis. Cases have been reported in California, Minnesota, Wisconsin, Massachusetts, Connecticut, New York, and Florida.

PATHOGENESIS

Once the organism is inoculated into the skin by the tick, it enters the lymphatic system and bloodstream. *E. chaffeensis* prefers to invade macrophages and monocytes, less commonly entering lymphocytes and rarely PMNs. Once phagocytosed by these cells, *E. chaffeensis* remains in the phagosomes, where it survives by inhibiting fusion of lysosomes that release toxic products that normally kill invading pathogens. In addition this organism blocks the signal transduction pathways that enhance interferon-γ production and simultaneously upregulates cytokine genes important for generation of the inflammatory response. Finally, the pathogen induces clustering of transferrin receptors in the phagolysosome membrane, allowing it to compete effectively for iron, a vital nutrient for bacterial growth. As the bacteria divide by binary fusion, they cluster together, forming intracellular inclusions called morulae. *E. phagocytophila* primarily invades PMNs and utilizes strategies similar to those of *E. chaffeensis* to survive within these cells. Both pathogens not only invade peripheral leukocytes but also infect the bone marrow, causing disruption of the normal maturation processes and blocking production of leukocytes, red blood cells, and platelets.

KEY POINTS

Epidemiology and Pathogenesis of Ehrlichiosis

1. Human monocytotropic ehrlichiosis is caused *E. chaffeensis:*
   a. Transmitted by the Lone Star tick found on the white-tailed deer,
   b. Common S.E. USA; hikers, outdoor workers, and golfers at risk.
2. Human granulocytotropic ehrlichiosis is caused by *E. phagocytophila:*
   a. Transmitted by *Ixodes* tick, same tick that transmits Lyme disease and Babesiosis,
   b. Found in California, Minnesota, Wisconsin, Massachusetts, Connecticut, New York and Florida.

CLINICAL MANIFESTATIONS

◆ CASE 13.4

A 49-year-old Caucasian male presented to the hospital with a two-week history of fever and malaise. Fever came on gradually and was associated with generalized headaches. He was given trimethoprim-sulfamethoxazole by his primary physician for presumed sinusitis but failed to improve. Fever increased to 103–104°F, generalized headache persisted, and he developed a nonproductive cough.

Epidemiology: He was an avid hunter and had been hunting with his father on several occasions during the last two months. He reported extensive tick exposure. His father developed "influenzae pneumonia" at the same time and had died in the hospital.

Physical examination: In the emergency room he was noted to have a fever of 103°F, heart rate 96, respiratory rate 22, blood pressure 144/60. He appeared toxic, somewhat lethargic, and inattentive. Conjunctiva were injected with bilateral hemorrhages, tender cervical lymphadenopathy was noted, neck was supple. Skin: a few hyperpigmented macular lesions over the anterior shins, no evidence of tick bites.

Laboratory findings: Hct 34, platelets 61K, peripheral WBC 3.6K (66% PMNs, 17% lymphocytes, 16% monocytes), smear: no morulae noted. Serum Na 125 mEq/l, AST 185, ALT 151, blood cultures × 2 no growth. CSF: WBC 205 (2% PMNs, 78% lymphocytes, 20% monocytes), RBC 0, TP 139, glucose 153, chest X-ray: within normal limits.

Treatment: He was treated with doxycycline and defervesced within 48 hours. One week after hospital discharge, serum IgG and IgM titers returned and were positive for *E. chaffeensis*.

Case 13.4 represents a classic presentation of human monocytotropic ehrlichiosis. Both forms of ehrlichiosis have incubation periods of approximately 7 days. Ehrlichia varies in its severity, and fatality rates of approximately 5% have been reported in both diseases. Manifestations tend to be more severe in the elderly and in immunocompromised patients. Like rickettsiosis, ehrlichiosis is a multisystem disease. Both forms of Ehrlichia present with the gradual onset of fever, chills, headache, myalgias, anorexia, and malaise. The monocytotropic form can result in respiratory insufficiency, renal insufficiency, and

meningoencephalitis. It is very possible that the patient's father in Case 13.4 died of respiratory complications from ehrlichiosis. Neck stiffness, depressed mental status, coma, and seizures are accompanied by CSF lymphocytosis and elevated CSF protein. Case 13.4 had a depressed mental status and typical CSF findings. The granulocytotropic form can also be associated with respiratory insufficiency. Rhabdomyolysis has also been described. Meningoencephalitis has not been described in granulocytotropic ehrlichiosis. Some patients with HGE have developed fatal opportunistic infections. Hypotension can develop with either infection and may mimic other forms of Gram-negative sepsis. A macular, maculopapular, or petechial rash is observed in 30–40% of patients with HME but in only 2–11% of patients with HGE.

Thrombocytopenia is a prominent finding in both diseases, and this finding combined with the epidemiology strongly suggested the diagnosis of ehrlichiosis in Case 13.4. The platelet count is depressed ($50,000–140,000/mm^3$) in the majority of patients. Platelet counts can drop below $20,000/mm^3$ in severe disease and can be associated with gastrointestinal bleeding. Leukopenia ($1,300–4,000/mm^3$) is also a frequent finding, peripheral neutrophil and/or lymphocyte counts being depressed in HME. In the granulocytotropic form, neutropenia predominates and is commonly associated with a left shift and relative lymphocytosis. As is observed in Case 13.4, elevated transaminase values (AST and ALT) are found in nearly all patients.

DIAGNOSIS AND TREATMENT

If the diagnosis of Ehrlichia is being considered, a Wright stain of the peripheral blood as well as a buffy coat smear should be carefully examined for the presence of morulae. These intracellular inclusions are seen in peripheral monocytes of only a small percentage of patients with HME; however, in HGE, granulocyte morulae can be identified in 25–80% of patients (see Figure 13.2). The percentage of granulocytes containing

Figure 13.2

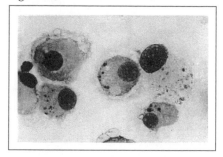

Granulocyte morulae found in human granulo-cytotropic ehrlichiosis. See also Color Plate 2.

morulae varies from 1% to 44%, higher levels of intracellular invasion being seen in the elderly.

Culture techniques are impractical and insensitive, and PCR methods remain experimental. As in rickettsiosis, serologic testing of acute and convalescent serum is the usual method for diagnosis. Antibodies usually take two to three weeks to reach detectable levels. Immunofluorescence assays are available through the state laboratories and the CDC. Titers above 1:64 combined with a fourfold rise between acute and convalescent serum is considered diagnostic.

Doxycycline (100 mg po or iv BID) is the treatment of choice (see Table 13.1), and in vitro testing confirms that Ehrlichia species are sensitive to tetracyclines. Clinical experience suggests that chloramphenicol (500 mg po or iv QID) is also effective; however, in vitro testing has demonstrated no significant anti-Ehrlichia activity. Because of these concerns doxycycline (4 mg/kg QD divided into two doses) is preferred over chloramphenicol in children despite the potential problems of dental staining.

KEY POINTS

Clinical Manifestations, Diagnosis, and Treatment of Ehrlichiosis

1. Incubation period 7 days, 5% mortality (elderly and immunocompromised):
   a. Gradual onset of fever, chills, headache, myalgias, anorexia, and malaise,
   b. Severe monocytic form: Respiratory insufficiency, renal insufficiency, and meningoencephalitis (with CSF lymphocytosis),
   c. Severe granulocytic form: Respiratory insufficiency, rhabdomyolysis, neutropenia resulting in Gram-negative sepsis,
   d. Macular, petechial rash in 30–40% of monocytic form but only 2–11% of granulocytic form.
2. Diagnosis presumptive in most cases:
   a. Thrombocytopenia and leukopenia common (neutropenia in granulocytic form),
   b. Moderate transaminase elevations,
   c. Peripheral smears: Morulae rare in monocytic form, common in granulocytic form,
   d. Retrospective serologies.
3. Treat with doxycycline. Chloramphenicol no activity in vitro therefore doxycline also recommended for children.

Coxiella burnetii (Q fever)

Potential Severity: Q fever is usually a self-limited disease; however, the rare patient who develops Q fever endocarditis often dies.

EPIDEMIOLOGY

The main reservoirs for *Coxiella burnetii,* the cause of Q fever, are farm animals: sheep, goats, and cows. Pet cats and dogs may also carry the organism. Mammals shed the pathogen in their urine, feces, and birth products. Transmission most commonly occurs in association with birthing, organisms being aerosolized from the placenta and inhaled by humans. *C. burnetii* is resistant to drying and can survive for long periods in the environment, and wind-borne particles can be inhaled weeks after parturition. Q fever is rare in the United States, 20–60 cases being reported annually. Outbreaks occur worldwide but may be missed because of the disease's nonspecific symptoms and signs. Significant numbers of cases have been reported in Spain, France, England, Australia, and Canada. In some areas the incidence of Q fever has been estimated to be 50 per 100,000.

PATHOGENESIS

Coxiella burnetii is a small pleomorphic rod (0.3–1 μm long) whose cell wall has many similarities to that of Gram-negative rods. Although this pathogen was originally classified in the rickettsial family, DNA sequencing indicates that the organism is more closely related to Legionella and Francisella and is a Proteobacteria. This organism is capable of varying its lipopolysaccharide antigens in response to environmental conditions. In the external environment the organism usually has Phase II lipopolysaccharide antigens; however, on invading the host, there is a shift to Phase I antigens.

Coxiella burnetii primarily infects the host through the respiratory tract. Infectious particles are inhaled and are then phagocytosed by pulmonary macrophages, surviving and growing within the acidic environment of the phagolysosome. The ability of the organism to hide within these acidic compartments may account for the great difficulty in curing chronic Q fever with antibiotics. Pulmonary infection induces a mononuclear cell infiltration and can cause areas of focal necrosis and hemorrhage. Infection can spread to the liver, causing granuloma formation. In patients with damaged heart valves *C. burnetii* can survive prolonged periods and cause chronic infection.

KEY POINTS

Epidemiology and Pathogenesis of Q Fever

1. Rare in the U.S., more commonly seen in Spain, France, England, Australia, and Canada.

2. Most commonly transmitted by farm animals: sheep, goats, and cows:
   a. Excreted in their urine, feces, birth products,
   b. Placenta highly infectious, and aerosolized organisms survive for prolonged periods.
3. *Coxiella burnetii* is a small, pleomorphic Gram-negative rod, changes its outer lipopolysaccharides:
   a. Phase II outer antigens in the environment,
   b. Phase I outer antigens when infecting the host.
4. Enters the host through the respiratory tract, survives within phagolysosomes of macrophages:
   a. Induces mononuclear cell infiltration, granuloma formation in the liver,
   b. Produces areas of focal necrosis and hemorrhage.

CLINICAL MANIFESTATIONS

The incubation period is approximately three weeks in most cases. Symptoms are often very mild or even absent. When symptoms are reported, most patients develop a self-limited flulike illness. Onset of fever is usually abrupt and associated with headache and myalgias. Others complain of a nonproductive cough, and a few rales may be detected on pulmonary exam. Chest X-ray is suggestive of a viral pneumonia with mild bilateral lower lobe infiltrates. Rarely, patients can develop acute respiratory distress syndrome or pleural effusions. Hepatitis may be asymptomatic or be associated with anorexia and malaise. Transaminase values are elevated; however, jaundice is very uncommon. Liver biopsy typically reveals doughnutlike granulomas consisting of a lipid vacuole surrounded by a fibrinoid ring. Other, less common manifestations include a maculopapular rash (10% of patients), myocarditis and pericarditis (1%), and meningitis or encephalitis (1%). A chronic infection persisting longer than six months develops in about 5% of patients and primarily involves the heart, causing symptoms of subacute bacterial endocarditis; however, conventional blood cultures are negative. Vegetations are rarely seen on cardiac echo, and this negative result often delays the diagnosis. Embolic phenomena and digital clubbing may be observed in the late stages of the infection. Valve replacement is commonly required as a consequence of severe valve dysfunction, and mortality in Q fever endocarditis is high (45–65%). Less commonly, chronic infection can develop in an aneurysm, vascular graft, the liver, lungs, joints, or bone.

DIAGNOSIS AND TREATMENT

The organism can be readily grown using cell culture techniques; however, cultures are not performed in most facilities because of the danger to lab personnel and the need for a P3 containment facility. PCR has been successfully used but is not commercially available. IFA testing is the primary method for diagnosis. Anti-Phase I and Phase II IgG, IgM, and IgA antibody titers should be tested. Elevated IgG (titer ≥ 1:200) and IgM (titer ≥ 1:50) antibody titers against Phase II antigens indicate acute disease, while elevated IgG (≥ 1:800) and IgA (≥ 1:100) antibody titers against Phase I antigens are diagnostic of chronic Q fever.

Antibiotics are less effective in Q fever than in other rickettsial diseases, and acute disease is usually self-limited, lasting two weeks. Tetracyclines have been shown to shorten the duration of fever in acute disease by 1–2 days. Doxycycline (100 mg po or iv BID × 2 weeks) is the treatment of choice. Fluoroquinolones are considered a reasonable alternative. In patients with Q fever, endocarditis cure rates have been improved by combining doxycycline with hydroxychloroquine (200 mg po TID) (see Table 13.1). Therapy for endocarditis must be very prolonged, 18 months to four years, to sterilize the valves. In some patients antibiotics have been continued for life.

KEY POINTS

Clinical Manifestations, Diagnosis, and Treatment of Q Fever

1. Incubation period three weeks, usually causing an abrupt flulike illness with cough.
2. Less commonly causes a maculopapular rash (10% of cases), other rarer complications:
   a. Severe respiratory compromise with adult respiratory distress syndrome,
   b. Hepatitis with elevated transaminases but minimal elevations in bilirubin,
   c. Myocarditis and pericarditis,
   d. Meningitis,
   e. Chronic endocarditis: Negative echo early in the disease, high mortality.
3. Diagnosis by IgG and IgM antibodies against Phase I and II antigen (blood cultures negative):
   a. IgG (titer ≥ 1:200) and IgM (titer ≥ 1:50) anti-Phase II antigens = acute disease,
   b. IgG (≥ 1:800) and IgA (≥ 1:100) anti-Phase I antigens = chronic disease.
4. Treatment not as effective as for rickettsial infections:
   a. Doxycycline × two weeks for acute disease; fluoroquinolones may also be helpful,
   b. Doxycycline and hydroxychloroquine × 18 months to four years or life for chronic endocarditis.

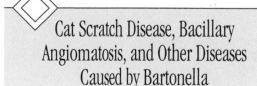

Cat Scratch Disease, Bacillary Angiomatosis, and Other Diseases Caused by Bartonella

Potential Severity: Cat scratch disease and bacillary angiomatosis are usually localized diseases that rarely cause serious illness.

Epidemiology

Young people under the age of 21 years most commonly contract cat scratch disease. This disease is distributed broadly throughout North America and is found worldwide. The incidence in the United States has been estimated to be 9–10 per 100,000. Cat scratch disease is most common in warm, humid climates. As the name implies, all epidemiologic data point to the cat as the primary vector for disease. Young cats are most commonly implicated. Kittens have a very high incidence of asymptomatic bacteremia with *Bartonella henselae* and are more likely to scratch humans. In addition to cat scratches, this disease may be transmitted to humans by fleas, and the flea is also responsible for spread from cat to cat. In addition to causing cat scratch disease, *B. henselae* is one cause of bacillary angiomatosis. The other species that causes this disease, *B. quintana,* is also globally distributed. It is transmitted by human body lice (*Pediculus humanus)* and causes disease in areas where sanitation and personal hygiene are poor. A third pathogenic strain, *B. bacilliformis,* causes Oroya fever and Verruga peruana, diseases that are found only in the Andes Mountains of South America, where the disease is transmitted by the sandfly. Other potentially pathogenic species of Bartonella have been identified; their relationship to disease is currently under active investigation.

KEY POINTS

Epidemiology of Bartonella Infections

1. Cat scratch disease is caused by *Bartonella henselae:*
   a. Transmitted primarily by young cats and less commonly by cat fleas,
   b. Common throughout North America, higher incidence in warm, humid areas.
2. Bacillary angiomatosis is caused by *B. henselae* and by *B. quintana:*
   a. *B. quintana* transmitted by human body lice,
   b. Spread in areas with poor sanitation, persons with poor personal hygiene.
3. *B. bacilliformis* transmitted by the sandfly in the Andes Mountains of South America.

Pathogenesis

Bartonella species are pleomorphic Gram-negative bacilli that stain poorly by Gram stain. The organism takes up silver and can be identified by Warthin-Starry stain. Bartonella enter the host through a break in the skin caused by a cat scratch or insect bite. The bacteria multiply at this site and subsequently spread to the local lymphatic system and adjacent lymph nodes. The bacteria contain flagella that allow them to move within the host. Flagellar and other surface proteins mediate attachment to red blood cells and endothelial cells. The attached bacteria can enter red cells, where they can multiply in vacuoles or in the cytoplasm. Bartonella are ingested by endothelial cells and multiply within a vacuole, forming intracellular clusters similar to Ehrlichia morulae. Certain species of Bartonella, including *B. bacilliformis, B. henselae,* and *B. quintana,* induce the formation of new vessels, and a Bartonella angiogenesis factor has been identified. Because Bartonella grows in both the intracellular and extracellular environments of the host, it induces both a granulomatous reaction consisting of macrophages and histiocytes and an acute inflammatory response consisting primarily of PMNs. This vigorous mixed immune response usually limits the spread of infection, a feature explaining why most Bartonella infections remain localized. In individuals with depressed immunity, such as AIDS patients, this bacteria can cause bacteremia and disseminate throughout the body.

Pathogenesis of Bartonella Infections

1. Pleomorphic Gram-negative rods, weakly take up Gram stain, silver stain preferred.
2. Enter via the skin, spread to the local lymphatics, rarely disseminate except in AIDS patients.
3. Survive within host cell intracellular vacuoles as well as extracellularly.
4. Produce an angiogenesis factor that stimulates the growth of new blood vessels.
5. Induce both granulomatous and acute PMN inflammatory reactions that prevent dissemination.

Clinical Manifestations

CASE 13.5

A 21-year-old Caucasian male was admitted with a 2-hour history of severe right lower abdominal pain, nausea, vomiting, and loose stools. In the emergency room his temperature was 39.7°C, pulse 133, blood pressure 101/40. His abdomen was soft and nontender with normal bowel sounds. A 1.5 × 1.5 × 6 cm warm, very tender mass was palpated in the right inguinal area. Genitalia were normal, without ulcers. CT scan demonstrated a soft tissue mass. Peripheral WBC 12,000 (54% PMNs, 34% band forms), Hct 43, chlamydia and GC urethral swabs were negative. Emergency surgical exploration revealed enlarged, matted right inguinal lymph nodes. Histopathology demonstrated an acute inflammatory response, and silver stain identified multiple rods. He defervesced within 3 days following po ciprofloxacin. On further questioning, this college student reported that he had been playing with wild cats near his apartment over the two weeks prior to his admission but did not recall being scratched.

CAT SCRATCH DISEASE

This disease usually presents as a single enlarged, warm, and painful lymph node near the site of skin inoculation. Lymph node swelling usually occurs within two weeks of inoculation. The patient in Case 13.5 developed unusually acute lymph node swelling that caused the sudden onset of severe pain, raising the possibility of a strangulated hernia and precipitating surgical exploration. The node can enlarge to 8–10 cm in diameter; however, in most cases the involved node expands to a diameter of 1–5 cm. Enlargement of a single node is the rule (85% of cases); however, as is observed in Case 13.5, some patients develop enlargement of a cluster of nodes or, less commonly, experience lymph node enlargement in two distinct anatomic sites. Generalized lymphadenopathy is rare. The site of lymph node enlargement depends on the site of inoculation. Axillary node involvement is most common. Epitrochlear, supraclavicular, submandibular, and inguinal nodes are other sites of lymphadenopathy. In addition to being painful, warm, and erythematous, about 10–15% of the lymph nodes drain pus. The lymphadenopathy usually resolves over one to four months but can persist for several years if not treated with antibiotics.

On careful questioning, the patient may report a skin lesion in the region where the lymph node drains. Within 3–10 days after inoculation a vesicular lesion develops that becomes erythematous and then papular. The skin lesions usually persist for one to three weeks, and by the time the patient seeks medical attention, the site of the scratch may be overlooked. However, if actively searched for, the primary lesion is detected in two thirds of patients. A primary lesion was not identified in Case 13.5. When questioned, a significant percentage of patients do not recall a cat scratch; however, nearly all patients provide a history of contact with a cat or, less commonly, a dog.

Low-grade fever and malaise accompany lymphadenopathy in about half of cases. Conjunctivitis occasionally develops when the eye is the portal of entry, and the combination of conjunctivitis and preauricular lymphadenopathy has been termed the oculoglandular syndrome of Parinaud. Less common manifestations include optic neuritis, encephalopathy that can result in seizures and coma, lytic bone lesions, granulomatous lesions of the liver and spleen, pneumonia, erythema nodosum, and thrombocytopenic purpura.

KEY POINTS

Clinical Manifestations of Cat Scratch Disease

1. Presents with a warm, tender, swollen lymph node 2 weeks after the scratch:
   a. Axillary node most common, involved node depends on the site of inoculation,
   b. The primary scratch can often be identified,
   c. Low grade fever is common.
2. Rarer manifestations include conjunctivitis, encephalopathy, and lesions in the liver and spleen.

BACILLARY ANGIOMATOSIS

This disease develops predominantly in indigent AIDS patients who have body lice, the primary vector for spread of *Bartonella quintana*. Bacillary angiomatosis is also seen in other immunocompromised patients and develops when the CD4 count drops below 100/mm³. The skin lesions usually begin as a cluster of small reddish papules that can enlarge to form nodules. Lesions appear vascular and bleed profusely when traumatized. They can be mistaken for Kaposi's sarcoma, pyogenic granuloma, cherry angiomas, or hemangiomas. Skin biopsy reveals multiple small blood vessels, enlarged endothelial cells, and PMN infiltration. *B. henselae* has also been identified as a cause of bacillary angiomatosis. Like this species, *B. quintana* can infect the liver and less commonly the spleen, resulting in the formation of discrete blood-filled cystic structures. This disease has been called bacillary peliosis.

BACTEREMIC ILLNESS

Bartonella quintana can seed the bloodstream and cause trench fever. This disease was common during World Wars I and II but is rare today, being seen primarily in homeless individuals with poor hygiene. Cases have been reported in the homeless in Seattle, Washington, and in Marseilles, France. Symptoms of fever, malaise, and bone pain involving the anterior shins usually begin 5–20 days after exposure. Splenomegaly is common, and in some patients a maculopapular rash may be seen. Recurrent fever every 5 days (quintan fever) is the most common presentation and is the basis for the organism's name. After the primary episode patients continue to have asymptomatic bacteremia lasting weeks to months. Both *B. quintana* and *B. henselae* can cause bacterial endocarditis, and these pathogens should be considered in cases of culture-negative bacterial endocarditis.

KEY POINTS

Clinical Manifestations of *Bartonella quintana*

1. The major cause of bacillary angiomatosis (*B. henselae,* a less common cause):
   a. Seen in indigent AIDS patients with body lice, CD4 usually < 100/mm³,
   b. Small, reddish papules that coalesce into nodules, bleed profusely,
   c. Histopathology: Multiple small vessels, enlarged endothelial cells, and PMN infiltration.
2. Bacteremic illness rare, seen in some homeless, recurrent 5-day fever, shin pain, malaise.

Diagnosis

Bartonella grows slowly on fresh blood agar, rabbit-heart-infusion agar, and chocolate agar. If Bartonella is suspected, the physician should contact the clinical microbiology laboratory to ensure that all cultures are incubated for prolonged periods (at least 21 days) in 5–10% CO_2 and high moisture. Because the organism adheres to the sides of glass blood culture flasks, the liquid media will not appear turbid. The bacteria's slow rate of growth also impairs recognition by standard CO_2-detection methods. Staining of broth with Warthin-Starry stain or acridine orange has been used to overcome these limitations.

Biopsies of lymph nodes and skin lesions are generally not required for diagnosis, and the histopathology of mixed granulomatous and acute inflammatory reaction is not specific. Palisading epithelioid cells are commonly seen, and a positive Warthin-Starry silver stain demonstrating black bacilli provides strong evidence for the diagnosis. However, organisms may be difficult to detect in chronically infected lymph nodes. Bacillary angiomatosis lesions demonstrate characteristic plump endothelial cells, neovascularity, and clusters of bacteria on silver staining.

An indirect IFA and enzyme immunosorbent assay are available to detect antibodies directed against Bartonella, and these tests have now replaced the cat scratch skin test. The skin test was previously considered a useful diagnostic tool but is no longer recommended. Unlike antibody titers, which have been ineffective at differentiating between species, PCR probes have proven to be more specific and are now commercially available.

Treatment

Azithromycin (500 mg followed by 250 mg × 4 days) is effective in patients with lymph node disease. Clarithromycin (500 mg po BID), doxycycline (100 mg po BID), or ciprofloxacin (500 mg po BID) for 10–14 days may also be effective (see Table 13.1). In severe cases intravenous azithromycin (500 mg QD) combined with rifampin (600 mg po or iv QD) is likely to be the most effective regimen. However, the ef-

ficacy of combined therapy has not been proven. In patients with bacteremia due to *Bartonella quintana,* therapy should be continued for four to six weeks, and if endocarditis has developed, six months of therapy is advised to reduce the risk of relapse. Patients with bacillary angiomatosis should be treated for two to four months, and four months of therapy is recommended for patients with bone, hepatic, or splenic lesions.

KEY POINTS

Diagnosis and Treatment of Bartonella Infections

1. Grow on conventional media, slow growing, clinical laboratory must be alerted.
2. Blood cultures frequently falsely negative because organisms adhere to sides of the flask.
3. Biopsies frequently unnecessary; Warthin-Starry stain showing black rods helpful.
4. Antibody titers using IFA or enzyme immunosorbent assay, as well as PCR now tests of choice.
5. Treatment: Azithromycin, clarithromycin, doxycycline, or ciprofloxacin × 10–14 days:
   a. Severe cases: iv azithromycin and rifampin (efficacy not proven),
   b. Bacteremia with *Bartonella quintana* treat four to six weeks, endocarditis six months,
   c. Bacillary angiomatosis treat two to four months, tissue abscesses four months.

Brucellosis

Potential Severity: This febrile illness is often difficult to diagnose but is rarely fatal.

Epidemiology

This bacteria is primarily transmitted to humans by infected wild and domestic animals. Direct animal contact, contact with animal products, and ingestion of unpasteurized dairy products are the most common ways in which humans contract brucellosis. Cattle, buffalo, camels, yaks, goats, and sheep are the most common domestic animals responsible for disease transmission. In the wild, swine, fox, caribou, antelope, and elk have been implicated. Bacteria enter the host through abrasions or cuts, the conjunctiva, or the gastrointestinal tract. Persons at risk are farmers, hunters, and those who ingest unpasteurized cheeses or other unpasteurized dairy products. The disease is found worldwide, being most common in the Mediterranean region, the Arab Gulf basin, the Indian subcontinent, Mexico, and Central and South America. In the United States brucellosis is most frequently reported in the South and Southwest. As a consequence of a rigorous farm animal screening and vaccination program and pasteurization of all dairy products, the overall incidence of brucellosis in the United States is low, 0.05 per 100,000, most cases being contracted by travelers who visit endemic areas.

Pathogenesis

Brucella are small, aerobic, Gram-negative coccobacilli. The three most common strains to cause human disease are *B. abortis, B. suis,* and *B. melitensis.* The organism expresses lipopolysaccharide (LPS) on its surface, and expression of the smooth form (S-LPS) enhances intracellular survival and is an important virulence factor. Brucella is a facultative intracellular pathogen. After entering the skin, the bacteria quickly attract PMNs. These cells ingest the pathogen, where it happily survives within the phagolysosome by neutralizing toxic oxygen byproducts through the production of a superoxide dismutase. The bacteria subsequently invade the lymphatic system and bloodstream, disseminating primarily to organs with rich reticuloendothelial systems (liver, spleen, and bone marrow). Here the bacteria are ingested by resident macrophages and survive in these cells by blocking phagosome-lysosome fusion, as observed with Ehrlichia.

KEY POINTS

Epidemiology and Pathogenesis of Brucellosis

1. Transmitted to humans by infected domestic and wild animals:
   a. Cattle, buffalo, camels, yaks, goats, and sheep,
   b. Swine, fox, caribou, antelope, and elk.
2. Most common in the Mediterranean region, Arab Gulf basin, Indian subcontinent, Mexico, Central and South America. U.S. uncommon, mainly in the South and Southwest.
3. Enters via skin break or ingestion of unpasteurized dairy products (milk, cheeses).
4. Aerobic Gram-negative coccobacilli, three pathogenic strains: *Brucella abortis, B. suis,* and *B. melitensis.*
5. Survives in phagolysosomes of PMNs and macrophages by producing superoxide dismutase and blocking phagosome-lysosome fusion.

Clinical Manifestations

CASE 13.6

A 40-year-old Caucasian male was seen in the emergency room complaining of right-sided chest pain for 4 days. Pain was sharp, very severe, and made worse by taking a deep breath. Pain was localized to the right chest and right upper quadrant and occasionally radiated to the shoulder. His chest pain was preceded by two weeks of low-grade intermittent fever accompanied by sweating. He noted a mild cough with minimal yellow sputum production.

Epidemiology: He periodically hunts wild pigs and had been hunting 5 weeks prior to his hospitalization.

Past medical history: Renal transplant 4 years earlier, on prednisone and Imuran.

Physical examination: Temperature 36.7°C, pulse 102, respiratory rate 24, blood pressure 126/94. Ill-appearing, breathing shallowly. No palpable lymph nodes. Bilateral inspiratory rales at the lung bases, right = left side. Small area of dullness, right lower lung field. Abdomen: no organomegaly or tenderness, extremities 2+ edema.

Laboratory findings: Chest X-ray: small right pleural effusion. Hct 37.5, WBC 13.7 (69% PMNs, 17% band forms), AST 84, ALT 32, Alk phosphatase 482, total bilirubin 2.4 (1.5 direct). Pleural fluid: 250 WBC (92% PMNs), LDH 741, TP 3.8, glucose 69, pH 7.38. Blood cultures × 2 positive for *Brucella suis*. He was treated with doxycycline and rifampin × 6 weeks and fully recovered.

Usually two to four weeks after inoculation or ingestion of Brucella, fever, chills, malaise, anorexia, headache, and back pain develop. In Case 13.6 the history of intermittent low-grade fever and sweats is typical. These nonspecific symptoms can persist for weeks, making the diagnosis difficult to ascertain. As a result brucellosis is one of the listed infectious causes of fever of undetermined origin (see Chapter 3). Physical exam is usually unimpressive; in most cases, the only positive findings are lymphadenopathy and splenomegaly. As is observed in Case 13.6, approximately one third of patients develop a focal infection. Localized disease is more likely in patients who have had untreated infection for 30 or more days. It is likely that immunosuppression predisposed the patient in Case 13.6 to develop a localized pleural infection as well as moderate hepatic involvement. Sites where Brucella may localize include:

1. **Bones and joints**. Septic arthritis is associated with mononuclear cells in the joint fluid, and Brucella can be cultured in half of the cases. Sacroiliitis is particularly common. Osteomyelitis is rare and usually involves the vertebral bodies and mimics tuberculous osteomyelitis.

2. **Liver**. This organ is probably always infected. Mild elevations of liver function tests are noted, and granulomas may be found on liver biopsy, particularly with *Brucella abortus*. Purulent abscesses are rare but may be seen with *B. suis* and, less commonly, with *B. melitensis*.

3. **Central nervous system**. Meningitis is the most frequent CNS complication and is associated with a CSF lymphocytic pleocytosis, elevated protein, and normal or depressed glucose. Encephalitis and brain abscess are rare.

4. **Cardiovascular system**. Endocarditis is rare but can be fatal. Generally, valve replacement must be combined with prolonged antibiotic therapy.

5. **Genitourinary system**. Brucella can often be recovered from the urine; however, invasion of the kidney is rare. Orchitis is reported in up to 20% of men with brucellosis, the testes being infiltrated with lymphocytes and plasma cells.

6. **Bone marrow**. Granulomas are detected in up to 75% of cases. Infection of the marrow can lead to anemia, leukopenia, and thrombocytopenia.

7. **Respiratory tract**. Pulmonary involvement is rare but can form discrete granulomas and rarely produces bronchopneumonia.

KEY POINTS
Clinical Presentation of Brucellosis

1. Two- to four-week incubation period: fever, chills, malaise, anorexia, headache, and back pain.
2. Important cause of FUO, lymphadenopathy and splenomegaly only positive physical findings.
3. Focal infection more common if treatment is delayed:
   a. Osteomyelitis and arthritis, particularly sacroiliitis,
   b. Hepatic involvement is common,

  c. Lymphocytic meningitis,
  d. Endocarditis usually requires valve re-
     placement,
  e. Positive urine culture common, orchitis
     in 20% of men,
  f. Bone marrow suppression, granulomas
     found,
  g. Pulmonary disease is rare.

Diagnosis

Blood cultures should be drawn in all patients
who are suspected of having brucellosis and are
positive in up to 70% of patients. However, the
organism is slow growing and can take up to 35
days to grow; but blood cultures usually take
7–21 days to turn positive. The clinical microbiology laboratory should be alerted so that cultures are held beyond 7 days. Bone marrow culture is also a high-yield diagnostic test and
should be considered in patients with negative blood cultures. Serologic diagnosis is the
most common method for making the diagnosis.
Serum agglutination titers measure IgG and IgM
antibodies against the three major pathogenic
Brucella strains but do not detect *Brucella
canis,* a rare cause of disease. A titer of >1:160
in the presence of appropriate symptoms is supportive of the diagnosis, as is a fourfold or
greater titer rise between acute and convalescent sera. IgG and IgM ELISA assays are also
available and demonstrate similar sensitivity and
specificity to the serum agglutination tests.

Treatment

Because Brucella survives within phagocytes antibiotics with good intracellular penetration are
recommended. The treatment of choice is doxycycline (100 mg po BID) and rifampin (600–900
mg po QD) for six weeks (see Table 13.1).
Single-drug therapy is not recommended because of the high likelihood of relapse. Doxycy-

cline combined with streptomycin (1 gm im QD
for the first three weeks) or gentamicin (5
mg/kg iv QD for the first three weeks) are useful alternatives. For children trimethoprim-sulfamethoxazole (10–12 mg/kg of the trimethoprim component per day divided into two
doses) and rifampin (20 mg/kg/day) are recommended. In cases of meningitis or endocarditis a
three-drug regimen consisting of doxycycline, rifampin, and trimethoprim-sulfamethoxazole has
been used. Therapy for these diseases must be
prolonged (several months to over a year). In
patients with endocarditis, replacement of the
infected valve is usually required for cure.

KEY POINTS
Diagnosis and Treatment of Brucellosis

1. Blood cultures are positive in 70% of cases,
   hold for 21 days.
2. Bone marrow cultures are often positive.
3. Serological diagnosis is frequently helpful:
   a. Serum agglutination or ELISA, IgM and
      IgG antibody titers,
   b. Titer of > 1:160 or fourfold rise between
      acute and convalescent samples.
4. Treatment: Doxycycline + rifampin or doxycycline + gentamicin or streptomycin × 6
   weeks:
   a. Alternative for children: Trimethoprim-
      sulfamethoxazole + rifampin
   b. Meningitis or endocarditis: Doxycycline +
      rifampin + trimethoprim-sulfamethoxa-
      zole × months to years.
   c. Never use a single drug, high risk of re-
      lapse.

Additional Reading

Lyme Disease
Kalish, R.A., Kaplan, R.F., Taylor, E., Jones-Wood-
   ward, L., Workman, K., and Steere, A.C. Evaluation
   of study patients with Lyme disease, 10-20-year
   follow-up. *J Infect Dis* 183:453-460, 2001.

Klempner, M.S., Hu, L.T., Evans, J., et al. Two controlled trials of antibiotic treatment in patients with persistent symptoms and a history of Lyme disease. *N Engl J Med* 345:85-92, 2001.

Massarotti, E.M. Lyme arthritis. *Med Clin North Am* 86:297-309, 2002.

Nadelman, R.B., Nowakowski, J., Fish, D., et al. Prophylaxis with single-dose doxycycline for the prevention of Lyme disease after an *Ixodes scapularis* tick bite. *N Engl J Med* 345:79-84, 2001.

Sigal, L.H. Lyme disease: a clinical update. *Hosp Pract* (Off Ed) 36:31-32, 35-37, 41-42, 47, 2001.

Smith, R.P., Schoen, R.T., Rahn, D.W., et al. Clinical characteristics and treatment outcome of early Lyme disease in patients with microbiologically confirmed erythema migrans. *Ann Intern Med* 136:421-428, 2002.

Leptospirosis

Centers for Disease Control and Prevention. Update: outbreak of acute febrile illness among athletes participating in Eco-Challenge-Sabah 2000—Borneo, Malaysia, 2000. *JAMA* 285:728-730, 2001.

Ko, A.I., Galvao Reis, M., Ribeiro Dourado, C.M., Johnson, W.D., Jr., and Riley, L.W. Urban epidemic of severe leptospirosis in Brazil. Salvador Leptospirosis Study Group. *Lancet* 354:820-825, 1999.

Rickettsial Diseases

Comer, J.A., Diaz, T., Vlahov, D., Monterroso, E., and Childs, J.E. Evidence of rodent-associated Bartonella and Rickettsia infections among intravenous drug users from Central and East Harlem, New York City. *Am J Trop Med Hyg* 65:855-860, 2001.

Holman, R.C., Paddock, C.D., Curns, A.T., Krebs, J.W., McQuiston, J.H., and Childs, J.E. Analysis of risk factors for fatal Rocky Mountain Spotted Fever: evidence for superiority of tetracyclines for therapy. *J Infect Dis* 184:1437-1444, 2001.

Paddock, C.D., Greer, P.W., Ferebee, T.L., et al. Hidden mortality attributable to Rocky Mountain spotted fever: immunohistochemical detection of fatal, serologically unconfirmed disease. *J Infect Dis* 179:1469-1476, 1999.

Watt, G., Kantipong, P., Jongsakul, K., Watcharapichat, P., Phulsuksombati, D., and Strickman, D. Doxycycline and rifampicin for mild scrub-typhus infections in northern Thailand: a randomised trial. *Lancet* 356:1057-1061, 2000.

Ehrlichiosis

Glushko, G.M. Human ehrlichiosis. *Postgrad Med J* 101:225-230, 1997.

Ijdo, I.J., Meek, J.I., Cartter, M.L., et al. The emergence of another tickborne infection in the 12-town area around Lyme, Connecticut: human granulocytic ehrlichiosis. *J Infect Dis* 181:1388-1393, 2000.

Wallace, B.J., Brady, G., Ackman, D.M., et al. Human granulocytic ehrlichiosis in New York. *Arch Intern Med* 158:769-773, 1998.

Q Fever

Bernit, E., Pouget, J., Janbon, F., et al. Neurological involvement in acute Q fever: a report of 29 cases and review of the literature. *Arch Intern Med* 162:693-700, 2002.

Caron, F., Meurice, J.C., Ingrand, P., et al. Acute Q fever pneumonia: a review of 80 hospitalized patients. *Chest* 114:808-813, 1998.

Raoult, D., Houpikian, P., Tissot Dupont, H., Riss, J.M., Arditi-Djiane, J., and Brouqui, P. Treatment of Q fever endocarditis: comparison of 2 regimens containing doxycycline and ofloxacin or hydroxychloroquine. *Arch Intern Med* 159:167-173, 1999.

Bartonella Infections

Brouqui, P., Lascola, B., Roux, V., and Raoult, D. Chronic *Bartonella quintana* bacteremia in homeless patients. *N Engl J Med* 340:184-189, 1999.

Fournier, P.E., Lelievre, H., Eykyn, S.J., et al. Epidemiologic and clinical characteristics of *Bartonella quintana* and *Bartonella henselae* endocarditis: a study of 48 patients. *Medicine* (Baltimore) 80:245-251, 2001.

Loutit, J.S. Bartonella infections: diverse and elusive. *Hosp Pract* (Off Ed) 33:37-38, 41-44, 49, 1998.

Zangwill, K.M., Hamilton, D.H., Perkins, B.A., et al. Cat scratch disease in Connecticut. Epidemiology, risk factors, and evaluation of a new diagnostic test. *N Engl J Med* 329:8-13, 1993.

Brucellosis

Chomel, B.B., DeBess, E.E., Mangiamele, D.M., et al. Changing trends in the epidemiology of human brucellosis in California from 1973 to 1992: a shift toward foodborne transmission. *J Infect Dis* 170:1216-1223, 1994.

Colmenero, J.D., Reguera, J.M., Martos, F., et al. Complications associated with *Brucella melitensis* infection: a study of 530 cases. *Medicine* (Baltimore) 75:195-211, 1996.

Chapter 14

Bioterrorism

Recommended Time to Complete: 1 day

Guiding Questions

1. What are the key characteristics that are required for the ideal bioterrorist agent?

2. What can physicians do to help in the early phases of a bioterrorist attack?

3. What clinical clues should raise the possibility of an anthrax attack?

4. How is bubonic plague normally transmitted and what are the usual clinical manifestations?

5. What groups are normally at risk for developing tularemia?

6. How does the clinical presentation of smallpox differ from chickenpox?

Potential Severity: Biological weapons are intended to kill and terrorize their victims. Treatment must be immediate, and public health measures need to be instituted quickly and efficiently to prevent additional casualties.

What we now call bioterrorism was once called biological warfare; the older term should be avoided because it implies that such biological agents are legitimate weapons for defeating a true or perceived enemy. In 1975 these weapons were rightfully condemned as inhumane and cowardly, and the majority of the civilized world agreed to ban biological weapons. Such agents cause great

pain and suffering and have the potential to kill large numbers of innocent bystanders. They subvert science that was generated to save lives and use it instead to kill and maim.

A biological weapon is defined as the use of "microbial...agents...for hostile purposes or in armed conflict." (USAMRIID's *Medical Management of Biological Casualties Handbook*, February 2001)

"Ideal" biological agents should be:

1. Able to reliably cause permanently debilitating or fatal disease in a high percentage of victims. Although agents that temporarily incapacitate in some circumstances may be use-

430

ful and leave intact the infrastructure to sustain an invading enemy.
2. Capable of being targeted precisely to the enemy and not cause a worldwide epidemic that could harm friendly soldiers or civilians.
3. Capable of being produced in large quantities at reasonable cost.
4. Capable of being stored for prolonged periods without losing potency.
5. Capable of being readily aerosolized to allow rapid delivery over a broad geographic area or rapid dissemination within closed environments such as tunnels or subways.

Only a restricted number of biological pathogens fulfill most of these criteria. Four agents are of particular concern at the present time. However, new "advances" that create superpathogens, genetically designed to fit the needs of the bioterrorist, are likely to add new organisms to the "most wanted" list. At the present time experts usually list anthrax, plague, tularemia, and smallpox as the top four potential biological weapons. Other organisms that could be used as biological weapons include botulinum toxins, brucellosis, Q fever, alpha viruses (Venezuelan equine encephalitis, Eastern and Western encephalitis), and viral hemorrhagic fevers (Ebola virus and Marberg agent).

Medical personnel must be aware of the clinical manifestations, modes of transmission, appropriate diagnostic tests, and available treatment and prophylactic options for managing a biological attack. The U.S. Army Medical Research Institute of Infectious Diseases (USAMRIID) recommends a ten-step approach (adapted from USAMRIID's *Medical Management of Biological Casualties Handbook*, February 2001, *www. usamriid.army.mil/education/bluebook.html*):

1. **Maintain a high index of suspicion**. Whenever possible, these diseases should be treated in the early phase of illness, when symptoms tend to be nonspecific. Without a high index of suspicion treatment may be delayed, and mortality may be greatly increased.

2. **Protect thyself**. Use of HEPA filters or even a surgical mask is warranted when a contagious respiratory illness is suspected or an aerosolized pathogen has been released. Appropriate immunizations should be up to date in all health care workers.

3. **Assess the patient**. History of recent symptoms; epidemiologic clues (see #9 below); vital signs; pulmonary, cardiovascular, and skin exam; and assessment of motor function should be quickly obtained.

4. **Decontaminate when necessary**. Patients usually present several days after exposure to biological agents, making decontamination unnecessary. Decontamination is more commonly required after exposure to chemical agents.

5. **Establish a diagnosis**. The approaches to diagnosis depend on the agent and will be reviewed below. Where appropriate, nasal and throat swabs (rayon rather than cotton swabs should be used) and blood, urine, and sputum cultures should be obtained, and environmental samples should be analyzed. Improved rapid diagnostic tests are currently under development, and samples should be provided to the Centers for Disease Control (CDC) (emergency contact number 1-770-488-7100), USAMRIID (1-888-USARIID), or Emergency Operations Center (EOC) Special Pathogens Branch (1-301-619-4728).

6. **Render prompt treatment**. Therapy is most effective in the prodrome period, at a time when clinical signs might not allow a specific diagnosis. Delay of treatment until the clinical manifestations are more developed often results in serious complications or death. In the proper setting, empiric therapy should be strongly considered in patients with an undifferentiated febrile illness or pneumonia. Doxycycline is particularly useful when a bioterrorist agent is being considered because this antibiotic treats anthrax, plague, tularemia, Q fever, and brucellosis. Fluoroquinolones also may have a potential role in empiric therapy.

7. **Practice good infection control**. For the majority of agents standard precautions provide adequate protection. The three exceptions are smallpox (strict airborne precautions are recommended), pneumonic plague (requires droplet precautions), and viral hemorrhagic fevers (require contact precautions).

8. **Alert the proper authorities**. Public health officials as well as the clinical laboratory should be immediately notified of a potential biological attack. Simultaneous reports of multiple infections in a discrete geographical area will serve to raise the alarm that a possible bioterrorist attack has occurred. Rapid action on the part of public health officials to deliver stockpiles of appropriate medications, establish appropriate triage and management teams, and assess the extent of the attack will reduce casualties and save lives.

9. **Assist in epidemiologic investigation**. It is critical that all health care personnel have a fundamental knowledge of epidemiologic principles. Whenever possible, occupation and travel history, immunizations, exposure to contaminated foods or water, and history of friends or co-workers becoming ill should be obtained, and this data should be provided to public health personnel.

10. **Maintain proficiency**. During the time of increased threat, health care personnel are inundated with facts concerning the various biological agents. However over time knowledge and proficiency can wane. It is critical that each person maintain proficiency in dealing with this low probability, but high consequence, problem.

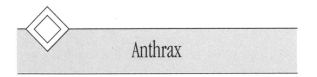

Anthrax

Anthrax is a natural infection of animals, primarily herbivores. Humans can contract the disease from infected animals or animal products. With the advent of domestic animal vaccinations this disease is now rarely encountered in the developed countries. As a consequence most health professionals are unfamiliar with the clinical manifestations of this potentially deadly organism. The United States, the Soviet Union, and Iraq have all manufactured anthrax spores. For the first time in our history anthrax spores were used to kill and injure innocent people in the United States. This attack has underscored the importance of early recognition and treatment of pulmonary and cutaneous anthrax.

Microbiology and Pathogenesis

Bacillus anthracis is a Gram-positive rod that can be easily grown on conventional nutrient media. On blood agar plates, the colonies are gray-white in color with ragged edges and are nonhemolytic. Colonies tightly adhere to the media and cannot be easily displaced by a culture loop. When this bacterium encounters unfavorable environmental conditions, it readily forms endospores. The spores are highly resistant to adverse conditions and are able to survive extreme temperatures, high pH and salinity levels, and disinfectants. In order to cause pulmonary infection, spores must be delivered as single particles, and weapons-grade anthrax spores are treated with an agent or agents that allows them to be disbursed as single particles rather than as clusters.

When individual spores are inhaled, their small size allows them to reach small bronchioles and alveoli. There macrophages phagocytose and carry the spores to the hilar and perihilar lymph nodes. Under the favorable environmental conditions of the host, the spores then germinate, and bacteria begin to quickly multiply and produce three exotoxins: protective antigen, lethal factor, and edema factor. Protective antigen binds to specific receptors on the cell surface and forms a channel that allows the entry of edema and lethal factor. These two agents result in cell swelling and death as well as extensive acute inflammation. Lethal factor has a protease activity that cleaves specific kinases, causing cell lysis. Spores can also be rubbed into the skin, where they germinate beneath the skin surface. In addition to infecting the lung mediastinum and skin, once the bacillus begins actively growing in the lymph nodes, it can then enter the bloodstream, causing septic shock and meningitis.

Epidemiology

In the past most cases of anthrax in the United States occurred as a result of contact with animal products imported from Asia, the Middle East, and Africa. Wool, goat hair, and animal hides are the most common sources of infection. Persons who worked in the early stages of processing these materials were exposed to the highest inoculum of spores and were most likely to contract disease. Processed materials have also caused human disease. Cases have been traced to shaving-brush bristles, wool coats, yarn, goatskin bongo drums, and heroin preparations. The largest recent outbreak of anthrax occurred in Sverdlovsk (now Yekaterinburg), Russia, in 1979, resulting in approximately 96 inhalation cases and 64 deaths. The accidental release of anthrax spores from a germ warfare facility is suspected, and recent polymerase chain reaction (PCR) analysis of tissue samples from 11 victims has confirmed this suspicion.

The introduction of anthrax spores into letters sent through the U.S. Postal Service recently caused multiple cases of inhalation as well as cutaneous anthrax. Postal workers were at particular risk because spores can be released from sealed envelopes during mail processing. Cross-contamination of mail also occurred. As a consequence of these events all mail recipients have been instructed to avoid opening suspicious mail. If powder is found in an envelope, the letter should be gently set down, the room quickly vacated, and appropriate authorities immediately notified. These recent events emphasize the importance of training public health and law enforcement personnel in proper handling of potentially contaminated samples, decontamination, and prophylaxis.

KEY POINTS

Pathogenesis and Modes of Spread of Anthrax

1. *Bacillus anthracis* is an aerobic Gram-positive rod, nonhemolytic on blood-agar plates.
2. Under poor nutrient conditions spores:
   a. Resist heat, high salinity, alkaline pH, and many disinfectants,
   b. When aerosolized, spores enter the lung, are ingested by macrophages, and are transported to the mediastinum.
3. Spores germinate in the mediastinum, and bacteria produce three exotoxins:
   a. Protective antigen, which binds to host cell receptors, allows lethal and edema factor entry,
   b. Lethal factor and edema factor, which cause cell lysis and tissue necrosis.
4. Naturally transmitted by animal products: wool, goat hair, and animal hides.
5. Spores can be purposely aerosolized as a bioterrorist weapon. Transmitted by mail. Postal workers and other mail handlers are at high risk.

Clinical Manifestations

CASE 14.1

A 63-year-old man was taken by his wife to the emergency room with a four-day history of fever, myalgias, and malaise. His wife reported that he had a sore throat, rhinorrhea, or other upper respiratory tract symptoms. He awoke confused and disoriented the morning of admission. Medical history included mild hypertension and placement of a coronary stent for atherosclerotic heart disease.

Epidemiology: Employed as a photo editor for a major tabloid newspaper in Florida, where he spent most of the day reviewing photographs submitted by mail or over the Internet. Physical examination showed him to be lethargic and disoriented. Temperature 39°C (102.5°F), blood pressure 150/80 mm Hg, pulse 110, respiratory rate 18/min. ENT: no pharyngeal erythema or exudate. No nuchal rigidity. Lungs: bibasilar rhonchi without rales. Heart: no murmurs, rubs, or gallops. Abdomen: soft, nontender, no organomegaly. Skin: clear. Neurologic exam: no focal deficits.

Laboratory findings: Hct: 46, peripheral WBC 9,400/mm³ (77% PMNs, 15% lymphocytes, 8% monocytes); chest X-ray: basilar infiltrates and a widened mediastinum. Lumbar puncture: cloudy, RBC 1375/mm³, WBC 4,750/mm³ (81% PMNs, 19% monocytes), protein 666 mg/dl, glucose 57 mg/dl CSF Gram stain: many PMN and many large Gram-positive bacilli, both singly and in chains). Blood and CSF cultures grew *Bacillus anthracis*. (See Figure 14.2.)

Outcome: Despite high-dose penicillin he suffered grand mal seizures, hypotension, acidosis, and renal failure and had an asystolic arrest on the third hospital day. Autopsy revealed no pulmonary parenchymal consolidation. 50 ml of gross blood was found in the mediastinum and several enlarged lymph nodes (1–2 cm in diameter) were also noted; on cross-sectional examination, the lymph nodes were hemorrhagic. (Adapted from Bush, L.M., Abrams, B.H., Beall, A., and Johnson, C.C. Index case of fatal inhalational anthrax due to bioterrorism in the United States. *N Engl J Med* 345:1607–1610, 2001.)

It is critical that health care personnel be familiar with the clinical manifestations of anthrax. An exposure and occupational history may be particularly helpful in focusing on the possibility of anthrax in patients with a febrile illness or cutaneous lesions of unclear etiology. During the recent bioterrorist attack in the United States the early recognition of the index case (Case 14.1) in South Florida by an infectious disease specialist led to the rapid institution of antibiotic prophylaxis and saved many lives. Unfortunately, several other physicians failed to recognize the early manifestations of inhalation anthrax in postal workers, and these patients later returned with full-blown fatal disease. Finally, the earlier recognition of several cutaneous anthrax cases could have alerted the authorities in New York in a more timely manner that a bioterrorist attack had also been launched in that state.

CUTANEOUS ANTHRAX

Skin disease is the most common manifestation of anthrax. One to seven days after spores are inoculated into the skin, a small papule develops. Over the next 3–4 days the lesion progresses to a vesicle, 1–3 cm in diameter. Erythema and nonpitting edema often surround the vesicle. Initially, the vesicular fluid is serous and contains large numbers of organisms. The vesicle subsequently ruptures, and a black eschar becomes evident at the base of the ulcer (see Figure 14.1). The name anthrax (Greek for "coal") refers to this characteristic black eschar. Despite the erythema and swelling, lesions are not painful but may be mildly pruritic. Lymphangitis, lymphadenopathy, fever, and malaise may accompany infection of the skin. After several weeks the skin lesion dries, and a permanent scar is formed. Lesions occur primarily on exposed regions of the body. The arms are the most frequent site of infection; the face and neck are also commonly involved. A single lesion is usually found, although multiple sites may become infected as a result of simultaneous inoculations.

KEY POINTS
Cutaneous Anthrax

1. Usually a single lesion develops on an exposed area of the body, arm most common.
2. Develops 1–7 days after inoculation; begins as a papule.
3. Progresses over 3–4 days to a vesicle filled with organisms, margin edematous.

Figure 14.1

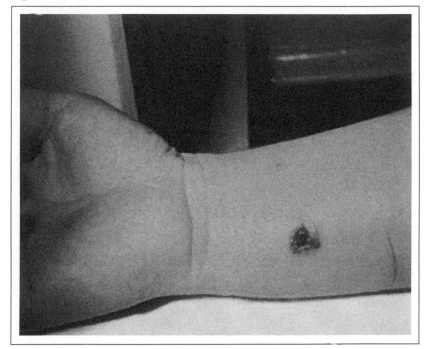

Typical cutaneous anthrax lesion. Note the black eschar and the edematous margins. See also Color Plate 3.

4. Lesion then ruptures and forms a black eschar.
5. Not painful, often itches.
6. Spontaneously heals over several weeks, leaving a scar.

INHALATION ANTHRAX (WOOLSORTERS' DISEASE)

It is important that the clinician be aware of the biphasic presentation of inhalation anthrax. It is likely that the patient in Case 14.1 had inhaled spores from a contaminated letter sent to his newspaper. Recognition and treatment during the first phase can be life saving. In Case 14.1 a flu-like illness was present for 4 days prior to the onset of fulminant mediastinal involvement, bacteremia, and meningitis. Because the patient failed to seek medical attention during the early phase of his illness, his fatal outcome could not have been prevented.

FIRST PHASE   From 1 to 5 days after inhalation of spores, the patient has symptoms suggestive of a viral syndrome: nonproductive cough, malaise, fatigue, myalgia, and mild fever. Occasionally, the sensation of chest heaviness is reported. Rhonchi may be heard on examination, but aside from fever no other abnormal physical findings are observed. As is observed in Case 14.1, pharyngitis and rhinitis do not usually accompany inhalation anthrax. Unless a careful exposure and occupational history is obtained and inhalation anthrax is included in the differential diagnosis, patients are often sent home with antipyretics for a presumed viral syndrome. It is during this period that spores are being transported by pulmonary macrophages from the lung parenchyma to the mediastinal lymph nodes. At this stage antibiotic treatment should prevent progression to the second phase.

SECOND PHASE Within 2–4 days symptoms temporarily resolve but are rapidly followed by the second, more severe stage of the disease. At this time spores have germinated in the mediastinal lymph nodes, and protective antigen, lethal factor, and edema factor are being produced by rapidly multiplying anthrax bacilli. Necrosis and hemorrhagic inflammation quickly develop, causing the sudden onset of severe respiratory distress with dyspnea, cyanosis, and diffuse diaphoresis, accompanied by fever, tachycardia, and tachypnea. On pulmonary auscultation, moist, crepitant rales are evident, and findings may be consistent with pleural effusions. Chest X-ray demonstrates a widened mediastinum without a definite parenchymal infiltrate and often also reveals pleural effusions. (Figure 14.2A). Thoracentesis reveals hemorrhagic fluid, and Gram stain as well as culture are usually positive. As described in Case 14.1, in about half of cases confusion followed by lethargy and coma may develop as a consequence of meningitis. On lumbar puncture, the CSF contains polymorphonuclear lymphocytes (PMNs), and large box-car-like Gram-positive rods are usually seen on Gram stain (Figure 14.2B). Death usually occurs within 24 hours and may be accompanied by septic shock. In the terminal stages of the illness blood cultures are usually positive. Death can be very sudden, and patients have been reported to die "in midsentence."

KEY POINTS
Inhalation Anthrax

> 1. First phase: Flu-like syndrome. No pharyngitis or rhinitis, chest heaviness may be described. Treatment can abort the second, lethal phase.

> 2. Second phase: Follows first phase after a brief asymptomatic period:
>   a. Sudden onset of severe respiratory distress, fever, tachycardia, and tachypnea,
>   b. Rales on chest exam and chest X-ray: widened mediastinum +/- pleural effusions,
>   c. Thoracentesis: hemorrhagic fluid (+) Gram stain and culture,
>   d. Confusion in half of cases and CSF: PMNs and (+) Gram stain and culture,
>   e. Death within 24 hours, blood culture (+), death can occur "in midsentence."

GASTROINTESTINAL ANTHRAX

Gastrointestinal infection has not been reported in the United States and is not an expected clinical consequence of a bioterrorist attack. This disease occurs primarily in developing countries, usually after ingestion of contaminated meat. The incubation period is usually 3–5 days. Patients initially have nausea, vomiting, anorexia, and fever. These symptoms are rapidly followed by acute abdominal pain, hematemesis, and bloody diarrhea. Findings on examination suggest an acute surgical abdomen, and there is moderate leukocytosis with immature band forms. Rapid progression to toxemia and shock leads to death within 2–5 days after the initial onset of symptoms. An oropharyngeal form of anthrax has also been described. Inflammatory lesions that resemble the cutaneous lesions develop on the posterior pharynx, hard palate, or tonsils. Tissue necrosis and edema are accompanied by sore throat, dysphagia, fever, regional lymphadenopathy, and toxemia.

Diagnosis

A careful epidemiologic history is the single most important means of suggesting the diagnosis of anthrax. In natural cases a history of contact with herbivores or products from these animals,

Figure 14.2

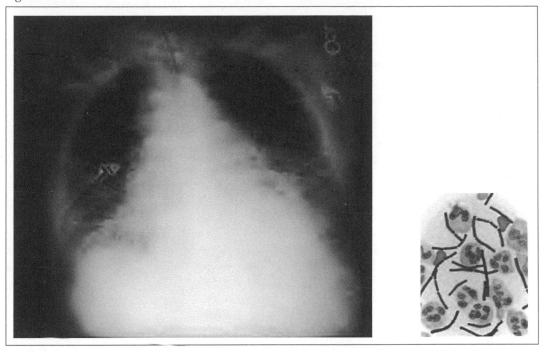

A   B

Pulmonary anthrax. (A) Chest X-ray showing a widened mediastinum. (B) CSF Gram stain demonstrating boxcar-like Gram-positive rods. (from N Engl J Med 345: 1607–1610, 2001).

particularly if the products come from outside the United States, should raise the possibility of anthrax. In the setting of a possible bioterrorist attack an employment history and history of being present in a contaminated area are important clues. By the time Gram stains and cultures of the blood and CSF are positive, the illness has progressed to the second, fatal phase. Diagnosis therefore must be presumptive, and the threshold for treatment must be low to prevent progression from mildly symptomatic to life-threatening disease. For epidemiologic purposes samples from the nose and face can be obtained by using rayon-tipped swabs. Cultures from these sites are specific but insensitive and in an individual patient cannot be used to decide whether or not to begin treatment. Nasal samples can be used to determine the physical

perimeters of exposure, and this data can be used to determine who should receive prophylactic antibiotics. The physical appearance of the skin lesions is characteristic, and Gram stains and cultures of the ulcer base are frequently positive. Enzyme-linked immunosorbent assays are available that measure antibody titers against lethal and edema toxin. A fourfold rise in titers over four weeks or a single titer of 1:32 is considered positive.

KEY POINTS

Diagnosis of Anthrax

1. Epidemiologic history is important, and diagnosis is often presumptive.

2. Nasal swabs are helpful for determining the physical parameters of exposure but not for deciding individual prophylaxis.
3. Gram stain and cultures of skin lesions are often positive.
4. Positive blood and CSF cultures usually accompany a fatal outcome.
5. ELISA assays for antibodies against lethal and edema toxin are available.

Treatment

Although penicillin has been recommended as the treatment of choice for naturally occurring anthrax, penicillin-resistant natural strains have been reported. Penicillin-resistant strains of anthrax have also been genetically engineered as bioterrorist weapons, and the military protocol recommends ciprofloxacin (400 mg iv Q12H) or doxycycline (200-mg loading dose, followed by 100 mg iv Q12H) as first-line therapy (see Table 14.1). Penicillin (4 million units iv Q4H) is recommended as an alternative once sensitivities have been obtained. Because penicillin treatment induces β-lactamase activity, penicillin should be combined with an additional antibiotic. Other antibiotics that demonstrate activity against anthrax and in the seriously ill patient may be combined with any of the above agents, including rifampin, vancomycin, imipenem, clindamycin, and clarithromycin. Treatment should be continued for 60 days, and the patient should be switched to oral antibiotics as the clinical condition improves. Excision of skin lesions is contraindicated because of the increased risk of precipitating bacteremia. However, after appropriate antibiotic therapy, excision and skin grafting may be necessary.

Before antibiotics became available, cutaneous disease resulted in a mortality rate of 10–20%. With appropriate antibiotic treatment, fewer than 1% of patients die. Despite appropri-

ate antibiotics and respiratory support, inhalation anthrax is frequently fatal. In the recent U.S. bioterrorist attack, half of the patients with inhalation anthrax survived, proving that the rapid institution of antibiotic can be life saving in early second-phase pulmonary anthrax. Gastrointestinal anthrax is also associated with high mortality (25–100%).

Prophylaxis

A vaccine derived from a component of the exotoxin is available and is recommended for all industrial workers who are at risk for exposure to contaminated animal products. As a result of increased concerns about biological warfare and bioterrorism, military personnel are now vaccinated. To date, surveillance studies have not detected any serious or unexpected adverse reactions. The vaccination series consists of six 0.5-ml subcutaneous injections given at 0, 2, and 4 weeks followed by doses at 6, 12, and 18 months. A yearly booster is also recommended. In cases of suspected exposure to *Bacillus anthracis*, antibiotic prophylaxis and vaccination are recommended. The regimens of choice are oral fluoroquinolones (ciprofloxacin, 500 mg BID; levofloxacin, 500 mg QD; or ofloxacin, 400 mg BID) or, if fluoroquinolones are contraindicated, doxycycline (100 mg BID). Prophylaxis should be continued until exposure is excluded. If exposure is confirmed, prophylaxis should be continued for four weeks in individuals who have received three or more doses of the vaccine and for 60 days in the unvaccinated patient. Because spores may remain in the body for prolonged periods before germinating, prophylaxis needs to be prolonged, and patients should be closely observed after completion of antibiotics. Within the first several days, exposed skin should be washed extensively with soap and water, and personal items should be decontaminated with 0.5% hypochlorite (one part household bleach to 10 parts water).

Table 14.1

Antibiotic Treatment of Bioterrorist Bacterial Agents

DRUG	DOSE	RELATIVE EFFICACY	COMMENTS
Anthrax	Duration 60 days		
Prophylaxis			
Ciprofloxacin	500 mg po BID	First-line	
Doxycycline	100 mg po BID	Alternative	
Treatment	Duration 60 days		
Ciprofloxacin (or)	400 mg iv Q12H	First-line	
Doxycycline	200 mg, followed by 100 mg iv Q12H		
In serious disease can be combined with:		Alternatives (see text)	
Penicillin G (or)	4 million units iv Q4H		
Rifampin (or)	600 mg po or iv QD		
Vancomycin (or)	1 gm iv Q12H		
Imipenem (or)	500 mg iv Q6H		
Clindamycin (or)	600–900 mg iv Q8H		
Clarithromycin	500 mg po BID		
Plague			
Prophylaxis			
Doxycycline	100 mg BID × 7 days		
Treatment	Treat 10-14 days		
Streptomycin (or)	15 mg/kg im Q12H	First-line	Equally effective
Gentamicin (or)	5 mg/kg iv QD		
Doxycycline	200 mg, then 100 mg iv Q12H		
Ciprofloxacin	400 mg iv BID	Alternatives	Likely to be effective, but little clinical experience
Chloramphenicol	500 mg iv Q6H		Treatment for meningitis
Tularemia			
Prophylaxis	Take for 2 weeks		
Ciprofloxacin	500 mg po BID		
Doxycycline	100 mg po BID		
Treatment	Treat 10–14 days		
Gentamicin	5 mg/kg iv QD	First-line	
Streptomycin	10-15 mg/kg im Q12H	Alternatives	
Doxycycline	200 mg, followed by 100 mg iv Q12H		

Treatment and Prevention of Anthrax

1. Treatment: Threshold must be very low in the setting of a bioterrorist attack:
   a. Intravenous ciprofloxacin or doxycycline, alternative: penicillin + second antibiotic,
   b. Combination therapy recommended for the seriously ill patient: Rifampin, vancomycin, imipenem, clindamycin, or clarithromycin can be added to the above regimens,
   c. Avoid excision of skin lesions, danger of precipitating bacteremia,
   d. Continue therapy × 60 days, danger of newly germinating spores and relapse
2. Prophylaxis for all individuals suspected of exposure:
   a. Fluoroquinolone (ciprofloxacin, levofloxacin, or ofloxacin), alternative doxycycline × 60 days,
   b. Vaccine, inactivated exotoxin: Military personnel and workers at risk of exposure, 6 doses for immunity followed by annual booster,
   c. Decontaminate exposed areas and personal items with 0.5% hypochlorite.

Plague (*Yersinia pestis*)

Like anthrax, plague is primarily a disease of animals. *Yersinia pestis* primarily infects rodents. In the United States the most common reservoirs are squirrels and prairie dogs. The disease is transmitted to humans by infected rodent fleas. Approximately 10 human cases are reported annually in the southwestern United States during the late spring, summer, and early fall. Disease outbreaks frequently occur in developing countries throughout the world. This agent was used as a biological weapon during World War II when the Japanese released plague-infected fleas in China. However, the spread of disease proved to be unpredictable and ineffective. Subsequently, both the United States and the Soviet Union developed reliable and effective methods of aerosolizing this agent.

Microbiology and Pathogenesis

Yersinia pestis is a Gram-negative bacillus that grows aerobically on standard nutrient plates, including blood and MacConkey agar. The organism grows slowly, often requiring 48 hours to become apparent, and colonies are small and grayish. When an infected flea bites a human, it regurgitates thousands of organisms into the skin, where they are phagocytosed by PMNs and monocytes. *Y. pestis* is usually killed by PMNs but is able to survive and replicate within monocytes, evading the host's immune system. Infected monocytes carry the organism to lymph nodes, where the pathogen actively replicates, causing marked acute inflammation and tissue necrosis. Regional lymph nodes become enlarged, forming buboes. *Y. pestis* can also quickly enter the bloodstream. Like other Gram-negative bacteria, it produces endotoxin and also possesses other virulence factors, including a coagulase and a fibrinolysin.

Epidemiology and Pathogenesis of *Yersinia pestis*

1. Usually spread by rodent fleas, rare cases in the Southwestern U.S.
2. Soviet Union and the U.S. developed methods to aerosolize.
3. Ingested by PMNs and monocytes, able to replicate in monocytes:

> a. Results in acute inflammation and tissue necrosis,
> b. Spreads to regional lymph nodes to form fluctuant buboes,
> c. Readily enters the bloodstream.

Clinical Manifestations

When infection is spread by fleas *Yersinia pestis* causes bubonic plague. The incubation period is usually 2–8 days, followed by the abrupt onset of fever, chills, weakness, and headache. Within hours the patient notes an enlarged, extremely painful cluster of regional lymph nodes termed a bubo. Marked swelling is noted, and pain is so severe that the patient avoids moving the infected area. Buboes are usually egg shaped and 1–10 cm in length. Within 2–4 days the patient dies of septic shock. Thrombosis of small vessels can develop, causing peripheral tissue necrosis and gangrene that may require amputation. In some patients a bubo is not present, and the patient presents in a moribund state caused by high-grade bacteremia. Meningitis may develop in a small percentage of patients.

If bioterrorists were to introduce *Yersinia pestis* as microdroplets into the air, the primary clinical presentation would be pneumonic plague. After an incubation period of 2–4 days there is a sudden onset of fever, chills, and myalgias. Within 24 hours patients begin coughing up blood as a result of bacterial production of coagulase, fibrinolysin, and tissue necrosis. Sputum can also be mucopurulent or watery. Chest pain, abdominal pain, nausea, vomiting, and diarrhea are other common symptoms. If antibiotics are not begun within 18 hours, the outcome is fatal. Patients experience increasing dyspnea, stridor, and cyanosis followed by respiratory arrest and circulatory collapse.

KEY POINTS

Clinical Manifestations of *Y. pestis* Infection

> 1. Flea-transmitted form, incubation of 2–8 days associated with:
>   a. Fever, chills, weakness, and headache,
>   b. Followed by bubo formation, nodes very painful,
>   c. Within 2–4 days septic shock leads to peripheral gangrene and death.
> 2. Pulmonic form expected in a bioterrorist attack:
>   a. Incubation period 2–4 days, chills, fever, myalgias,
>   b. Within 24 hours bloody sputum production, chest pain, followed by dyspnea and cyanosis,
>   c. Death within 18 hours without antibiotic treatment.

Diagnosis

The possibility of a biological attack with *Yersinia pestis* should be considered if multiple patients begin presenting to the emergency room with hemoptysis and severe rapidly progressive pneumonia. Sputum Gram stain frequently reveals Gram-negative rods. A presumptive diagnosis can also be made by finding bacilli on peripheral blood smear. Chest X-ray demonstrates bilateral bronchopneumonia. Definitive diagnosis is made by sputum and blood cultures, which often take over 48 hours because of the organism's slow growth rate. PCR detection is under development and promises to be rapid, specific, and highly sensitive (can detect ≥10 organisms).

Treatment

If pneumonic plague is not considered and conventional antibiotic treatment for community-acquired pneumonia is mistakenly begun, the infection will quickly progress, resulting in death. Streptomycin (15 mg/kg im Q12H), gentamicin (5 mg/kg/day iv), and doxycycline (200-mg loading dose followed by 100 mg iv Q12H) are the treatments of choice and should be continued for 10–14 days (see Table 14.1). Ciprofloxacin (400 mg iv Q12H) is another potentially effective regimen; however, clinical experience with this agent is limited. Chloramphenicol (25-mg/kg loading dose followed by 15 mg/kg Q6H) is recommended for the treatment of meningitis. Surgical debridement of buboes should not be performed because of the risk of spreading the infection to others. Lymph node needle aspiration may provide some relief and provides material for culture and Gram stain. The lymph nodes usually slowly shrink on antibiotic therapy. The overall mortality for pneumonic plague is 60%; however, if appropriate therapy is delayed for ≥24 hours, mortality is nearly 100%. The fatality rate for bubonic plague is 14%; however, with early therapy all patients should survive.

Prophylaxis

Person-to-person spread of *Yersinia pestis* does occur. Patients with pneumonic plague cough and aerosolize the organism, leading to secondary cases of pneumonia. Therefore patients with pulmonary disease require strict isolation with droplet precautions for at least 48 hours after the start of antibiotic therapy. Individuals who have had face-to-face contact with patients with plague pneumonia should receive doxycycline prophylaxis (100 mg po BID) for 7 days or for the duration of potential exposure plus 7 days. In patients with bubonic plague only standard precautions are required, and prophylaxis is unnecessary. Contacts should be observed for 7 days. A vaccine is not currently available. Production of a licensed killed vaccine was discontinued in 1998. This vaccine was effective for the prevention of the bubonic form but not

inhalation disease. However, a new vaccine, shown to be effective for inhalation disease in mice, has been developed and is currently being tested in primates.

KEY POINTS

Diagnosis, Treatment, and Prevention of Plague

1. Readily diagnosed by sputum or lymph node aspirate. Gram stain, cultures usually require 48 hours. A sensitive PCR method is under development.
2. Treatment with streptomycin, gentamicin, or doxycycline × 14 days, delay > 24 hours = death:
   a. Ciprofloxacin may be effective,
   b. Chloramphenicol for meningitis.
3. Prevention:
   a. Respiratory precautions for pneumonic plague × 48 hours of antibiotic treatment,
   b. Doxycycline × 7 days for respiratory exposure,
   c. Vaccine under development.

Tularemia
(*Francisella tularensis*)

Francisella tularensis is another zoonotic pathogen that under natural conditions incidentally infects humans. Infection is usually contracted following contact with rabbits, muskrats, beavers, squirrels, and birds. Hunters develop disease following skinning, dressing, and eating infected animals. Less commonly, the infection can be spread to humans by ticks, biting flies, and mosquitoes. Aerosol droplets of contaminated water or mud and animal bites can also transmit the disease. Tularemia is most commonly encountered in temperate climates during the summer months due to insect transmission and in December during hunting season. The United States and possibly other countries have weaponized this agent. Both dry and wet forms have been created. As with anthrax and plague, the most efficient way to deliver lethal doses of *F. tularensis* is by aerosol.

Microbiology and Pathogenesis

Francisella is a small, aerobic, Gram-negative coccobacillus. This bacterium does not routinely grow on standard media, requiring cysteine or cystine for growth. Glucose-cystine blood agar supports growth; however, selective media are often required to isolate this pathogen from normal skin and mouth flora. Its cell wall has a high fatty acid content capsule that resists serum bactericidal activity. The organism produces no known exotoxins but expresses a lipopolysaccharide (LPS) endotoxin that is 1000 times less potent than *Escherichia coli* LPS.

Most natural infections result from bacteria gaining entry through a small break in the skin. The organism is phagocytosed by monocytes and is able to survive intracellularly. *Francisella tularensis* can also grow in hepatocytes and endothelial cells. As the organisms grow and lyse cells, they induce an acute inflammatory reaction, and tissue necrosis is followed by granuloma formation. Cell-mediated immunity plays a critical role in controlling this intracellular pathogen. Only 10–50 bacteria are required to cause skin and pulmonary infection, making this organism extremely dangerous to laboratory workers.

KEY POINTS

Mode of Spread and Pathogenesis of Tularemia

1. Usually cutaneously spread from infected rabbits, muskrats, beavers, squirrels, and birds.

2. An aerosolized form can be manufactured for bioterrorism.
3. Gram-negative coccobacillus, requires cysteine-supplemented media:
   a. High fatty-acid content cell wall, LPS endotoxin, less potent than *E. coli*,
   b. Intracellular pathogen induces acute inflammation and granuloma formation,
   c. Low inoculum causes disease (10–50 organisms), very dangerous.

Clinical Manifestations

The clinical picture of tularemia is very similar to that of plague. The incubation period is usually 3–5 days and is followed by the abrupt onset of high fever, chills, malaise, myalgias, chest discomfort, vomiting, abdominal pain, and diarrhea. A severe generalized headache is often a prominent complaint. Natural disease is most commonly the ulceroglandular form. At the site of bacterial entry a painful ulcer with raised borders develops that is associated with painful regional adenopathy. Approximately 20% of patients may develop a febrile illness without lymphadenopathy and may become hypotensive. Watery diarrhea may be a prominent complaint, and the disease may be mistaken for salmonella typhoid fever.

The pneumonic form is rare under natural circumstances but can occur in sheep shearers, farmers, and laboratory workers. The pneumonic form would be the expected presentation after an aerosol bioterrorist attack. The clinical presentation is identical to that of pneumonic plague with the exception that cough is usually dry and hacking rather than productive. Hemoptysis can occur but is rare. In some patients respiratory complaints may not be prominent, and primary complaints may mimic typhoid fever.

KEY POINTS

Clinical Manifestations of Tularemia

> 1. Similar clinically to plague, incubation period 3–5 days:
>   a. Abrupt onset of fever, headache, malaise, myalgias, abdominal pain, and diarrhea,
>   b. Ulceroglandular form: Painful ulcer with raised borders, regional lymphadenopathy,
>   c. 20% present with typhoid fever–like illness without lymphadenopathy.
> 2. Bronchopneumonia expected with a bioterrorist attack, similar to plague except dry, hacking cough, hemoptysis rare. May present with typhoid fever–like symptoms.

Diagnosis

The presentation of multiple patients with severe bronchopneumonia associated with a nonproductive cough should raise the possibility of a bioterrorist attack with *Francisella tularensis*. Chest X-ray demonstrates changes consistent with a bronchopneumonia in 50% of cases after inhalation. Pleural effusions may be noted in 15% of those with pneumonia. Aspiration of the pleural fluid usually reveals lymphocytes, suggesting tuberculosis. Sputum and wound Gram stains are usually negative. The organism can be identified in lymph nodes by silver stain. Blood cultures and tissue sample cultures may be positive, but the organism must be grown by using media containing a sulfhydryl compound. The organism should be handled in a BSL-3 containment facility because of the risk to laboratory personnel. Diagnosis is usually made by testing for antibodies to the organism. Two weeks are required before significant antibody titers of >1:160 develop.

Treatment

Effective treatment regimens include streptomycin (10-15 mg/kg im Q12H) and gentamicin (5 mg/kg iv or im QD) (see Table 14.1). Gen-

tamicin is preferred over streptomycin for a presumed bioterrorist attack because a streptomycin-resistant strain was developed in the 1950s and may have been obtained by other countries. This strain was sensitive to gentamicin. The mortality from tularemia pneumonia is 30%, making this a less deadly bioterrorist weapon than anthrax or plague.

Prevention

Person-to-person transmission is not reported with tularemia. Therefore standard contact precautions are sufficient. Prophylaxis should be administered within 24 hours of exposure. Ciprofloxacin (500 mg po BID) or doxycycline (100 mg po BID) for two weeks are recommended. There is an investigational live-attenuated vaccine given by scarification. This vaccine provides significant protection against the inhalation and typhoidal forms of disease.

KEY POINTS

Diagnosis, Treatment, and Prevention of Tularemia

> 1. Gram stain of sputum and skin ulcers usually negative and culture requires special media.
> 2. May be identified in lymph nodes by silver stain.
> 3. Diagnosis is usually presumptive, antibody titers rise after two weeks.
> 4. Treatment and prevention:
>   a. Gentamicin the drug of choice, ciprofloxacin and streptomycin are alternatives,
>   b. Respiratory precautions are not required,
>   c. Prophylaxis within 24 hours of exposure with ciprofloxacin or doxycycline × 14 days,
>   d. Vaccine is under development.
> 5. Mortality rate is 30%; lower than those for pulmonary anthrax or plague.

Smallpox

Smallpox was eradicated worldwide in 1977. As a result smallpox vaccinations were discontinued for civilians in 1980 and for military recruits in 1989, leaving a high percentage of the world's population without immunity to this deadly virus. Although there are only two known repositories of the variola virus, the CDC in Atlanta and the Institute of Viral Preparations in Moscow, stockpiles of the virus may be in the hands of others.

Epidemiology

Smallpox is spread from person to person and has no other animal reservoirs. The incubation period before symptomatic illness is 7–17 days (average: 12 days). The period of communicability begins with the onset of rash and continues until all scabs separate from the skin, three to four weeks after the onset of illness. The virus is shed from lesions in the oropharynx and on the skin, producing airborne droplets and skin fragments that can be inhaled. Patients are most infectious if they are coughing or have the hemorrhagic form of disease. The communicability of smallpox is low in comparison to that of chickenpox and measles, secondary cases occurring most commonly in household contacts and hospital personnel. The virions are relatively resistant to drying and to many disinfectants and can remain infectious for months at room temperature. Autoclaving, chlorine preparations, iodophores, and ammonia inactivate them.

A number of factors make variola a potentially dangerous biological weapon:

1. Infection can be spread via aerosol, and the virions survive in the environment.
2. Person-to-person transmission allows continued spread after the attack.

3. Routine vaccination was discontinued, creating large susceptible civilian and military populations.
4. The potency of stored vaccine may be declining.
5. The disease causes severe morbidity and mortality.
6. Health care personnel have no clinical experience with this disease; therefore delays in diagnosis, treatment, and prevention would be expected.

KEY POINTS
Epidemiology of Smallpox

1. Humans are the only reservoir for disease.
2. Incubation period 7–17 days.
3. Infectious with the onset of the rash until scabs separate from the skin:
   a. Transmitted from person to person by coughing or skin particles,
   b. Spread within households and to hospital personnel,
   c. Virions can survive in the environment, inactivated by chlorine, ammonia, iodine, and heat.

Virology and Pathogenesis

Variola is a large, double-stranded DNA virus. The virus replicates in the cytoplasm of cells, and new viral particles are released by bud formation on the cell surface. Virus-containing airborne droplets and dust particles are inhaled. The virus then spreads from the upper respiratory tract to the regional lymph nodes, enters the bloodstream, causing transient viremia, and then invades virtually all body tissues. Epithelial cells are particularly susceptible, accounting for the prominent skin lesions. Initially, edema develops at infected sites in the skin, accompanied by perivascular infiltration with mononuclear and plasma cells, causing the formation of macular skin lesions. Subsequently, the epithelial cells undergo ballooning degeneration, and spherical inclusion bodies containing clusters of virions (Guarnieri's bodies) form in the cell cytoplasm. These changes are accompanied by the formation of papular skin lesions. Cell necrosis follows, accompanied by the formation of skin vesicles. Viral replication then ceases, and the skin lesions become crusted and dry, eventually healing and forming prominent scars.

KEY POINTS
Pathogenesis of Smallpox

1. Variola is a double-stranded DNA virus.
2. Replicates in the cytoplasm of host cells, infectious particles bud from the cell surface.
3. Enters the lung via airborne droplets, spreads to regional nodes then to the bloodstream:
   a. Disseminates to all tissues,
   b. Epithelial cells very susceptible, skin develops perivascular infiltration,
   c. Ballooning degeneration and inclusion body formation, followed by cell necrosis.

Clinical Manifestations

The first clinical manifestations of the disease are nonspecific and consist of the acute onset of fever, rigors, malaise, headache, backache, and vomiting. Delirium develops in approximately 15% of cases, and a transient erythematous rash may appear. This clinical prodrome lasts 2–4 days and is caused by high-level viremia. During this period virus can be readily cultured from the blood. Next the exanthem becomes apparent. Lesions begin on the face, hands, and forearms, subsequently spreading to the lower extremities and over the next week spreading to the trunk (see Figure 14.3). The distribution of skin lesions is centrifugal (i.e., peripheral greater than central). Initially, macules are seen that subsequently form papules and then progress to pustular vesicles. Finally, after about two weeks the lesions form dry scabs that fall off, leaving

Figure 14.3

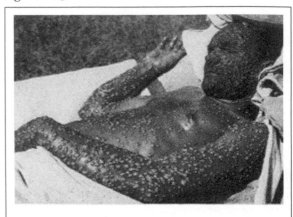

A

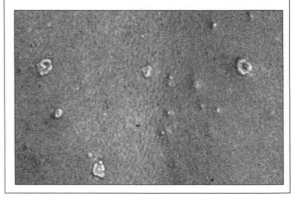

B

A. Adult with severe smallpox skin lesions (from www. coldcure.com). B. Close up of individual raised skin lesions all at a similar stage of progression. (From Henderson, D.A. Smallpox: Clinical and epidemiologic features. *Emerg Infect Dis* 5:537-539, 1999.) See also Color Plate 3.

scars. The skin lesions progress in a synchronous fashion; that is, at any one time, all skin lesions are at a similar stage.

The clinician must be able to differentiate smallpox from chickenpox (varicella-zoster virus), a common naturally occurring infection. Three clinical characteristics are most helpful in differentiating the two diseases. First, chickenpox is usually not associated with a significant prodrome. Patients often feel well prior to the onset of skin lesions. Second, the lesions of chickenpox begin in different locations than those of small-pox. In chickenpox lesions are first seen on the trunk and often spare the face. Subsequently, lesions spread to the arms and legs. Chickenpox lesions have a centripetal distribution (i.e., central greater than peripheral) rather than the centrifugal distribution of smallpox. Third, the morphology of the skin lesions differs. Skin lesion development is asynchronous in chickenpox. Macules, papules, vesicles, and scabs can all be seen at the same time on an individual patient. Chickenpox lesions are irregular in shape and size and are usually superficial, while smallpox lesions have smooth borders, are of similar size, and are deep, often extending to the dermis. The vesicles of smallpox feel shotty, while chickenpox vesicles are soft and collapse easily.

KEY POINTS
Clinical Manifestations of Smallpox

1. The clinician must be able to differentiate from chickenpox.
2. Febrile prodrome for 2–4 days associated with high-level viremia (no prodrome with chickenpox).
3. Skin lesions are centrifugal (extremities to trunk) versus centripetal in chickenpox.
4. Synchronous development versus asynchronous in chickenpox.
5. Progress from macular to papular to vesicular to crusting, leaves scars, lesions feel shotty; chickenpox lesions are softer and usually do not scar.

Diagnosis

Full-blown disease can be readily diagnosed clinically. The diagnosis can be confirmed by viral culture on chorioallantoic membrane. PCR diagnostic techniques are under development and will allow more rapid diagnosis. A particular problem from an epidemiologic standpoint is the potential failure to recognize relatively mild cases of smallpox in persons with partial immunity. These patients may shed virus from the oropharynx in the absence of skin lesions.

Treatment and Prognosis

At the present time no treatment other than supportive care is available. Cidofovir is active against poxviruses and may be considered for treatment. The overall mortality for smallpox is 30% in unvaccinated patients and 3% in vaccinated patients. Mortality rates are highest in the very young and very old.

Prevention

The identification of a smallpox victim represents a public health emergency, and public health officials should be immediately notified. Vaccination of all exposed persons is recommended as quickly as possible, and vaccination within 7 days is protective. The vaccine contains vaccinia virus (cowpox virus) and is administered by intradermal inoculation using a bifurcated needle. Successful vaccination should result in a vesicle formation at the site of inoculation followed by scar formation (scarification). Side effects include low-grade fever and axillary adenopathy. Disseminated vaccinia occurs in approximately 3 per 10,000 vaccinations. The vaccine is contraindicated in persons with HIV infection, immunosuppression, or history or presence of eczema or in persons who have close contact with individuals having one of these conditions. Vaccinia immune globulin (VIG) may be protective, but the large volume required for intramuscular administration (0.6 mlc/kg im or 42 ml in a 70-kg person) makes this an impractical tool for mass prophylaxis.

Infected patients must be strictly isolated. Placement in a negative air pressure room with the door closed is recommended. Masks, gowns, and gloves must be worn by persons entering the room. Transport of the patient should be limited. All surfaces and supplies must be treated as contaminated. Large numbers of patients would quickly overwhelm isolation facilities and would necessitate separate temporary isolation facilities.

KEY POINTS

Diagnosis, Treatment, and Prevention of Smallpox

1. Readily diagnosed clinically, can be confirmed by viral culture.
2. Minimally symptomatic patients may spread disease and need to recognized and isolated.
3. Infected patients should be strictly isolated: Negative pressure rooms, masks, gloves, gowns.
4. Cidofovir may prove helpful, but there is no clinical experience with this agent.
5. Vaccine protective if given within 7 days of exposure:
   a. Live vaccinia virus given by intradermal inoculation,
   b. Contraindicated in HIV infection, immunosuppression, history or presence of eczema,
   c. Vaccinia immune globulin protective but impractical for large numbers of patients.

Additional Reading

General
USAMRIID Medical Management of Biological Casualties Handbook. U.S. Army Medical Research Institute of Infectious Diseases, Fort Detrick, Maryland, February 2001.

Anthrax
Borio, L., Frank, D., Mani, V., et al. Death due to bioterrorism-related inhalational anthrax: Report of 2 patients. *JAMA* 286:2554–2559, 2001.

Bush, L.M., Abrams, B.H., Beall, A., and Johnson, C.C. Index case of fatal inhalational anthrax due to bioterrorism in the United States. *N Engl J Med* 345:1607–1610, 2001.

Centers for Disease Control and Prevention. Investigation of bioterrorism-related anthrax and interim guidelines for clinical evaluation of persons with possible anthrax. *JAMA* 286:2392–2396, 2001.

Inglesby, T.V., O'Toole, T., Henderson, D.A., et al. Anthrax as a biological weapon, 2002: Updated recommendations for management. *JAMA* 287: 2236–2252, 2002.

Mayer, T.A., Bersoff-Matcha, S., Murphy, C., et al. Clinical presentation of inhalational anthrax following bioterrorism exposure: Report of 2 surviving patients. *JAMA* 286:2549–2553, 2001.

Plague
Boisier, P., Rahalison, L., Rasolomaharo, M., et al. Epidemiologic features of four successive annual outbreaks of bubonic plague in Mahajanga, Madagascar. *Emerg Infect Dis* 8:311–316, 2002.

Gabastou, J.M., Proano, J., Vimos, A., et al. An outbreak of plague including cases with probable pneumonic infection, Ecuador, 1998. *Trans R Soc Trop Med Hygiene* 94:387–391, 2000.

Gage, K.L., Dennis, D.T., Orloski, K.A., et al. Cases of cat-associated human plague in the Western US, 1977–1998. *Clin Infect Dis* 30:893–900, 2000.

Human plague—United States, 1993–1994. *MMWR* 43:242–246, 1994.

Tularemia
Feldman, K.A., Enscore, R.E., Lathrop, S.L., et al. An outbreak of primary pneumonic tularemia on Martha's Vineyard. *N Engl J Med* 345:1601–1606, 2001.

Limaye, A.P., and Hooper, C.J. Treatment of tularemia with fluoroquinolones: Two cases and review. *Clin Infect Dis* 29:922–924, 1999.

Perez-Castrillon, J.L., Bachiller-Luque, P., Martin-Luquero, M., Mena-Martin, F.J., and Herreros, V. Tularemia epidemic in northwestern Spain: Clinical description and therapeutic response. *Clin Infect Dis* 33:573–576, 2001.

Tularemia—Oklahoma, 2000. *MMWR* 50:704–706, 2001.

Smallpox
Frey, S.E., Couch, R.B., Tacket, C.O., et al. Clinical responses to undiluted and diluted smallpox vaccine. *N Engl J Med* 346:1265–1274, 2002.

Frey, S.E., Newman, F.K., Cruz, J., et al. Dose-related effects of smallpox vaccine. *N Engl J Med* 346:1275–1280, 2002.

Joklik, W.K., Moss, B., Fields, B.N., Bishop, D.H., and Sandakhchiev, L.S. Why the smallpox virus stocks should not be destroyed. *Science* 262:1225–1226, 1993.

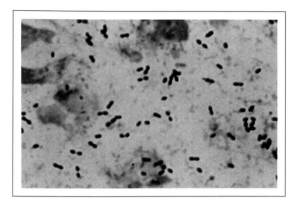

Figure 4.1B Lobar pneumococcal pneumonia: sputum Gram stain

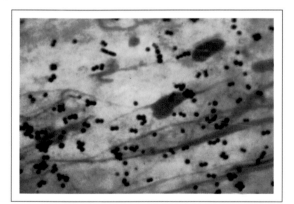

Figure 4.3B Bronchopneumonia due to *Staphylococcus aureus:* sputum Gram stain

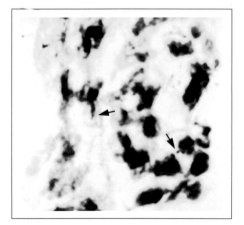

Figure 4.4B Bilateral apical infiltrates due to *Mycobacterium tuberculosis:* sputum AFB smear showing acid-fast bacilli (arrows)

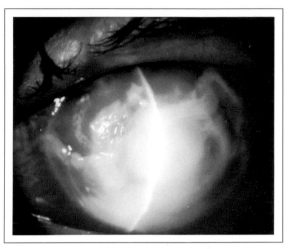

Figure 5.1 *Pseudomonas aeruginosa* keratitis

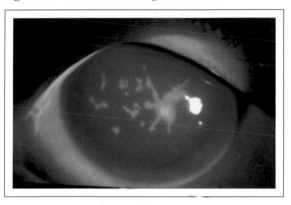

Figure 5.2 Herpes keratitis: fluorescein stain

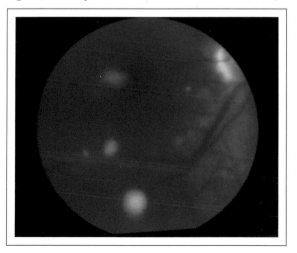

Figure 5.3 Candida retinitis

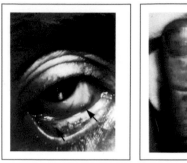

A   **B**

Figure 7.1 A. Infectious endocarditis: conjunctival hemorrhages **B.** Infectious endocarditis: nailbed splinter hemorrhage

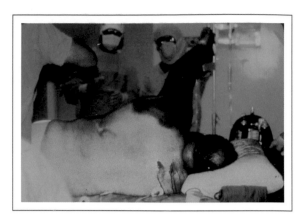

Figure 10.2A Patient from Case 10-3 with clostridium myonecrosis

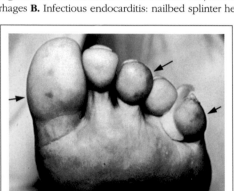

Figure 7.1C Infectious endocarditis: Osler nodes

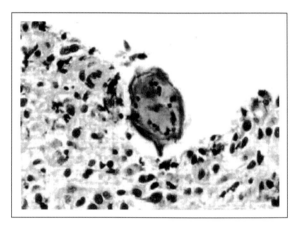

Figure 12.9 Bladder biopsy showing *S. haematobium* egg

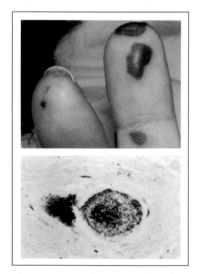

Figure 7.1D Infectious endocarditis: Janeway lesions

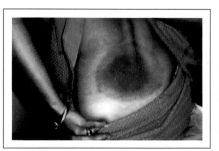

Figure 13.1 Erythema migrans

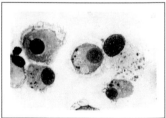

Figure 13.2 Granulocyte morulae of human granulocytotropic ehrlichiosis

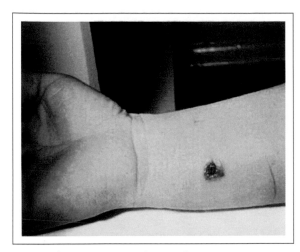

Figure 14.1 Cutaneous anthrax eschar

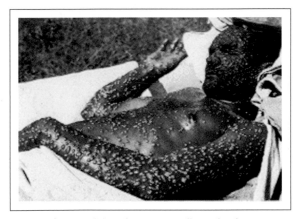

Figure 14.3A Adult with severe smallpox skin lesions

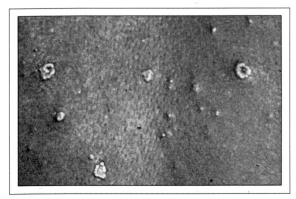

Figure 14.3B Close up of individual raised smallpox skin lesions

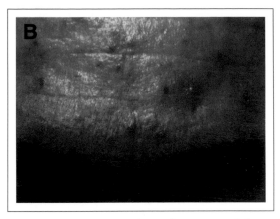

Figure 17.1B Seroconversion and acute retroviral syndrome: acneiform lesions

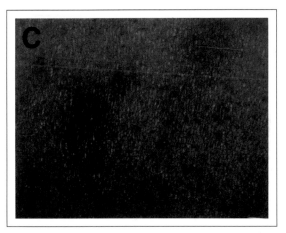

Figure 17.1C Seroconversion and acute retroviral syndrome: macules on the chest

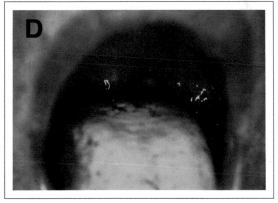

Figure 17.1D Seroconversion and acute retroviral syndrome: ulcerations in the oral cavity

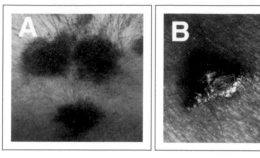

Figure 17.3 **A.** Kaposi's sarcoma: macular lesions **B.** Kaposi's sarcoma: tumorlike lesions

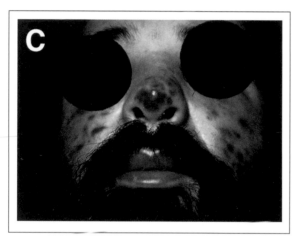

Figure 17.3C Kaposi's sarcoma: lesions have a purple color

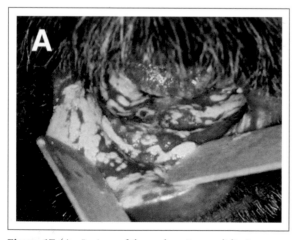

Figure 17.4A Lesions of the oral cavity: candidiasis

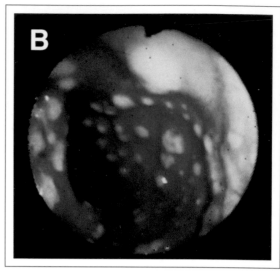

Figure 17.4B Lesions of the oral cavity: candida esophagitis

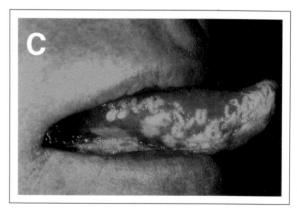

Figure 17.4C Lesions of the oral cavity: oral "hairy" leukoplasia

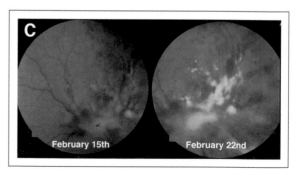

Figure 17.6C Retinitis due to cytomegalovirus

Sankar Swaminathan

Serious Adult Viral Illnesses Other Than HIV

Recommended Time to Complete: 1 day

Guiding Questions

1. Who is most likely to become ill with a serious adult viral illness?

2. What presenting features and laboratory tests are useful in making a diagnosis?

3. What are the major complications of each serious adult viral disease?

4. What treatments are available for each viral illness?

5. Which patients should be treated?

6. What preventive measures are available?

Potential Severity: Most adult viral illness with the exception of varicella and influenza virus can cause severe illness, but are not life threatening.

Varicella in the Adult

Varicella-zoster virus (VZV), a double-stranded DNA herpesvirus, causes two diseases: chickenpox and herpes zoster, or shingles. Chickenpox is a manifestation of primary infection, whereas herpes zoster is caused by reactivation of latent infection.

Epidemiology

Approximately 3–4 million cases of chickenpox and 500,000 cases of zoster occur each year in the United States. However, dramatic reductions in chickenpox incidence have recently been reported and may be due to the introduction of varicella vaccine in 1995. Chickenpox is primarily a disease of childhood. Nevertheless, 10% of the adult population is estimated to be at risk for infection, and 10% of cases occur in patients over the age of 13 years. For unclear reasons chickenpox occurs more frequently in adults who reside in tropical regions. VZV circulates exclusively in humans, and there are no other known reservoirs of infection. The disease becomes epidemic in the susceptible population in winter and early spring, affecting both genders and all races equally. Transmission is via the respiratory route and requires close contact, although the virus is highly infectious, with attack rates of 70–90% in susceptible family members.

In contrast, herpes zoster affects primarily the elderly. Zoster is caused by reactivation of latent VZV in those who have previously had chickenpox. Zoster occurs in up to 1% of people over 60 years of age, and 75% of cases occur in those over age 45. The development of zoster is not associated with exposure to others with chickenpox or zoster, although patients with zoster may themselves be capable of transmitting the virus to susceptible individuals. Zoster does occasionally occur in younger individuals, particularly those who are immunosuppressed.

Pathophysiology and Clinical Manifestations

Chickenpox is popularly thought to be a benign childhood rite of passage. Nevertheless, there are approximately 250 deaths each year in the United States due to chickenpox and its complications. The overall risk of death is about 15-fold higher in adults and is estimated to be more than 3 per 10,000 cases. Most deaths in adults are due to the development of visceral complications, as discussed below.

The disease begins by infecting the respiratory tract. VZV then replicates at local sites, which have not been clearly identified, and infects the reticuloendothelial system. Viremia ensues, followed by diffuse seeding of the skin as well as internal organs and the nervous system. Replication of the virus occurs in the corium and dermis, leading to degenerative changes and the formation of multinucleated giant cells, resulting in the characteristic diffuse vesicular rash. There is usually a mild prodrome of fever and malaise of 3–5 days, followed by a rash. The rash initially appears on the trunk and spreads outward (centrifugal rash, see Chapter 14), and may also be present on the oral mucosa. The rash begins as small, erythematous papules less than 1 cm in diameter that rapidly evolve into vesicles. As viral replication proceeds and infiltration by polymorphonuclear leukocytes occurs, the lesions appear purulent. A hallmark of chickenpox is that lesions are simultaneously found at all stages of development: maculopapules, vesicles, and scabs. The lesions appear umbilicated in the center as they evolve. Successive crops of lesions occur over several days, with complete healing by 10–14 days in uncomplicated cases. Lifelong latent infection in the dorsal root ganglia is then established by VZV.

Reactivation of VZV can result in herpes zoster, also known as shingles. Zoster presents as a localized eruption along the course of one or more dermatomes, most commonly the thoracic or lumbar dermatomes. The rash, which is often preceded by localized pain, begins as erythematous papules, which evolve into vesicles. The vesicles may coalesce into large confluent blisters with a hemorrhagic component. Healing occurs over the course of 2 weeks, although permanent skin changes such as discoloration and scarring may occur. When zoster affects the first branch of the trigeminal nerve, herpes zoster ophthalmicus may occur, with involvement of the cornea and potentially sight-threatening complications. Involvement of other branches of the trigeminal or facial nerves may result in unusual presentations with intraoral vesicles. The constellation of lesions in the external auditory canal, loss of taste, and facial palsy is referred to as the Ramsay Hunt syndrome and is caused by infection of the fifth, ninth, and tenth cranial nerves.

KEY POINTS

Epidemiology, Pathogenesis, and Clinical Manifestations of Varicella Zoster Infection

1. Chickenpox infects 3–4 million/year in the U.S., 10% adults; zoster 500,000/year.
2. Highly infectious, spreads person to person by air droplets, zoster represents reactivation.
3. Double-stranded DNA virus, enters via the respiratory tract, then disseminates.
4. Primarily infects the skin in chickenpox:
   a. Lesions begin on the trunk, spread outwardly (centrifugal),
   b. Lesions in all stages (maculopapules, vesicles, and scabs) are present at the same time.
5. Reactivation from the ganglion affects a single dermatome, pain precedes rash:
   a. Ophthalmicus infects the cornea, can be sight-threatening,
   b. Ramsay Hunt syndrome: Facial palsy, loss of taste, lesions in external auditory canal.

Diagnosis

The diagnosis of chickenpox can usually be made on clinical grounds, on the basis of the characteristics described above. Since the eradication of all known natural human reservoirs of smallpox and the discontinuation of universal vaccination, the clinical diagnosis of chickenpox has been relatively straightforward. Nevertheless, the possibility of smallpox as a biological warfare agent and resumption of vaccination of larger segments of the population may necessitate considering smallpox or disseminated vaccinia in the differential diagnosis of a diffuse vesicular rash in an adult. Smallpox lesions, in contrast to those of chickenpox, classically begin at the periphery, involve the palms and soles, and spread centrally (see Chapter 14). A diffuse vesicular eruption, Kaposi's varicelliform eruption, occasionally occurs in patients with eczema. This syndrome may be caused either by vaccination with vaccinia virus or by herpes simplex virus. The diagnosis can be made on the basis of the history and identification of the virus in vesicle fluid. Occasionally, enteroviral infection may cause diffuse cutaneous vesicular lesions that mimic early chickenpox. These lesions are often found on the palms and soles as well as the oral mucosa and do not progress like those of chickenpox.

The diagnosis of herpes zoster may sometimes be more difficult, the primary alternative diagnosis being herpes simplex virus. Culture of the virus from unroofed vesicles remains the most reliable method of differentiating viral agents in this situation, although polymerase chain reaction (PCR)–based tests are also highly specific and sensitive. Antibody-based assays performed on lesion scrapings or vesicle fluid may also be useful depending on availability.

KEY POINTS

Diagnosis of Varicella Zoster Infection

1. Diagnosis is generally made on the basis of skin rash morphology.
2. Rarely, herpes zoster can be mistaken for herpes simplex infection.
3. Vesicles can be cultured for virus.
4. PCR is highly specific and sensitive.

Complications

◆ **CASE 15.1**

A 36-year-old mother of two presented to the emergency room with complaints of shortness of breath. She had noted the onset of skin lesions and low-grade fever 2 days before admission. Her son was recovering from a recent bout of chickenpox. Aside from her skin rash, she had been feeling well until the day of admission, when she began experiencing a dry cough and increasing shortness of breath. On exam she had a temperature of 38.5°C and respiratory rate of 30/min. She appeared in moderate respiratory distress. Skin: extensive rash primarily involving the trunk and face. Lesions varied in character, being vesiculopustular as well as nodular. A few crusted lesions were also noted. Pulmonary exam revealed a few rales. Chest X-ray: bilateral lower lobe infiltrates with a fine reticulonodular pattern. Arterial blood gas: pH 7.45, pCO$_2$ 35, pO$_2$ 70 mm Hg on room air. Intravenous acyclovir was begun. New crops of skin lesions were noted over the first 24 hours; however, she then defervesced, and her respiratory status slowly improved. She did not require intubation and was discharged on oral acyclovir.

The major complications of varicella result from involvement of the pulmonary and nervous systems. Varicella pneumonitis is more common in adults and the immunocompromised than in children. It has been estimated that as many as 1 in 400 adults with chickenpox have some pulmonary involvement, although most cases appear to be subclinical. When clinical varicella pneumonitis occurs in the adult, it is often associated with high morbidity and mortality. Fortunately, the patient in Case 15.1 responded quickly to acyclovir and did not suffer severe respiratory compromise. Pneumonitis can be particularly severe in pregnant women during the later stages of pregnancy. This may be due both to the respiratory impairment due to a gravid uterus and immunologic changes associated with pregnancy. Smoking and the presence of a large number of skin lesions have been identified as risk factors for the development of

varicella pneumonia. As is illustrated in Case 15.1, tachypnea, dyspnea, and fever with nodular or interstitial markings on chest X-ray are typically observed. Development of encephalitis in association with chickenpox in adults is relatively uncommon, occurring in up to 0.1–0.2% of patients, with mortality as high as 20%. Seizures are common and are accompanied by headache, fever, and progressive obtundation.

The major complications of herpes zoster are also neurologic. Involvement of the central nervous system (CNS) can almost always be demonstrated in relatively asymptomatic sufferers from zoster when the CSF is examined. The most common complication is postherpetic neuralgia, especially in those over 50 years of age. As many as half of these patients will have persistent, severe pain in the area of the lesions. Encephalitis, transverse myelitis, and Guillain-Barré syndrome can also accompany an episode of herpes zoster. A specific complication of zoster, particularly of ophthalmic zoster, is the subsequent development of granulomatous cerebral angiitis, which may result in stroke. Ophthalmic zoster may result in keratitis, iridocyclitis, and, in severe cases, loss of vision.

Chickenpox and zoster in the immunosuppressed patient present special problems. Bone marrow transplant recipients and children with hematologic malignancies are especially prone to visceral dissemination from both chickenpox and zoster, with high mortality.

KEY POINTS

Complications Associated with Varicella Zoster Infection

1. Pneumonia in adults can be fatal:
   a. More severe in pregnant women,
   b. Severity often correlates with extent of the skin lesions,
   c. Worse in smokers.
2. Encephalitis is rare, associated with seizures, headache, obtundation, 20% mortality.

3. Herpes zoster is associated with multiple complications:
   a. Postherpetic neuralgia in up to 50% of patients. More common if > 50 yo,
   b. Guillain-Barré syndrome, transverse myelitis, and encephalitis,
   c. Ophthalmic branch keratitis, iridocyclitis, blindness, also granulomatous cerebral angiitis.
4. Dissemination in immunosuppressed patients is often fatal.

Treatment

The mainstay of treatment for VZV is acyclovir and related nucleoside analogues that inhibit the viral DNA polymerase. Acyclovir therapy is recommended for adults and adolescents with chickenpox. Treatment reduces the number of total lesions and shortens the duration of lesion formation by about 1 day. It is unknown whether treatment reduces the likelihood of serious complications in adults such as those described above. The recommended adult dosage is 800 mg orally five times per day. The minimum inhibitory concentration of acyclovir for VZV is 2–6 µM, which is difficult to achieve by oral administration. Intravenous treatment is indicated in cases of varicella pneumonia and should be considered in other cases of visceral or CNS involvement. The usual dosage is 5–10 mg/kg given every 8 hours. Prompt infectious disease consultation should be obtained in all cases of complicated varicella or varicella in the immunocompromised patient.

Antiviral treatment of herpes zoster reduces acute neuritis and accelerates healing. Treatment of zoster in the immunosuppressed patient prevents dissemination. Ophthalmic zoster is usually treated with oral acyclovir or with the more bioavailable valacyclovir and famciclovir. The latter are prodrugs of acyclovir and penciclovir, respectively (see Chapter 1). Treatment of cutaneous zoster may also reduce the incidence or duration of postherpetic neuralgia, but the data supporting these effects has been questioned. Nevertheless, oral famciclovir and valacyclovir are approved for this indication and are more convenient than acyclovir, as they can be administered less frequently. The concurrent administration of corticosteroids to treat postherpetic neuralgia is also controversial, but some studies claim improvement in the quality of life when steroids are added to antiviral therapy.

KEY POINTS

Treatment and Prevention of Varicella Zoster Infections

1. Acyclovir is recommended for adolescents and adults with chickenpox. Serious infection should receive high-dose intravenous therapy.
2. Antiviral treatment for all cases of herpes zoster (acylovir, famciclovir, or valacyclovir):
   a. Reduces acute neuritis and accelerates healing,
   b. Prevents dissemination in the immuno-compromised host,
   c. May reduce postherpetic neuralgia,
   d. Efficacy of concurrent treatment with corticosteroids to reduce postherpetic neuralgia is controversial.
3. Live attenuated vaccine is highly efficacious:
   a. Recommended for all susceptible individuals > 12 months of age,
   b. Impact on herpes zoster not clarified.
4. Varicella zoster immune globulin effective at preventing active disease:
   a. Give within 96 hours of exposure,
   b. Recommended for all exposed pregnant women and immunocompromised patients.

Prevention

A live attenuated varicella vaccine has been available since 1995. It is close to 100% effective in preventing serious disease and has a low incidence of side effects. Immunity has been persistent over the period since initial licensure. Varicella vaccination is recommended for all susceptible individuals older than 12 months of age. The long-term effects of vaccination on the incidence of herpes zoster are still unclear. Although rates of zoster are lower in vaccinated individuals, the vaccine strain may actually reactivate more frequently but subclinically. Furthermore, a decrease in circulating wild-type virus may result in less frequent natural boosting of immunity and therefore lead to an increased incidence of zoster in previously infected individuals. There have also been concerns among parents and pediatricians that early vaccination might not be the best policy. Decision analyses support vaccination, however, and indicate that vaccination reduces the risk of morbidity and mortality. Vaccination also becomes more important as its acceptance rate increases because herd immunity is likely to reduce infection during childhood, increasing the risk of adult disease.

Varicella zoster immune globulin is effective in preventing disease in susceptible individuals when administered within 96 hours of exposure. Its use should be considered in all immunocompromised patients and susceptible pregnant women who have been exposed.

Epstein-Barr Virus

Epidemiology

Infection with Epstein-Barr virus (EBV) is ubiquitous, 90–95% of all adults displaying serologic evidence of past infection. In the United States approximately 50% of children are seropositive by age 5, with a second period of seroconversion occurring in early adulthood. Infection occurs earlier in developing countries and in cer-

tain areas of the United States. Most cases of EBV infection are transmitted by the presence of virus in oropharyngeal secretions of asymptomatic shedders. Blood transfusions and transplantation of solid organs or bone marrow may also be associated with EBV transmission.

Pathophysiology and Clinical Manifestations

◆ CASE 15.2

An 18-year-old freshman college student presented to student health with fever and sore throat for 1 week. His temperature was 102°F, his tonsils were enlarged, and he had diffuse lymphadenopathy. The possibility of mononucleosis was raised, and a VCA IgG was 1:20 and VCA IgM 1:80 at that time. Over the next week he became increasingly ill, developing scleral icterus and fever to 105°F. On exam he was noted to have a tender, enlarged liver and palpable spleen; multiple petechiae were noted on both lower legs. Liver transaminases were elevated: GOT 950, GPT 1000, LDH 4000, bilirubin total 6.0, direct 4.8. Hct 25, WBC 860 (3% PMNs, 19% band forms, 70% lymphocytes, 10% monocytes), numerous atypical lymphocytes seen on smear. Platelets 23,000, ESR 12. Repeat serologies revealed a VCA IgM of 1:160 and VCA IgG 1:640. Glucocorticoid therapy was considered; however, over the next two weeks his fever spontaneously resolved, liver function tests returned to normal, his Hct increased to 35, WBC improved to 3,000 with 70% PMNs, and platelets rose to 100,000/mm³. His spleen remained enlarged, and he was warned to avoid contact sports for the next few months.

EBV is associated with a variety of clinical disorders arising from different pathogenic mechanisms. Infection during childhood is often asymptomatic or associated with nonspecific symptoms. Infection during adolescence or adulthood more commonly results in the syndrome of acute infectious mononucleosis, characterized by a vigorous humoral and cellular immune response to rapidly proliferating EBV-infected B cells. The most common signs and symptoms of mononucleosis include fever, sore throat, malaise, and lymphadenopathy. The pharyngitis may be exudative and severe. The enlarged lymph nodes are usually not tender. Other findings, in order of decreasing likelihood, include splenomegaly, hepatitis, palatal petechiae, jaundice, and rash. The rash, when seen, is nonspecific and may be transient. Administration of ampicillin during early EBV-associated mononucleosis very commonly results in a maculopapular rash.

Many aspects of this clinical syndrome, for example, fever, lymphadenopathy, splenomegaly, and atypical lymphocytosis, are due to the vigorous T and NK cell proliferation and cytokine response of the immune system rather than direct viral infection, replication, and cytolysis. As is illustrated in Case 15.2, individuals occasionally develop a chronic active infection characterized by ongoing lytic EBV replication and multiple organ system disease, such as pneumonitis, hepatitis, pancytopenia, and iritis. Individuals with a rare, inherited X-linked immunodeficiency, known as X-linked lymphoproliferative syndrome (XLP) or Duncan's syndrome, are prone to overwhelming lethal primary infection with Epstein-Barr virus. Survivors are at risk for the subsequent development of lymphoma and agammaglobulinemia. The genetic defect in these patients has been mapped to a small cytoplasmic protein SAP, which is implicated in regulation of T and NK cell signaling. After resolution of primary infection, EBV persists for life as a latent infection in B cells and as a lytic infection in the oropharynx. Persistent EBV infection is controlled by a virus-specific immune response and is asymptomatic in most humans. However, immunosuppression associated with HIV infection, transplantation, or congenital immunodeficiencies can result in uncontrolled oligoclonal or monoclonal B cell proliferation of latently infected cells. Uncontrolled lytic infection in the oropharynx is manifested as oral hairy leukoplakia in immunosuppressed hosts. Persistent, latent EBV infection is also associated with development of Burkitt's lymphoma, nasopharyngeal carcinoma,

certain types of Hodgkin's disease, gastric adenocarcinoma, and leiomyosarcomas in immunosuppressed hosts. Infection of NK cells by EBV has recently been associated with hypersensitivity to mosquito bites and the development of NK cell leukemia.

Complications

Occasional serious and life-threatening complications of EBV infection occur and include autoimmune hemolytic anemia, erythrophagocytic syndrome, thrombocytopenia, splenic rupture, and neurologic syndromes. The latter, although rare, include encephalitis and Guillain-Barré syndrome. The most common causes of death from EBV-associated mononucleosis in healthy adults are neurologic complications, splenic rupture, and airway obstruction. It should be emphasized that mononucleosis-associated encephalitis is rare and usually benign. Nevertheless, any of these complications may be the presenting sign of mononucleosis, and "atypical" cases are not unusual.

KEY POINTS
Epidemiology, Pathogenesis, and Clinical Manifestations of Epstein-Barr Virus

1. Spread by oral secretions, 95% of adults carry the virus.
2. Infects B cells, manifestations due to a vigorous T and NK cell inflammatory response.
3. Fever, sore throat and lymphadenopathy are the classic triad of mononucleosis.
4. The differential diagnosis includes acute HIV infection.
5. Ampicillin almost always causes a rash.
6. Acute complications: Splenic rupture, neurologic involvement, and airway obstruction. Less commonly, hepatitis, hemolytic anemia, thrombocytopenia, and neutropenia.

7. Chronic complications: Hairy leukoplakia, B cell lymphoma, NK cell lymphoma, gastric adenocarcinoma, and leiomyosarcomas.

Diagnosis

Diagnosis of mononucleosis is usually based on clinical suspicion confirmed by laboratory testing. The clinical diagnosis in the typical adolescent or young adult is usually not too difficult. However, many cases occur in which few or none of the classic signs are evident at the initial presentation. Other causes of infectious mononucleosis syndrome that should be considered in the young adult are cytomegalovirus, acute HIV infection, human herpesvirus 6, toxoplasmosis, cat-scratch disease, and lymphoma. Laboratory confirmation of EBV infection is primarily achieved by serologic testing. Heterophile antibodies directed against sheep erythrocyte agglutinins are positive in about 90% during the primary infection. Commercially available Monospot testing for heterophile antibodies is less sensitive in children, and sequential Monospot testing or determination of EBV-specific antibodies is indicated when the clinical findings are suggestive of EBV infection and the initial Monospot is negative. The presence of IgM antibodies to viral capsid antigen (VCA) is the most sensitive and specific indicator of acute infection. These are usually detectable at the initial presentation, along with IgG VCA antibodies. IgM VCA antibodies (IgM VCA Abs) decline and are absent by four to eight weeks, however, whereas IgG VCA Abs persist for life. Antibodies to EBV nuclear antigens (EBNAs) do not develop until approximately four weeks after onset of symptoms and persist for life. Seroconversion to anti-EBNA positivity is therefore indicative of recent EBV infection. Although antibodies to EBV early antigens are often elevated during acute infection, they may persist for variable periods and are occasionally detectable in healthy convalescent patients many years after infection and are therefore of limited utility in diagnosing acute infection.

Quantifying peripheral blood viral load by polymerase chain reaction is being evaluated for its ability to identify immunosuppressed patients with, or at high risk for developing, EBV-associated B cell lymphomas. However, this new technology is not yet considered standard care owing to lack of standardized methodologies, validated clinical cutoffs, and documentation of clinical utility.

KEY POINTS
Diagnosis of Epstein-Barr Virus

1. Heterophile antibody agglutination test (+) 90% of primary disease.
2. Monospot less sensitive in children, often needs to be repeated.
3. IgM antibody to VCA (viral capsid antigen) most sensitive and specific:
   a. Often elevated at the time of presentation,
   b. Declines quickly, absent by four to eight weeks, positive IgM VCA = recent EBV infection,
   c. IgG VCA persists for life.
4. EBNA (nuclear antigen) begins to rise after four weeks, rising titer = recent EBV infection.
5. Antibodies to early EBV antigens are usually not helpful.
6. Quantitative PCR viral load is primarily experimental.

Treatment

Treatment of EBV-associated diseases is closely linked to the underlying pathogenesis of the disease. The usual treatment for EBV-associated malignancies is based on cancer chemotherapy and radiation therapy rather than antiviral strategies; however, these options will not be discussed here.

INFECTIOUS MONONUCLEOSIS

Supportive treatment is generally indicated, since more than 95% of infectious mononucleosis cases resolve uneventfully without specific therapy. Acetaminophen can be used to reduce fever. Use of concomitant antibiotics for possible bacterial pharyngitis should be judicious and be supported by positive culture results, owing to the high incidence of allergic reactions to antibiotics such as ampicillin during acute infectious mononucleosis. The use of corticosteroids for uncomplicated infectious mononucleosis is still controversial. Corticosteroids have been shown to reduce fever and shorten the duration of constitutional symptoms. However, adverse drug complications can arise from even short courses of corticosteroid use, and corticosteroid use is probably best avoided in routine infectious mononucleosis, a self-limited disease. Corticosteroids are generally reserved for infectious mononucleosis cases that are complicated by potential airway obstruction from enlarged tonsils, severe thrombocytopenia, or severe hemolytic anemia. These complications result from the excessive immune response to virus infection rather than uncontrolled viral infection, and a short course of corticosteroids at 1 mg/kg/day of prednisone with tapering over one to two weeks can be effective for treating the excessive tonsillar proliferation or autoimmune symptoms. Corticosteroids might also be used for other autoimmune complications that are rarely associated with infectious mononucleosis such as CNS involvement, myocarditis, or pericarditis.

As was described above, acyclovir provides no significant clinical benefit for treatment of uncomplicated infectious mononucleosis. The combination of acyclovir and corticosteroids for uncomplicated infectious mononucleosis inhibits oral viral replication but provides no clinical benefit. In rare, complicated cases of primary EBV infection and infectious mononucleosis in which the patient is immunosuppressed or severely ill, acyclovir or ganciclovir treatment may be rational, given the safety profile of these drugs, their ability to inhibit EBV replication in vitro and in vivo, and anecdotal reports of clinical response in unusual cases in which excessive EBV replication may have been pathogenic.

CHRONIC ACTIVE EBV INFECTION/CHRONIC FATIGUE SYNDROME

Rare patients have an unusual clinical course following infectious mononucleosis with severe illness and evidence of chronic active EBV infection. These patients typically have extremely high antibody responses to EBV early antigens, lack antibodies to EBNA-1, and exhibit severe disease with end organ involvement or evidence of increased viral load in affected tissues. Both clinical responses and failures with acyclovir or corticosteroids have been noted in anecdotal reports of these unusual patients with chronic active EBV infection.

EBV infection has also been implicated as a cause of the much more common chronic fatigue syndrome. However, seroepidemiologic studies have argued against a pathogenic role for EBV in chronic fatigue syndrome. In addition, a placebo-controlled study with acyclovir has shown no efficacy for patients with chronic fatigue syndrome.

ORAL HAIRY LEUKOPLAKIA

Oral hairy leukoplakia is an unusual lesion of the tongue found in HIV-infected patients. Vigorous EBV lytic replication is present in the excessively proliferating epithelium. This is the only instance in which disease appears to be a direct consequence of lytic EBV replication and oral acyclovir therapy (3.2 gm/day) can temporarily reverse the lesions. However, since nucleoside analogues have no effect on persistent, latent EBV infection, lytic EBV replication and oral hairy leukoplakia frequently recur on withdrawal of therapy. Topical application of podophyllotoxin can also be used to control progression of the lesions.

KEY POINTS

Treatment of Epstein-Barr Virus

1. Acute mononucleosis is generally given supportive care:
   a. Avoid antibiotics when possible,
   b. Prednisone for airway obstruction, thrombocytopenia, or hemolytic anemia,
   c. Acyclovir or ganciclovir may be helpful in very severe cases.
2. Chronic active EBV infection:
   a. Very high antibodies to early antigens, no EBNA antibody production,
   b. Severe end organ involvement,
   c. May benefit from antiviral therapy.
3. Chronic fatigue syndrome: Antiviral therapy of no benefit.
4. Oral hairy leukoplakia in HIV-infected patients due to lytic EBV infection:
   a. Acyclovir can control the infection,
   b. Relapse often occurs when treatment is discontinued.

Hantavirus

◆ **CASE 15.3**

A 19-year-old man who had been in excellent health and was a marathon runner presented to a local emergency room in New Mexico complaining of fever, myalgia, chills, headache, and malaise. He did not have dyspnea or cough. His fiancee had died 2 days earlier of a respiratory illness that was not characterized. The patient had a temperature of 39.4°C, blood pressure of 127/84, heart rate of 118, and respiratory rate of 24. The remainder of the physical exam was normal. Laboratory examination revealed a hematocrit of 49.6 percent, a WBC of 7100 with 66% segmented neutrophils and 10% band forms, a platelet count of 195,000, a creatinine level of 1.1 mg/dl, a serum lactate dehydrogenase level of 195 IU/l, and an oxygen saturation of 91% on room air. He had a normal urinalysis and chest X-ray. He was dis-

charged after treatment with acetaminophen, antibiotics, and amantadine. Two days later, the patient returned to a clinic complaining of persistent symptoms as well as vomiting and diarrhea. He was discharged with no change in diagnosis or therapy. Over the following day a cough productive of blood-tinged sputum and worsening respiratory distress developed. The patient suffered cardiopulmonary arrest and could not be resuscitated. Chest X-ray during the terminal illness revealed diffuse alveolar and interstitial infiltrates.

This case, taken from the description of the outbreak of hantavirus pulmonary syndrome (HPS) in the Four Corners region of New Mexico, Arizona, Colorado, and Utah in 1993, dramatically illustrates almost every characteristic of this devastating illness spread by rodents.

Epidemiology

Hantaviruses are carried by chronically infected rodents that shed the virus in their saliva and urine. Humans become infected when they inhale aerosols of these infected fluids. Risk factors thus include cleaning or entering any buildings that harbor rodents. There are mice that harbor hantavirus strains and readily enter human dwellings in many areas of the United States. Since 1993 cases of HPS have been reported in New England and the Midwest as well as other areas, and dozens of cases occur annually.

Pathophysiology and Clinical Manifestations

As was described in Case 15.3, HPS begins with fever and myalgias that may be associated with abdominal complaints. Initially, the patient does not appear extremely ill. Over the next few days respiratory symptoms develop. These are initially mild, and cough and dyspnea may be minimal. Fever, tachycardia, mild hypotension, and hypoxia are usually present. Hemoconcentration, presence of immature white blood cells, mild thrombocytopenia, increased partial thromboplastin time (PTT), and lactate dehydrogenase are all typical. A pulmonary vascular leak syndrome occurs, and hypoxia, shock, and pulmonary edema (adult respiratory distress syndrome) may develop rapidly. Little inflammation is seen in autopsies or biopsies of the affected lung.

Diagnosis

Hantavirus serology is almost always positive in patients at the time of admission. Virus can also be demonstrated in tissue by PCR-based methods and by immunohistochemical staining. If HPS is suspected, infectious disease consultation should be obtained immediately, and the Centers for Disease Control and Prevention should be notified.

Treatment and Prevention

If the patient can be supported through the period of hypoxia and shock, recovery can be complete. It is important to realize that in HPS the vascular permeability of the lung is abnormal, and fluid administration should be performed with this in mind. Intravenous ribavirin has been used investigationally for HPS, although its efficacy has not yet been demonstrated.

Prevention of HPS consists of personal precautions to avoid inhalation of aerosolized material contaminated by rodents and general measures to decrease rodent infestation.

KEY POINTS
Hantavirus

1. Spread by rodents that excrete the virus in their saliva and urine, aerosol inhaled.

2. Found in the New Mexico, Arizona, Colorado, Utah Four Corners area, New England, and the Midwest.
3. Initially mild febrile illness with abdominal pain to fulminant respiratory failure:
   a. Virus causes a pulmonary capillary leak syndrome with ARDS,
   b. Severe hypoxia, hemoconcentration, increased PTT and LDH.
4. Diagnosis: Serologies, PCR, and immunohistochemical stains are available.
5. Supportive care, cautious fluid administration, full recovery if survive the ARDS.

Influenza

Epidemiology

Influenza virus is a major cause of morbidity and mortality worldwide. Influenza A and B both cause epidemic illnesses, and influenza A can cause worldwide pandemics such as the one in 1918–1919, when over 20 million people died. Influenza routinely causes epidemics every one to three years. The number of cases always increases in the winter months. The virus changes the structure of its hemagglutinin and neuraminidase proteins by genetic mutation, a process known as antigenic drift. This allows production of variant strains to which there is less protective antibody in the population. Occasionally, influenza A virus acquires a completely different set of antigens by a process known as antigenic shift. These large changes in surface antigens allow the virus to infect large segments of the population who lack cross-reactive or protective antibody, thus leading to a pandemic. The virus is thought to undergo antigenic shift by reassortment, or exchange of segments of its genome with avian influenza species. The process of reassortment and production of virulent human species may occur in pigs that can be infected with both human and avian species.

Influenza has the highest attack rates among the very young but causes the greatest morbidity and mortality among the elderly. It is also particularly dangerous to those who have underlying pulmonary disease or who are immunocompromised. In the United States influenza causes about 15 million excess respiratory illnesses per year in young people and about 4 million cases per year in older adults. It is transmitted efficiently by aerosols of respiratory secretions generated by coughing, sneezing, and talking.

KEY POINTS
Epidemiology of Influenza

1. Influenza A and B cause epidemics, influenza A also causes pandemics.
2. Epidemics every one to three years, occur in the winter.
3. Antigenic drift = changes in hemagglutinin and neuraminidase proteins by genetic mutation.
4. Antigenic shift = reassortment, or exchange of genomic segments with avian influenza species:
   a. Occurs in influenza A,
   b. Causes pandemics,
   c. Reassortment may occur in pigs.
5. Virus is spread by aerosols from respiratory secretions.
6. In U.S., 15 million infections annually in the young, 4 million in older adults.

Pathophysiology and Clinical Manifestations

The onset of influenza is abrupt. The patient can often tell you exactly when he or she fell ill with fever, headache, shaking chills, and myalgias. The fever may be quite high, stays up for at least 3 days, and is usually resolved within one week. Fever and systemic symptoms predominate in the clinical picture, but a dry cough is invariably present and usually lasts after the fever has gone down. Rhinorrhea, cervical adenopathy, and nonexudative pharyngitis are common. Recovery can be prolonged, taking up to three weeks or even longer, during which period the patient suffers from cough and persistent fatigue.

Once influenza virus infects the respiratory epithelium, it kills the host cell as it replicates. The virus multiplies rapidly, leading to the production of large numbers of infectious virus in the respiratory secretions, as well as causing diffuse inflammation and damage. In severe cases there is extensive necrosis. Pulmonary function is abnormal even in normal hosts and may remain abnormal for a period of weeks after recovery.

Complications

The major complications of influenza are viral pneumonia and secondary bacterial pneumonia. In influenza pneumonia there is rapid progression to dyspnea and hypoxia. The clinical and radiographic picture is that of adult respiratory distress syndrome, and antibiotics are ineffective. The mortality rate in this situation is very high. The lungs are hemorrhagic, and there is diffuse involvement but little inflammation. This complication was a major cause of death among young adults during the 1918–1919 pandemic but is rarely seen today. However, the possibility remains that new strains could cause an increased number of such cases. Secondary bacterial pneumonia is caused by the usual bacterial causes of pneumonia, particularly *Staphylococcus aureus, Haemophilus influenzae,* and *Streptococcus pneumoniae* species. The patient appears to be recovering from influenza but then has a relapse with fever and typical signs of pneumonia (see Case 4.1). In this case the clinical picture is typical of bacterial pneumonia.

As with varicella, aspirin use during influenza has been associated with the development of Reye's syndrome. Reye's syndrome is characterized by fatty infiltration of the liver and mental status changes such as lethargy or even delirium and coma. There is no specific treatment other than correction of metabolic abnormalities and reduction of elevated intracranial pressure.

KEY POINTS
Pathogenesis and Clinical Manifestations of Influenza

1. Infects the respiratory epithelium, causing cell necrosis and acute inflammation.
2. Abrupt onset of high fever, shaking chills, headache, myalgias, pharyngitis, and rhinorrhea.
3. Complications:
   a. Viral pneumonia can progress to fatal ARDS and pulmonary hemorrhage,
   b. Superinfection with *Staphylococcus aureus, Haemophilus influenzae,* or *Streptococcus pneumoniae,*
   c. Reye's syndrome associated with aspirin use.

Diagnosis

The most useful distinguishing characteristic in influenza in contrast to other respiratory illnesses is the predominance of the systemic symptoms. In addition, the epidemic nature of the disease in the community is helpful in making a diagnosis. When influenza is circulating in a community, an adult displaying the symptoms described above is highly likely to have influenza. Rapid serologic tests are now available, and some can detect both type A and B influenza in throat and nasal swabs. However, the sensitivity of such tests is somewhat variable, depending on the source and quality of the specimen as well as other factors and may be as low as 60%. Culture and immunodetection of

antigens also allow more sensitive determination of virus in secretions in 1–2 days.

Treatment

Amantadine and rimantadine are drugs that inhibit influenza virus A infection by binding to a virus membrane protein. They are more effective when given early in infection, although treatment is usually instituted in complicated cases regardless of the time since onset of illness. A major side effect of amantadine is CNS symptoms, particularly in the elderly. Two neuraminidase inhibitors, zamanavir and oseltamivir, are highly effective in inhibiting both type A and B influenza. Zamanavir has to be administered by inhalation, whereas oseltamivir is given orally (see Chapter 1).

KEY POINTS
Diagnosis and Treatment of Influenza

1. Early diagnosis with commercial immunodetection methods, viral culture confirmatory.
2. Amantadine and rimantandine bind the viral membrane and block influenza A infection; give to all influenza A–infected patients, early treatment is more effective.
3. Neuraminidase inhibitors zamanavir and oseltamivir effective for A and B influenza. Give early.

Prevention

Influenza vaccine is a trivalent inactivated vaccine directed against both types A and B influenza. The strains are selected for each year's vaccine on the basis of what was circulating worldwide last year. Vaccine effectiveness depends to some degree on the success of the match between the vaccine and the currently circulating strains. Vaccination decreases disease severity as well as the infection rate. The groups to be targeted for influenza vaccination are listed below; the list is taken from the recommendations of the Advisory Committee on Immunization Practices.

KEY POINTS
Groups to Target for Influenza Immunization

1. Groups at increased risk for influenza complications:
   a. Persons 65 or older,
   b. Residents of nursing homes or other chronic care facilities,
   c. All persons with chronic pulmonary or cardiovascular disease (including asthma),
   d. All those under 18 on chronic aspirin therapy,
   e. Women who will be in the second or third trimester of pregnancy during the influenza season.
2. Those with increased risk of transmitting influenza to high-risk individuals:
   a. Health care personnel,
   b. Employees of nursing homes or other chronic care facilities who have patient contact,
   c. Home care providers and household contacts of those at high risk.

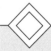

Herpes Simplex Virus

Epidemiology

Herpes simplex virus (HSV) is a ubiquitous human pathogen. There are two distinct types: HSV-1 and HSV-2. HSV-1 causes primarily orolabial lesions, whereas HSV-2 causes genital lesions. More than 90% of adults worldwide exhibit serologic evidence of infection with HSV-1. The prevalence of HSV-2 infection, which causes primarily genital infections, is considerably lower but ranges from at least 10% to 80%, depending on the population studied. The likelihood of contracting HSV-2 infection closely correlates with sexual activity; the higher the number of sexual partners and other sexually transmitted diseases, the higher is the likelihood of HSV-2 infection. Transmission of HSV is usually person to person and occurs by direct contact with infected secretions or mucosal surfaces.

Pathophysiology and Clinical Manifestations

Once the virus enters a mucosal or skin surface, it replicates in the epithelium and infects a nerve ending. It is then transported to the nerve ganglia, where it establishes a latent infection that persists for the lifetime of the host. The trigeminal and sacral ganglia are the most common sites of HSV-1 and HSV-2 latency. Viral replication occurs in the ganglia during initial infection. Initial infection with HSV-1 is often subclinical, and many people never experience clinical reactivation, although they are clearly seropositive. Others experience gingivostomatitis, especially small children. The lesions are usually ulcerative and exudative and may involve extensive areas of the lips, oral cavity, pharynx, and perioral skin. Healing occurs over a period of several days to two weeks and is usually complete, without scarring. Secondary episodes result in fever blisters, typical vesicular, and ulcerative lesions. These occur most commonly at the vermilion border of the lips but may also occur on other sites on the face or in the mouth. Many environmental factors may trigger a recurrence, such as sunlight exposure, stress, and viral infections. Secondary episodes are usually much less severe.

HSV-2 causes genital herpes in both women and men. Lesions may be vesicular, pustular, or ulcerative, involving the penis in men and the vagina and cervix in women. Typical symptoms are pain, itching, dysuria, and vaginal or urethral discharge. Symptoms of primary infection tend to be more severe in women. Primary infection not uncommonly results in aseptic meningitis and mild systemic symptoms such as fever. Occasionally, inflammation is severe enough to lead to temporary bladder or bowel dysfunction.

HSV-1 and HSV-2 can also affect many other sites of the body where they have been inoculated. Whitlow is HSV infection of the finger, resulting from the inoculation of virus into abraded skin. This condition may be seen in health care workers as well as those who have been exposed to virus either from autoinoculation or person-to-person transmission. The lesions are vesicular and pustular with local erythema, pain, and drainage. They are often mistaken for bacterial infections, resulting in unnecessary drainage and antibiotics. Herpes gladiatorum is the name given to HSV infection acquired by wrestlers in which the virus is inoculated into breaks in the skin as a result of competition.

Complications

HSV keratitis is a potentially dangerous consequence of HSV infection of the cornea. It may be caused by either HSV-1 or HSV-2, more commonly by HSV-1. Once HSV keratitis has occurred, the patient remains at risk for recurrences. HSV keratitis is one of the most common causes of blindness in the United States. Symptoms consist of tearing, pain, erythema, and conjunctival swelling. Dendritic corneal lesions are easily visualized by fluorescein staining. Involvement of deeper structures or corneal scarring can lead to blindness (see Chapter 5).

HSV encephalitis occurs in approximately 1 per 250,000–500,00 people per year. The vast majority of cases are due to HSV-1, and concurrent skin lesions are usually not present. Although encephalitis may be the result of primary infection, most patients can be shown to have been previously infected. HSV encephalitis is characterized by fever, altered mentation, and focal neurologic signs. Personality changes and bizarre behavior are common, and many patients have seizures. The disease process typically affects the temporal lobe and is usually unilateral. It may progress in a fulminant manner with frank hemorrhagic necrosis of the affected areas of the brain. With antiviral treatment mortality has been reduced but still remains above 15%, and the majority of survivors exhibit long-term cognitive impairment (see Chapter 6).

Widespread cutaneous dissemination (eczema herpeticum) can be seen in those with eczema. Visceral dissemination of HSV is rare in the normal host. However, herpetic tracheobronchitis is often seen in the debilitated, intubated hospitalized patient and may occasionally progress to pneumonitis.

KEY POINTS

Epidemiology, Pathogenesis, and Clinical Manifestations of Herpes Simplex Virus

1. HSV-1 causes herpes labialis; over 90% of individuals worldwide have been infected.
2. HSV-2 causes genital herpes; the incidence varies from 10% to 80% depending on sexual activity.
3. Transmitted from person to person by contact with infected surfaces or mucosa.
4. Virus replicates in nerve ganglia, periodically reactivates, causing recurrent infection:
   a. HSV-1 resides in the trigeminal ganglion,
   b. HSV-2 resides in the sacral ganglion.
5. Lesions are vesiculopustular, moderately painful.
6. Less common forms of skin infection:
   a. Herpetic whitlow, usually found in health care workers, mistaken for a bacterial infection,
   b. Herpes gladiatorum, develops in wrestlers at sites of skin abrasions.
7. Complications can be serious:

a. Herpes encephalitis (HSV-1): Personality changes, obtundation, seizures, 15% mortality,
b. Herpes keratitis: A leading cause of blindness,
c. Cutaneous dissemination in eczema patients, bronchopneumonia in debilitated patients.

Diagnosis

Diagnosis of labial or genital herpes is usually not difficult on clinical grounds. The typical vesicle on an erythematous base, the "dewdrop on a rose petal," is not always present, however. Culture of vesicle fluid is highly sensitive and specific. HSV can also be demonstrated by direct staining for HSV antigens. Staining of lesion scrapings and examination for giant cells (the Tzanck test) is quick but nonspecific and insensitive. The diagnosis of HSV encephalitis can be difficult, especially early in the course of the illness. A mild lymphocytic CSF pleocytosis is common, as are red blood cells and elevated protein levels. However, none of these findings are diagnostic. CSF PCR for HSV is highly sensitive and specific and is the optimal laboratory test to confirm the diagnosis. MRI of the brain and EEG often show abnormalities localizing to the temporal areas even early in the disease.

Treatment

First episodes of all types of HSV infection benefit from treatment. For both orolabial and genital herpes, oral acyclovir, famciclovir, and valacyclovir are all effective. Treatment of recurrent episodes of HSV-1 or HSV-2 is somewhat unsatisfactory. Although treatment may reduce the duration of symptoms somewhat, especially in HSV-2, the results are not dramatic. Some patients find early institution of therapy, as soon as prodromal symptoms such as tingling or itching

appear, to be helpful. For patients with frequent, severe, recurrent genital herpes, suppressive therapy can be helpful, and any of the three antivirals mentioned above may be used. HSV encephalitis should be treated with acyclovir 10 mg/kg Q8H intravenously for a minimum of 14 days. Disseminated HSV infection, particularly in the immunosuppressed host, usually requires high-dose intravenous therapy.

KEY POINTS

Diagnosis and Treatment of Herpes Simplex Virus

1. Diagnosis clinically, immunofluorescence, and viral culture. CSF PCR for encephalitis.
2. Treatment for primary skin infections (acyclovir, famciclovir, or valacyclovir).
3. Recurrent episodes more controversial, can treat during the prodrome, suppressive therapy may be used for recurrent genital herpes.
4. High-dose intravenous acyclovir for encephalitis or disseminated disease.

Cytomegalovirus

Epidemiology

Human cytomegalovirus (CMV) is a common infection worldwide. Prevalence of the infection varies greatly based on socioeconomic factors, although there is no clear link to hygienic practices. In the United States anywhere from 40% to 80% of children are infected by puberty. Young children may be a major source of infection for adults, and caretakers of young children have a 20-fold increased risk of infection. Person-to person spread can occur by contact with almost any human body fluid or substance, such as blood, urine, saliva, cervical secretions, feces, breast milk, or semen. The virus is also therefore spread by sexual contact and by blood and organ transfusion.

Pathophysiology and Clinical Manifestations

Most human CMV infections are thought to be subclinical, but occasionally, primary infection in the normal host results in a mononucleosis syndrome. CMV is thought to cause approximately 10% of mononucleosis cases and is the major cause of heterophile (Monospot)-negative mononucleosis. CMV mononucleosis is more common in slightly older adults but can be difficult to distinguish clinically from EBV-associated mononucleosis. Although it has been suggested that pharyngitis and cervical adenopathy are less common with CMV, both may be observed with CMV mononucleosis. The fever in CMV mononucleosis lasts on average for more than three weeks. Rash is present in about 30% of patients, and ampicillin provocation of rash has been noted. Other complications of CMV infections in the normal host include hepatitis, pneumonitis, and Guillain-Barré syndrome. Many of the laboratory findings of EBV mononucleosis are also seen in CMV infection.

CMV infection in the immunocompromised host produces most of the morbidity and mortality associated with CMV. CMV infects and produces severe disease in several organ systems, and syndromes include retinitis, hepatitis, pneumonitis, GI disease (gastric and esophageal ulcers and colitis), and polyradiculopathy. Further details of the management of these complications are discussed elsewhere (see Chapter 17).

Diagnosis

Culture of virus is not a useful test for diagnosing CMV infection in the normal host. Virus may be shed for long periods in the urine and intermittently by persons infected in the past. The most reliable test is a fourfold rise in IgG titer to CMV. IgM detection also provides strong evidence for acute infection, although this can occasionally be seen in normal hosts during reactivation. Diagnosis of the various manifestations of CMV disease in the immunocompromised host is discussed elsewhere.

Treatment

Antiviral treatment of CMV infection is almost never required in the normal host, and spontaneous resolution is almost invariable, even after a lengthy illness. However, corticosteroids may be used for the same autoimmune or hematologic complications as in EBV infection. In those rare cases in which CMV appears to be causing specific organ-system disease such as esophagitis, in the normal host ganciclovir may be administered. In the immunocompromised host ganciclovir or foscarnet is frequently required to control end organ CMV infections.

KEY POINTS
Cytomegalovirus Infection

1. A common worldwide infection. In the U.S. 40–80% of children positive.
2. Young children are the primary source of infection for adults.
3. Transmitted by blood, urine, saliva, cervical secretions, semen, feces, and breast milk.
4. Many infections are subclinical, leading cause of heterophile-negative mononucleosis.
5. In immunocompromised host causes retinitis, hepatitis, pneumonitis, GI disease (gastric and esophageal ulcers and colitis), and polyradiculopathy.
6. Diagnosis by IgM anti-CMV titer in the normal host.
7. Self-limited disease in the normal host, ganciclovir or foscarnet treatment for the immunocompromised patient.

Additional Reading

Cohen, J.I., and Corey, G.R. Cytomegalovirus infection in the normal host. *Medicine* 64:100–114, 1985.

Couch, R.B. Drug therapy: Prevention and treatment of influenza. *N Engl J Med* 343:1778–1787, 2000.

Duchin, J.S., et al. Hantavirus pulmonary syndrome: A clinical description of 17 patients with a newly recognized disease. *N Engl J Med* 330:949–955, 1994.

Swaminathan, S., and Wang, F. Antimicrobial therapy of Epstein-Barr virus infections. In Yu, V., Merigan, T.C., Barriere, S., et. al. (Eds.), *Antimicrobial Therapy and Vaccines.* Lippincott Williams & Wilkins, Baltimore, 2002.

Vazquez, M., LaRussa, P.S., Gershon, A.A., Steinberg, S.P., Freudigman, K., and Shapiro, E.D. The effectiveness of the varicella vaccine in clinical practice. *N Engl J Med* 344:955–960, 2001.

Reuben Ramphal

Chapter

16

Infections in the Immunocompromised Host

Time Recommended to Complete: 1 day

Guiding Questions

1. How should immunocompromised hosts be classified and why?
2. What pathogens most commonly infect neutropenic patients?
3. What pathogens are responsible for infection in patients with defects in cell-mediated immunity?
4. How should bone marrow transplant patients be classified?
5. Do all immunocompromised hosts with fever require empiric antibiotics?

Potential Severity: Rapid evaluation and empiric antibiotics are required in the febrile neutropenic patient. High-grade life-threatening bacteremia is common.

Introduction

Medical advances in the management of malignancies and organ failure have given rise to a population of patients that is now commonly called the immunocompromised host. Immunocompromised hosts are patients with leukemias, lymphomas, and solid tumors who are receiving cytotoxic chemotherapy or other chemotherapy, bone marrow transplants including stem cell transplants, and all solid organ transplants. Additionally, the use of a number of immunosuppressive agents and immune modulators for inflammatory disorders has added to this expanding number of patients whose major host defense mechanisms are in some way not optimally functioning to combat environmental as well as endogenous organisms. These failures result in infections by both normally accepted human pathogens and human saprophytes but also by environmental organisms of low intrinsic virulence.

One of the most striking examples of this type of host is the patient with AIDS who advances from being susceptible to virulent organisms such as *Mycobacterium tuberculosis* that are controlled by cell-mediated immunity to being susceptible to organisms that are relatively avirulent such as *Pneumocystis carinii* and later, as the patient's immunity wanes even further, to saprophytic mycobacteria, latent viruses, and parasites. Many of the ideas discussed in this chapter apply to the AIDS patient (see Chapter 17). However, the AIDS patient does not generally demonstrate the other major defect, loss of mucosal barriers and circulating neutrophils, that is seen following cytotoxic chemotherapy. Another type of immunocompromised host that should be kept in mind is the patient with an immunodeficiency syndrome that has a genetic basis. Most of these become apparent in childhood, presenting with histories of recurrent sinopulmonary infections or skin infections, most often due to bacterial agents. The management of such patients is best discussed in the pediatric literature. Thus in the truest sense, the population under discussion should be called the "medically or iatrogenically compromised host," since compromise results mainly from treatment of an underlying disease. Finally, careful attention must be paid to the splenectomized patient, who is compromised in his or her ability to make opsonic antibody against encapsulated

bacteria and is susceptible to overwhelming sepsis caused mainly by pneumococci and *Haemophilus influenzae*.

Immunocompromised patients can be divided into three main types, although there may be overlaps in the populations, as will be discussed:

1. Patients whose major defect is caused by cytotoxic therapy or irradiation and for whom the major defect is neutropenia and mucosal barrier damage
2. Patients whose major defect is suppression of cell-mediated immunity due to truly immunosuppressive agents to control organ rejection or inflammation
3. Patients who show both forms of compromise

It is absolutely essential that these distinctions be made at the initial patient encounter, since important decisions about diagnostic approaches and the need for immediate empiric therapy and its type need to be made on the basis of this assessment. Stated another way, one must distinguish between neutropenia and immunosuppression as the cause of the host compromise, since they predispose to different types of infections. The categorization of common medically compromised patients is shown in Figure 16.1. It becomes evident that some defects will be temporary, until repair mechanisms are fully functional, for example, until the bone marrow recovers, mucosal regeneration has occurred, or immunosuppressive agents have been stopped. Some will be lifelong, since immunosuppression may be required to maintain organ function or control inflammation. A full understanding of these classifications and their application to specific populations will provide a firm foundation in managing the immunocompromised host.

KEY POINTS
Classification of Immunocompromised Patients

1. Neutropenic patients are defined as having a neutrophil count of <500 mm³:

Figure 16.1

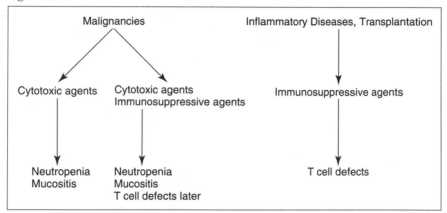

Pathways leading to the immunocompromised host.

a. Risk of infection increases as the cell number decreases further,
    b. Caused by cancer chemotherapy that depresses the bone marrow.
2. Cell-mediated immune deficiencies:
    a. Associated with corticosteroids,
    b. Follows immunosuppression for organ transplantation.
3. Mixed defects:
    a. Bone marrow transplant patients in the early stages are neutropenic,
    b. After the bone marrow repopulates, they have depressed cell-mediated immunity.

◆ **CASE 16.1**

A 51-year-old Caucasian male received high Ara C induction for relapse of his acute lymphocytic leukemia. Two days after completion of his 7-day course of chemotherapy his absolute neutrophil count was 0 cells/mm³. He developed a fever 1 day later and was begun on mezlocillin and gentamicin. Over the next 48 hours he remained febrile and developed a 2 × 2 cm black skin lesion on his right thigh. The lesion was dark black and necrotic in appearance and was mildly painful to the touch. Tissue biopsy revealed sheets of Gram-negative rods and four of four blood cultures drawn at the onset of fever were positive for *Pseudomonas aeruginosa*, *E. coli*, and *Klebsiella pneumoniae*. His antibiotic regimen was switched to ceftazidime and gentamicin. Over the next week his neutrophil count increased, and he defervesced.

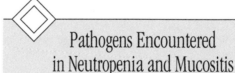

Pathogens Encountered in Neutropenia and Mucositis

Bacteria

Neutrophils and mucosal barriers are the principal mechanisms for preventing the majority of bacteria from entering the bloodstream via the skin, gut, oral cavity, and respiratory tract. Practically, neutropenia is defined as a circulating neutrophil count of <500 neutrophils/mm³ of blood. The lower the numbers of circulating neutrophils, the higher is the incidence of infections, and the more severe and more difficult they are to treat, especially if tissue is involved. While neutrophils are capable of ingesting all bacteria, they are ineffective in killing facultative intracellular parasites such as Salmonella, Listeria, and Nocardia. Therefore a reduction in the number of neutrophils does not predispose to infections by these bacteria. It is generally accepted that such organisms are not among the primary pathogens to be found in the neutropenic patient. Instead, it is the plethora of common bacteria that are found as commensal or saprophytic organisms on the host and in the environment that are the chief offenders. The sources of the organisms in this setting will be mainly the skin, oral cavity, and gastrointestinal (GI) tract and any organisms that are introduced by cross-contamination from environmental sources. Examples of environmental cross-infection are organisms ingested in food at a time when the gut has been denuded by cytotoxic chemotherapy. The bacteria that are most commonly reported are listed with their probable sources in Table 16.1. In Case 16.1 it is likely that the patient's bacteremia originated from the GI tract. As in this case, polymicrobial bacteremia is commonly encountered with severe neutropenia. There are, of course, many more species found in these environments, any of which may be found in the neutropenic patient. Remarkably, anaerobic Gram-negative rods such as Bacteroides are not frequent causes of bacteremias in neutropenic patients despite their large numbers in the GI tract.

Fungi

Bacteria are not the only members of the human or environmental flora that infect the neutro-penic patient. Organisms that exist in lower numbers and that are resistant to antibacterial agents, yeasts and molds, for example, also play a significant role in infection in the neutropenic patient, since neutrophils are also the first line of defense against some of these agents. However, it should be borne in mind that some of these organisms are also held in check by cell-mediated immunity, and they also appear in patients in whom this arm of host defenses is compromised. In patients with neutropenia and mucositis fungi are generally not among the earliest pathogens to accompany fever in the neutropenic patient (febrile neutropenic patient). Early in neutropenia bacteria are the main pathogens, but when neutropenia is prolonged and profound, because fungi are resistant to conventional antibiotics, they have a selective advantage and overgrow as the normal bacterial flora is eliminated. Hence fungal infections are often referred to as "superinfections," because they occur while patients are receiving antibacterial agents. Occasionally, when a patient has received antibiotics in the recent past and the level of fungal colonization in the gut is high, fungi may emerge as primary pathogens early in neutropenia before antibiotics are given, or they may infect a central venous catheter from the skin, particularly Candida species. Some fungi, such as Aspergillus species, may be acquired early by inhalation from the environment but not become symptomatic until much later, after the organism has multiplied sufficiently in the lung and has invaded lung parenchyma and blood

Table 16.1

Sources of Bacteria That Commonly Infect Neutropenic Patients

SKIN	ORAL CAVITY	GUT
Coagulase-negative staphylococci	Viridans streptococci	*E. coli,* Klebsiella
		Other enteric bacteria
S. aureus	Oral anaerobes	Gut anaerobes
		Enterococci
		Pseudomonas aeruginosa

vessels, thus appearing to be a superinfection. Fungi that may appear early in neutropenia are *Candida albicans, C. tropicalis, C. krusei, C. glabrata,* other Candida species, and rarely Aspergillus species. Certain fungi that cause severe infections in other populations, such as Mucor species, are infrequently encountered in the neutropenic patient.

KEY POINTS

Infections Associated with Neutropenia and Mucositis

1. Infecting organisms primarily arise from the skin, oral cavity, and GI tract.
2. Bacteria include *Staphylococcus epidermidis, S. aureus, S. viridans,* enterococcus, enteric Gram-negatives, Pseudomonas; anaerobes less common.
3. Fungal infections develop after antibiotic therapy has had time to reduce the bacterial flora; Candida and Aspergillus species are most common.

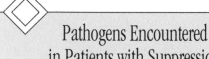

Pathogens Encountered in Patients with Suppression of T Cell Functions

These patients make up an increasing large number of individuals with a variety of underlying diseases. Initially, patients receiving corticosteroids were the major group of patients falling into this category. However, with the increased popularity of organ transplantation and the use of antirejection therapies directed primarily against T cells, transplant patients have become an important population in this category. Bone marrow transplant recipients receiving allogeneic cells represent a mixed group of patients who initially are neutropenic until the bone marrow is reconstituted and also develop T cell defects

as immunosuppression is continued to prevent rejection or to treat graft-versus-host disease.

Bacteria

Patients whose main defect is immunosuppression have increased susceptibility to only a few bacterial agents. These include Mycobacteria species, *Listeria monocytogenes,* and Nocardia species; rarely, they may have a Salmonella species. While they may become infected with common bacteria, this is not normally the result of their immunosuppression but is usually due to other medical interventions such as an indwelling catheter. Community-acquired infections caused by common bacterial agents should not be neglected as possible sources of fever.

Fungi

In addition to unusual bacteria, patients with T cell defects resulting from immunosuppression are susceptible to many species of fungi, both yeast and filamentous forms. The most common fungal organism is *Cryptococcus neoformans,* which is encountered during chronic immunosuppression in the transplant population. The filamentous fungi that are most important are Aspergillus species, Fusarium species, and the Mucor/Rhizopus group. Depending on geographic location *Histoplasma capsulatum* and *Coccidioides immitis* are also important pathogens in these patients. Increasingly, there are also reports of the so-called black, or dematiaceous, fungi causing infections. A wide variety of fungal pathogens have been reported, and listing all of the offending pathogens is beyond the scope of this chapter. The basic principle that needs to be remembered is that patients with depressed T cell function become infected with fungal organisms that are generally of low virulence in a normal host. Remarkably, the most common yeastlike species such as Candida do not cause infection in this population, a finding suggesting that these species are primarily controlled by neutrophils. The role of filamentous fungal infections in organ transplantation cannot be overemphasized; when they occur, cure is extremely difficult in the face of continued immunosuppression, and death is a common outcome.

Viruses

T cells and antibodies are the most important arms of the host defense mechanisms in defending against viral infections. In most instances cell-mediated and humoral immunity function together to prevent and control active viral infections. The patient with T cell defects following immunosuppression is likely to have pre-existing antibody against many viruses unless there has been total ablation of existing T cells and reconstitution with immunologically naive cells. Usually, reconstituted donor populations contain memory cells to make antibody, although the response may be blunted. Therefore transplant patients tend to be more susceptible to viruses that are latent in the body rather than becoming infected with new viruses. Loss of cell-mediated immunity allows latent viruses to reactivate. Additionally, patients may acquire such infections from transfused blood components or a transplanted organ. The main viruses that are seen as a result of reactivation are cytomegalovirus (CMV), herpes simplex, herpes zoster, Epstein-Barr virus, and hepatitis B and C viruses. Those most often acquired by transfusion or donor organ are CMV and Epstein-Barr virus. Other uncommon viruses such as HHV-6 have also been implicated as a cause of active infection in these patients.

The vast majority of viral syndromes in transplant patients are due to reactivation or acquisition of CMV. The hallmark of CMV reactivation is their late onset after transplantation, active infection usually developing from four to six weeks to more than 12 months after transplantation. The clinical presentation is often fever, but pneumonia, hepatitis, and colitis are also seen.

CMV retinitis is rare in this population compared to its incidence in AIDS patients.

Other Organisms Seen in Patients with T Cell Defects

This population is also at risk from a variety of other unusual agents. Among these are *P. carinii*, a fungus that is latent in the lungs and that was particularly prevalent in children treated for acute lymphocytic leukemia and organ transplant patients on corticosteroid therapy. Currently, this infection is highly associated with undiagnosed AIDS, since antibiotic prophylaxis with trimethoprim-sulfamethoxazole has dramatically reduced the incidence among patients with malignancies and transplantation. Another unusual organism that is encountered to a lesser degree is *Toxoplasma gondii,* a parasite that is primarily reactivated from an old infection (see Chapter 17). Rarely, disseminated Strongyloides, a worm, has also been seen in patients on chronic corticosteroid therapy (see Chapter 12).

KEY POINTS
Infections in Patients with Defective Cell-Mediated Immunity

1. Can be infected with the same community-acquired pathogens as normal hosts.
2. Increased risk of bacterial infections with Mycobacteria species, *Listeria monocytogenes,* Nocardia species, and Salmonella species.
3. Fungal infection is often life threatening and may be difficult to diagnose:
   a. Cryptococcus most common,
   b. Aspergillus species, Fusarium species, and the Mucor/Rhizopus group,
   c. Histoplasmosis or coccidiomycosis depending on geographical location,
   d. Dematiaceous fungi, or black mold.
4. Reactivation of old viral infections a major concern:

a. CMV most common, due to reactivation, blood transfusion, or infected organ transplant,
b. EBV less common.
5. Other pathogens include Pneumocystis, toxoplasmosis, disseminated strongyloidiasis.

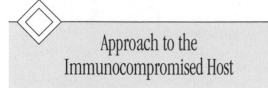

Approach to the Immunocompromised Host

In approaching the febrile compromised host or even a compromised host who has a site of infection, one should refrain from generalizations about the medical urgency required for treatment until the patient is properly classified. The guiding principle to be followed is that the type of infecting organism and hence empiric therapy and need for urgency is chiefly governed by the type of host compromise. Not every compromised host requires empiric antibiotic therapy. The following questions and algorithm are therefore suggested.

The Febrile Neutropenic Patient

Is the patient neutropenic from recent cytotoxic chemotherapy?

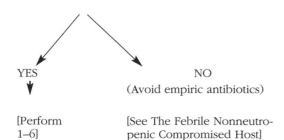

YES

[Perform 1–6]

NO
(Avoid empiric antibiotics)

[See The Febrile Nonneutropenic Compromised Host]

1. Physical examination for sites of infection: lungs, skin, biopsy new skin lesion.
2. Blood, urine, and any other suspicious sites cultured.
3. Chest radiograph: If infiltrate is detected, bronchoscopy with lavage is usually indicated because of the wide variety of potential pathogens and the common occurrence of a nonproductive cough in the neutropenic patient.
4. Begin empiric antibiotic therapy with a single antibiotic or combination therapy, generally an antipseudomonal cephalosporin with good Gram-positive activity (cefepime or ceftazidime), a carbapenem alone (imipenem), or an antipseudomonal beta-lactam plus an aminoglycoside (ticarcillin-clavulanate or piperacillin tazobactam + gentamicin or tobramycin or amikacin). The outcomes of therapy are identical. Vancomycin as empiric therapy is indicated only if there is clinical evidence of a line-associated infection or heavy colonization with methicillin-resistant *Staphylococcus aureus* (MRSA).
5. Further management will depend on response to therapy and culture results.
6. Antifungal agents are rarely needed within the first 96 hours after the institution of antibiotics.

Most patients with fever and neutropenia will fit into the category of fevers of unknown origin; that is, all cultures will be negative. However, it should be borne in mind that the absence of neutrophils blunts the inflammatory response, and such patients may have a site of infection that is not obvious. Such patients may have an abscess without "pus." Therefore all suspicious complaints must be thoroughly explored. One such infection is perirectal abscess. Management with antibiotics alone is generally unsuccessful. Proper management requires that a clinical diagnosis be made and surgical drainage be performed. Careful examination of the skin must be repeated daily. As is illustrated in Case 16.1, disseminated infection often seeds the skin, producing discrete lesions. All new skin lesions, no matter how benign in appearance, should be biopsied for histopathology and culture, and these often provide the diagnosis before blood cultures turn positive. In Case 16.1 the skin lesion appearance was characteristic of ecthyma gangrenosum, a septic lesion that is commonly associated with *Pseudomonas aeruginosa* bacteremia.

Following initiation of empiric antibiotics the patient should be reassessed after receiving antibiotics for 96 hours. If fever of greater than 38°C (100.4°F) persists, antifungal therapy is recommended. In the past amphotericin B was empirically initiated; however, recently, voriconazole has been shown to achieve similar outcomes with reduced infusion-related reactions and reduced nephrotoxicity. Transient visual changes and hallucinations, however, develop in a significant percentage of voriconazole-treated patients (see Chapter 1). Another advantage of voriconazole is the ability to switch to an oral preparation after the patient has improved, allowing earlier discharge from the hospital.

Increasingly, the febrile neutropenic patient is being managed as an outpatient, particularly if he or she is expected to have a short duration of neutropenia and does not have other serious illnesses. These are generally patients with solid tumors or lymphomas. Oral antibiotics are administered at home for a fever in these low-risk patients; if their fevers do not respond, they are then hospitalized for further care. One can expect that such management will become more commonplace in the future.

KEY POINTS

Management of the Neutropenic Patient

1. Careful physical exam: Careful exam of lungs, perirectal area, and skin, biopsy new skin lesions.
2. Culture all sites, including blood cultures.

3. Chest X-ray: If infiltrate, consider bronchoscopy with lavage.
4. Empiric antibiotics:
   a. Monotherapy with cefepime, ceftazidime, or imipenem,
   b. Dual therapy with ticarcillin-clavulanate or piperacillin-tazobactam + aminoglycoside,
   c. Catheter-related infection, colonized with MRSA, add vancomycin.
5. Reassess at 96 hours; if fever persists, add antifungal therapy (amphotericin B or voriconazole).
6. Outpatient management of fever is increasing in popularity.

The Febrile Nonneutropenic Compromised Host

The number of possible organisms that can infect this patient population is so large that empiric therapy is *not* recommended unless a specific site of infection is identified or unless after evaluation a specific pathogen is thought to be the most likely cause. Even cellulitis may have a nonbacterial origin. Empiric therapy may be given for central catheter or urinary tract infections because these tend to be the usual organisms. These patients are also susceptible to the usual community-acquired infections, both bacterial and viral, and often come from the community for evaluation of an infectious illness. Therefore a thorough history should be obtained, including details of onset of the fever, family illnesses, the underlying reason for immunosuppression, and the dose and length of time on immunosuppressive therapy. Patients who have lived in certain geographic areas may have activation of latent infections or succumb to specific infections, for example, histoplasmosis in the Ohio River valley and coccidioidomycosis in the Southwest. However, none of the specific infections in this patient population require immediate empiric therapy. Emergent anti-infective therapy is usually not life saving in this patient population. Certain sites of infection, however, do require urgent diagnostic action:

1. Patients with a headache or other central nervous system complaints should have a lumbar puncture performed if this can be done safely. Cryptococcal meningitis and Listeria meningitis are the most urgent diagnoses and do require immediate treatment.
2. Any suspicious sites should be cultured, along with blood and urine. A urinalysis is helpful, since these patients are not neutropenic
3. An inflamed central line may be treated presumptively for Gram-positive infection
4. If chest X-ray is abnormal and the patient is producing sputum, a sample should be cultured and sent for Gram, acid-fast, and silver stains. If there is no sputum, urgent pulmonary and infectious diseases consultations should be requested for a diagnostic evaluation. Because the number of possible causes of pulmonary infection is so large in this population, empiric therapy is not recommended unless there is respiratory failure.
5. If the patient is febrile but none of the above yields a diagnosis, obtain an infectious diseases consultation. The entities causing fever in the setting of a normal initial evaluation are so diverse that much time and resources can be easily wasted.

While the approach outlined above is most applicable to the transplant population, it must not be forgotten that the greatest numbers of immunosuppressed patients are those receiving corticosteroids. While there has been much debate about what dosages of these agents predispose to infection, a useful general rule is to assume that any dose above physiologic maintenance may be immunosuppressive. Doses as low as 10 mg/day of prednisone have led to invasive pulmonary aspergillosis. Therefore when

the physician is faced with a febrile nontransplant patient on corticosteroids for an inflammatory disorder, the points discussed above should be kept in mind. Finally, since immunosuppressive agents may blunt an inflammatory response, the clinician should consider that even low-grade temperatures may indicate the presence of a serious infection.

Patients with Mixed Deficits

Hematologic transplantation, of which there are now many varieties, presents a mixed picture. The complexity of the care of these patients requires the early input of a subspecialist. Immediately after transplantation the physician is faced with the problems of the neutropenic patient. Later, after bone marrow or cell engraftment has occurred, the patient suffers from the same infections as the organ transplant patient: fungi, viruses, and facultative intracellular bacteria. Of note, however, patients with graft-versus-host disease demonstrate an increased incidence of invasive pneumococcal infections and suffer a high fatality rate from three months to years after transplantation. This predisposition is attributable to several factors: functional hyposplenism due to total body irradiation and chronic graft-versus-host disease, decreased IgG2, and decreased specific pneumococcal antibody production.

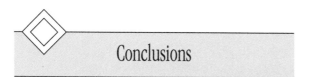

Conclusions

There will continue to be a large population of medically compromised hosts with advances in the treatment of malignancies and transplantation. These patients fit into two general categories that predispose them to infections that are controlled by either neutrophils or T cells. The bone marrow or stem cell transplant fits into both categories depending on the time after transplantation. The febrile neutropenic patient can be considered a near medical emergency and requires empiric antibacterial therapy with one or two broad-spectrum antibiotics. The patient with immunosuppression as opposed to neutropenia requires a thorough evaluation and does not require urgent empiric antibiotic therapy unless the cause of the fever is known on presentation. It is advisable that these patients be cared for by specialists in the area of infections. One can expect that outpatient management of these patients will become increasingly common.

Additional Reading

Bodey, G.P., Buckley, M., Sathe, Y.S., and Freireich, E.J. Quantitative relationships between circulating leukocytes and infection in patients with acute leukemia. *Ann Intern Med* 64:328–340, 1966.

Fishman, J.A., and Rubin, R.H. Infection in organ-transplant recipients. *N Engl J Med* 338:1741–1751, 1998.

Hughes, W.T., Armstrong, D., Bodey, G.P., Bow, E.J., Brown, A.E., Calandra, T., Feld, R., Pizzo, P.A., Rolston, K.V., Shenep, J.L., and Young, L.S. 2002 guidelines for the use of antimicrobial agents in neutropenic patients with cancer. *Clin Infect Dis* 34:730–751, 2002.

Koh, A., and Pizzo, P.A. Empirical oral antibiotic therapy for low risk febrile cancer patients with neutropenia. *Cancer Invest* 20:420–433, 2002.

Sickles, E.A., Greene, W.H., and Wiernik, P.H. Clinical presentation of infection in granulocytopenic patients. *Arch Intern Med* 135:715–719, 1975.

Walsh, T.J., Pappas, P., Winston, D.J., et al. Voriconazole compared with liposomal amphotericin B for empirical antifungal therapy in patients with neutropenia and persistent fever. *N Engl J Med* 346:225–234, 2002.

Bernard Hirschel

HIV Infection

Recommended Time to Complete: 3 days

Guiding Questions

1. How is HIV primarily transmitted and how do genital ulcers increase the risk of HIV?
2. Which cells does the HIV virus primarily infect?
3. What are the symptoms and signs of primary HIV infection?
4. What is the preferred test for diagnosis of HIV and how is AIDS defined?
5. What is meant by the term "the window period"?
6. How is HIV activity monitored?
7. Below what level of CD4 count does the host begin to have opportunistic infections?
8. What are the indications for initiating antiretroviral therapy?
9. What are the goals for therapy and what factors increase the risk of developing resistance?

Potential Severity: Management of HIV is challenging and complex. The associated opportunistic infections are often difficult to diagnosis and are often life-threatening.

Epidemiology

Originating in Eastern Africa, possibly through transmission of a precursor virus from a chimpanzee between 1910 and 1950, HIV infection has now spread across the world. Sub-Saharan Africa remains the epicenter of the epidemic:

There are 3–4 million new infections per year in that region, 30 million Africans live with HIV, and more than 10 million have already died of the disease. Uganda alone has lost 2 million people to AIDS, with 300–400 deaths per day, every day from 1985 to 2002, in a country with a population of 20 million. In the sub-Saharan countries transmission occurs predominantly by heterosexual intercourse, as many women as men being infected. On average, infected women are younger than infected men, but the infection predominates in the most productive age strata, a feature that contributes to the disastrous socioeconomic impact of the AIDS epidemic.

North America's and Western Europe's problems pale in comparison with those of Africa. Nonetheless, the number of HIV-infected persons living in the United States has reached almost 1 million. Incidence figures are difficult to determine because most newly acquired infections are not diagnosed. Judging from the number of patients who had a first HIV-positive test (which may be due to an infection acquired years earlier), infection rates declined during the 1990s, reaching a plateau around 1998. Some reports claim that there has been a slight increase since 1998, perhaps due to an increase in sexual risk taking linked to a false sense of security created by the existence of highly active antiretroviral therapies (HAART). However, HAART may also decrease transmission of HIV by decreasing viremia.

The probability of HIV infection varies depending on the type of exposure. Transfusion with a unit of HIV-infected blood is almost certain to infect the recipient. In the absence of treatment the child of an HIV-positive mother has about a 30% chance of infection. The chance of infection after getting stuck by an infected needle is about 1 in 300.

Most infections occur by sexual exposure. The primary determinant of infectivity is the level of viremia. Local genital factors modulate that risk. Inflammation such as may be caused by sexually transmitted diseases attracts lymphocytes, which may harbor HIV and in the recipient may provide a reservoir of cells which are vulnerable to HIV infection.

Per act of vaginal or anal intercourse and compared to other sexually transmitted diseases, the risk of infection with HIV is quite low. Depending on the viremia, it varies from roughly 1% to 0.01%. In the presence of genital ulcers, infection rates as high as 10% have been reported. This compares with rates of 20–40% after exposure to syphilis or gonorrhea. Nonetheless, repeated sexual exposure, as occurs in a serodiscordant couple, entails substantial risk, typically reaching 1% per month. It is likely that the risk is higher during the first months of a sexual partnership than later; indeed, some studies show HIV-specific, potentially protective cellular immune response in seronegative sexual partners of seropositive persons. Absence of infection in the past is no guarantee for the future, however; increasing immune deficiency and viremia are part of the natural history of untreated HIV infection and carry with them an increased risk of transmission. Anal and vaginal intercourse are approximately equally effective in transmitting HIV. Some but not all studies have found that the risk of transmission from an HIV-infected man to a woman is higher than the other way around. In comparison to vaginal or anal intercourse, oral sex is certainly much less risky, that is, the risk is too low to be quantified. However, examples of transmission by oral sex are known in any sizable HIV center. Condoms are effective in preventing transmission. Transmission was never observed in a large series of couples who declared that they "always" used condoms. However, perfect compliance with using condoms and avoidance of slippage and breakage are difficult to achieve in practice.

Efforts regarding prevention have had varying success:

◆ HIV infection through infected blood products has almost been eliminated. Rare cases (fewer than one transmission in 500,000 blood transfusions) may still occur if blood is donated during the so-called window period.

◆ Use of antiretroviral therapy in the mother has the potential to decrease the mother-to-child transmission rate from more than 30% to less than 1%. Such transmission has now become very rare in Western Europe and the United States and is almost always the result of some procedural failure.

◆ Needle exchange programs and methadone or even heroin substitutions have decreased the incidence of HIV infection in intravenous drug users by more than 90%.

◆ As was noted above, condoms are effective in decreasing HIV transmission, particularly in stable couples. Incidence rates of HIV have decreased in homosexual communities practicing safer sex. The decrease in the prevalence of HIV may have contributed to a reduced rate of infection among younger gays even without necessarily perfect adherence to safer-sex guidelines. Among both homosexuals and heterosexuals subgroups persist with continuing high-risk practices and a high incidence of sexually transmitted diseases and HIV. From 1999 to 2001 several instances of small epidemics of syphilis were reported in Dublin, Bristol, Baltimore, Paris, and California.

In contemplating the use of scarce resources to fight HIV infection, it is important to realize that prevention is much more cost-effective than cure. Even with unrealistically favorable assumptions regarding efficacy and costs of HAART, costs per life year saved are 20–100 times less for condoms than for antiretroviral treatment. But it is the sick who are crying for help, not the healthy who are crying for condoms.

KEY POINTS
Epidemiology of HIV Infection

1. Highest incidence is in Africa, where the virus originated:
   a. 3–4 million new infections per year,
   b. 30 million living with AIDS,
   c. Heterosexual transmission, incidence in men = that in women.
2. North America and Europe have lower incidence and prevalence:
   a. U.S. is approaching prevalence of 1 million,
   b. Incidence has slightly increased since 1998 owing to a change in attitude caused by HAART.
3. Risk of HIV infection:
   a. Very high with a contaminated blood transfusion,
   b. 1/300 for needle stick,
   c. Mother-to-child without treatment = 30%,
   d. Vaginal or anal intercourse: 0.01–1%, genital ulcers increase risk 10×, condoms prevent transmission.
4. Preventive measures are very cost-effective in comparison to treatment.

Pathogenesis of HIV Infection

The primary targets of HIV are probably the dendritic cells in the mucosa of the genital tract. HIV attaches to these cells through a specific receptor called DC-SIGN. The dendritic cells transport HIV into lymph nodes, where HIV infects lymphocytes. The receptors for HIV are mainly the CD4 molecules on the surface of a subpopulation of T lymphocytes. A coreceptor is also necessary for infection. Viruses that preferably interact with the coreceptor CCR5 are called R5 viruses (or monocytotrophic or nonsyncytium-inducing) and predominate in early infection. Later on, HIV often acquires the capacity to interact with the CXCR4 receptor; such viruses are called X4 (syncytium-inducing or lymphocytotrophic). CD4 lymphocytes whose T cell receptor is specific for HIV proteins proliferate and are preferentially infected. This preferential infection followed by destruction may explain the specific immune deficiency toward HIV (see below).

More than 98% of lymphocytes are localized in the lymph nodes and spleen. Nonetheless, the HIV that is produced by the newly infected lymphocytes floods the blood and is transported into all tissues within a matter of days. Viremia reaches high levels, up to millions of HIV genomcs per milliliter. During this time many patients become symptomatic with fever, skin lesions, pharyngitis, and swollen lymph nodes. This self-limited disease (see Figure 17.1), lasting usually a few days to a few weeks, is called primary HIV infection, the acute retroviral syndrome, or seroconversion syndrome. The im-

Figure 17.1

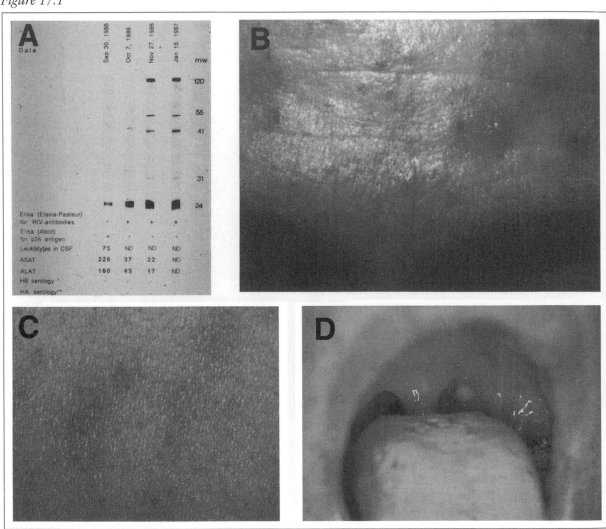

Seroconversion and the acute retroviral syndrome. (A) Appearance of bands on successive Western blots. Note the CSF pleocytosis and elevated transaminase levels. (B) Acneiform lesions during the acute retroviral syndrome. (C) Macules on the chest. The photograph shows about 1 square inch of skin. (D) Ulcerations in the oral cavity during the acute retroviral syndrome. See also Color Plate 3.

mune response kicks in; antibodies directed against HIV appear in the blood, and cytotoxic T cells, specific for HIV-infected cells, proliferate. This HIV immune response rapidly achieves partial control of HIV infection. Viremia levels decrease by several orders of magnitude and stabilize at a lower level, called "plateau level." This level may vary from fewer than 50 to several hundred thousand copies of HIV RNA per milliliter and correlates closely with further evolution toward immune deficiency: The higher the level, the faster is the development of AIDS.

A progressive decrease in the level of CD4 T-cells is the hallmark of HIV-induced immune deficiency. A fall from the normal levels of approximately 1,000 CD4 cells/µl occurs during acute HIV infection. After seroconversion the level of CD4 lymphocytes again rises but rarely returns to normal values. Later, during the chronic phase of HIV infection, there is a progressive loss of about 70 cells/µl per year. However, the speed at which immune deficiency progresses is extremely variable among individuals. In rare cases AIDS may appear as early as one or two years after infection. An incubation period of 10 years is more typical, whereas rare patients, called long-term nonprogressors, show no evidence of damage to the immune system at all and survive many years with low viremia and a normal number of CD4 cells.

An enormous amount of research has been conducted to find factors that influence the rate of progression. Table 17.1 is a summary of genetic traits that are thought to correlate with faster or slower development of immune deficiency. The patient's age at the time of infection also plays a role: The older you are, the more likely it is that progression will be rapid. (The late fetal and perinatal period is an exception; neonatally acquired HIV may progress very rapidly.) Unfortunately, we can change neither our age nor our parents, and no easily influenced factors for progression (e.g., "Drink carrot juice, and you'll never get AIDS") have been found so far.

CD4 cells are the conductor of the immunologic orchestra; they are critical for some of the most important functions, including the development of specific CD8 T cell cytotoxic response and the production of neutralizing antibodies. When the number of CD4 cells decreases below a critical level of about 200/µl, the so-called AIDS-defining diseases start to appear. The list of these diseases (see Table 17.2) is relatively short and very specific: *Pneumocystis carinii* pneumonia rather than aspergillosis and Kaposi's sarcoma and lymphoma rather that many other tumors. Some of these infections are highly suggestive of HIV infection, such as *Pneumocystis carinii* pneumonia, whereas others also occur in patients with normal immune systems or with immune deficiencies other than AIDS, such as pneumococcal pneumonia, Candida stomatitis, and tuberculosis. Most of the opportunistic diseases are caused by the reactivation of latent herpes viruses (e.g., cerebral lymphoma due to Epstein-Barr virus, retinitis due to cytomegalovirus), fungi (*Pneumocystis carinii* pneumonia), or bacteria (tuberculosis). Other infections may be newly acquired, such as salmonella or cryptococcosis.

We noted above that the nascent HIV immune response controls the runaway viral proliferation that is observed during acute HIV infection. How do we explain the eventual failure of this immune response? Despite thousands of papers written on the subject, a clear answer is not at present available. While long-term nonprogressors tend to have a vigorous HIV-specific cytotoxic immune response, the overlap with populations showing progression is considerable. The role of antibodies to HIV is also unclear; in individual cases there is no clear correlation between the existence of neutralizing antibodies and progression. The extreme mutability of HIV leads to the emergence of HIV quasi-species that are no longer recognized by the immune response (the so-called immune escape phenomenon). In addition, HIV infects preferably proliferating lymphocytes, but the lymphocytes that proliferate in response to HIV infection are precisely those whose receptors recognize HIV-derived peptides. Infection of

Table 17.1

Genes That Influence HIV-1 Disease or Response to Treatment

GENE/GENETIC REGION	PROTEIN FUNCTION	INFLUENCE OF POLYMORPHISM[†]
Susceptibility to infection		
CCR5	Chemokine receptor	Decreased susceptibility to infection
RANTES	Chemokine	Decreased susceptibility to infection
Natural history		
CCR5	Chemokine receptor	Delayed (D32) or accelerated (promoter) progression
CCR2	Chemokine receptor	Delayed progression
CX3CR1	Chemokine receptor	Controversial
SDF1	Chemokine	Controversial
MIP-1a	Chemokine	Accelerated progression
RANTES	Chemokine	Controversial
Interleukin-10	Cytokine	Accelerated progression
MBL	Mannose-binding lectin	Controversial
Class I HLA	MHC	Accelerated progression (homozygosity)
HLA-B*5701	MHC	Delayed progression
HLA-B*35	MHC	Accelerated progression
HLA-Cw*04	MHC	Accelerated progression
Response to treatment		
CCR5	Chemokine receptor	Virologic response
MDR1	Drug transporter (PGP)	Drug concentrations and immunologic response
CYP2D6	CYP450 isoenzyme	Drug concentrations
Treatment toxicity		
SREBP-1c	Cholesterol/triglyceride regulator	Hyperlipidemia
*Haplotype HLA-B*5701, DR7, DQ3*	MHC	Hypersensitivity to abacavir

From Telenti, A., Aubert, V., and Spertini, F. Individualising HIV treatment—pharmacogenetics and immunogenetics. *Lancet* 359:722, 2002.
[†]Polymorphism or allele may exert influence not directly but through linkage disequilibrium with other alleles.
MHC = major histocompatibility complex; PGP = P-glycoprotein.

these lymphocytes eventually leads to their destruction.

Effective therapy reverses most of the immune deficiency. CD4 cell counts recover even in patients who had practically no cells left when treatment started. The cell counts continue to increase for several years, finally reaching a plateau of 500–1,000 cells in most patients. The immune response to the most important

pathogens recovers, as can be seen by the disappearance of opportunistic diseases. There is one exception, however: The immune response to HIV itself remains deficient even after successful treatment.

In North America and Western Europe most patients come to medical attention during the so-called latent or plateau period of chronic HIV infection, when clinical signs and symptoms are

Table 17.2

Indicator Conditions in the Case Definition of AIDS (Adults)

Candidiasis, of esophagus, trachea, bronchi, or lungs: 3,846 (16%)

Cervical cancer, invasive: 144 (0.6%)

Coccidioidomycosis, extrapulmonary: 74 (0.3%)

Cryptococcosis, extrapulmonary: 1,168 (5%)

Cryptosporidiosis with diarrhea >1 month: 314 (1.3%)

Cytomegalovirus of any organ other than liver, spleen, or lymph nodes; eye: 1,638 (7%)

Herpes simplex with mucocutaneous ulcer >1 month or bronchitis, pneumonitis, esophagitis: 1,250 (5%)

Histoplasmosis, extrapulmonary: 208 (0.9%)

HIV-associated dementia: disabling cognitive and/or other dysfunction interfering with occupation or activities of daily living: 1,196 (5%)

HIV-associated wasting: involuntary weight loss >10% of baseline plus chronic diarrhea (≥2 loose stools/day ≥30 days) or chronic weakness and documented enigmatic fever ≥30 days: 4,212 (18%)

Isospora belli infection with diarrhea >1 month: 22 (0.1%)

Kaposi's sarcoma: 1,500 (7%)

Lymphoma, Burkitt's: 162 (0.7%), immunoblastic: 518 (2.3%), primary CNS: 170 (0.7%)

Mycobacterium avium, disseminated: 1,124 (5%)

Mycobacterium tuberculosis, pulmonary: 1,621 (7%), extrapulmonary: 491 (2%)

Nocardiosis: <1%

Pneumocystis carinii pneumonia: 9,145 (38%)

Pneumonia, recurrent bacterial (≥2 episodes in 12 months): 1,347 (5%)

Progressive multifocal leukoencephalopathy: 213 (1%)

Salmonella septicemia (nontyphoid), recurrent: 68 (0.3%)

Strongyloidosis, extraintestinal: none

Toxoplasmosis of internal organ: 1,073 (4%)

The numbers and percentages behind the diagnoses indicate the frequencies of occurrence in the database of the Swiss HIV cohort study, an ongoing registry of more than 11,000 patients.

rare or absent. Nonetheless, the infection remains active, with the production of 10^9–10^{11} viral particles per day. At the same time several billion CD4 cells are destroyed and replaced each day. A finding of 10^{11} virus per day means that there is a potential for mutation at every single nucleotide position. It is therefore not surprising that under the selective pressure of a partly effective immune response or of partly effective therapy, resistant mutations rapidly emerge. To obtain a durable antiviral effect, several drugs must be combined to completely abolish viral production. Once this goal has been achieved, emergence of resistance becomes much less likely, and in those circumstances patients may be treated for many years without viral breakthrough. Nonetheless, the virus persists in reservoirs that are not accessible to current treatment. These reservoirs may include nonproductive infection in pools of long-lived lymphocytes. Sensitive molecular techniques suggest that the half-life of this type of reservoir may reach several years, making eradication by continuous treatment unrealistic.

Clinical Manifestations of Primary HIV Infection

The incubation period for symptomatic infection is usually two to four weeks but can be as prolonged as 10 weeks. Onset of fever can be abrupt and is associated with diffuse lymphadenopathy and pharyngitis. The throat is usually erythematous without exudates or enlarged tonsils. Painful ulcers can develop in the oral and genital mucosa (see Figure 17.1). Gastrointestinal complaints are common, many patients experiencing nausea, anorexia, and diarrhea. A skin rash often begins 2–3 days after the onset of fever and usually involves the face, neck, and upper torso. Lesions are small, pink to red macules or maculopapules

(see Figure 17.1). Headache is another prominent symptom, and aseptic meningitis is noted in about one quarter of patients. Headache is often retro-orbital and made worse by eye movements. CSF findings are consistent with viral meningitis: lymphocytes, a normal glucose, and mildly elevated protein. Guillain-Barré syndrome as well as seventh cranial palsy have been reported. The peripheral leukocyte count may be normal or slightly below normal, with a decrease in CD4 lymphocytes, an increase in CD8 lymphocytes, and a CD4 to CD8 ratio commonly less than 1:0. Liver transaminase values may be moderately elevated. The illness is self-limited, severe symptoms usually resolving over two weeks. Lethargy and fatigue may persist for several months.

Laboratory Evaluation of HIV Infection

Diagnosis of HIV Infection

HIV infection is diagnosed by the detection of HIV-specific antibodies in the plasma or serum.

These antibodies appear a few weeks after infection, shortly before or after the symptoms of the acute retroviral syndrome. From studies in which the date of infection is precisely known, for instance, in those infected by a blood transfusion, the delay to the appearance of antibodies can be determined: About 5% of patients seroconvert within 7 days, 50% within 20 days, and more than 95% within 90 days.

There remains a period (called the "window period") during which antibodies cannot be detected in the plasma, although the patient is infected. During a few days the HIV-specific p24 antigen is detectable alone, without antibodies. Therefore some tests now combine the detection of antigen and antibody. The gene amplification (PCR, etc.) tests for the detection of viral genomes should not be used for early diagnosis, as they are both much more expensive and less specific than the antibody tests. The antibody tests remain positive for the lifetime of the HIV-infected person, except possibly in very rare cases in which treatment was started before seroconversion.

HIV antibody tests are among the most reliable of all medical tests, with specificity and sensitivity largely exceeding 99%. Nonetheless, in view of the importance of the diagnosis and the possibility of clerical errors (mislabeled tubes and such), it is recommended to confirm the diagnosis by a second blood sample. This is especially important when the pretest probability is low, raising the proportion of false-positives. Indeterminate test results are much more frequent than true false positives. These arise when substances in the patients' plasma interact with impurities in the HIV antigen preparations. Usually, in these cases the color reaction of the ELISA test is above the threshold for positivity but much below the results of a routine positive test. To diminish these indeterminate reactions, manufacturers are attempting to purify the HIV protein that is used, using recombinant technology. In the presence of an indeterminate test and particularly in the absence of risk factors for HIV infection, the patient should be reassured

that the result is negative, and the negativity should be confirmed by a second test using a different method. Such a method might involve use of the so-called Western blot. With the Western blot, the HIV proteins are first separated by electrophoresis and then blotted onto a nitrocellulose membrane (see Figure 17.1). This membrane is incubated with a dilution of the patient's serum. Specific antibodies fix to the respective HIV proteins, producing a colored band after a coloring reaction. From the position of the band it can be deduced whether the reaction is due to an HIV-specific protein or is nonspecific.

KEY POINTS
Diagnosis of HIV Infection

1. Diagnosis of HIV is made by measuring anti-HIV antibodies.
2. 5% seroconvert within 7 days, 50% within 20 days, and >95% within 90 days.
3. "Window period" = viremia + negative serology, lasts a few days to several weeks.
4. PCR-based tests not recommended for diagnosis.
5. HIV antibody tests highly specific and sensitive.
6. Indeterminant test is usually false positive, confirm by Western blot analysis.

Tests Used for Monitoring of Treatment and Prognosis

Levels of viremia and CD4 count are critical for assessing the need for and response to antiretroviral therapy. To determine the amount of virus, genomic tests are now almost universally used. These tests measure the quantity of HIV genomes per milliliter of plasma. Because the genomes consist of RNA, the RNA first has to be transcribed into DNA, which is then amplified, most often by the polymerase chain reaction (PCR). Patients with untreated HIV infection typically have 500 to 1,000,000 copies of HIV-RNA per milliliter; with treatment this number decreases to undetectability, which means, depending on the test being used, fewer than 5–50 copies of HIV-RNA per milliliter. Ideally, after two to six months of treatment all patients on modern antiretroviral therapy should have fewer than 50 copies of HIV-RNA per milliliter.

Many studies have shown that the long-term prognosis of untreated HIV infection depends on the viremia. However, within this broad correlation there are large interindividual variations, with patients remaining in good health for many years despite a viremia exceeding 100,000 copies per milliliter. For short-term prognosis the CD4 count is more useful. The occurrence of opportunistic infections and tumors is unusual with CD4 counts above 200. Below this value the incidence rises exponentially. It is very unusual for patients to die of AIDS with CD4 counts above 50/ml.

KEY POINTS
Tests for Monitoring Treatment and Prognosis

1. Level of viremia correlates with speed of progression; copies of RNA/ml usually measured by PCR.
2. RNA copies/ml varies from 500 to 1 million; treatment should reduce to < 50 within 6 months.
3. Undetectable varies depending on the sensitivity of the test used, individual test varies by 2×.
4. CD4 count < 200, at risk of opportunistic infections and tumors.
5. CD4 count varies up to 10–30% between counts.

Tests for Antiretroviral Resistance

Although antiretroviral combination therapy is effective in the majority of patients, resistance may occur, and the treatment may need to be adjusted. To guide the choice of therapy, tests measuring antiretroviral resistance have been developed. Two types of tests are in use:

1. Genotypic tests are those that determine the sequence of the relevant viral genes: the reverse transcriptase and the protease genes. The sequence shows the presence or absence of mutations that are associated with antiretroviral resistance. However, with rare exceptions the occurrence of a specific mutation does not predict a specific resistance phenotype. Rather, the combination of many mutations must be considered. The prediction of resistance from such a combination of mutations is called the virtual phenotype.
2. Phenotypic tests excise the relevant gene from amplified patient virus and insert the excised portion into a standard virus of known growth properties. This recombinant virus is then exposed to various drugs, and its resistance is ascertained. Phenotypic tests are more expensive than genotypic tests and take one to three weeks to complete.

The value and use of resistance tests are continued subjects of controversy. It has been difficult to show that these tests improve the outcome of treatment, but they may allow discontinuation of ineffective drugs, thus sparing side effects and expense. The use of resistance testing is discussed further in the section on HIV therapy.

Laboratory Tests in the Management of HIV Infections: Caveats

Modern antiretroviral treatment would be impossible without the use of laboratory tests. However, physician and patient need to be aware of the limits and, in particular, need to avoid overinterpretation of small changes. Thus the precision of the measurement of the viral load is only about 0.3 log (twofold). This means that values of 200 and 400 may actually be the same. Another problem with the interpretation of HIV viremia is the expression "undetectable viremia." Of course, detectability depends on the assay used. Experimental assays with sensitivities of as low as one or three copies per milliliter actually show viremia in almost all patients who have started their treatment during chronic HIV infection. It is unknown whether very low viremias (e.g., fewer than 10 copies per milliliter) are better for the patients than viremias that are detectable but between 10 and 50 copies per milliliter.

In patients whose viremias are low on treatment, some values may nonetheless exceed 50 or 100 copies from time to time. These "blips" of viremia are of no great prognostic significance and should not prompt a change in treatment, whereas values above 500 are clearly predictive of subsequent resistance and escape.

The CD4 count is not a very precise measure. It results from the multiplication of two percentages (the percentage of lymphocytes among leukocytes and the percentage of CD4 positive lymphocytes among all lymphocytes). The number of lymphocytes varies during the day, depending on such things as food, physical activity, and steroid levels. In addition, laboratories and lab technicians vary in their interpretation of the morphology of leukocytes. Therefore CD4 counts may vary as much as 10–30% when counts are repeated at frequent intervals within the same individual.

KEY POINTS
Tests for HIV Drug Resistance

1. Genotype testing detects specific mutations, used to predict resistance.
2. Phenotypic testing inserts viral genes into a standardized viral strain and measures sensitivities; time consuming and expensive.
3. Allows discontinuation of ineffective drugs.

Opportunistic Diseases

◆ CASE 17.1

A 28-year-old African American male was admitted to the hospital with a three-week history of progressive shortness of breath accompanied by a nonproductive cough. Two weeks earlier he was seen by his local doctor for the same complaints and was given an oral antibiotic. He noted no improvement in his symptoms.

Epidemiology: He reported that he had had multiple episodes of unprotected homosexual intercourse 3 years earlier but had been abstinent over the past few months. He denied intravenous drug use and had never smoked cigarettes.

Physical examination: He appeared anxious and short of breath. Vital signs: Temperature 38.2°C, pulse 120/min, blood pressure 110/60, respiratory rate 34/min. He had no lymphadenopathy. Throat: White plaques on his posterior pharynx consistent with thrush. Chest: Clear breath sounds, no rales or rhonchi. Heart: II/VI systolic ejection murmur, no rubs or gallops. Abdomen: No organomegaly. Genitalia: within normal limits. Extremities without edema. Skin clear.

Laboratory findings: ABG on room air, pH 7.44, pCO_2 32, pO_2 62, HCO_3 20. Chest X-ray: Diffuse bilateral interstitial, fluffy infiltrates forming a butterfly pattern. Bronchial lavage Giemsa stain revealed *Pneumocystis carinii*. (See Figure 17.2.)

He was begun on iv solumedrol and trimethoprim-sulfamethoxazole. His shortness of breath gradually improved over the next 3 days, and he was discharged on oral trimethoprim-sulfamethoxazole. HIV antibody was positive and was confirmed by Western blot. CD4 count was 150 cells/μl.

Introduction

Case 17.1 represents a typical example of the primary episode of symptomatic AIDS. Opportunistic infections are a consequence of reactivation of latent infection or acquisition of a new infection, often caused by microorganisms of intrinsically low virulence. Cytomegalovirus, *Toxoplasma gondii,* viruses of the herpes group, *Pneumocystis carinii* (PCP), papovavirus JC (the agent of progressive multifocal leukoencephalopathy), and *Mycobacterium tuberculosis* were usually acquired years before, but they lie dormant as long as the immune response is intact. Once immune deficiency is profound, these microorganisms may start to proliferate. Some of these agents can be isolated long before clinical signs appear. However, progressively, organ damage and symptoms will occur, such as stomatitis and symptomatic esophagitis due to *Candida albicans.* In advanced stages of immune suppression, agents that are usually nonpathogenic can have devastating consequences. Examples include destruction of the retina by CMV and cachexia caused by *M.*

avium, which is present in the blood of 25% of patients with CD4 counts below 10/µl. Several infections can be present at the same time, greatly complicating diagnosis and treatment. Even before HAART, the prevention of opportunistic infections by antibiotics and antivirals prolonged survival and improved the quality of life. Since 1996 HAART has made an enormous difference. Advanced stages of AIDS with chronic diarrhea, cachexia, and central nervous system and pulmonary manifestations have become rare in the United States and Western Europe.

Classification of HIV Infection

The stages of HIV infection are defined by clinical events and by the CD4 lymphocyte count (Table 17.3). This classification, established in

Table 17.3

Stages of HIV Infection

	CLINICAL CATEGORIES*		
CD4 CELL CATEGORIES	**A** ASYMPTOMATIC, OR PGL OR ACUTE HIV INFECTION	**B** SYMPTOMATIC (NOT A OR C)	**C** AIDS INDICATOR CONDITIONS (1987)
>500/mm³ (≥29%)	A1	B1	C1
200–499/mm³ (14–28%)	A2	B2	C2
<200/mm³ (<14%)	A3	B3	C3

Clinical signs associated with clinical stage A
    Primary HIV infection
    Persistent generalized lymphadenopathy (PGL)
    Lack of symptoms (asymptomatic patients)
Clinical signs and symptoms associated with clinical stage B
    Oral candidiasis
    Relapsing vaginal candidiasis
    Herpes zoster
    Localized neoplasia of the cervix
    Any other clinical manifestations not defined by categories A and C
Clinical category C
    Corresponds to the occurrence of a so-called AIDS-defining opportunistic disease as listed in Table 17.2

*Dark shaded areas represent the stages that are defined as AIDS in the United States.

1992, indicates clearly whether the patient is immunosuppressed and whether he or she is symptomatic. The meaning of the word "AIDS" is not the same on both sides of the Atlantic. In the United States every person with a CD4 count below 200 is considered to have "AIDS" (darker shaded area in Table 17.3); alternatively, patients may have AIDS because they have a so-called AIDS-defining opportunistic infection. In Europe the CD4 count does not enter into the definition of AIDS, which remains synonymous with the occurrence of an opportunistic disease as defined in Table 17.2. The stage of HIV infection is defined by the CD4 lymphocyte count (biological stage 1, 2, or 3) and clinical events (A, B, or C). Occurrence of a type C disease defines AIDS. As noted above, in the United States AIDS is also defined by a CD4 count of less than $200/mm^3$ (categories C1, C2, C3, A3, or B3).

KEY POINTS

Classification of HIV Infection

1. Classification is based on CD4 count and clinical symptoms.
2. U.S. and Europe have different definitions of AIDS:
   a. U.S. = CD4 < 200 or an AIDS-defining illness,
   b. Europe = AIDS-defining illness.

Primary and Secondary Prophylaxis

Primary prophylaxis prevents the first occurrence of a disease; secondary prophylaxis prevents relapses after a first episode. Many opportunistic infections in AIDS can be prevented. Patients who should receive such prevention are identified by their CD4 lymphocyte count and by serologic tests with evidence of previous exposure to the infectious agent. For instance, the presence of IgG against *Toxoplasma gondii* in a patient whose CD4 count is below 100 identifies a high risk of cerebral toxoplasmosis. Regular

measures of the CD4 count combined with serologic tests done at the beginning of the follow-up are necessary for a timely start of prevention.

Opportunistic infections have a tendency to relapse. Therefore as long as the underlying immune deficiency is not corrected, secondary prevention is often necessary.

Of course, preventive therapy has risks and side effects such as allergies, resistance development, and drug interactions, but the risk-to-benefit ratio has been proven favorable especially for prevention of PCP and cerebral toxoplasmosis by trimethoprim-sulfamethoxazole. On the other hand, once antiretroviral therapy is efficacious and the CD4 count has risen durably above 200, these preventive measures can be discontinued. Table 17.4 summarizes the common preventive regimens.

KEY POINTS

Prophylaxis

1. Latent infections often activate as cell-mediated immunity wanes.
2. Serologic and skin testing are used to detect latent infections on initial evaluation.
3. Prophylaxis is recommended for CD4 < 200.
4. After treatment of active infections, secondary prophylaxis is often necessary to prevent relapse.
5. Prophylaxis can be discontinued after HAART, when the CD4 is durably > 200.

Pulmonary Infections

The differential diagnosis of pulmonary disease in HIV-infected patients depends on the patient's history (presence of intravenous drug abuse, previous episodes of bacterial pneumonia, exposure to tuberculosis), the CD4 lymphocyte count, and the use of preventive therapy (see Table 17.5). PCP was the initial opportunistic infection in one third of the cases of AIDS during the early years of the epidemic. It re-

Table 17.4

Prophylaxis of Opportunistic Infections

DISEASE	INDICATIONS	DRUGS AND DOSAGE	COMMENTS
Pneumocystis carinii pneumonia (PCP)	Primary prophylaxis if CD4 counts less than 200/μl or after an episode of PCP	Trimethoprim-sulfamethoxazole 800/160 mg one double-strength tablet 3 times a week or 400/80 mg QD	Most effective Protects also against cerebral toxoplasmosis
		Pentamidine aerosols 300 mg once monthly	Doesn't protect against cerebral toxoplasmosis
		Dapsone 50 mg/day plus pyrimethamine 50 mg/day	Add folinic acid 15 mg 2 times per week
Cerebral toxoplasmosis	Primary prophylaxis if CD4 count below 100	Trimethoprim-sulfamethoxazole 800/160 mg 3 times weekly or 400/80 mg QD	Protects also against pneumocystosis
	Secondary prophylaxis	Sulfadiazine 2 gm per day or clindamycin 600 mg TID **plus** pyrimethamine 25 mg QD	
Mycobacteria other than tuberculosis	Primary prophylaxis if CD4 count less than 50/μl	Azithromycin 1200 mg/ week **or** rifabutin 300 mg/day	Rifabutin has many drug interactions, in particular with protease inhibitors
Tuberculosis	Primary prophylaxis if more than 5 mm skin induration with a 5 U tuberculin test	Isoniazid 5 mg/kg/day (maximum 300 mg/day) during 6 month with 40 mg/day of vitamin B6 po	The skin reaction is difficult to interpret with moderate to advanced immune deficiency
Cryptococcosis	Primary prophylaxis if CD4 count is below 50 Secondary prophylaxis after an episode of cryptococcosis	Fluconazole 400 mg per week **or** 200 mg 3 times weekly Fluconazole 200 mg/day	Only in regions with a high incidence
Cytomegalovirus retinitis	Primary prophylaxis if CD4 count below 50 and secondary prophylaxis after an episode of retinitis	Valganciclovir 450 mg/day po	

Table 17.5

Lung Diseases Linked to HIV

DIAGNOSIS	SIGNS AND SYMPTOMS	LABORATORY RESULTS	RADIOLOGY	INITIAL TREATMENTS
Bacterial pneumonia due to *Streptococcus pneumoniae*	Rapid onset of fever, dyspnea, cough, and sputum production	Leukocytosis with neutrophilia, blood cultures often positive	Lobar or diffuse infiltrate	Amoxiclav or cephalosporin
Pneumocystis carinii pneumonia	Fever, dyspnea, cough for several weeks. Auscultation is usually normal	Hypoxemia, elevated LDH, diagnosis through bronchoalveolar lavage	Diffuse reticulonodular interstitial infiltrate	Trimethoprim-sulfamethoxazole
Tuberculosis	Weight loss, fever, cough, night sweats, lymphadenopathy	Positive sputum smear by Ziehl stain; positive sputum and blood cultures; typical histopathology of lymph nodes	Mediastinal adenopathy; variable pulmonary infiltrate; cavitary upper lobe lesions are rare	Isoniazide + rifampin + pyrazinamide + ethambutol
Kaposi's sarcoma	Usually associated with skin or mucosal lesions	Typical lesions seen on bronchoscopy	Nodular infiltrates with perihilar location	Treatment for HIV, rarely radiotherapy or chemotherapy
Interstitial lymphoid pneumonia	Transitory fever and dyspnea	No specific findings	Reticulonodular infiltrates	Possibly steroids; diagnosis by exclusion

mains frequent, but the incidence has greatly decreased through the use of trimethoprim-sulfamethoxazole and HAART. Compared to HIV-negative patients, bacterial pneumonia, in particular that due to *Streptococcus pneumoniae,* is 10–100 times more frequent in HIV-positive patients. Tuberculosis can occur at any degree of immune deficiency but is particularly frequent in patients who have grown up in developing countries.

With a CD4 count above 200 and a lobar infiltrate, the presumptive diagnosis is bacterial pneumonia, and empiric treatment should be started with amoxicillin-clavulanate, a cephalosporin, or one of the quinolones active against Gram-positive bacteria. If immune deficiency is more profound (CD4 count below 200/mm^3), PCP is most likely unless the patient has faithfully taken trimethoprim-sulfamethoxazole prophylaxis. The chest X-ray pattern is helpful in narrowing the diagnostic possibilities (see Table 17.6). However, in all patients, whatever the degree of immune suppression, a definite diagnosis usually requires bronchoalveolar lavage.

Table 17.6

Chest X-Ray and Possible Etiologies

CHEST X-RAY	ETIOLOGY
Normal	Bronchitis
	PCP
Lobar or other focal infiltrates	Bacterial pneumonia
	TB, PCP, cryptococcosis
Diffuse interstitial infiltrates	PCP
	TB
	Bacterial pneumonia
	Atypical pneumonia
	Interstitial lymphocytic pneumonia
Pleural effusion	Bacterial pneumonia
	TB
	Kaposi's sarcoma
Mediastinal adenopathy	TB
	Atypical mycobacteria
	Lymphoma
	Kaposi's sarcoma
Cavities	Lung abscess
	Mycobacterium kansasii
	Rhodococcus equi
	TB
	Staphylococcus aureus
Cysts or bullae	PCP

PNEUMOCYSTIS CARINII PNEUMONIA

DIAGNOSIS AND TREATMENT   As is illustrated in Case 17.1, PCP is a subacute disease. With rare exceptions its occurrence is limited to immunosuppressed patients with a CD4 count of less than 200/µl. Symptoms originate in the respiratory tract (dry cough, dyspnea) and are accompanied by fever (always), weight loss, and fatigue. A prominent symptom is dyspnea on exertion. Initially, patients experience shortness of breath with exercise but do not complain of shortness of breath at rest. Alveolar fluid accumulation associated with pneumocystic infection interferes with oxygen exchange, and patients quickly outstrip the ability of their lungs to supply arterial oxygen. Lung auscultation is usually normal. The chest X-ray (see Figure 17.2), which can be normal, typically shows a reticulonodular bilateral infiltrate that can be asymmetric. Classically, the infiltrates form a butterfly pattern, mimicking pulmonary edema associated with left-sided congestive heart failure. Rarely, the standard chest X-ray shows cystic lesions or a pneumothorax. In cases of PCP prophylaxis by pentamidine inhalations the chest X-ray is often atypical with asymmetrical infiltrates limited to the lung apex. Tests of the peripheral blood are usually nonspecific; however, the LDH is found to be elevated in over 90% of patients with pneumocystic infection. Higher values and a persistent elevation despite appropriate therapy are associated with a poorer prognosis. The Gallium-67 citrate scan is very sensitive and demonstrates increased uptake in infected areas of the lung. However, this test is expensive, time consuming (usually takes 2 days to complete), and nonspecific. Gallium scan is most useful in patients with suspected PCP who have a normal chest X-ray.

The diagnosis of PCP is established by special stains of bronchoalveolar lavage fluid or of sputum induced by the inhalation of 3% NaCl during 30 minutes. If clinical suspicion of PCP is high, it is recommended that treatment be started before confirmation of the diagnosis because PCP can still be found in bronchoalveolar lavage fluid 1–3 days later. In rare cases the diagnosis may necessitate a transbronchial biopsy; this is particularly true if pentamidine inhalations have been used. More sensitive methods have been published, but they have not displaced staining in clinical practice.

Treatment modalities will depend on the gravity of PCP. If the patient is very short of breath, with a pO$_2$ of less than 70 mm, patients will usually be admitted to hospital and treated intravenously. If signs of gravity are absent and if the patient is not nauseated, outpatient treatment is possible. The drug of choice is high-dose trimethoprim-sulfamethoxazole, two dou-

Figure 17.2

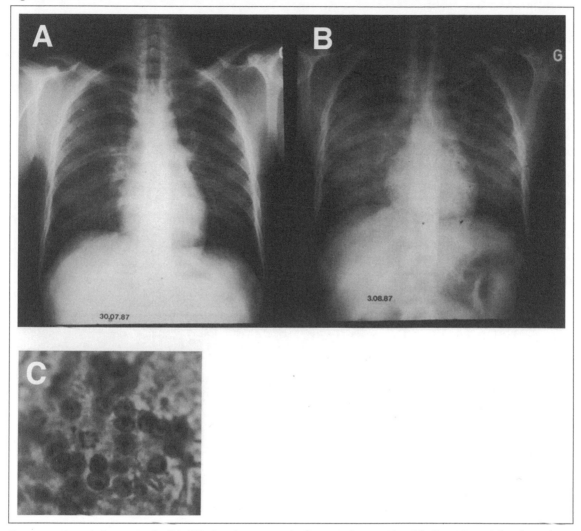

Pneumocystis carinii pneumonia. (A) CXR showing symmetric, fine reticular opacities. (B) Chest X-ray 4 days later showing the typical worsening on therapy. (C) *Pneumocystis carinii* revealed by silver staining in bronchoalveolar lavage sample.

ble-strength (DS) tablets (1,600 mg of sulfamethoxazole and 320 mg of trimethoprim, Q8H for 21 days), followed by secondary prevention using 400 mg of sulfamethoxazole and 80 mg of trimethoprim daily until the CD4 count durably exceeds 200/mm³. Intravenous therapy is indicated in gravely ill patients, particularly those with nausea or vomiting.

Trimethoprim-sulfamethoxazole has numerous side effects, of which drug rashes are the most frequent. If the skin lesions are extensive and in particular if there is mucosal involvement, if leukopenia and thrombocytopenia is severe, or if renal or hepatic toxicity or serious vomiting occurs, alternative treatment is necessary. The addition of folinic acid has been attempted to decrease the incidence of bone marrow suppression; however, it diminishes the efficacy of treatment and is not recommended. There are many alternatives to trimethoprim-sulfamethoxazole, but their efficacy is in general inferior, and many have other serious side effects, which are summarized in Table 17.7.

At the start of the AIDS era patients with PCP, even if correctly treated, often experienced increased respiratory distress and worsening lung infiltrates during the first few days. In many cases this initial degradation necessitated intubation or caused death. Severe respiratory compromise that necessitates intubation can be prevented by giving steroids (1 mg/kg prednisone per day for 5 days, then 40 mg/day for 5 days, followed by 20 mg/day for 11 days) in cases of severe pneumocystosis with a pO_2 below 70 mm Hg. Prednisone should be given prior to or simultaneously with initiation of antipneumocystis therapy.

KEY POINTS

Clinical Manifestations, Diagnosis, and Treatment of PCP

1. A subacute disease that develops in HIV-infected patients with CD4 < 200.

2. Fever, dyspnea on exertion, dry cough, weight loss, and fatigue are the primary symptoms.
3. Pulmonary exam is usually normal.
4. Chest X-ray may be normal but usually demonstrates an interstitial butterfly pattern.
5. LDH is usually elevated, and pO_2 is usually depressed.
6. Treatment: Trimethoprim-sulfa is the drug of choice.
7. Prednisone if pO_2 < 70 mm, given before anti-PCP therapy.

PREVENTION In populations with CD4 counts below 200/mm^3, the risk of PCP is roughly 20% per year; the risk of a relapse after a first episode is even higher: 40% after 6 months. Primary prevention diminishes the risk of pneumocystis; however, if severe immunosuppression persists without highly active antiretroviral therapy, the risk is still 19% after three years of prevention by trimethoprim-sulfamethoxazole and 33% after three years of pentamidine aerosols. Primary and secondary prevention strategies use the same treatment options:

◆ Trimethoprim-sulfamethoxazole DS (800/160 mg) three times per week or one single-

Table 17.7

Treatment of *Pneumocystis carinii* Pneumonia: Trimethoprim-Sulfamethoxazole and Alternatives

SUBSTANCES	DOSAGE	SIDE EFFECTS
Trimethoprim-sulfamethoxazole	Two 800/160 mg pills Q8H or 20 mg/kg/iv/day Q6H	Skin rash, nausea, vomiting, anemia, and leukopenia
Dapsone plus	100 mg po QD	Rash, nausea, and vomiting. Hemolytic anemia in patients with G6PD deficiency
trimethoprim	1.2 gm po QD	
Clindamycin plus	3 × 600 mg po QD	
Primaquine	30 mg po QD	
Atovaquone	2 × 750 mg po QD	Skin lesions, nausea, vomiting, and diarrhea; less efficacious but better tolerated than sulfonamides.

strength (400/80 mg) daily. Trimethoprim-sulfamethoxazole has the advantages of great efficacy, protection against cerebral toxoplasmosis, and low price. However, almost 50% of patients will develop signs of cutaneous intolerance. Desensitizing permits readministration in the majority of cases, but this has been mostly used in cases of treatment, when alternatives to trimethoprim-sulfamethoxazole are clearly less satisfactory. The mechanisms of trimethoprim-sulfamethoxazole intolerance are not well understood. Dose dependency is one of the features that argues against "allergy," as is the observation that up to 60% of patients who have shown cutaneous intolerance do not develop a skin rash when reexposed.

◆ Dapsone, 100 mg/day. This treatment does not protect against cerebral toxoplasmosis. If IgG antitoxoplasma antibodies are present, add pyrimethamine to dapsone. Daily schedules (50 mg dapsone + 50 mg of pyrimethamine QD) or weekly schedules (200 mg of dapsone + 75 of pyrimethamine QW) are equivalent.

◆ Pentamidine by inhalation (Respirgard nebulizer), 300 mg every four weeks. Some patients, particularly smokers, cannot tolerate inhaled pentamidine because of cough and asthma. Preventive use of a bronchodilator may be helpful.

◆ Atovaquone 750 mg/day BID. This treatment is well tolerated but expensive.

KEY POINTS
PCP Prophylaxis

> 1. 20% per year incidence of PCP in HIV patients with CD4 < 200 if not prophylaxed.
> 2. Trimethoprim-sulfa is the drug of choice, efficacious, inexpensive, and prevents toxoplasmosis.
> 3. Alternatives are not as effective:
>   a. Dapsone: Does not cover toxoplasmosis, must add pyrimethamine,
>   b. Pentamidine: Associated with cough and asthma,
>   c. Atovaquone: Expensive.

BACTERIAL PNEUMONIA

Bacterial pneumonia as a complication of HIV infection produces the same symptoms and signs as pneumonias in HIV-negative patients: sudden onset of fever, chills, cough, and dyspnea. By far the most frequent cause is *Streptococcus pneumoniae,* but *Haemophilus influenzae* (particularly in smokers), *Staphylococcus aureus,* and *Pseudomonas aeruginosa* may also be implicated. Bacteremia and relapses are frequent. Empirical treatment consists of amoxicillin-clavulanate or a second- or third-generation cephalosporin; treatment duration is 10–14 days (see Chapter 4).

TUBERCULOSIS

Tuberculosis (TB) usually presents as a subacute disease with weight loss, cough, fever, night sweats, and lung lesions. If immune suppression is very advanced, however, the chest X-ray may be atypical for TB. Interstitial infiltrates may predominate, without cavitary lesions; central nervous system tuberculosis becomes more frequent; mediastinal adenopathy is evident on the chest X-ray; and the blood culture is often positive. Diagnosis relies on the acid-fast stain of the sputum; however, this test is frequently negative in disseminated (miliary) tuberculosis. For culture, liquid media are recommended because results are more rapid; growth is usually evident by 10–14 days, and presumptive identification of the mycobacterium can be made by nucleic acid probes. Susceptibility testing should always be done because multiresistant tuberculosis is a serious threat to the HIV-positive person, the mortality rate exceeding 50%. Initial treatment should include four drugs: isoniazid 300 mg po per day (plus vitamin B6), rifampin 600 mg/day, pyrazinamide 20–30 mg/kg/day, and ethambutol 15 mg/kg/day. This quadruple therapy should be continued during the first two months, followed by isoniazid and rifampin for a further seven months. Patients respond well to classic antituberculous treatment, but without HAART and reversal of the underlying immune deficiency there is a high risk of persistent disease and death as a consequence of other complications of AIDS. In cases of isoniazid and/or rifampin resistance, specialized consultation is advised.

The coadministration of HAART and treatment for TB is a particular problem. On the one hand, protease inhibitors and rifampin modify each others' plasma levels; on the other hand, the concomitant administration of seven or more drugs may be toxic to the liver and gut. In addition, immune reconstitution disease caused by HAART is difficult to distinguish from paradoxic inflammatory reactions, which are sometimes observed at the start of anti-TB treatment. If immune suppression is not very advanced, it is often more reasonable to postpone HAART for a few months while anti-TB drugs take their effect.

KEY POINTS
Tuberculosis in AIDS

1. Usually a subacute disease with weight loss, cough, fever, night sweats, and lung lesions.
2. With severe immunosuppression can present as miliary disease:
   a. Interstitial lung disease,
   b. Meningitis,
   c. Negative sputum AFB smears, but positive blood cultures.
3. Susceptibility testing is critical, multiresistant TB is associated with 50% mortality in AIDS.
4. Four-drug therapy: INH, rifampin, pyrazinamide, and ethambutol. Delay HAART therapy when possible.

MYCOBACTERIUM KANSASII

In HIV-positive patients, *Mycobacterium kansasii* causes a disease that resembles classical TB with fever, cough, weight loss, and pulmonary infiltrates predominating at the apex; more rarely, apical cavities are observed. Classic antituberculous drugs such as isoniazid, rifampin, and ethambutol are efficacious.

Mycobacteria Other Than Tuberculosis (MOTT)

Mycobacterium avium intracellulare (and similar mycobacteria) do not usually cause pulmonary disease but rather a systemic illness with fever, weight loss, night sweats, and liver involvement. However, MOTT are frequently found in sputum, where their pathogenic significance remains uncertain.

PULMONARY KAPOSI'S SARCOMA

In patients with obvious cutaneous Kaposi's sarcoma (KS) (see Figure 17.3) the involvement of mucosal surfaces is frequent (30–50% of cases) and in general asymptomatic. When the lung is involved, the chest X-ray shows reticulonodular infiltrates with a perihilar distribution, hilar lymphadenopathy, and, more rarely, pleural effusions. Treatment by radiotherapy or chemotherapy is indicated for relief of cough or dyspnea. In general, lung lesions as well as other manifestations of Kaposi's sarcoma improve on antiretroviral combination therapy.

OTHER RARE PULMONARY DISEASES

INTERSTITIAL LYMPHOID PNEUMONIA Interstitial lymphoid pneumonia is usually a diagnosis by exclusion; it is particularly frequent in children and presents with fever and dyspnea. The chest X-ray shows reticulonodular infiltrates that may vary and disappear spontaneously. Pathogenesis is not clear; maybe HIV itself is implicated. Treatment relies on corticosteroids.

HISTOPLASMOSIS Contrary to the localized pulmonary disease that is observed in immuno-

Figure 17.3

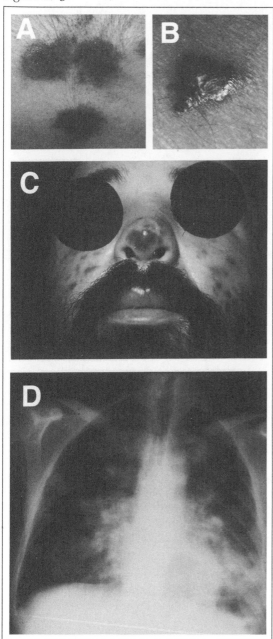

Kaposi's sarcoma. (A) Macular lesions. (B) Tumorlike lesion. (C) Lesions have a purple color. Note the preferential location on the tip of the nose or penis (not shown). (D) Pulmonary involvement with nodular central opacities and peripheral extension. See also Color Plate 4.

competent populations (see Chapter 4), histoplasmosis in AIDS is often disseminated with anemia, enlargement of liver and spleen, and positive blood cultures. Gastrointestinal involvement with ulcers, skin lesions, and lymphadenopathies are also frequent. The diagnosis is established by blood or bone-marrow culture. Treatment relies on amphotericin B or itraconazole.

COCCIDIOIDOMYCOSIS Coccidioidomycosis is restricted to the southwestern United States and Central America. Symptoms are fever, cough, and reticular nodular infiltrates. Diagnosis relies on culture of sputum or bronchoalveolar lavage fluid. Treatment is by amphotericin B (0.5–1 mg/kg/ day) or fluconazole (400–800 mg/day).

DISSEMINATED TOXOPLASMOSIS Rarely, and only in the presence of extreme immunosuppression (CD4 count below 20), *Toxoplasma gondii* can cause a devastating disseminated disease with prominent lung involvement. Typically, the lactate dehydrogenase (LDH) is extremely elevated. Toxoplasma organisms can be seen in the bronchoalveolar lavage. This form of toxoplasmosis is treated like cerebral toxoplasmosis.

NOCARDIA ASTEROIDES *Nocardia asteroides* is a cause of chronic pneumonia and nodular pulmonary lesions. Other organs, such as the kidney and the brain, can be involved. The disease is diagnosed by direct stain of the sputum, where delicate, Gram-labile, branched filaments are detected. Treatment relies on prolonged administration of high doses of trimethoprim-sulfamethoxazole; alternatives are imipenem and the newer fluoroquinolones.

INVASIVE ASPERGILLOSIS Invasive aspergillosis is often a terminal complication with disastrous prognosis in hospitalized patients who have received steroids and suffer from neutropenia. Cardiac and central nervous system lesions may be associated with pneumonia.

RHODOCOCCUS EQUII Rhodococcus causes cavitary acute pneumonias, which carry a very somber prognosis. A contact with horses is found in about half of the patients. Treatment relies on vancomycin that can be combined with ciprofloxacin. Other regimens include imipenem, amikacin, or rifampin.

Gastrointestinal System

Gastrointestinal infections are common in HIV infected patients (see Table 17.8), and can be the first manifestation of AIDS. Severe weight loss and chronic diarrhea are often problematic in end-stage AIDS patients and present a diagnostic and therapeutic challenge to the clinician. (Also see Chapter 8).

ORAL CAVITY AND ESOPHAGUS

CANDIDIASIS Candidiasis is the most frequent of the opportunistic infections, occurring in virtually all HIV-positive patients with severe immunosuppression. Usually, oral candidiasis presents with yellowish-white plaques on the oral mucosa (oral thrush) (see Figure 17.4); these plaques detach easily, revealing a reddish mucosa beneath. The erythematous form of candidiasis consists of brilliant red spots on the tongue or palate. Candidiasis can also present as angular cheilitis or perlèche. Clinical diagnosis is usually evident; cultures are difficult to interpret because Candida is found in the mouth of many people without stomatitis.

Often, Candida stomatitis is associated with esophagitis. This may cause dysphagia and retrosternal pain. Candida esophagitis is a so-called AIDS-defining opportunistic infection; patients with this complication are classified in CDC class C, whereas patients with stomatitis only are classified in class B. Oral imidazoles, especially fluconazole, have become the treatment of choice. In previously untreated patients, single doses of 150–400 mg are effective. Options for subsequent management vary. HAART with reversal of immune suppression prevents relapses. If this is not possible, some physicians prefer to wait for a relapse and retreat, whereas others favor preventive therapy, for instance, by 50 mg of fluconazole per day or 150 mg per week. After years of intermittent treatment or prevention, relapses become more frequent, and resistance of Candida is common. Such cases may present difficult problems of management. Other imidazoles, such as itraconazole solution, voriconazole, or ketoconazole, may remain effective. In other cases intravenous therapy with amphotericin B, at doses of 20–30 mg/day, are necessary. Newer agents such as echocandine (Cancidas®) are easier to administer.

KEY POINTS
Oral Candidiasis

1. Develops in all HIV patients with serious immunocompromise.
2. Typically see white plaques that detach when scraped, red spots on the tongue and palate.
3. Often accompanied by esophagitis, an AIDS-defining illness.
4. Fluconazole the treatment of choice.
5. Recurrent pharyngitis common, suppression often results in resistance

MOUTH ULCERS AND APHTHOUS STOMATITIS Superficial lesions of the oral esophageal mucosa cause pain and dysphagia. Differential diagnoses includes herpes simplex, cytomegalovirus, side effects of drugs (zalcitabine), and idiopathic ulcers. If the lesion persists, a biopsy with viral culture or immunofluorescence is often necessary for diagnosis.

ORAL HAIRY LEUKOPLAKIA Oral hairy leukoplakia is a whitish lesion with irregular borders in the lateral part of the tongue, due to Epstein-Barr virus (see Figure 17.4C). Often, the lesion is bilateral. Histology shows epithelial hyperplasia.

Table 17.8

Gastrointestinal Diseases in HIV

WHERE	DISEASE	ETIOLOGY	SIGNS AND SYMPTOMS	DIAGNOSIS
Oral cavity	Thrush	Candida stomatitis (*Candida albicans*)	Whitish plaques	Inspection
	Leukoplakia	Epstein-Barr virus	Whitish spots with irregular surface on margin of tongue	Inspection and biopsy
	Aphthous ulcers	Herpes simplex, CMV, idiopathic or unknown	Painful erosions around 5 mm in diameter	Culture or biopsy
Esophagus	Candida esophagitis	*Candida albicans*	Dysphagia, retrosternal pain with coexisting Candida stomatitis	Clinical signs and symptoms, endoscopy
	Ulcers and erosions	Cytomegalovirus or herpes simplex	Dysphagia and retrosternal pain	Endoscopy (longitudinal ulcers) and histology
Stomach	Gastritis	Candida, CMV, herpes, *Campylobacter*	Various signs and symptoms. Frequently, pH is elevated. Malabsorption	Endoscopy and biopsy
Small intestine	Ileitis	Cryptosporidium *Isospora belli* *Enterocytozoon bieneusii*	Chronic watery diarrhea Loss of weight Malabsorption	Examination of feces
		Salmonella, Shigella, Campylobacter	Acute or subacute diarrhea and fever	Culture of feces and blood
	Malignant lymphoma		Loss of weight Intestinal obstruction Perforation	CT scan and biopsy
Biliary system	Cholangitis	CMV Cryptosporidium HIV Microsporidium	Epigastric pain, nausea, anorexia, weight loss	Endoscopy or X-ray examination showing segmental stenosis without gallstones
Liver	Hepatitis	*Mycobacterium avium intracellulare*	Fever, weight loss Diarrhea	Biopsy or blood culture
Colon	Colitis	CMV or herpes simplex	Abdominal pain Tenesmus	Biopsy

Figure 17.4

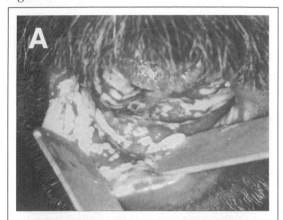

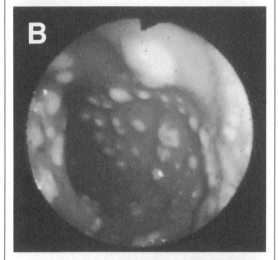

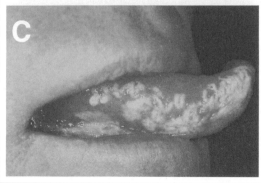

Lesions of the oral cavity and esophagus. (A) Candidiasis, oral thrush. (B) Candida esophagitis. (C) Oral hairy leukoplakia. See also Color Plate 4.

Usually, treatment is not necessary, but in resistant cases, topical application of podophyllotoxin can be effective. Acyclovir can also be administered but usually causes only temporary regression of the lesions (see Chapter 15).

TUMORS   Kaposi's sarcoma frequently involves the oral cavity. It produces painless macules or nodules with characteristic purple coloration on the palate, gingivae, or tongue.

SALIVARY GLANDS   Benign lymphoepithelial lesions and cystic hyperplasia involve mostly the parotid gland; they can be associated with xerostomia. The clinical picture is similar to that of Sjögren's syndrome. The parotid lesions are particularly frequent in children and are attributed to HIV itself.

DIFFERENTIAL DIAGNOSIS OF ESOPHAGITIS   As was noted above, the most frequent cause of esophagitis is infection by *Candida albicans*. However, when esophageal symptoms occur in a patient who does not have clear evidence of Candida stomatitis, other causes must be sought:

♦ Cytomegalovirus causes longitudinal ulcers. The lesion can be diagnosed only by biopsy, showing the characteristic viral inclusions in endothelial, epithelial, or smooth muscle cells.
♦ Involvement of the esophagus by herpes is most often caused by herpes simplex type I and less commonly by herpes simplex type II or by herpes zoster. Lesions are typically small. Diagnosis is made by biopsy plus immunofluorescence and/or culture.
♦ Idiopathic ulcers. This is a diagnosis by exclusion. Treatment by thalidomide may bring relief.

KEY POINTS

Esophagitis in HIV

1. *Candida albicans* is most common.
2. CMV is less common, causes longitudinal ulcers, viral inclusions on biopsy.

3. Herpes type I is moderately frequent, HSV-2 and herpes zoster are less common, diagnosis by culture or immunofluorescence.
4. Thalidomide may help idiopathic esophageal ulcers.

SMALL AND LARGE INTESTINE

DIARRHEA Diarrhea associated with weight loss is one of the hallmarks of AIDS, particularly in Africa, where AIDS, diarrhea, and weight loss are practically synonymous ("slim disease"). HIV itself, as well as many opportunistic pathogens and tumors, can involve the small and large intestine and cause diarrhea. For this reason the differential diagnosis is vast. In the text we will briefly comment on the most frequent causes (also see Chapter 8).

DRUGS Many of the antiretroviral drugs can cause diarrhea, in particular nelfinavir, ritonavir, amprenavir, lopinavir (Kaletra®), indinavir, and didanosine. Because patients with HIV often receive antibiotics, the possibility of colitis associated to *Clostridium difficile* must often be considered, and the *C. difficile* toxin must be sought in feces.

SALMONELLA, CAMPYLOBACTER, AND SHIGELLA These are frequent causes of acute gastroenteritis in both non-HIV and HIV-infected populations. In HIV infection bacteremia is extremely frequent, particularly bacteremia due to *Salmonella typhimurium* or *S. enteritidis*.

ABDOMINAL TUBERCULOSIS Abdominal tuberculosis presents with fever, pain, weight loss, or obstruction. These symptoms are difficult to distinguish from those of abdominal lymphoma. Often, the diagnosis is made only at laparoscopy.

MYCOBACTERIA OTHER THAN TUBERCULOSIS (MOTT) These infections are often caused by *Mycobacterium avium*, but other mycobacterial species cause similar clinical signs and symptoms and may be more difficult to diagnose because they grow poorly in cultures (for instance, *Mycobacterium genavense*). MOTT causes a systemic illness with fever, weight loss, and positive blood cultures. In biopsies of the gastrointestinal tract the submucosa may be filled with characteristic acid-fast microorganisms. Diarrhea and abdominal pain dominate the clinical picture.

CYTOMEGALOVIRUS COLITIS Diseases due to CMV are the result of reactivation of latent CMV infection (i.e., IgG antibodies against CMV were present before symptoms started) in immunosuppressed patients, usually with a CD4 count below 50. Symptoms may be severe, with diarrhea, abdominal pain, tenesmus, and fever. Colonoscopy shows multiple erosions, and biopsies reveal the characteristic intranuclear inclusions. CMV is also implicated in some cases of cholangitis and pancreatitis.

CRYPTOSPORIDIUM In immunocompetent individuals *Cryptosporidium parvum* causes asymptomatic infections and acute diarrhea. In immunosuppressed patients diarrhea becomes chronic, causing malabsorption. Oocysts can be found in the feces. No treatment has so far proven effective, although paromomycin (500–750 mg po TID) and macrolides such as azithromycin (1,250 mg po/day), clarithromycin (500 mg po BID), and albendazole (400 mg po/day) can be tried in addition to symptomatic treatment of diarrhea (loperamide, biphenoxilate, and narcotics).

MICROSPORIDIUM Three types of microsporidiae are found in cases of diarrhea: *Enterocytozoon bieneusii* (most frequent), *Encephalitozoon intestinalis* (which can also involve the biliary tract), and *Encephalitozoon cuniculi*. Some patients do not have symptoms; however, more often patients suffer with profuse diarrhea, abdominal pain, and weight loss. Thirty percent of cases of chronic diarrhea in immunosuppressed HIV-positive patients may be due to *Enterocytozoon bieneusii*. A special stain (modified trichrome stain) reveals the parasite in feces.

Previous treatments were not very effective, and eradication of the organism was usually impossible. Fumagillin (20 mg TID for 2 weeks) has recently been shown to clear the spores and prevent relapse in the majority of patients (see Chapter 8). Albendazole (400 mg BID) is useful in cases of *Encephalitozoon intestinalis* infection.

ISOSOPORA BELLI Diarrheas caused by *Isopora belli* are frequent in developing countries, for instance, in Africa and Haiti. The treatment of choice is trimethoprim-sulfamethoxazole, which is also effective in primary and secondary prevention.

KEY POINTS
HIV-Associated Diarrhea

1. HIV infection alone can cause diarrhea.
2. Antiretroviral drugs as well as antibiotics (*Clostridium difficile*) can cause diarrhea.
3. Salmonella gastroenteritis is more commonly associated with bacteremia in HIV patients.
4. *Mycobacterium tuberculosis* and atypical mycobacteria result in diarrhea.
5. CMV colitis in patients with CD4 < 50, diagnosed by biopsy.
6. Protozoa include cryptosporidium, microsporidia, and *Isospora belli*, search for oocysts, trichrome stain for microsporidia.

RECTUM AND ANUS

Many HIV-infected patients are at risk for other sexually transmitted infections such as gonococcal proctitis, syphilis, and venereal warts. Herpes simplex can cause rectitis with tenesmus and bleeding; in addition, in severely immunosuppressed patients, herpes simplex may cause persistent and debilitating ulcerations. Such lesions may necessitate admission to hospital and parenteral therapy with high-dose acyclovir. Resistance to acyclovir may develop; the alternative treatment is foscarnet. Less commonly, such ulcerations can be caused by cytomegalovirus.

Anal and rectal carcinoma is particularly frequent in homosexual patients. The development of these tumors is probably related to the human papilloma virus. Screening programs for this virus in homosexual patients have been considered, in analogy to screening for cervical cancer, but are not part of routine clinical practice.

TUMORS OF THE DIGESTIVE SYSTEM

KAPOSI'S SARCOMA When patients with cutaneous Kaposi's sarcoma undergo endoscopy, gastric or intestinal involvement is found in about one half of the cases. However, such involvement is usually asymptomatic, and involvement of the gastrointestinal tract without involvement of skin is rare. Rare complications include bleeding, obstruction, invagination, and perforations.

LYMPHOMA AIDS-associated lymphomas involve preferentially the gastrointestinal tract (and the brain) and cause diarrhea, abdominal pain, fever, and weight loss. Therefore symptoms of lymphoma are difficult to distinguish from those of opportunistic infections. Chemotherapy is theoretically effective but often very difficult to administer to these severely immunosuppressed patients.

Liver

Liver disease can develop as a consequence of antiretroviral therapy. In addition the same behaviors that lead to HIV infection also increase the risk of contracting hepatitis B and hepatitis C (see Chapter 8).

VIRAL HEPATITIS

Coinfection with HIV and hepatitis B virus (HBV) or hepatitis C virus (HCV) is very frequent. Both HCV and HIV are transmitted parenterally; that is why HIV-HCV coinfection is particularly frequent in IV drug addicts and hemophiliacs. HBV is transmitted sexually, with increased incidence in men who have sex with men. HIV and HCV infection influence each other mutually. Coinfected patients tend to have unfavorable prognostic indices for hepatitis C: higher incidence of infection with HCV type 1, of cirrhosis, and of high levels of HCV viremia. On the other hand, HCV influences HIV infection; notably, the CD4 response to highly active retroviral treatment is less vigorous in coinfected patients than in those infected with HIV only. Experience with interferon treatment of HIV-HCV coinfection was long disappointing. However, this may be changing as a consequence of HAART for HIV and of combination therapy with interferon and ribavirin for hepatitis C. Nevertheless, the treatment of hepatitis C in coinfected patients remains a challenge. Interactions between liver disease and HAART are frequent and unfavorable, and contraindications to the use of interferon (for instance, a history of depression) and of ribavirin (anemia) are frequent.

KEY POINTS
Coinfection with HIV and Hepatitis C

1. Coinfection is frequent in iv drug abusers and hemophiliacs.
2. HIV-infected patients tend to have more severe hepatitis C: infected with HCV type 1, higher incidence of cirrhosis, high levels of HCV viremia.
3. Hepatitis C–infected patients have a reduced response to HAART.
4. HAART combined with interferon and ribavirin demonstrates increased responsiveness.

HEPATITIS B

Lamivudine (3-TC) is active against both HIV and hepatitis B. In HBV-HIV coinfected patients HAART using lamivudine diminishes HBV viremia. After years of therapy, however, the risk of development of lamivudine resistance is high. Tenofovir may be used in this situation (see Chapter 8).

LIVER DAMAGE INDUCED BY ANTIRETROVIRAL DRUGS

Almost all antiretroviral drugs may cause liver damage. However, the nature of that damage differs:

◆ The nucleoside reverse transcriptase inhibitors (NRTIs) rarely cause severe steatosis associated with elevated plasma lactate levels. This side effect is more frequent with stavudine than with other NRTIs.
◆ The protease inhibitors indinavir and BMS-632232 cause asymptomatic hyperbilirubinemia (pseudo-Gilbert's syndrome). Ritonavir and nelfinavir can rarely cause cholestasis and hepatitis.
◆ Nonnucleoside retrotranscriptase inhibitors are also associated with toxic hepatitis. Severe cases, with death and liver transplantation, have been reported after use of nevirapine, particularly in women. Such severe cases have not been reported with efavirenz.

Central Nervous System

Central nervous system disease develops commonly in HIV-infected patients. Morbidity and mortality are frequent and the clinician should always investigate HIV patients with new-onset headache or unexplained neurological symptoms (see Table 17.9, Figure 17.5, and Chapter 6).

PRIMARY HIV INFECTION

About half of patients with the acute retroviral syndrome complain of headaches, and in 5–20% clinical signs of meningitis such as neck stiffness or photophobia are evident. Encephalitis, with symptoms ranging from confusion to coma, is

Figure 17.5

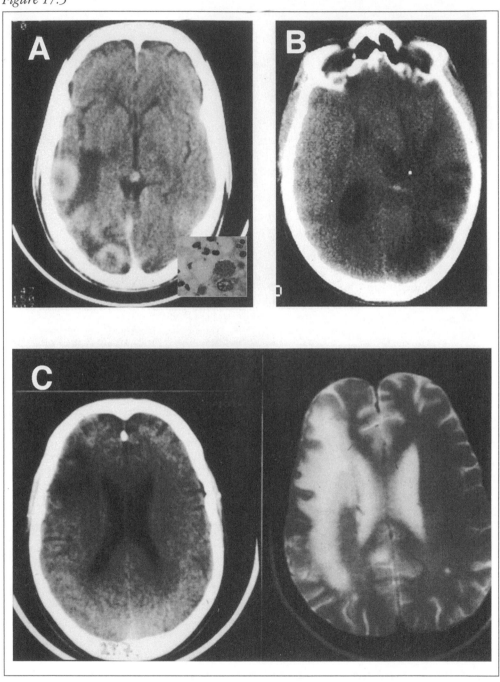

Neurologic complications of AIDS (A) Toxoplasma encephalitis. Note the typical ring enhancing lesions. Insert: Toxoplasma cyst in a brain biopsy. (B) Brain lymphoma. (C) Progressive multifocal leukoen-cephalopathy. Left: CT scan, Right: MRI scan.

Table 17.9

Central Nervous System in HIV

DIAGNOSIS	SYMPTOMS AND SIGNS	LABORATORY/ CSF FINDINGS	CT/MRI/ PET-SPECT	TREATMENT OF CHOICE
Cerebral toxoplasmosis	Focal deficit, headache, fever, seizures	<200 CD4 cells. Presence of IgG antitoxoplasma antibodies. PCR possible if untreated	Multiple corticomedullary lesions with contrast enhancement and edema. PET scan: hypodense lesions	Sulfadiazine + pyrimethamine + folinic acid
Primary cerebral lymphoma	Slow onset of ↓ consciousness, headache, or focal deficits	<100 CD4. CSF: PCR always positive for Epstein-Barr virus. Rarely cytology +	Variable number of lesions, periventricular contrast enhancement, lesions are + in the PET scan	Radiotherapy ± chemotherapy
Progressive multifocal leukoencephalopathy	Progressive ↓ of superior cerebral functions, focal lesions	<100 CD4 cells. CSF: usually positive for papovavirus JC	CT: ↓ density of white substance, no contrast enhancement or edema. MRI: ↑ T2 signal without gadolinium enhancement	No specific treatment; cidofovir? Intensify anti-HIV treatment
Cryptococcal meningitis	Fever, headache. Meningeal signs can be present or absent	<100 CD4. Blood and CSF + for cryptococcal antigen. Direct stain of CSF	CT: basilar contrast-enhancement, enlarged ventricles	Amphotericin B ± flucytosine, or fluconazole
HIV encephalopathy and dementia	Cognitive and motor impairment	<200 CD4 HIV ↑ in the CSF. Moderate ↑ in CSF cells and proteins	Corticosubcortical atrophy. MRI shows ↑ signal in T2	Intensify the anti-retroviral treatment
Aseptic meningitis	Headache, neck stiffness, photophobia, nausea during PHI	Moderate or no immunosuppression. CSF: moderate cell ↑	Normal	No specific treatment
CMV encephalitis	Confusion, lethargy, cranial nerve palsies, nystagmus	<50 CD4 PCR in CSF is positive	Periventricular contrast enhancement	Foscarnet and ganciclovir

PET/SPECT = positron emission tomography/single photon emission computed tomography. CSF = cerebrospinal fluid; PHI = primary HIV infection.

rare. In the cerebrospinal fluid (CSF), lymphocytes predominate with a cell count of 5–200/μl. Cranial nerve involvement may occur. Symptoms usually disappear spontaneously.

HIV ENCEPHALOPATHY

HIV encephalopathy is synonymous with HIV dementia or AIDS-related dementia. This syndrome includes cognitive, behavioral, and motor symptoms and signs. HIV-related dementia is often a diagnosis of exclusion after neuroradiologic examinations and CSF examination have failed to show an opportunistic disease. Problems with memory, mental slowness, and lack of precision are usually the first signs. Apathy and withdrawal may be interpreted as a depressive reaction. Clinical examination shows difficulties in comprehension and coordination, abnormal gait, nystagmus, and archaic reflexes. Without treatment, dementia progresses within a few months. Convulsions may appear. Neuroradiologic investigation usually shows cerebral atrophy. In the MRI scan, the T2 signal is increased in the subcortical white matter, preferentially in the parasagittal regions.

The CSF shows a variable increase in proteins and mononuclear cells. Since the introduction of HAART, the incidence of HIV dementia has greatly decreased. In established dementia the effect of HAART is variable, but spectacular improvements are noted in some patients.

KEY POINTS
HIV Encephalopathy

1. A diagnosis of exclusion.
2. Dementia symptoms accompanied by apathy and withdrawal can be mistaken for depression.
3. MRI: Increased T2 signal in the subcortical white matter in parasagittal regions.
4. HAART has dramatically decreased the incidence of HIV dementia.

FOCAL CNS LESIONS

Cerebral toxoplasmosis, primary cerebral lymphoma, and progressive multifocal leukoencephalopathy cause some 90% of focal lesions of the central nervous system. Differential diagnosis relies on the CT scan, nuclear magnetic resonance imaging, and the PCR to amplify DNA of putative infectious agents in the CSF. Cerebral biopsy remains an option in exceptional cases.

TOXOPLASMA ENCEPHALITIS Toxoplasma encephalitis follows reactivation of latent toxoplasma infection (see Figure 17.5A). Such latent infection is present in 10% (in the United States) to more than 90% (in developing countries) of HIV-infected persons. Toxoplasma encephalitis usually starts with a focal deficit, for instance, hemiplegia, convulsions, headaches, fever, or confusion. In the vast majority of cases the CD4 count is below 200, and if toxoplasma IgG antibodies have been sought, they were usually present in the past or are present at the time of presentation. Another diagnosis should be considered first if these antibodies are absent or if the patient has taken trimethoprim-sulfamethoxazole prophylaxis. The CT or MRI scans show abscesses, which are usually multiple and preferentially located at the corticomedullar junction and in the basal ganglia. Annular contrast or gadolinium enhancement is typical, as is marked edema.

If the antibodies are positive and the images are typical, empiric treatment is warranted. If the diagnosis is in doubt, *Toxoplasma gondii* DNA can be amplified from the CSF. The rate of DNA positivity decreases when PCR is tried after treatment has already started. The treatment of choice is dual treatment with sulfadiazine (1–1.5 gm po QID) and pyrimethamine (200 mg po the first day, then 50 mg Q6D) associated with folinic acid (10 mg/day) to prevent bone marrow toxicity. Steroids (dexamethasone 4 mg iv Q6H) may be administered to diminish the cerebral edema. Sulfadiazine and pyramethamine should be continued for four to six weeks. After two weeks brain CT or MRI scans should be repeated, and improvement is expected. On completing therapy, secondary prevention is indicated with sulfadiazine 2 gm/day po and pyrimethamine 25 mg/day po. This will also prevent PCP. Often, the treatment of toxoplasmosis is not well tolerated because of cutaneous, renal, or hepatic toxicity of sulfadiazine and bone marrow toxicity due to both sulfadiazine and pyrimethamine. Alternatively, clindamycin (600 mg Q6H, then 600 mg Q12H) can be combined with pyrimethamine; tolerance is usually better, but the efficacy is reduced. Another alternative is atovaquone suspension (750 mg Q12H or Q8H) combined with pyrimethamine.

KEY POINTS
CNS Toxoplasmosis

> 1. Usually presents with focal findings, occurs with CD4 < 200, IgG toxoplasma antibody (+).
> 2. MRI or CT scan demonstrates multiple contrast-enhancing ringlike lesions.
> 3. Empiric treatment indicated if symptoms and MRI findings are typical, CSF PCR confirmatory.
> 4. Sulfadiazine and pyrimethamine plus folinic acid.
> 5. Follow-up CT or MRI at 2 weeks should demonstrate improvement.
> 6. After treatment, secondary prophylaxis is required.

PRIMARY BRAIN LYMPHOMA This type B lymphoma, which has a high malignancy rate, is constituted of large immunoblastic lymphocytes (see Figure 17.5B). It always contains the genome of Epstein-Barr virus. Clinical signs usually progress rapidly during a few weeks with confusion, focal signs, and headache. CT or MRI scans show one or several lesions, with irregular contrast enhancement and preferred periventricular localization. Rarely, lymphomatous cells can be seen in the CSF, where PCR for Epstein-Barr virus is almost always positive. Newer techniques such as single photon emission computed tomography (SPECT) and positron emission tomography (PET) show hyperactivity in the lesions and are useful to differentiate lymphoma from cerebral toxoplasmosis and from progressive multifocal leukoencephalopathy. Although these tumors are sensitive to radiation and chemotherapy, the prognosis is poor. Long-term survivors are predominantly those with CD4 counts > 200/μl at diagnosis.

KEY POINTS
CNS Lymphoma in HIV

> 1. Caused by EBV, B cell lymphoma.
> 2. Rapid progression of headache, focal signs, and confusion.
> 3. MRI or CT scan shows 1–2 irregular enhancing lesions, CSF PCR (+) EBV. PET and SPECT scans helpful in differentiating from toxoplasmosis and PML.
> 4. Sensitive to radiation and chemotherapy, but prognosis poor if CD4 < 200.

PROGRESSIVE MULTIFOCAL LEUKOENCEPHALOPATHY Progressive multifocal leukoencephalopathy follows reactivation of papovavirus JC, to which 75% of the population is seropositive (see Figure 17.5C). The virus infects oligodendrocytes; these are localized in the white matter, and their destruction causes demyelinization. The disease starts insidiously with loss of memory or dysphasia or visual disturbances, aphasia, or motor signs, more rarely with convulsions. CT and MRI scans show one or several lesions; these are subcortical, do not show contrast enhancement or edema, and are MRI hyperintense in T2 scans. Usually, the PCR in the CSF is positive for the papovavirus JC. There is no specific treatment (cidofovir and cytosine arabinoside have been tried, with inconsistent results), but highly active antiretroviral therapy is usually followed by stabilization and even clinical improvement.

KEY POINTS
Progressive Multifocal Leukoencephalopathy

1. Caused by reactivated JC papovavirus, infects oligodendrocytes, demyelinization.
2. Dementia, aphasia, motor deficits.
3. MRI hyperintense T2 images of subcortical regions.
4. PCR (+) for JC papovavirus.
5. Treatment with highly active antiretroviral therapy.

MENINGITIS *Cryptococcus neoformans*, a yeast, is the most frequent cause of meningitis in HIV infection. It occurs in profoundly immunosuppressed patients and is particularly frequent in Africa and the United States. The disease usually starts with headaches and fever; curiously, meningeal signs can be absent. The diagnosis can be made on direct examination of CSF stained with India ink, by cryptococcal antigen in the CSF or in the blood, or by CSF or blood culture. The CSF shows moderate pleocytosis and an increase in protein; however, in some cases the CSF formula is minimally abnormal. CT and MRI scans may not be helpful. (See Chapter 6 for a complete discussion.)

Treatment in severe cases consists of amphotericin B iv (0.7 mg/kg) for at least two weeks. Some recommend the addition of flucytosine (25 mg/kg Q6H), but the drug is difficult to handle because of gastrointestinal and bone marrow toxicity. After two weeks fluconazole, 400 mg per day for six to ten weeks, followed by 200 mg/day until immune function recovers, replaces amphotericin. In less severe cases (without intracranial hypertension, normal mental status, cryptococcal antigen in the CSF at less than 1:1000 dilution), fluconazole can be used from

the start. Itraconazole is not a good choice because it does not penetrate well into the CSF.

KEY POINTS
Cryptococcal Meningitis in HIV

1. The most common cause of meningitis in HIV-infected patients.
2. Headache and fever are the most common complaints, neck stiffness absent.
3. CSF lymphocytosis is usual, but CSF formula may be minimally abnormal:
   a. India ink positive, + CSF antigen,
   b. Culture frequently positive, as are blood cultures.
4. Treatment: Amphotericin B +/− flucytosine × two weeks followed by fluconazole.

CNS INFECTION BY CYTOMEGALOVIRUS Cytomegalovirus can cause various nervous system diseases in HIV infection: polyradicular myelitis, peripheral neuropathy, and encephalitis. Patients with encephalitis are usually profoundly immunosuppressed, with fewer than 50 CD4 cells/ml. Diagnosis is difficult and is usually made after exclusion of other, more frequent etiologies in patients who are confused, lethargic, and have cranial nerve palsies and nystagmus. Typical findings in the MRI or CT scan are periventricular contrast enhancement. PCR in the CSF is more than 80% sensitive and specific. Although foscarnet and ganciclovir should theoretically be effective, the prognosis is unfavorable.

CEREBROVASCULAR ACCIDENTS Cerebrovascular accidents are much more frequent in HIV-infected patients than in comparable populations of the same age. The pathogenesis is uncertain, but a direct involvement of HIV in vasculitis is suspected. Transient ischemic attacks have also been described.

OTHER RARE CEREBRAL DISORDERS Rare focal diseases include cryptococcoma (in these cases the cryptococcal antigen test in CSF and blood can be negative), tuberculoma, varicella-zoster virus encephalitis, and secondary or tertiary syphilis. In drug addicts septic emboli may be associated with cerebral abscesses and mycotic aneurysms.

PERIPHERAL NEUROPATHY

DISTAL SYMMETRIC POLYNEUROPATHY This may cause painful paresthesia and dysesthesia in hands and feet, associated with diminished reflexes and motor weakness in the legs and autonomic dysfunction. Such polyneuropathies can be very difficult to manage. Amitriptyline or carbamazepine may be useful. Aggravating circumstances include concomitant vitamin deficiencies, diabetes, and alcohol abuse, as well as drugs such as dapsone, vincristine, and isoniazid. Among antiviral drugs, stavudine and zalcitabine cause neuropathy, as do, more rarely, didanosine and lamivudine. These drugs can usually be replaced by other nucleosides if necessary.

INFLAMMATORY DEMYELINATING POLYNEUROPATHY This disease usually occurs during early stages of HIV infection. Presentation is similar to that of Guillain-Barré syndrome. Evolution is usually favorable with steroids, plasmaphereses, or intravenous immunoglobulins. In some cases CMV infection is involved.

MONONEURITIS MULTIPLEX Sudden nerve palsies of one or several nerves, including cranial and laryngeal nerves, can occur at any stage of HIV infection. Varicella-zoster virus can be the cause in cases of advanced immunodeficiency.

MYELOPATHY Myelopathy presents with gait disturbance, ataxia, spastic paraparesis, and urinary or fecal incontinence. The MRI scan is usually normal, but edema or even enhancing lesions may be seen. Autopsy findings show vacuolization of myelin and an accumulation of macrophages. There is no specific treatment, but potentially reversible causes of myelopathy such as epidural abscess; toxoplasmosis; infections

with HTLV1, herpes simplex, herpes zoster, or cytomegalovirus; and a deficit in vitamin B12 should be excluded.

KEY POINTS
Peripheral Neuropathies in HIV

> 1. Distal symmetrical polyneuropathy is associated with paresthesias and weakness, drugs that cause neuropathy should be discontinued. Treatment with amytriptyline or carbamazepine.
> 2. Inflammatory demyelinating polyneuropathy: Plasmapheresis or CMV treatment.
> 3. Mononeuritis multiplex can be caused by varicella zoster.
> 4. Myelopathy can lead to spastic paraparesis, look for reversible causes.

Ophthalmology

All HIV-infected patients should be warned to report changes in vision or other eye symptoms to their physician immediately. Eye disease in a patient infected with HIV all too frequently leads to significant and permanent visual impairment if not treated emergently (see Chapter 5).

HIV RETINOPATHY

HIV retinopathy is frequent and benign and does not necessitate treatment. Cotton wool exudates are characteristically observed; these correspond to focal lesions of ischemia. Other than exudates, there may be intraretinal hemorrhages, telangiectasis, and microaneurysms; these must be distinguished from retinal lesions caused by diabetes or hypertension. HIV retinopathy does not interfere with vision.

CYTOMEGALOVIRUS RETINITIS

Chorioretinitis due to CMV occurs in patients with profound immunosuppression and fewer than 50

CD4 cells/ml; IgG CMV antibodies are invariably present (see Figure 17.6C). Before HAART became available, 25–30% of patients with AIDS developed retinitis before death. All patients with HIV should be repeatedly questioned about changes in vision, more specifically, blurring of vision, loss of central vision or other blind spots, floaters, or flashing lights. CMV retinitis is a subacute disease with visual deficits progressing within a few weeks. The diagnosis is easily made by examining the retina, where there is a charac-

teristic mix of exudates, hemorrhages, and atrophy. Exudates often sheath the vessels. Without treatment lesions invariably progress, with retinal detachment and progressive loss of vision. Often, both eyes are involved, as well as other organs such as the colon, the esophagus, or the brain.

Treatment starts with high doses of medication, followed by secondary prevention, using the same drugs at lower doses. Three drugs are available: ganciclovir, foscarnet, and cidofovir. Their use is as follows:

Figure 17.6

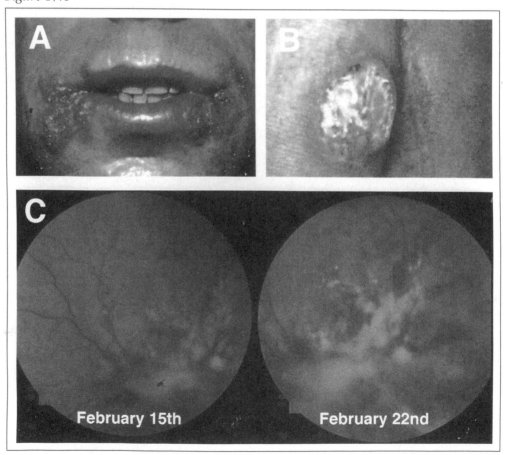

Herpesvirus group infections. (A) Herpesvirus type 1. Chronic perioral lesions that have become resistant to acyclovir. (B) Ulcer due to herpesvirus type 2, diameter 5 cm. (C) Retinitis due to cytomegalovirus. Note the rapid progression over 7 days. See also Figure 17.6C on Color Plate 4.

◆ Ganciclovir is administered at 5 mg/kg iv Q12H. Its main side effects are leukopenia and thrombocytopenia. Ganciclovir accumulates in patients with renal failure, and the doses have to be adapted. Oral ganciclovir is available but is poorly absorbed and is recommended only for primary and secondary prophylaxis (see Chapter 1). A newer oral preparation, valganciclovir, has improved bioavailability and may be efficacious for treatment (450 mg BID) as well as for maintenance therapy.

◆ Foscarnet is administered at 60 mg/kg Q8H. It is nephrotoxic (hydration with 1 liter of 0.9% NaCl is necessary) and causes numerous electrolyte disturbances (hypocalcemia, hypokalemia, hypophosphatemia, and hypomagnesemia), convulsions, and genital ulcers.

◆ Cidofovir has the advantage of infrequent administration (5 mg/kg once weekly for two weeks, then 5 mg/kg every two weeks), but it is also nephrotoxic (in 25% of patients) and may cause neutropenia. Nephrotoxicity can be diminished, but not eliminated, by administering probenecid 2 gm po before cidofovir and 1 gm after 1 and 8 hours, in conjunction with intravenous NaCl.

After an initial treatment course lasting at least two weeks, doses can be lowered: valganciclovir 450 mg per day, foscarnet 100 mg/kg/day 5 days per week, cidofovir 5 mg/kg every two weeks. Treatment with intravenous ganciclovir and/or foscarnet necessitates use of a permanent catheter. Secondary prevention of CMV retinitis is onerous. In patients with a good response to HAART and a durable rise of CD4 counts above 100, treatment can be discontinued without risk of relapse.

Patients with persistently low CD4 counts should be regularly examined to detect cytomegalovirus retinitis and to prevent loss of vision by early treatment. Preventive administration of oral ganciclovir diminishes the incidence of CMV retinitis by about 50%. However, because of expense, inconvenience, and side effects, such prevention has not commonly been used. Of course, the best prevention of all is the correction of the underlying immunodeficiency by effective HAART.

KEY POINTS
CMV Retinitis

1. Prior to HAART therapy 25–30% of AIDS patients developed this infection.
2. Subacute onset of visual symptoms: Blurred vision, scotomas, floaters, or flashing lights.
3. Characteristic retinal findings: Mix of exudates, hemorrhages and atrophy, vascular sheathing.
4. Treatment required to prevent progression to retinal detachment and blindness:
   a. Ganciclovir is the drug of choice, causes bone marrow toxicity, correct dosing for renal dysfunction.
   b. Foscarnet is associated with renal failure; iv NaCl protective.
   c. Cidofovir, once-a-week therapy, is associated with renal failure in 25% of patients; probenecid and iv NaCl are helpful protective measures.
5. Maintenance therapy is required if CD4 < 100, primary prophylaxis reduces incidence but is expensive and associated with side effects.

RETINAL NECROSES

These are medical emergencies necessitating treatment within hours, and they are caused by varicella-zoster virus. Two clinical presentations can be distinguished

ACUTE RETINAL NECROSIS (ARN) ARN causes orbital pain and inflammation visible in the anterior ocular segment with hypopyon. At the same time there is peripheral retinal necrosis with vasculitis. Without treatment progression is rapid, with retinal detachment and blindness.

PROGRESSIVE OUTER RETINAL NECROSIS (PORN)
Unlike ARN, PORN does not cause pain. However, the patient notices a brutal loss of visual acuity. Often, these patients have had herpes zoster recently. The anterior segment does not show evidence of inflammation; however, there are peripheral lesions of retinal necrosis. Again, there is a major risk of rapid loss of vision. For both ARN and PORN treatment involves high doses of intravenous acyclovir and possibly ganciclovir if there is a possibility of CMV retinitis.

KEY POINTS
Retinal Necrosis

> 1. Caused by varicella-zoster virus, can follow a bout of herpes zoster.
> 2. Acute retinal necrosis is accompanied by acute pain and inflammation, hypopyon may be seen.
> 3. Progressive outer retinal necrosis is painless but associated with marked visual loss.
> 4. High-dose iv acyclovir must be started emergently or ganciclovir if CMV possible.

OTHER INFECTIOUS EYE DISEASES

Pneumocystis carinii may rarely involve the retina. Cryptococcal meningitis may be complicated by papillary edema. Particularly in drug addicts, *Candida albicans* and other bacteremia may cause retinitis. Uveitis is a complication of the use of rifabutin, particularly when rifabutin levels are boosted by coadministration of macrolides or protease inhibitors.

Skin Diseases

It is important to recognize skin diseases during HIV infection (see Table 17.10). The development of a new skin rash often warrants immediate action. For instance, new acneiform lesions accompanied by fever suggest primary HIV infection. New onset of a maculopapular total body rash is indicative of a drug rash. New crops of macular, papular, pustular, or vesicular lesions may represent the first manifestation of an opportunistic infection. Even benign skin diseases may have a major psychological impact when they reveal the patient's HIV status to the outside world.

PRIMARY HIV INFECTION

Primary HIV infection causes erythematous macules or papules with ill-defined limits and symmetric distribution on the front and back, the face, and sometimes the palms and soles. The skin lesions neither itch nor hurt. They resemble pityriasis of Gilbert or the lesions of secondary syphilis, which are the principal differential diagnoses. Other differential diagnoses are a viral exanthema due to Epstein-Barr virus, cytomegalovirus, or rubella or a toxic or allergic reaction to drugs. The lesions persist for a median of two weeks, than fade spontaneously. Less commonly, painful mucosal ulcers occur (see Figure 17.1).

OPPORTUNISTIC INFECTIONS WITH SKIN OR MUCOSAL INVOLVEMENT

CHRONIC HERPES SIMPLEX In severely immunosuppressed patients herpes simplex type I or II may cause persisting genital, perianal, or perioral ulcerations (see Figure 17.6). Although herpes simplex is by far the most likely etiologic agent, there is a large differential diagnosis, including infections by fungi, mycobacteria, cytomegalovirus, varicella-zoster virus, and malignant skin tumors; confirmation is obtained by biopsy and immunofluorescence or by culture of virus. The preferred treatment is valacyclovir 500 mg Q12H or famciclovir 125 mg Q12H. Herpes simplex virus may become resistant to acyclovir and its derivatives, necessitating alternative treatment with foscarnet.

HERPES ZOSTER Herpes zoster is caused by reactivation of varicella-zoster virus; it occurs almost

Table 17.10

Skin Diseases in HIV

INFECTION	SIGNS AND SYMPTOMS	DIAGNOSIS	TREATMENT	COMMENTS
Acute HIV infection	Reddish macules on the trunk, the face, palms and soles of feet	↑ viremia and P24 antigenemia	HAART	Standard screening test for HIV can still be negative
Oral leukoplakia	Whitish plaques on the lateral aspect of the tongue	Clinical aspect	No treatment	Associated with advancing immunodeficiency
Kaposi's sarcoma (due to HHV8)	Macules, papules, or nodules of purple to dark blue color. Edema and ulcers are possible	Inspection and histology	HAART. Local treatment. Cryotherapy, radiotherapy, and systemic chemotherapy	
Bacillary angiomatosis (*Bartonella henselae*)	Red to violet papule or nodule	Histology (culture is difficult)	Antibiotics (macrolides, quinolones, and tetracyclines)	Rare, associated with advanced immunodeficiency
Herpes zoster	Vesicles on a red surface, necrosis, dermatomal distribution	Through inspection possibly confirmed by culture and immunofluorescence	Valacyclovir or famciclovir or acylovir po, in serious cases iv acyclovir	Chronic and disseminated forms are possible in advanced immunodeficiency
Seborrheic dermatitis (mold *Malassezia*)	Red and squamous plaques on the face and trunk	Inspection	Topical ketoconazole	Prevalence >30%
Acute condylomata	Wartlike papules resembling a rooster's comb	Inspection or histology and typing of HPV	Curettage, podophyllin, electrocoagulation or laser	Treat sexual partner at the same time
Molluscum contagiosum (pox virus)	Umbilicated papules	Inspect and histology	Curettage or electrocoagulation	
Herpes simplex	Painful vesicles or ulcers, which can become very large	Inspection, culture, and immunofluorescence	Valacyclovir or famciclovir; possibly acylovir iv	The lesions are primarily perianal, vulvar, or peribuccal
Prurigo nodularis	Isolated, very itchy squamous papules	Histology	Symptomatic treatment	Possibly with UV irradiation

20 times more frequently in HIV-positive patients than in HIV-negative patients of the same age, and can present at any stage of immunosuppression. In the severely immunosuppressed patient herpes zoster may extend beyond one or two dermatomes and cause atypical, ulcerated, and painful lesions that are difficult to treat. In cases in which the skin lesions are not typical, biopsy with direct immunofluorescence establishes the diagnosis. Particularly in cases in which immune suppression is severe, treatment is indicated, by valacyclovir 1 gm Q8H or famciclovir 500 mg Q12H. In patients with severe immune suppression, intravenous acyclovir may be preferred.

KAPOSI'S SARCOMA Kaposi's sarcoma (KS) is a very unusual "tumor." Infection by a virus, human herpes virus 8 (HHV-8), is a necessary but not sufficient condition. KS appears in patients who are HHV-8 seropositive and have a variable degree of immunosuppression. Very often, KS is multifocal from the start. Karyotypic anomalies have not been described. Lesions resemble reactive hypoplasia more than typical malignancies.

In the United States and in Europe this is essentially a disease of those who acquired their HIV infection by homosexual contact. Although cases do occur in patients with nearly normal CD4 counts, immune suppression greatly increases the risk. The lesions of Kaposi's sarcoma are macules, papules, or nodules of characteristic purple color. Preferred locations are the extremities, the tip of the nose, and the palate (see Figure 17.3). Often, the lesions are only slowly progressive and do not cause pain. In rare cases, KS may run an aggressive course with nodular, ulcerated lesions, limb edema, and gastrointestinal and pulmonary involvement. KS is easy to recognize; when in doubt, a skin biopsy showing vascular proliferation and fusiform cells will yield the diagnosis.

The incidence and severity of Kaposi's sarcoma is favorably influenced by highly active antiretroviral therapy, which has become the mainstay of treatment. If the lesions persist or enlarge, local treatment by cryotherapy or radiotherapy is recommended. Systemic treatment is necessary

in cases with edema of the extremities, genitalia, or the face or in case of massive visceral involvement. As a rule, many chemotherapeutic agents produce remissions, but these are rarely of long duration. For reasons of relative lack of side effects and good efficacy, liposomal preparations of Adriamycin, used at the dose of 40 mg/m² every two to three weeks, are currently the most popular. Treatment with a combination of bleomycin 10 mg/m² and vincristine (2 mg) is also effective, as is high-dose α-interferon (up to 50 × 10⁶ units iv 5 days per week) in patients with more than 200 CD4 cells/ml.

KEY POINTS

Kaposi's Sarcoma

1. Associated with HHV-8 virus, in U.S. and Europe found in HIV-infected homosexual men.
2. Macules, papules, or nodules; purple color, usually on extremities, the tip of the nose, and the palate.
3. Rarely aggressive with limb edema, GI, and pulmonary involvement.
4. Histopathology: Vascular proliferation and fusiform cells.
5. Treatment: May be refractory to therapy:
   a. HAART usually induces remissions,
   b. Local disease: Cryotherapy or radiotherapy,
   c. Severe disease: Liposomal Adriamycin or vincristine and bleomycin or α-interferon.

BACILLARY ANGIOMATOSIS Bacillary angiomatosis is caused by *Bartonella henselae*, the same agent that is responsible for cat-scratch disease (see Chapter 13) and *Bartonella quintana*. In HIV infection Bartonella causes papules and nodules with red to violet color. These are present in variable numbers, are not painful, and may be ulcerated. Patients are usually febrile and extremely immunosuppressed. In addition to the skin, the liver (peliosis hepatis) and bone may be involved. A biopsy with silver impregnation stains can show the Bartonella and differentiate the disease from Kaposi's sarcoma. A serologic test is also available. Prolonged treatment with clarithromycin 500 mg Q12H, azithromycin 250 mg Q24H, or ciprofloxacin 500 mg Q12H is necessary.

SEBORRHEIC DERMATITIS Seborrheic dermatitis is frequent in the general population. However, in HIV-infected patients the disease may be particularly severe. Reddish plaques covered by small scales appear on the face (nose, between the eyebrows), the scalp, and on the sternum. Ketoconazole creams and shampoos are efficacious.

MOLLUSCUM CONTAGIOSUM These lesions are caused by poxvirus. There are multiple umbilicated, painless, flesh-colored papules or nodules, particularly on the face and on the genitalia. In immunosuppressed patients they can persist for months and become extremely numerous. The lesions can be destroyed by curettage, electrocoagulation, or cryotherapy. Cidofovir may be effective in extreme cases.

SEXUALLY TRANSMITTED DISEASES The occurrence of sexually transmitted diseases in an HIV-positive patient is a reminder of unsafe sexual practices and an occasion to reinforce educational messages about the need to prevent transmission of HIV (see Chapter 9). These diseases commonly have cutaneous manifestations.

Syphilis has a high prevalence in HIV infected patients and the presence of a syphilitic chancre increases the risk of contracting HIV infection. The treatment of syphilis in the HIV-infected person has elicited a great deal of controversy. Contrary to widespread beliefs, serologic tests for syphilis are as valid in the HIV-infected patient as in the HIV-noninfected patient. The recommended treatment regimens are 2.4 million units of benzathine penicillin intramuscularly at weeks 0, 1, and 2 in cases of secondary or latent tertiary syphilis and a prolonged course of high-dose intravenous penicillin or ceftriaxone in cases of suspected neurosyphilis.

DRUG REACTIONS Drug rashes are very frequent during HIV infection and can constitute an emergency. Alarming signs are conjunctivitis or lesions of the buccal mucosa, generalized erythrodermia, and detachment of the skin; these necessitate hospitalization and specialized consultation. Often, however, drug rashes are mild and will disappear even if the drug is continued; this is particularly true of early reactions to efavirenz and to nevirapine. Because alternative treatments often have disadvantages of their own, an effort should be made to "treat through" drug eruptions that are not severe.

KEY POINTS
Drug Rashes in HIV-Infected Patients

1. Danger signs: Conjunctivitis, buccal mucosa lesions, erythroderma, skin detachment.
2. Treat through milder drug eruptions.

SKIN DISEASES THAT ARE AGGRAVATED BY HIV

Many common skin diseases seem to be more severe in patients who also have HIV infection. These include dryness of the skin, psoriasis, reactions to insect stings, and dermatomycosis.

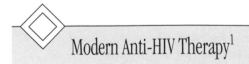

Modern Anti-HIV Therapy[1]

Introduction: The Ten Commandments of Antiviral Treatment

Highly active antiretroviral therapies (HAART), usually consisting of two NRTIs plus an HIV protease inhibitor, have been widely used since 1996. They produced durable suppression of

[1]This section was written with the help of Markus Flepp, Véronique Schiffer, and Rainer Weber.

viral replication with undetectable plasma levels of HIV-RNA in more than half of the patients. Immunity recovered, and morbidity and mortality fell by more than 80%. Treatment was thought to be particularly effective when started early; therefore HAART was recommended for essentially all HIV-infected persons who were willing to commit themselves to lifelong therapy.

Besides these successes, however, HAART also produces problems. HIV is not eradicated by present-day drugs, and often, patients cannot comply with long-term combination treatment. Moreover, HAART causes unexpected and ill-understood side effects. The dogma of earliest possible treatment has therefore come under attack.

The 10 principles governing antiretroviral treatment are summarized in Table 17.11. The process of starting and maintaining HAART is complex. Within the last few years the numbers of antiretrovirals, their known and potential interac-

Table 17.11

10 Principles for HAART

1. Indication

The presence of HIV infection establishes theoretically the indication for treatment, but treatment does not usually start until subclinical immune deficiency is apparent.

2. Combination

Antiretroviral treatment consists of at least three drugs.

3. First chance = best chance

The choice of drugs during a first treatment course determines what possibilities still remain when a second and different treatment becomes necessary later on. Chances for success are best first. Later on, alternatives are limited by selection of resistant mutants.

4. Complexity

Antiretroviral treatment is complex, in particular because of drug interactions and side effects.

5. Resistance

Selection of resistant quasi-species occurs frequently. Within substance classes, cross-resistance is complete among available NNRTIs and partial among PIs and NRTIs.

6. Information

Starting and maintaining an effective antiretroviral treatment is time consuming because the information needs of physician and patients are considerable.

7. Motivation and compliance

The patient's willingness to take the drugs regularly at prescribed times and dosages will largely determine the success of treatment. Patients must understand the relationship between insufficient compliance and drug resistance.

8. Monitoring

Efficacy of antiretroviral treatment is established by regular measures of viral RNA and of CD4 counts.

9. Goals of treatment

The goal of treatment is durable suppression of viral RNA below 50 copies/ml of plasma. Such suppression minimizes selection of resistant mutants, causes immune reconstitution, and improves avoidance of morbidity and mortality.

10. Studies

Antiretroviral treatment continues to evolve toward greater simplicity and efficacy. Patients should be encouraged to participate in clinical studies that aim to optimize therapy.

tions with each other and with non-HIV drugs, and the list of their side effects have all increased exponentially. Usually, a physician specializing in HIV care should be consulted whenever HAART is started or changed. It is that physician's job to guarantee that the treatment chosen is optimal for the particular patient. Mismanagement of antiretroviral therapy can lead to untoward toxicities and the development of resistant virus that can no longer be treated.

KEY POINT

Starting or Changing HAART

> A physician specializing in HIV should be consulted whenever HAART is started or changed. Mismanagement of antiretroviral therapy can lead to untoward toxicities and resistant virus.

Indications for Starting Treatment

The progression of HIV infection to AIDS has been compared to a train speeding toward an accident. The CD4 count represents the distance from the locomotive to the site of the train wreck, and the viral load represents the speed of the moving train. The CD4 count indicates the degree of immune deficiency and predicts short-term risk of opportunistic disease. Without treatment this risk is below 1% per year when the CD4 counts are above 500/ml but rises to 30% with CD4 counts below 100. In the long term, prognosis is also determined by the viral load, that is, the number of HIV RNA copies per milliliter of plasma. Elevated viral load predicts more rapid progression toward AIDS in population-based studies, although interindividual variations are enormous. While HIV destroys CD4 cells and the lymph node architecture, causing progressive immunodeficiency, antiretroviral treatment suppresses viral replication, prevents further destruction of the immune system, and even allows for considerable repair in patients who start treatment while already immunosuppressed.

Treatment must be adapted to each patient, taking into account the speed of progression, the patient's acceptance of treatment, the likelihood of compliance, and possible side effects. The recommendations in Table 17.12 are only approximations because individual factors, though often decisive, do not lend themselves to abstractions in a table. Possible advantages and disadvantages of early start of treatment are outlined in Table 17.13.

The course of HIV infection has been compared to a train speeding toward an accident. The CD4 count represents the distance from

Table 17.12

Indications for Starting Antiretroviral Treatment

CLINICAL STAGE ACUTE HIV INFECTION	LABORATORY VALUES IRRELEVANT	RECOMMENDATIONS CONSIDER HAART, OBTAIN SPECIALIZED CONSULTATION	
	CD4 count	*Viral load*	
Chronic asymptomatic HIV		< 50000	>50000
infection (stage A)	>500	Wait	Wait
	350–500	Wait	Consider HAART
	< 350	Treat	Treat
Symptomatic chronic HIV infection (CDC stage B or C)	Irrelevant	Treat	

Table 17.13

Potential Advantages and Disadvantages of Early Antiretroviral Treatment

POSSIBLE ADVANTAGES OF STARTING TREATMENT EARLY	POSSIBLE DISADVANTAGES OF STARTING TREATMENT EARLY
Maximal suppression of viral replication; as a consequence, lesser risk of selection of resistant mutants	Risk of resistance as a consequence of suboptimal compliance
Prevention of immune deficiency and more complete immune reconstitution	Duration of efficacy of treatment may be limited
Less risk of side effects in patients whose general state of health is excellent	Loss of quality of life through short-term side effects and possible long-term toxicity
	Cost
Healthy carriers are less contagious when treated; lesser number of new infections?	Transmission of new infections with drug-resistant viruses

the locomotive to the site of the train wreck, and the viral load represents the speed. In the absence of symptoms these parameters are used to determine the timing of antiretroviral therapy to prevent AIDS.

Three different classes of drugs are currently available (see Table 17.14):

1. Nucleoside reverse transcriptase inhibitors (NRTI), such as abacavir (ABC), didanosine (ddI), lamivudine (3TC), stavudine (d4T), zalcitabine (ddC), and zidovudine (AZT)
2. Nonnucleoside reverse transcriptase inhibitors (NNRTI), such as efavirenz (EFV) and nevirapine (NVP)
3. Protease inhibitors (PI), such as amprenavir (APV), indinavir (IDV), lopinavir/ritonavir (LPV/r), nelfinavir (NFV), ritonavir (RTV), and saquinavir (SQV)

Optimal suppression of viral replication requires the use of at least three drugs, that is, one or two NRTIs with one or two PIs or with an NNRTI or possibly three NRTIs. The choice of drugs is determined by several factors, including drug interactions, dosage intervals (e.g., by the need to accommodate professional activity), future therapeutic options, or possible pregnancy.

At the present time there are no clear criteria for choosing between protease inhibitors and NNRTIs in initial treatment. Treatment experience with PIs is greater. Some advantages and disadvantages of the two classes of drugs are shown in Table 17.15.

The following treatment options are not recommended:

◆ Therapy with only one or two drugs
◆ Combinations of ddI plus ddC or ddC plus d4T (added toxicity), zidovudine plus d4T (antagonism), or ddC plus 3-TC (no data)
◆ Use of saquinavir, particularly the hard-gel capsule (Invirase) without concomitant ritonavir (insufficient drug levels)
◆ Use of Agenerase or saquinavir, without concomitant ritonavir, in combination with efavirenz (insufficient drug levels)

Treatment Monitoring

TOLERANCE AND SIDE EFFECTS

NRTIs can be toxic to mitochondria, producing liver damage, lactic acidosis, lipoatrophy, and polyneuropathy. PIs cause nausea, vomiting, and diarrhea; elevate plasma cholesterol and triglyc-

Table 17.14

Anti-HIV Drugs Available in 2002

Generic Name (Abbreviation)	Trade Name	Usual Dosage in the Absence of Renal Failure	Class
Abacavir (ABC)	Ziagen	300 mg BID	NRTI
Didanosine (ddI)	Videx	300-400 mg QD*	NRTI
Lamivudine (3-TC)	3-TC	150 mg BID	NRTI
Stavudine (d4T)	Zerit	40 mg BID†	NRTI
Tenofovir (TFV)	Viread	300 mg QD	NRTI
Zalcitabine (ddC)	Hivid	0.75 mg TID	NRTI
Zidovudine (AZT)	Retrovir	250 mg BID	NRTI
AZT + 3-TC	Combivir	1 tab BID	NRTI
AZT + 3-TC + ABC	Trizivir	1 tab BID	NRTI
Efavirenz (EFV)	Stocrin	600 mg once daily	NNRTI
Nevirapine (NVP)	Viramune	200 mg BID	NNRTI
Amprenavir (APV)	Agenerase	900 mg BID‡	PI
Indinavir (IDV)	Crixivan	800 mg BID‡	PI
Lopinavir/ritonavir (LPV/r)	Kaletra	400/100 mg BID§	PI
Nelfinavir (NFV)	Viracept	1250 mg BID	PI
Ritonavir (RTV)	Norvir	100 mg BID‖	PI
Saquinavir hard gel (SQVh)	Invirase	400 mg BID‡	PI
Saquinavir soft gel (SQVs)	Fortovase	1600 mg BID	PI

NRTI = nucleoside reverse-transcriptase inhibitor; NNRTI = nonnucleoside reverse-transcriptase inhibitor; PI = protease inhibitor.
*250-300 mg QD if weight < 60 kg; adjust dose in case of renal failure.
†30 mg BID if weight < 60 kg; adjust dose in case of renal failure.
‡When coadministered with RTV.
§533/133 mg BID (4 pills BID) when coadministered with efavirenz.
‖100 mg BID when coadministered with APV, IDV, or SQVs; 400 mg BID when coadministered with SQVh.

erides; induce insulin resistance and glucose intolerance; and contribute, together with NRTIs, to the redistribution of fatty tissue (atrophy in the face and extremities contrasting with fat accumulation in breasts and abdomen). Treatment of dyslipidemia with statins is problematic because of the potential for drug interactions.

All drugs produce various specific side effects; an overview is presented in Table 17.16. Light shading means that the corresponding side effect has been reported in more than 5% of patients, and dark shading designates the drug's principal side effect. Because the drugs have usually been tested in combination, assignment of a particular side effect to a particular drug is often uncertain; this is particularly true of the various aspects of the lipodystrophy syndrome. Lipoatrophy and lactic acidosis seem to be more strongly associated with d4T than with other NRTIs, while fat accumulation may be particularly frequent when the combination of saquinavir and ritonavir is used. The potential side effects necessitate regular patient visits. Our usual schedule requires a visit after one, two, and four weeks of treatment; if all goes well, the intervals may then lengthen to every two to three months. For surveillance of toxicity we ask for a complete blood count, liver enzymes, lactates, and serum cholesterol and triglycerides.

Table 17.15

PIs Compared to NNRTIs in Initial Treatment When Combined with NRTIs

	ADVANTAGES	DISADVANTAGES
Protease inhibitors	• Well-documented clinical efficacy • Relatively slow selection for resistance when treatment is suboptimal • Partial cross-resistance only; possible efficacy of a second PI in case of failure	• Heavy pill burden • GI side effects • Elevation of serum cholesterol and triglycerides • Glucose intolerance • Lipodystrophy • Osteopenia?
Nonnucleosides	• Only a few pills to swallow • Better compliance • Possibly less lipodystrophy	• Data concerning surrogate markers only • Rapid development of resistance when treatment is suboptimal • Cross-resistance among currently used NNRTIs • Cutaneous side effects, including rare cases of Stevens-Johnson syndrome

KEY POINTS

Monitoring Drug Toxicity

1. Follow-up visits should be scheduled 1, 2, and 4 weeks after initiation of a new treatment.
2. If all goes well, the intervals may then lengthen to every two to three months.
3. Tests for surveillance of toxicity: Complete blood count, liver enzymes, lactates, serum cholesterol, and triglycerides.

DRUG INTERACTIONS

PIs and NNRTIs are preferably metabolized by cytochrome P3A. Therefore there exists a great potential for drug interactions. Drugs such as rifamycins or hypericum (St. John's wort) may lower PI and NNRTI concentrations by inducing cytochrome P3A. Other drugs may accumulate because they compete for cytochrome P3A with NNRTIs and PIs. Such is the case, for instance, for ergot alkaloids (dramatic cases of ergotisms with amputations have been published) and for many benzodiazepines. Hardly a week goes by without new interactions being reported; we recommend consulting Internet resources for up-to-date information. Among the best of these sites are those produced by the Department of Pharmacology and Therapeutics of the University of Liverpool (www.hiv-druginteractions.org) and the electronic journal Medscape (http://medscape.com/home/topics/aids/aids.html).

Ritonavir deserves special mention. It is the most powerful inhibitor of cytochrome P3A known in medical therapeutics. Its capacity to inhibit metabolism of other PIs can be put to good use; increasingly, other PIs, such as indinavir, lopinavir, saquinavir, and amprenavir, are combined with small doses of ritonavir (100 mg twice daily) to boost plasma drug levels and to lengthen intervals between dosages.

Ritonavir is the most powerful inhibitor of cytochrome P3A known in medical therapeutics. It can be used to boost plasma levels of other protease inhibitors.

Table 17.16

Frequent Side Effects of Anti-HIV Drugs

| | REVERSE TRANSCRIPTASE INHIBITORS | | | | | | | | PROTEASE INHIBITORS | | | | | |
| | NRTIs | | | | | | NNRTIs | | | | | | | |
CLINICAL SYMPTOM	ABC	AZT	DDC	DDI	D4T	3TC	EFV	NVP	APV	IDV	LPV	NFV	RTV	SQV
Abdominal pain										▨				▨
Alterations of taste									▨				▨	▨
CNS symptoms							■							
Diarrhea	▨		■						▨	■	■	■	■	■
Drug rash	■						■	■	▨					
Fat accumulation							?	?	▨	▨	▨	▨	▨	▨
Fat loss	▨				■	▨	?	?						
Fatigue		▨												
Fever	■							■						
Headaches		▨				▨	▨	▨						
Hypersensitivity syndrome	■					▨		■						
Kidney stones										■				
Myalgia		▨												
Nausea	▨	▨	▨	▨	▨	▨			■	▨			▨	■
Pancreatitis				■										
Paresthesias														
Polyneruopathy			■	■	■									
Sleep disturbances	▨						■							
Stomatitis			▨											
Vertigo							■							
Vomiting									■	▨				
Laboratory tests														
Amylase ↑				■										
Bilirubin ↑										▨				
Cholesterol ↑							▨				■		■	▨
Creatinine ↑														
Cytopenias		■												
Glucose ↑									▨	▨	▨	▨	▨	▨
GOT/GPT ↑				▨	▨			▨						
Lactate ↑	▨	▨			■	▨								
Macrocytosis		▨												
Triglycerides ↑									▨	▨	▨	▨	▨	▨

Key: Black = principle side effect; gray = side effect in > 5% of patients.

Compliance

Compliance largely determines the long-time success or failure of HAART. The demands made by compliance are greater than those in most other diseases because more than 95% of dosages need to be taken correctly to guarantee optimal results. Patients must acquire adequate understanding of HIV pathogenesis, the goals of HIV treatment, and pharmacokinetics. They should be able to recognize the most frequent side effects and know how to manage them.

Aids to improve compliance abound, although few have been tested rigorously. Pillboxes are popular; these contain all the drugs taken during one week in separate compartments. The establishment of a detailed written schedule, showing how and when to take the drugs in relation to meals and drinks, is recommended. More elaborate and expensive procedures involve the use of electronic pillboxes, in which a device records each time the bottle cap is unscrewed; the information can be downloaded into a computer and discussed with the patient. Directly observed therapy is becoming a possibility with once-a-day regimens; this may be particularly appropriate in combination with methadone maintenance.

KEY POINT
Compliance

> For HIV therapy 95% of dosages need to be taken correctly to guarantee optimal results.

Efficacy

Viral suppression is measured by lowering of the viral load, rise of CD4 counts, and clinical efficacy, which are all closely related. Above approximately 20–50 copies/ml, the nadir of viral load reached through treatment predicts duration of viral suppression. Time to optimal viral suppression depends on the initial viral load and on the sensitivity of the viral load test that is used. Combination treatment must produce a rapid fall in viral load, which should drop to fewer than 400 copies/ml after 12 weeks and to fewer than 50 copies/ml after 24 weeks. Viral load measurements and CD4 counts are recommended every three months.

KEY POINT
Efficacy

> Viral load should drop to <400 copies/ml after 12 weeks and to <50 copies/ml after 24 weeks.

Resistance Tests

Suboptimal treatment, lack of compliance, insufficient bioavailability, or drug interactions can result in prolonged periods of low drug concentrations with continued viral replication and selection of resistant mutants. The presence of resistance genotypes and phenotypes can be detected by using commercially available methods. Studies show that these tests are mainly useful for excluding drugs to which the virus is resistant but are less helpful for finding drugs to which the virus is sensitive. Resistance tests are recommended in patients who are yet untreated but who have been likely infected since 1997 because they may harbor a primarily resistant HIV variant. They are also recommended after early treatment failure.

KEY POINTS
Resistance Testing

> 1. Resistance tests are mainly useful for excluding drugs.
> 2. Order before treating patients who are likely to have been infected in 1997 or later.

Measurement of Plasma Drug Concentrations

In prospective studies, trough concentrations of protease inhibitors correlated well with degree and duration of viral suppression. However, the utility of these measures in clinical practice has not been established. They are recommended in cases of unexpected toxicity, in cases of suspected problems with compliance that cannot be investigated otherwise, or when multiple medications may produce unforeseeable pharmacokinetic interactions.

Treatment Modification and Simplification

Once a complicated drug regimen has suppressed viremia, patients and physicians would like to simplify treatment. It is risky to replace triple therapy (with a PI and two NRTIs) with just two drugs. However, when the PI is replaced by an NNRTI, viral suppression persists for at least two years. It is also possible to replace the PI/2NRTI combination with the three NRTIs ABC/AZT/3-TC, provided that the patient had been antiretroviral drug-naive when he or she started triple therapy. Insulin resistance and serum cholesterol and triglycerides tend to normalize, but fat redistribution is usually irreversible. Strategic treatment interruptions are being evaluated in clinical trials, but they cannot yet be recommended in routine practice.

Procedures in Case of Failure

Treatment must often be changed because of intolerance, drug interactions, or side effects. If viremia is below 50 copies/ml, a single offending drug can be replaced. The procedure is different in cases of virologic failure, that is, when viremia does not decrease to fewer than 50 copies/ml after six months (nine months if the initial viremia exceeded 1,000,000 copies/μl), or if viremia rises to more than 200 copies after transient suppression. In this situation a new combination should be chosen, containing, if possible, a drug from a class that had not been used previously. At least one additional drug should also be replaced by one to which the patient is unlikely to be resistant on the basis of his or her drug history and resistance tests.

However, such changes to new therapy are not automatic, especially in patients who have experienced long-standing failure with exposure to many drugs. Such patients often maintain CD4 counts at relatively high levels and are thus protected against clinical complications. On the other hand, salvage regimens might be ineffective and/or toxic, and drug holidays may produce falling CD4 counts. Maintenance of a virologically failing regimen is therefore often the best option.

KEY POINTS
Failing Regimens

1. A new combination should be chosen, containing, if possible, a drug from a class that had not been used previously.
2. At least one additional drug should also be replaced by one to which the patient is unlikely to be resistant.
3. A virologically failing regimen should be maintained if there is no alternative, often preserves the CD4 count.

Start and End of Prophylaxis for Opportunistic Infections

Efficacious antiretroviral treatment, provided that it is started in time, prevents immune deficiency and obviates the need for prophylaxis of opportunistic infections. Even if started late, HAART is usually followed by immune reconstitution. Prophylaxis of opportunistic infections can be discontinued after the CD4 count has risen above certain levels for at least three months. This level is 100 CD4 cells/µl for stopping prophylaxis of cytomegalovirus and nontuberculous mycobacteria, and 200 CD4 cells/µl for stopping prophylaxis of *Pneumocystis carinii* pneumonia and toxoplasma encephalitis.

Conclusions and Outlook

Antiretroviral treatment has profoundly changed the prognosis of HIV infection. However, such treatment is complex. Chances for success are best in those who were previously untreated; therefore everything possible must be done to optimize the first treatment given. A specialized colleague should be consulted when a physician is starting or changing antiretroviral treatment. Compliance remains essential for treatment success. All drugs must be taken as prescribed. In asymptomatic patients with CD4 counts above 350, it is better to abstain than to risk failure through insufficient treatment. Furthermore, it doesn't make sense to talk reluctant patients into accepting drugs; refusal of HAART must be respected.

Treatments continue to evolve. Triple therapy with two combination pills a day is already available. A once-a-day, one-pill protease inhibitor is in phase 3 trials. Drugs for new targets will follow. Within five years judicious use of strategic treatment interruption and of immune stimulation may permit survival in good health, without drugs, at least for some patients.

Additional Reading

Some of the best (certainly the most up-to-date) resources can be accessed via the Internet, for instance:

http://hivinsite.ucsf.edu/InSite or http://medscape.com/home/topics/aids/aids.html for general information

http://www.hiv-druginteractions.org is particularly useful for information about drug interactions

http://www.hivatis.org/trtgdlns.html for the latest treatment guidelines

http://www.unaids.org for the latest statistics on epidemiology

Index

Page numbers in *italics* denote figures; those followed by "t" denote tables.